Hot Topics in Acute Care Surgery and Trauma

Series Editors
Federico Coccolini, General, Emergency and Trauma Surgery Department
Pisa University Hospital, Pisa, Italy

Raul Coimbra, Riverside University Health System Medical Center
Riverside, USA

Philip Stahel, Denver, USA

Michael Sugrue, Letterkenny, Ireland

George Velmahos, Boston, USA

Dieter Weber, Perth, Australia

Endorsed by the World Society for Emergency Surgery (WSES) and the American Association for Trauma Surgery (AAST), the series covers the most debated topics in acute care and trauma surgery, from perioperative management to organisational and health policy issues, to the complex management of acute and trauma surgical patients. It is a valuable resource for both trainees and acute surgical professionals.

Belinda De Simone • Fausto Catena
Andrew A. Gumbs
Haytham M. A. Kaafarani
Andrew W. Kirkpatrick
Editors

New Technologies, Precision Medicine, and AI in Emergency General Surgery

Revolutionizing Surgical Practice for Optimal Patient Care

Springer

Editors
Belinda De Simone
Department of Emergency and General Minimally Invasive Surgery
Level I Trauma Center
Bufalini Hospital, AUSL Romagna
Cesena, Italy

Department of Theoretical and Applied Sciences
eCampus University
Novedrate, Como, Italy

Andrew A. Gumbs
Department of General-, Visceral-, Vascular and Transplantation Surgery
University of Magdeburg
Magdeburg, Germany

Service de Chirurgie Digestive Minimale Invasive, Hôpital Antoine Béclère, Assistance Publique-Hôpitaux de Paris
Clamart, France

Fausto Catena
Department of Medical and Surgical Sciences
University of Bologna
Bologna, Italy

Haytham M. A. Kaafarani
Department of Surgery
Massachusetts General Hospital, Harvard University
Boston, MA, USA

Andrew W. Kirkpatrick
Departments of Surgery and Critical Care Medicine
The TeleMentored Ultrasound Supported Medical Interventions (TMUSMI) Research Group: The University of Calgary
Calgary, AB, Canada

ISSN 2520-8284 ISSN 2520-8292 (electronic)
Hot Topics in Acute Care Surgery and Trauma
ISBN 978-3-032-09356-1 ISBN 978-3-032-09357-8 (eBook)
https://doi.org/10.1007/978-3-032-09357-8

This Springer imprint is published by the registered company Springer Nature Switzerland AG
The registered company address is: Gewerbestrasse 11, 6330 Cham, Switzerland

To my Mother Lucienne and my Father Nicola,

to the family that flows in my blood

and to the family that lives in my heart.

To my Mentors

To all those who support me with love,

understanding, and unconditional acceptance

—Belinda De Simone

Forewords

Over the past quarter century, the practice of emergency general surgery (EGS) has evolved from a reactive, procedure-oriented discipline to a structured, data-informed specialty focused on systems-based care and outcomes. In the late 1990s and early 2000s, the growing burden of acute surgical disease and variability in care prompted the development of dedicated EGS services, modeled in part on the trauma and critical care paradigms. This shift enabled around-the-clock surgical coverage, standardized triage pathways, and integration with critical care and interventional radiology. Concurrently, the field matured through multicenter collaborations which facilitated large-scale outcomes research and the establishment of disease severity grading systems.

Today, EGS is positioned at the intersection of acute care surgery, systems science, and data-driven precision medicine. The emphasis has shifted from simple operative decision-making toward risk stratification, resource optimization, and multidisciplinary coordination. Innovations in perioperative care, damage-control strategies, and minimally invasive approaches have improved survival and functional recovery, while structured performance metrics and national benchmarking have elevated the quality and accountability of care delivery.

Looking forward, the potential to redefine EGS lies in the integration of advanced analytics, artificial intelligence (AI), and precision health technologies. Predictive algorithms and real-time clinical decision support systems could transform diagnosis, triage, and operative timing—reducing unwarranted variation and enabling individualized care based on physiologic and genomic data. Machine learning applied to continuous physiologic monitoring, imaging interpretation, and outcomes forecasting promises earlier recognition of decompensation and smarter allocation of resources. Combined with innovations in telemedicine, robotics, and digital health infrastructure, AI-driven precision EGS could mark the next major paradigm shift—transforming emergency surgery from an episodic, high-intensity intervention into a proactive, data-informed continuum of acute surgical care.

Walter L. Biffl, MD, FACS
Professor of Acute Care Surgery
Department of Surgery
Scripps Clinic/Scripps Clinic Medical Group, La Jolla, CA, USA

Acute care physicians should be prepared to handle the fast advancements in technology including artificial intelligence (AI) and robotics that will impact future healthcare. AI is anticipated to penetrate vital clinical areas like emergency radiology, critical care, and emergency surgery. AI can be used in the four general P domains including Prediction of outcome, timely Participation in decisions, Prevention of diseases, and in tailoring medicine to be Personalized. Continuous accumulative data collection, including electronic health records, medical machine outputs, images, and videos, and their analysis is important to make appropriate timely critical clinical decisions. This will be refined overtime improving our knowledge, understanding, and wisdom in using AI in emergency surgery and critical care medicine.

Healthcare providers should be part of the development of AI by understanding its potential and limitations. They should be familiar with AI types of data, its sources, and principles of their management in the era of AI to be prepared for using it in their future clinical practice. Multiple challenges will be faced when adopting AI in healthcare which can be economical, legal, technical, administrative, or ethical. These cannot be addressed without proper knowledge and understanding of AI. Surgery is not just a craft but science and art. We hope that this book, *New Technologies, Precision Medicine, and AI in Emergency General Surgery*, will help acute care surgeons to understand, evaluate, and grasp important concepts of AI and digest it to aid them in using this fast-developing technology wisely and properly. This knowledge may help them overcome the multiple barriers to be faced when implementing AI.

Fikri M. Abu-Zidan, MD, FRCS, PhD, FACS,
Dip Applied Statistics
Professor of Acute Care Surgery and Disaster Medicine
Department of Surgery, College of Medicine and Health Sciences,
United Arab Emirates University, Al-Ain, United Arab Emirates

The future delivery of Emergency General Surgery will be guided by Artificial Intelligence (AI). Our academic responsibility is to generate the underlying data to develop well-informed AI systems to optimize patient outcome.

Ernest E. Moore, MD
Director of Surgery Research, Ernest E. Moore Shock Trauma Center
Distinguished Professor of Surgery, University of Colorado,
Boulder, CO, USA

Preface

Emergency and trauma surgery have long represented one of the most complex and unpredictable frontiers of modern medicine. Every day, surgeons face critically ill and fragile patients, often with multiple comorbidities, incomplete clinical information, and limited time to act. Decisions must be made in seconds, decisions that can change the course of a life. In this demanding environment, precision, adaptability, and judgment are the surgeon's most trusted allies.

Unlike elective surgery, emergency general surgery does not allow patient selection, optimal preparation, or complete control over risk factors. What remains within the surgeon's control is the decision-making process, the ability to interpret limited data, to act under uncertainty, and to translate experience into safe, effective care. It is precisely in this space that new technologies, precision medicine, and artificial intelligence can bring transformative change.

This book was conceived from the belief that innovation should serve those working in the most challenging conditions. Advanced imaging, fluorescence-guided surgery, robotics, telemedicine, simulation, and data-driven decision support systems are no longer optional tools, they are essential extensions of the surgeon's eyes, mind and hand. Their integration into emergency surgery promises to reduce complications, shorten hospitalization, and, most importantly, enhance the safety and dignity of patient care.

The journey toward AI-augmented emergency surgery is not only technological but also cultural. It requires a new way of thinking where human intuition and digital intelligence coexist to support real-time, context-aware decisions. It also calls for ethical reflection, multidisciplinary collaboration, and continuous education to ensure that innovation remains patient-centered and equitable.

This volume gathers the collective expertise of surgeons, scientists, and educators who share a common vision: to redefine emergency surgery as a discipline equal in scientific depth, technological sophistication, and intellectual rigor to any subspecialty in modern medicine.

As the Editor, this project represents both a professional milestone and a deeply personal journey. It reflects the conviction that even in the most acute and chaotic scenarios, technology and humanism can converge, empowering surgeons to decide better, act safer, and heal faster.

I am profoundly grateful to all contributors for their enthusiasm, their trust, and their pioneering spirit. Together, we hope to inspire a new generation of emergency surgeons ready to embrace the future, one that is intelligent, compassionate, and guided by innovation.

Belinda De Simone, MD, PhD(c)
World Society of Emergency Surgery
Novedrate (CO), Italy

The field of emergency general surgery stands at the threshold of a profound transformation. Once defined by rapid decision-making under uncertainty and limited resources, it is now being reshaped by the integration of new technologies, precision medicine, and artificial intelligence (AI). These innovations are not merely incremental improvements—they represent a paradigm shift in how we understand, diagnose, and treat time-dependent surgical disease. For decades, emergency surgery has been driven by clinical acumen, experience, and intuition. Today, these timeless skills are being complemented by data-driven insights, digital platforms, and intelligent systems capable of learning from millions of clinical encounters. Artificial intelligence is helping acute care surgeons predict complications before they occur; precision medicine is enabling tailored perioperative care based on genetic, metabolic, and physiological signatures; and robotic and minimally invasive technologies are redefining the boundaries of what can be safely achieved in the most critical settings. This book, *New Technologies, Precision Medicine, and AI in Emergency General Surgery*, offers a comprehensive and forward-looking exploration of this evolving landscape. It brings together world leading experts, innovators, and clinicians from across the world who share a common vision: to integrate technology into surgical emergency care not as a replacement for the surgeon, but as an extension of their capability, judgment, and compassion. The chapters that follow address the full spectrum of modern emergency general surgery—from robotic and image-guided interventions to machine learning algorithms that enhance triage, diagnosis, and risk prediction. They explore how new technologies can personalize perioperative pathways. Most importantly, they discuss how these innovations can improve outcomes, equity, and sustainability in healthcare systems. One principle remains unchanged: the centrality of the emergency surgeon. Technology must serve a human purpose: it should empower rather than replace, and clarify rather than complicate. The ethical challenges accompanying this digital revolution are as significant as the technical ones. Surgeons must therefore remain not only skilled operators but also informed leaders, capable of guiding the responsible adoption of innovation for the benefit of their patients and society. This volume represents an essential contribution to the ongoing dialogue between surgery and technology.

Fausto Catena, MD, PhD, FRCS
Bologna, Italy
Founder of the World Society of Emergency Surgery

Artificial intelligence holds unique promise in the field of emergency surgery, where decisions often need to be made in minutes or even seconds. Unlike cancer surgery, where surgeons may have weeks to analyze imaging, review pathology, and plan interventions, emergency surgeons must rapidly diagnose, prioritize, and act under extreme pressure. In such high-stakes environments, AI systems can provide real-time data interpretation, image analysis, and clinical decision support, helping surgeons recognize life-threatening patterns faster than traditional methods.

Despite these clear advantages, emergency surgery has often been viewed as "the neglected sibling" in the development and application of surgical AI. Much of the research and investment has focused on elective or oncologic procedures, where data are cleaner and outcomes more predictable. Yet it is precisely in the unpredictable and time-sensitive world of trauma, acute care, and transplant surgery that AI could have the most transformative impact.

In transplant surgery, for example, AI could also optimize donor-recipient matching, predict graft viability, and guide intraoperative management during time-critical procedures. By enhancing both the speed and accuracy of surgical decision-making, AI has the potential to elevate emergency and other time-sensitive surgical fields into data-driven disciplines where every second truly matters.

Andrew A. Gumbs, MD, MSc (AI), FACS
Magdeburg, Germany

> Whatever I know, I owe solely to my assiduous reading of books of the ancients, to my desire to understand them and to appropriate this science; then I have added the observation and experience of my whole life.

These were the words of Albucasis, the father of surgery, more than ten centuries ago, as he roamed the hallways of Andalusia.

We are today witnessing a new era in Surgery. The era of artificial intelligence (AI). Make no mistake, we will need to change in Surgery the way we think, the way we decide, the way we teach, the way we learn, the way we document, and the way we operate.

I dedicate this book, led by the unstoppable Belinda de Simone, who was gracious enough to include many of us, to the patients we take care of everyday in the emergency room, in the trauma bay, in the intensive care unit, in the ward, and in the clinic, and to the future generations of Trauma and Emergency Surgeons. One day, we hope to be their ancients.

Haytham M. A. Kaafarani, MD, MPH, FACS
Boston, MA, USA

It is an immense honor to be included among the established surgical luminaries and rising innovative stars of Global Surgery, who have championed and labored to produce this disruptively brilliant textbook titled *New Technologies, Precision Medicine, and AI in Emergency General Surgery*. This work reflects our shared vision to redefine the practice of emergency general surgery through innovation, precision, and artificial intelligence systems. Our personal toehold in this complex Global Scientific effort has been to try to understand the Human Factors of remotely guiding less experienced or even naïve responders required to perform beyond normal practice boundaries through catastrophic necessity. The TeleMentored Ultrasound Supported Medical Interventions Research Group (TMUSMI) thus constitutes a resuscitative paradigm that prioritizes augmenting human resilience (augmented intelligence) as a baseline capability to compare to all other autonomous technologies (artificial intelligence) too.

Andrew W. Kirkpatrick, CD, MD, MHSc, FRCSC, FACS
Calgary, AB, Canada

Contents

Part I

Evolution of Surgical Technologies in Acute Care and Emergency Surgery to Precision Medicine and Personalised Treatment in Acute Care and Emergency Surgery

Historical Development of Surgical Technologies

1

Andrey Litvin

1.1 Introduction

The historical development of new technologies in acute care and emergency surgery is inextricably linked with progress in surgery and medicine in general [1–3]. The first operations were performed thousands of years ago, before the invention of anesthesia and before the understanding of infection prevention measures. Since then, extraordinary advances have been made in how surgeries are performed and what types of surgeries are now possible. New surgical techniques have resulted in better results, faster recovery, less pain, and longer survival for patients [1].

For emergency surgery, the progress that has occurred in surgical techniques and surgical instruments is crucial [4]. Also, one of the most notable advances in surgery is the introduction of minimally invasive surgical techniques, including robotic laparoscopic surgery, which have been shown to reduce morbidity and mortality in emergency general surgery patients [5]. The development of institutional robotics programs has further increased access to these technologies, allowing the use of trained surgeons around the clock [6]. Integration of decision support systems, including the use of artificial intelligence (AI), in emergency surgery settings can improve decision-making and operating room management [7]. Precision medicine is another emerging field with significant potential to improve diagnosis, prognosis, and personalized care in acute care settings [8]. Technologies for imaging, telemedicine, and remote monitoring in emergency surgery are also rapidly evolving and require historical description [9].

Overall, these technological advances and strategic implementations have collectively contributed to the historical development and improvement of acute care and emergency surgery.

A. Litvin (✉)
Gomel State Medical University, University Clinic, Gomel, Belarus

B. De Simone et al. (eds.), *New Technologies, Precision Medicine, and AI in Emergency General Surgery*, Hot Topics in Acute Care Surgery and Trauma,
https://doi.org/10.1007/978-3-032-09357-8_1

1.2 Historical Development of New Surgical Techniques and Instruments

The historical development of surgical techniques and instruments in emergency surgery has been marked by several key milestones, reflecting advances in both technology and surgical techniques [10]. Initially, primitive tools such as blades made of flint, jade, and obsidian were used for cutting, and the human hand was the main tool for various surgical maneuvers [11]. The evolution of surgical instruments began with the adaptation of everyday devices and advanced significantly with the development of specialized instruments such as the scalpel, which advanced materials from bone and ivory to sterilizable metals. The introduction of hemostatic forceps by Celsus in the first century AD marked significant advances in the control of bleeding during surgery. This practice has evolved over the centuries with the development of atraumatic forceps for vascular repair [12]. The lithotomy procedure, which dates back to ancient Greece, led to the development of specialized instruments such as stone hooking instruments and pathfinders, which improved the accuracy and safety of bladder stone removal. In the twentieth century, tangential occlusion clamps developed by Friedrich Trendelenburg made it possible to partially clamp vessels, facilitating complex vascular operations [13].

Continuous improvements in surgical techniques and instruments, driven by technological advances and the need for more effective and safe procedures, highlight the dynamic nature of surgical practice and its critical role in emergency medicine [4].

1.3 History of Minimally Invasive Technologies in Emergency Surgery

The historical development of minimally invasive technologies in emergency surgery has been a progressive process marked by significant achievements and challenges. The origins of these technologies go back more than 2000 years, and their concept and development span the period from antiquity to modern times [5]. Over the past 30 years, minimally invasive surgery (MIS) has revolutionized modern surgical practice, becoming the standard of care for many diseases due to its benefits, such as reduced surgical trauma, shorter hospital stays, reduced postoperative pain, and faster recovery [5]. Despite these advantages, the adoption of MIS in the acute care setting has been slow compared to elective surgery. For example, a study found that only 28.7% of surgeons used laparoscopy in more than half of primary emergency care cases, highlighting the need for specialized training and increased surgeon confidence [14].

Table 1.1 History of minimally invasive emergency surgery

Year	Event
1901	German Dr. Georg Kelling pioneered laparoscopy with an advanced fiber-optic lens system
1959	Endoscopy to visualize the common bile duct and for gallstone removal was greatly improved through application of the Hopkins rod-lens system
1987	The 1st video-cholecystectomy was performed by Dr. Philippe Mouret in France
1992	Dr. Camran Nezhart reported the first laparoscopic radical hysterectomy and lymphadenectomy
2007	First trans-gastric cholecystectomy and first trans-vaginal appendectomy

The development of robotic surgical technologies has further expanded the application of MIS in emergency situations, allowing for increased precision and 24-hour access to minimally invasive techniques [15]. In elderly patients, MIS is recommended for acute conditions such as cholecystitis and appendicitis, although its use is often limited by comorbidities rather than age [16]. Mastering the skills to treat MIS in emergency situations poses significant challenges. Research shows that proficiency is typically achieved after an average of 30 procedures, highlighting the need for structured training programs and credentialing systems [5]. Overall, although MIS technology has gained widespread use in elective surgery, its implementation in emergency surgery continues to evolve, driven by technological advances and the ongoing need for specialized training and system support [17].

Table 1.1 shows the main historical milestones in the development of minimally invasive emergency surgery [4].

1.4 History of Surgical Robotics and Automation in Surgery and Emergency Surgery

The historical development of surgical robotics and automation in emergency surgery has been marked by several key milestones. The term "robot" was first coined by Karel Capek in 1920 [6]. The first documented use of a robot in surgery occurred in 1985 using the PUMA 560 robotic arm, which was used for CT-guided neurosurgical biopsies [6]. The development of MIS has led to the development of the robotic MIS system, providing improved three-dimensional vision, increased instrument precision, and improved surgeon ergonomics [18]. In recent years, the possibility of implementing robotic surgery in acute care settings has been intensively studied, with institutions developing robotic emergency care programs that provide 24-hour access to minimally invasive surgical interventions, thereby reducing patient morbidity and mortality [18, 19].

Table 1.2 shows the historical steps in the development of robotic surgery [4].

Table 1.2 History of robotic surgery

Year	Event
1985	A robot, using software developed by Dr. Yik san Kwoh, assisted in performing a brain biopsy
1994	Dr. Camran Nezhart, considered the father of operative video-laparoscopy, used the 1st robotic arm to hold a camera/instrument
2000	Robot 1st assisted in the operations of the esophagus and pancreas
2001	First "Lindbergh operation": a robot did a cholecystectomy in Paris under the direction of a surgeon in New York
2006	First "un-manned operation": a robot placed a defibrillator in a patient in Milan using the logic of thousands of operative data stored in a computer in Boston
2008	Robot performed the resection of part of a liver donated by a person

1.5 History of Artificial Intelligence in Medicine and Emergency Surgery

The history of the development of AI in surgery is inextricably linked with the history of AI in medicine and the history of AI in general. The progressive growth and development of the AI platform in surgery is described below and organized by specific time periods of fundamental transformation.

In Table 1.3, we see the main milestones in the use of AI in medicine and surgery [20].

By decade, the history of AI development as a whole is as follows:

1930s. Emerging in the late 1930s, cybernetics, a discipline that studies the control and communication of living organisms and machines, began to form the first foundations of artificial intelligence. Cybernetics introduced an innovative lens through which machines were viewed not simply as inert tools but as objects capable of simulating complex processes observed in living organisms [21].

1940s. The 1940s brought together key elements of AI. An important moment came in 1943, when scientists Walter Pitts and Warren McCulloch explored artificial neural networks, laying the foundation for future technologies. Their work was continued by Marvin Minsky, who designed the first neural network machine, called SNARC, in 1951. This was a step toward machines with cognitive abilities [21].

1950s. Many trace the origins of AI discourse to a seminal paper published in 1950 by famed mathematician and computer scientist Alan Turing. Turing proposed cognitive machines and the Turing test, a method for assessing a machine's human-like intelligence. This innovative idea sparked an ongoing debate about AI. Thanks to Turing, the influence of AI began to permeate various industries, including medicine, in the early 1950s [21].

The term "artificial intelligence" was coined by John McCarthy in 1956 at a Dartmouth seminar, marking the academic birth of AI. The Dartmouth Workshop was a defining moment in the history of AI, defining the mission and scope of the field [21]. By the late 1950s, AI had moved from theory to practical experiments and applications, laying the foundation for future research and advancements. It was an

Table 1.3 History of the development of AI in medicine and surgery

Year	Event
1950	Alan Turing develops the "Turing test"
1952	Machine learning
1956	John McCarthy coins the term "AI"
1961	Unimate, the first industrial robot, joins the assembly line at GM
1964	First chatbot: Eliza
1966	Shakey, "first electronic person"
1971	Research Resource on Computers in Biomedicine was founded by Saul Amarel at Rutgers University
1972	MYCIN was developed
1973	SUMEX-AIM was created
1975	The first NIH-sponsored AIM Workshop Held
1976	CASNET was demonstrated at the Academy of Ophthalmology meeting
1980	Development of EMYCIN: expert rule-based system
1986	Release of Dxplain: a decision support system
2000	Deep learning
2007	IBM began the development of DeepQA technology (Watson)
2010	CAD applied to endoscopy
2011	Gastroenterology Apple's virtual assistant, Siri, is integrated into iPhones
2014	Amazon's virtual assistant, Alexa, is released
2015	Pharmabot was built
2017	Arterys: First FDA-approved cloud-based DL application in healthcare
2017	Chatbot Mandy: automated patient intake
2022	LLM, ChatGPT
1990s–present	AI trials in emergency surgery

era of boundless hope, a vision of a future in which machines could match or exceed human mental abilities [21].

1960s. Early AI focused on developing machines that could draw conclusions or make decisions that previously only humans could make. The first industrial robotic arm (Unimate; Unimation, Danbury, Connecticut, USA) performed automated injection molding on a General Motors assembly line in 1961. Unimate could execute step-by-step commands. A few years later (1964), Joseph Weizenbaum introduced Eliza. Using natural language processing, Eliza was able to communicate using pattern-matching methodology to mimic human conversation (shallow communication), which served as the basis for future chatbots [20]. In 1966, Shakey, the "first electronic man," was developed. Created at Stanford Research Institute, it was the first mobile robot capable of interpreting instructions. Instead of simply executing one-step commands, Shakey could process more complex instructions and perform appropriate actions. This was a major milestone for robotics and AI [20].

1970s. In 1975, the first AI physician assistant appeared. It was created by the future founder of biomedical informatics, Edward Shortliffe. His work was one of the early AI-based expert systems. An AI system with backward chaining, MYCIN. This AI assistant was supposed to help the doctor recognize pathogenic bacteria that cause dangerous conditions, such as meningitis or bacteremia, and then prescribe antibiotics and calculate their dosage based on the patient's body weight [20].

1980s. In 1986, the University of Massachusetts released the DXplain decision support system. This program uses the entered symptoms to make a differential diagnosis. It also serves as an electronic medical textbook containing detailed descriptions and additional references. When first released, DXplain provided information on approximately 500 diseases. It has since expanded to more than 2400 diseases [20].

By the late 1990s, there was renewed interest in machine learning, especially in healthcare, which, along with the aforementioned technological developments, set the stage for the modern era of AI in medicine.

2000–2020s—the modern era of AI in medicine and surgery.

AI has developed particularly rapidly in this millennium. New technologies in AI have included generative AI models, which run on a generative pre-trained transformer (GPT) model. Moreover, the most famous is the ChatGPT model, which has powerful tools for natural language processing (NLP). The main goal of NLP models is to enable computers to understand and process the natural language that people use to communicate with each other. NLP models include a wide range of tasks, including language translation, speech recognition, text synthesis, question answering, and more, all aimed at bridging the gap between human communication and computer understanding [22].

The emergence of reference model architectures, wearable technologies, and advanced surgical data infrastructures is driving rapid advances in AI in surgery. New multimodal AI baseline models can improve patient outcomes, facilitate surgical training, and optimize surgical care [23].

In emergency surgery, AI has begun to be used to diagnose and treat all surgical emergencies. Modern artificial neural networks are used to predict, diagnose, and treat emergency conditions of the abdominal cavity: acute appendicitis, acute pancreatitis, acute cholecystitis, perforated gastric or duodenal ulcer, acute intestinal obstruction, and strangulated hernia. Currently developed intelligent systems allow a surgeon in an emergency setting not only to check their diagnostic and prognostic assumptions but also to use AI in complex emergency clinical cases [24].

AI has come a long way from the Turing test to today. We are at the dawn of a new era in medicine as AI begins to be incorporated into everyday clinical practice. The potential applications of the role of AI in emergency surgery are currently limitless. These range from improving our diagnostic capabilities and increasing workflow efficiency, and even helping to more accurately risk-stratify patients with common abdominal emergencies [25].

Despite these advances, the implementation of AI in emergency surgery is still in its early stages, and research, training, and clinical validation are needed to fully realize its potential [26]. The COVID-19 pandemic has further accelerated the adoption of artificial intelligence technologies in emergency services, demonstrating their usefulness in crisis management and highlighting the need for integrated AI systems in emergency response [27]. Overall, the journey of AI in emergency surgery has been marked by significant technological advances and persistent challenges that continue to shape its development and application [27].

The opportunities and risks of different types of AI vary markedly, and when considered, there are 3 eras of AI. AI 1.0 includes symbolic AI, which attempts to encode human knowledge into computational rules as well as probabilistic models. The era of AI 2.0 began with deep learning, in which models are trained on examples labeled as truth. This era brought many advancements, both in people's daily lives and in healthcare. Deep learning models are task-specific, meaning they do one thing at a time, and they mainly focus on classification and prediction. AI 3.0 is the era of core models and generative AI. Models in AI 3.0 have fundamentally new (and potentially transformative) capabilities, as well as new types of risks, such as hallucinations. These models can perform many different types of tasks without retraining on a new dataset [28].

AI has proven itself well in a variety of emergency situations, especially in situations where consistent and high-quality decision-making is critical [20]. Early applications of AI in emergency medicine and surgery included predictive modeling and personalized risk assessment, which have shown promise in improving surgical outcomes and assisting in complex decision-making processes [20]. AI-based decision support systems have been developed to assist in the diagnosis and treatment of abdominal diseases such as acute appendicitis and acute pancreatitis [24]. The integration of AI in emergency medical care has expanded to predictive modeling, patient monitoring, and operational management, highlighting its broad applicability [27]. Surgical robots capable of performing tasks such as supervised suturing and anastomosis represent another milestone indicating the possibility of more automated emergency surgical procedures in the future [19]. The role of AI in trauma care has also evolved, with algorithms now being used to predict, triage, and predict injury outcomes, enabling the transformation of trauma care from the point of injury to hospital care [29].

1.6 Evolution of Precision Medicine and Personalized Treatment in Emergency Surgery

The understanding of precision medicine and personalized treatment in medicine and surgery has changed significantly over the years, based on the early twentieth-century vision of individualized treatment for patients rather than simply treating their diseases [30]. The concept of personalized medicine, which involves tailoring treatment strategies to patients' individual characteristics, has been part of medical practice since Hippocrates emphasized the importance of understanding the person with the disease more than 2400 years ago [30]. However, the modern era of precision medicine began with advances in genomic research and human genome mapping, which laid the foundation for personalized treatment approaches [31]. The National Institutes of Health initiative launched in 2015 further focused attention on precision medicine by emphasizing the use of genomic sequencing and population health data to develop prevention and treatment strategies [31]. In emergency surgery, the adoption of precision medicine has been slower compared to areas such as oncology, but recent studies have shown its potential benefits in acute care settings, such as improved diagnosis and personalized intensive care for diseases such as sepsis, trauma, and acute pancreatitis [8]. Technological advances in data mining, machine learning, and rapid PCR-based diagnostics have facilitated the integration of precision medicine into emergency care, enabling faster and more accurate patient stratification and treatment [32].

1.7 History of Telemedicine and Remote Monitoring in Emergency Surgery

The historical development of telemedicine and remote monitoring in emergency surgery was marked by several stages. The beginning of telemedicine dates back to March 10, 1876, when Alexander Graham Bell used his newly invented telephone to call for help after an accident. This was the first case of remote calling of emergency medical services [33]. The field has changed significantly since then, with NASA using telemedicine to provide real-time medical monitoring of astronauts in space [33]. The pandemic has further accelerated the adoption of telemedicine, as evidenced by the development of remote monitoring programs for patients with COVID-19, which used secure communication methods to track patient data and improve the efficiency of care when needed, including abdominal emergencies [34].

1.8 Conclusion

Thus, modern acute care and emergency surgery actively use advances in the fields of new technologies, precision medicine, and artificial intelligence, which can significantly improve the quality and speed of emergency medical care. New technologies being used in emergency surgery include new surgical instruments, imaging and intraoperative monitoring techniques, surgical robotics, telemedicine, improved operating rooms, and, of course, AI and personalized surgical care. The most rapid development of new technologies is currently occurring in the areas of AI, precision medicine, and robotics.

References

1. Britt LD. The establishment and evolution of acute care surgery. In: Siegler M, Rogers Jr S, editors. Violence, trauma, and trauma surgery. Cham: Springer; 2020. https://doi.org/10.1007/978-3-030-31246-6_20.
2. Kutcher ME, Peitzman AB. A history of acute care surgery (emergency surgery). In: Di Saverio S, Catena F, Ansaloni L, Coccolini F, Velmahos G, editors. Acute care surgery handbook. Cham: Springer; 2017. https://doi.org/10.1007/978-3-319-15341-4_2.
3. Yoon KW, Choi K, Yoo K, Gil E, Park CM. Clinical significance of acute care surgery system as a part of hospital medical emergency team for hospitalized patients. Ann Surg Treat Res. 2023;104(1):43–50. https://doi.org/10.4174/astr.2023.104.1.43.

4. Lee Y. Historical development of modern surgery in America. Adv Hist Stud. 2016;5:168–82. https://doi.org/10.4236/ahs.2016.54015.
5. de'Angelis N, Marchegiani F, Schena CA, Khan J, Agnoletti V, Ansaloni L, Barría Rodríguez AG, Bianchi PP, Biffl W, Bravi F, Ceccarelli G, Ceresoli M, Chiara O, Chirica M, Cobianchi L, Coccolini F, Coimbra R, Cotsoglou C, D'Hondt M, Damaskos D, et al. Training curriculum in minimally invasive emergency digestive surgery: 2022 WSES position paper. World J Emerg Surg. 2023;18(1):11. https://doi.org/10.1186/s13017-023-00476-w.
6. Morrell ALG, Morrell-Junior AC, Morrell AG, Mendes JMF, Tustumi F, DE-Oliveira-E-Silva LG, Morrell A. The history of robotic surgery and its evolution: when illusion becomes reality. Rev Colégio Bras Cir. 2021;48:e20202798. https://doi.org/10.1590/0100-6991e-20202798.
7. De Simone B, Abu-Zidan FM, Gumbs AA, Chouillard E, Di Saverio S, Sartelli M, Coccolini F, Ansaloni L, Collins T, Kluger Y, Moore EE, Litvin A, Leppaniemi A, Mascagni P, Milone L, Piccoli M, Abu-Hilal M, Sugrue M, Biffl WL, Catena F. Knowledge, attitude, and practice of artificial intelligence in emergency and trauma surgery, the ARIES project: an international web-based survey. World J Emerg Surg. 2022;17(1):10. https://doi.org/10.1186/s13017-022-00413-3.
8. Lee S, Lam SH, Hernandes Rocha TA, Fleischman RJ, Staton CA, Taylor R, Limkakeng AT. Machine learning and precision medicine in emergency medicine: the basics. Cureus. 2021;13(9):e17636. https://doi.org/10.7759/cureus.17636.
9. Giangola M, Havens JM. Imaging in emergency general surgery. In: Brown C, Inaba K, Martin M, Salim A, editors. Emergency general surgery. Cham: Springer; 2019. https://doi.org/10.1007/978-3-319-96286-3_3.
10. Lipka A. From knife to suture: an outline of the history of surgical instrument development. Q J Hist Sci Technol. 2023;68(2):135–73. https://doi.org/10.4467/0023589XKHNT.23.018.17880.
11. Jones CL. Surgical instruments: history and historiography. In: Schlich T, editor. The Palgrave handbook of the history of surgery. London: Palgrave Macmillan; 2018. https://doi.org/10.1057/978-1-349-95260-1_12.
12. Sachs M, Auth M, Encke A. Historical development of surgical instruments exemplified by hemostatic forceps. World J Surg. 1998;22:499–504. https://doi.org/10.1007/s002689900424.
13. Qayumi K. Surgical techniques: past, present and future. Surg Tech Dev. 2012;2(1):e9. https://doi.org/10.4081/std.2012.e9.
14. Ceresoli M, Pisano M, Abu-Zidan F, Allievi N, Gurusamy K, Biffl WL, Tebala GD, Catena F, Ansaloni L, Sartelli M, Kluger Y, Baiocchi G, WSES MIS working group, WSES MIS consortia, Coccolini F. Minimally invasive surgery in emergency surgery: a WSES survey. World J Emerg Surg. 2022;17(1):18. https://doi.org/10.1186/s13017-022-00419-x.
15. Byer A. The origins of minimally invasive and robotic surgery and their impact on surgical practice: a sociological, technological history. In: Gharagozloo F, Patel VR, Giulianotti PC, Poston R, Gruessner R, Meyer M, editors. Robotic surgery. Cham: Springer; 2021. https://doi.org/10.1007/978-3-030-53594-0_2.
16. Waha JE, Uranues S. Laparoscopic approaches to emergency general surgery. In: Latifi R, Catena F, Coccolini F, editors. Emergency general surgery in geriatrics. Hot topics in acute care surgery and trauma. Cham: Springer; 2021. https://doi.org/10.1007/978-3-030-62215-2_30.
17. Costa-Navarro D, Romero-Simó M. Laparoscopy in surgical emergencies. In: Di Saverio S, Catena F, Ansaloni L, Coccolini F, Velmahos G, editors. Acute care surgery handbook. Cham: Springer; 2016. https://doi.org/10.1007/978-3-319-15362-9_14.
18. Gharagozloo F, Tempesta B, Meyer M, Nguyen D, Gruessner S, Redan J. History of robotic surgery. In: Gharagozloo F, Patel VR, Giulianotti PC, Poston R, Gruessner R, Meyer M, editors. Robotic surgery. Cham: Springer; 2021. https://doi.org/10.1007/978-3-030-53594-0_3.
19. de'Angelis N, Khan J, Marchegiani F, et al. Robotic surgery in emergency setting: 2021 WSES position paper. World J Emerg Surg. 2022;17(1):4. https://doi.org/10.1186/s13017-022-00410-6.
20. Kaul V, Enslin S, Gross SA. History of artificial intelligence in medicine. Gastrointest Endosc. 2020;92(4):807–12. https://doi.org/10.1016/j.gie.2020.06.040.

21. Jean A. Une brève introduction à l'intelligence artificielle [A brief history of artificial intelligence]. Med Sci. 2020;36(11):1059–67. https://doi.org/10.1051/medsci/2020189.
22. Litvin AA, Stoma IO, Sharshakova TM, Rumovskaya SB, Kyovalev AA. New possibilities of artificial intelligence in medicine: a narrative review. Health Ecol Issues. 2024;21(1):7–17. (In Russ.). https://doi.org/10.51523/2708-6011.2024-21-1-01.
23. Varghese C, Harrison EM, O'Grady G, et al. Artificial intelligence in surgery. Nat Med. 2024;30:1257–68. https://doi.org/10.1038/s41591-024-02970-3.
24. Litvin A, Korenev S, Rumovskaya S, et al. WSES project on decision support systems based on artificial neural networks in emergency surgery. World J Emerg Surg. 2021;16:50. https://doi.org/10.1186/s13017-021-00394-9.
25. Rimmer L, Howard C, Picca L, et al. The automaton as a surgeon: the future of artificial intelligence in emergency and general surgery. Eur J Trauma Emerg Surg. 2021;47:757–62. https://doi.org/10.1007/s00068-020-01444-8.
26. Hunter OF, Perry F, Salehi M, et al. Science fiction or clinical reality: a review of the applications of artificial intelligence along the continuum of trauma care. World J Emerg Surg. 2023;18:16. https://doi.org/10.1186/s13017-022-00469-1.
27. De Simone B, Abu-Zidan FM, Gumbs AA, et al. Knowledge, attitude, and practice of artificial intelligence in emergency and trauma surgery, the ARIES project: an international web-based survey. World J Emerg Surg. 2022;17(1):10. https://doi.org/10.1186/s13017-022-00413-3.
28. Howell MD, Corrado GS, DeSalvo KB. Three epochs of artificial intelligence in health care. JAMA. 2024;331(3):242–4. https://doi.org/10.1001/jama.2023.25057.
29. Liu N, Zhang Z, Ho AF, Ong ME. Artificial intelligence in emergency medicine. J Emerg Crit Care Med. 2018;2:82. https://doi.org/10.21037/jeccm.2018.10.08.
30. Taher F, Hofmann A, Assadian A. Precision medicine in vascular and endovascular surgery. J Clin Med. 2023;2023(12):1031. https://doi.org/10.3390/jcm12031031.
31. Guillén DG. The historical background of personalized medicine. In: Barilan YM, Brusa M, Ciechanover A, editors. Can precision medicine be personal; can personalized medicine be precise? Oxford: online edn, Oxford Academic; 2022. https://doi.org/10.1093/oso/9780198863465.003.0002.
32. Strehlow M, Alvarez A, Blomkalns AL, Caretta-Wyer H, Gharahbaghian L, Imler D, Khan A, Lee M, Lobo V, Newberry JA, Riberia R, Sebok-Syer S, Shen S, Gisondi MA. Precision emergency medicine. Acad Emerg Med. 2024; https://doi.org/10.1111/acem.14962. Advance online publication.
33. Fung BM, Markarian E, Serper M, Tabibian JH. Current applications of telemedicine in gastroenterology. Am J Gastroenterol. 2022;117(7):1072–9. https://doi.org/10.14309/ajg.0000000000001761.
34. Gorincour G, Monneuse O, Ben Cheikh A, Avondo J, Chaillot PF, Journe C, Youssof E, Lecomte JC, Thomson V. Management of abdominal emergencies in adults using telemedicine and artificial intelligence. J Visc Surg. 2021;158(3S):S26–31. https://doi.org/10.1016/j.jviscsurg.2021.01.008.

2 Essential Surgical Tools and Imaging Techniques in Emergency Surgery: A Practical Overview

Silvia Jasmine Barbara, Carlo Vallicelli, Giulia Griggio, and Fausto Catena

2.1 Introduction

This chapter provides a practical overview of essential surgical tools and imaging techniques used in emergency surgery, with a particular focus on their role in minimally invasive emergency and trauma procedures. The objective is to support clinical decision-making by outlining indications, principles of use, and integration into emergency surgical workflows, rather than to deliver procedural step-by-step descriptions, which are addressed elsewhere in this volume. The content is intended as educational guidance rather than formal clinical recommendations. The choice of surgical tools and imaging modalities should be individualized according to patient condition, institutional resources, and surgeon expertise. The principles discussed apply primarily to haemodynamically stable patients undergoing surgery for abdominal trauma or emergency general surgical conditions. An understanding of surgical timing and prioritization is fundamental when selecting appropriate

S. J. Barbara
Department of Morphology, Experimental Medicine and Surgery, University of Ferrara, Ferrara, Italy

C. Vallicelli (✉)
General, Emergency and Trauma Surgery Department, Bufalini Hospital, Cesena, Italy
e-mail: carlo.vallicelli@auslromagna.it

G. Griggio
Department of General Surgery and Medical-Surgical Specialties, University of Catania, Catania, Italy

F. Catena
General, Emergency and Trauma Surgery Department, Bufalini Hospital, Cesena, Italy

Dipartimento di Scienze Mediche e Chirurgiche, Alma Mater Stodiorum, University of Bologna, Bologna, Italy
e-mail: faustocatena@gmail.com

B. De Simone et al. (eds.), *New Technologies, Precision Medicine, and AI in Emergency General Surgery*, Hot Topics in Acute Care Surgery and Trauma,
https://doi.org/10.1007/978-3-032-09357-8_2

technologies in emergency settings. The Institute for Healthcare Optimization proposed the Timing in Acute Care Surgery (TACS) classification, a colour-coded triage system that stratifies patients requiring operative intervention within 24 hours of emergency department admission [1, 2]. This system integrates haemodynamic status, disease severity, and the presence of sepsis as key determinants of surgical urgency [3]. According to the TACS classification, Red (Level 1) patients require immediate surgical intervention within 1 hour, and Orange (Level 2) patients within 2 hours. Yellow (Level 3) cases should access the operating room within 6 hours, Green (Level 4) within 12 hours, and Blue (Level 5) within 24 hours. A validated White (Level 6) category has been introduced to identify cancelled or delayed procedures that should be rescheduled within one week [4]. For practical purposes, Levels 1 and 2 are classified as emergency cases, while Levels 3 and 4 are considered urgent cases [5]. Operating room prioritization follows this stratification, with higher-acuity cases taking precedence. Ongoing clinical reassessment is essential, as changes in physiological status may necessitate escalation to a higher priority level [6]. Emergency and trauma surgical practice most commonly involves exploratory laparotomy, appendectomy, and abdominal wound exploration or debridement. Exploratory laparotomy is primarily indicated in blunt or penetrating abdominal trauma, while emergency operative management is also required for acute bowel ischemia, strangulated hernias, generalized peritonitis, and gastrointestinal perforations, typically classified as Level 2 conditions. Complicated appendicitis, complicated diverticulitis with sepsis, and gangrenous cholecystitis represent frequent Level 3 indications for urgent surgical intervention. For consistency throughout this chapter, the terms "emergency" and "urgent" will be used interchangeably unless otherwise specified.

2.2 Patient and Trocar Positioning as a Prerequisite for Effective Tool Use

Patients are generally positioned supine on the operating table, ideally using pressure-redistributing pads to reduce the risk of pressure-related injuries during prolonged or complex procedures [7]. Upper and lower limbs may be positioned alongside the body or abducted, depending on the surgical field of interest and the required range of instrument motion. Secure fixation of the trunk and extremities is recommended to prevent inadvertent displacement during table tilting or rotation, which is frequently required to optimize exposure and visualization [8]. The surgical team is positioned in relation to the operative field to ensure ergonomic instrument handling and unobstructed visualization, thereby reducing operator fatigue and improving precision during tool manipulation [9]. In minimally invasive emergency surgery, access to the abdominal cavity is achieved through the establishment of pneumoperitoneum using carbon dioxide, most commonly via the Veress needle or open (Hasson) technique. Adequate pneumoperitoneum is essential to create sufficient working space for the safe introduction of optical systems and operating trocars under direct vision. Correct trocar placement and triangulation are critical to maximize the efficiency and safety of energy devices, staplers, and imaging tools, facilitating controlled movements and reducing the risk of iatrogenic injury [10]. Standard trocar diameters typically range from 5 to 12 mm; however, reduced-diameter ports (2–4 mm) have been introduced and may offer comparable clinical outcomes in selected cases, while potentially reducing access-related trauma [11]. Technological advancements in minimally invasive surgery have progressively expanded the range and performance of available surgical tools. These innovations support faster, more accurate intraoperative decision-making in emergency and trauma settings, contributing to improved visualization, reduced operative time, and a lower risk of missed injuries—factors that are particularly relevant in time-critical scenarios [12–14].

2.2.1 Haemostasis and Energy Devices

In laparoscopic emergency surgery, pneumoperitoneum contributes to haemostasis by exerting a direct pressure effect on small vessels (baro-haemostasis) and through carbon dioxide–induced vasoconstriction. While this mechanism is often sufficient to control minor oozing, active bleeding from larger vessels typically requires dedicated haemostatic tools, including mechanical clips, energy-based coagulation devices, topical haemostatic agents, or conventional gauze compression [15, 16]. Maintenance of a bloodless operative field is essential not only for haemostasis but also for optimal visualization. Even limited bleeding can significantly impair image quality, as blood absorbs and darkens the laparoscopic light source, obscuring anatomical planes and increasing the risk of iatrogenic injury [17]. For this reason, tissue dissection and vascular control in emergency settings rely heavily on electrosurgical and energy-based devices. The choice of device is influenced by tissue characteristics, bleeding severity, surgeon experience, and the need for durable haemostasis to minimize postoperative haemorrhage [18]. Monopolar energy devices (e.g. curved hook) provide cutting and coagulation functions, reaching high temperatures (up to approximately 350 °C). Their use is associated with smoke production and a relatively wide lateral thermal spread, which may extend up to 22 mm [19]. Bipolar devices (e.g. bipolar forceps or scissors) deliver energy exclusively to the tissue grasped between the jaws, achieving coagulation without cutting and limiting maximum temperatures to approximately 100 °C, thereby reducing collateral thermal damage [19]. Advanced bipolar radiofrequency systems (e.g. LigaSure™, EnSeal™) deliver high-current, low-voltage energy that denatures collagen and elastin, allowing reliable vessel sealing—typically up to 7.5 mm in diameter. Newer-generation devices combine vessel sealing with integrated cutting functions, improving efficiency in emergency procedures [16]. Ultrasonic energy devices (e.g. Harmonic™) convert electrical energy into mechanical vibration, enabling precise dissection and coagulation while sealing vessels generally up to 3.5–5 mm. Prolonged activation may lead to jaw temperatures exceeding 150 °C, increasing the risk of lateral thermal injury [20]. Hybrid technologies combining bipolar and ultrasonic energy aim to optimize haemostasis while facilitating fine tissue dissection [21]. Laser-based systems (e.g. CO_2 or argon laser) convert electromagnetic energy into thermal energy for coagulation and tissue ablation, with limited collateral spread depending on tissue absorption and penetration depth [20]. In emergency laparoscopy, thermal injury represents a significant risk. Instruments cool more slowly than in open surgery due to the humid intraperitoneal environment, which also increases electrical conductivity. Excessive activation time, high temperatures, or inadvertent contact may result in blunt or thermal tissue injury and perforation, potentially worsening patient outcomes [22]. Tissue coagulation begins at approximately 60 °C; at higher temperatures, cellular water vaporizes, leading to membrane disruption, charring between 200 and 300 °C, and tissue vaporization beyond 500 °C [16]. The main characteristics, advantages, and limitations of energy-based haemostatic devices commonly used in emergency surgery are summarized in Table 2.1. Adjunct haemostatic tools complement energy-based techniques and include mechanical clip applicators (titanium or absorbable), topical active haemostatic agents based on fibrinogen and thrombin (e.g. fibrin glues, patches, or powders), and passive haemostatic matrices that promote platelet aggregation and clot formation [23–25]. Passive agents should be avoided in patients with coagulation disorders, while gelatin-based products should not be used in contaminated fields [26]. Synthetic and semi-synthetic sealants may also be employed to create a protective barrier over bleeding surfaces [27, 28]. Non–energy-based haemostatic tools and their main characteristics are summarized in Table 2.2.

2.2.2 Mechanical Stapling Devices

Mechanical staplers are devices designed to create an automatic suture by placing metal staples (double or triple shifted rows of U-shaped graphs) between tissues and vessels [29, 30]. *Linear staplers* (e.g. Covidien TA™, Ethicon Linear™) are the most common and come in lengths of 35, 45, and 60 mm. The latest models are more flexible and can be articulated. The cartridges vary in thicknesses and closure heights and are distinguished by different colours; a reduced thickness enhances the haemostatic effect, whereas an increased thickness reinforces tissue tightness. The surgeon selects the appropriate cartridge based on tissue characteristics, regardless of the surgical setting. *EndoLinear Cutting staplers* (e.g EndoGIA™, Echelon Flex™) include a cutting function after sealing the tissues with two or three rows of staples on each cutting border. *Circular staplers* (e.g. Ethicon Circular™, Covidien EEA™) place a double staple line circumferentially and simultaneously cut the tissue with a circular blade; their calibres comprise 21-25-29-31-33 mm staple-heads [31]. New-age staplers are powered by electrical motors that control activation, articulation, closing, and opening of the tool; tissue compression is sensed by transducers and visualized on small monitors mounted on the instrument's shaft [32].

2.2.3 Wound Protection and Access Devices

Wound infections occur frequently (up to 10%) in laparoscopic clean-contaminated or dirty procedures, prompting the introduction of surgical wound protectors to try to stem contamination and postoperative infection rates [33]. Early materials used

Table 2.1 Energy-based devices for haemostasis and dissection in emergency surgery

Energy modality	Examples	Mechanism of action	Temperature range	Vessel sealing capacity	Advantages	Limitations/Risks
Monopolar coagulation	Curved hook	Electrical current passes through tissue, producing cutting and coagulation	Up to ~350 °C	Not specific for vessel sealing	Versatile; effective cutting, and coagulation	Wide lateral thermal spread (up to 22 mm), smoke production, and higher risk of collateral thermal injury
Bipolar coagulation	Bipolar forceps, bipolar scissors	Energy delivered only between the jaws holding the tissue	Up to ~100 °C	Small vessels	Controlled coagulation; reduced thermal spread	No intrinsic cutting function (in conventional devices)
Advanced bipolar radiofrequency	LigaSure™, EnSeal™	High-current, low-voltage bipolar energy denatures collagen and elastin	Lower peak temperatures than monopolar	Vessels up to ~7.5 mm	Reliable haemostasis; some devices allow cutting	Higher cost; learning curve
Ultrasonic energy	Harmonic™	High-frequency mechanical vibration denatures collagen	Up to ~150 °C with prolonged activation	Vessels ~3.5–5 mm	Precise dissection; limited smoke	Risk of thermal injury with prolonged activation; lateral spread up to 2–10 mm
Hybrid bipolar + ultrasonic	Thunderbeat™	Bipolar energy for haemostasis + ultrasonic energy for cutting	Variable	Vessels up to ~7 mm	Combines effective haemostasis and fine dissection	Device cost; requires familiarity
Laser electrocautery	CO_2/Argon laser	Electromagnetic energy converted to thermal energy	Depends on tissue absorption	Small vessels	Precise coagulation; limited collateral damage	Limited availability; specialized equipment

Table 2.2 Non–energy-based haemostatic tools commonly used in emergency surgery

Haemostatic method	Examples	Composition/ Mechanism	Indications	Advantages	Limitations/ Contraindications
Mechanical clip applicators	Titanium or absorbable clips	Mechanical vessel occlusion	Small–medium vessel bleeding	Immediate haemostasis; no thermal injury; reusable or disposable options	Limited use in friable tissues; risk of clip displacement
Active adhesive haemostatic agents	Fibrin glues (Quixil™, Tisseel™, Evicel™, Surgiflo™, FloSeal™); fibrin patches/powders (TachoSil™, Takea™, Fibrin Pad™)	Human fibrinogen and thrombin form an adherent fibrin clot	Diffuse oozing; parenchymal bleeding; patients with coagulation disorders	Rapid action; fully resorbable; effective even with impaired coagulation	Higher cost; requires relatively dry field
Passive (mechanical) haemostats	Oxidized regenerated cellulose (TaboTamp™, Knu-nit, Surgicel™)	Matrix promotes platelet activation and clot formation; acidic pH denatures proteins	Capillary and low-pressure bleeding	Easy to use; bactericidal properties	Ineffective in coagulation disorders; swelling may cause compression
Gelatin-based haemostats	Porcine/bovine gelatins (FloSeal™)	Absorbable gelatin matrix promoting clot formation	Surface bleeding after compression	Conforms to irregular surfaces; effective with compression	Avoid in contaminated fields; requires wet gauze coverage
Synthetic and semisynthetic sealants	Hemopatch™, DuraSeal™	Polymerize to form a protective sealing barrier	Reinforcement of suture lines; low-pressure bleeding	Immediate sealing; no blood-derived components	Limited haemostatic power alone; cost

varied widely and included cloth, polyethylene, and plastic drapes [34]; the latest devices (e.g. Alexis™) are mainly composed of non-adhesive plastic sheaths attached to single or double rubber rings, which ease wound retraction by securing the rubber ring(s) to the incision's edges [35].

2.3 Imaging and Visualization Technologies

2.3.1 Intraoperative and Perioperative Imaging Modalities in Emergency Surgery

Imaging technologies play a pivotal role in emergency surgery by supporting diagnosis, operative planning, and intraoperative decision-making. Radiological imaging modalities represent the first level of assessment in acute and trauma settings. Ultrasound is a first-line, cost-effective tool that allows real-time visualization of soft tissues, vascular flow, organ margins, free peritoneal fluid, and possible vascular extravasation, enabling rapid identification of internal bleeding, organ injuries, and foreign bodies [37–39]. Conventional radiography of the chest, abdomen, and pelvis is frequently used to detect pneumothorax, hemothorax, pelvic instability, skeletal fractures, free intra-abdominal air, and retained foreign bodies, while providing rapid information with relatively low radiation exposure [40–42]. Computed tomography (CT) represents the second-line imaging modality in emergency and trauma surgery, offering high sensitivity and specificity for the detection of hollow-viscus and solid-organ injuries. Its ability to generate high-resolution cross-sectional and three-dimensional reconstructions facilitates comprehensive assessment of complex injuries and supports operative strategy selection, although its use must be balanced against radiation exposure, costs, and limited intraoperative availability [43–46]. Angiography provides advanced vascular imaging, enabling real-time evaluation of blood flow, identification of vascular injuries or pseudoaneurysms, and guidance for haemostatic interventions such as angioembolization or targeted surgical repair; however, its technical complexity, procedural duration, contrast-related risks, and radiation exposure must be carefully considered in emergency contexts [47–49]. Magnetic resonance imaging (MRI) plays a limited role in acute surgical decision-making due to longer acquisition times and reduced accessibility, despite its excellent soft-tissue contrast and diagnostic accuracy comparable to CT in selected indications [50, 51]. Within the operating room, intraoperative visualization systems constitute an essential surgical tool. Modern laparoscopic camera platforms provide high-definition two-dimensional imaging with advanced light balance, color fidelity, and magnification, reaching ultra-high-definition resolutions up to 8K. These systems significantly enhance precision and safety during minimally invasive emergency procedures. Although robotic platforms offer three-dimensional vision, contemporary laparoscopic imaging systems have achieved image quality sufficient for complex emergency interventions. Major videoendoscopic system providers include Olympus, Stryker, and Karl Storz [36]. Emerging technologies, such as head-mounted displays, immersive visualization systems, and retinal projection platforms, aim to further enhance depth perception and situational awareness [10]. Together, perioperative radiological imaging and intraoperative visualization technologies provide complementary, real-time anatomical and functional information, enabling surgeons to optimize operative strategies, reduce complication rates, and minimize inadvertent injury to adjacent structures in emergency surgical settings [52].

2.3.2 Fluorescent Imaging with Indocyanine Green

Indocyanine green (ICG) is a non-toxic, non-radioactive, water-soluble fluorophore that can be administered intravenously or interstitially, with a recommended dose not exceeding 2 mg/kg [53]. Other fluorescent contrast agents currently approved for medical use by the FDA and the European Medicines Agency include methylene blue and sodium fluorescein [54]. Following intravenous injection, ICG binds to plasma lipoproteins, whereas after interstitial administration, it accumulates in lymphatic tissues. When excited by near-infrared light (approximately 800 nm), it emits a green fluorescent signal that can be detected by dedicated imaging systems [55, 56]. This technology enables real-time assessment of bowel perfusion—particularly useful for evaluating intestinal anastomoses and transection margins—as well as visualization of vascular anatomy, clarification of extrahepatic biliary structures, and identification of lymphatic drainage pathways [57, 58]. In emergency and trauma surgery, fluorescence imaging with ICG represents an emerging adjunct that may prove valuable in assessing tissue perfusion in anatomically distorted or compromised areas, where inflammation, ischemia, or tissue damage may limit conventional visual assessment [59, 60]. Despite encouraging preliminary results, further studies are required to define standardized indications, optimal dosing, timing, and safety profiles in acute care settings before routine adoption in emergency surgery can be recommended [61, 62].

2.3.3 Intraoperative Cholangioscopy

In biliary disease, the implementation of intraoperative cholangioscopy during laparoscopic elective or urgent cholecystectomy has improved both diagnostic accuracy and therapeutic capability, reducing the need for a dedicated endoscopic team in the operating room [63]. A cholangioscope allows direct visualization of the biliary mucosa and exploration of the biliary tree (e.g. Olympus cholangioscope™, Boston Scientific SpyGlass™). When used intraoperatively, it may be introduced via the trans-cystic or trans-hepatic route and accommodates accessories such as biopsy forceps, retrieval baskets, dilation balloons, and lithotripsy devices, enabling interventions ranging from diagnostic sampling to stone fragmentation and biliary drainage [64, 65]. In emergency settings, intraoperative cholangioscopy is particularly useful during acute cholecystitis, where inflammatory changes may distort anatomy and conventional endoscopic approaches (EUS or ERCP) can be technically challenging or less readily available [66].

2.3.4 Robotic Surgery

Robotic surgery represents an important evolution of minimally invasive techniques, offering enhanced visualization, instrument dexterity, and ergonomic control [67–69]. Advanced three-dimensional imaging platforms and stable camera systems may improve precision during complex procedures. In addition, artificial intelligence–assisted technologies can analyse real-time video feeds to support instrument tracking and spatial awareness, potentially reducing inadvertent tissue injury [70]. However, the application of robotic-assisted surgery in emergency settings remains limited by higher costs, logistical constraints, technical complexity, and the requirement for specialized expertise and platform availability [71]. Current evidence suggests that artificial intelligence is unlikely to replace the surgeon; rather, a complementary role is anticipated, in which AI supports surgical decision-making by integrating intraoperative data while clinical judgment remains central [72]. A recent consensus statement from the World Society of Emergency Surgery has suggested that robotic technology may be considered in selected acute settings, provided that adequate experience, institutional support, and appropriate infrastructure are available [73–75].

2.4 Anastomosis, Drainage, and Tool-Driven Decision-Making

Following emergency abdominal surgery, surgeons are frequently required to decide whether to perform an intestinal anastomosis—manual or mechanical—or to divert the bowel with an enterostomy, as well as whether to place intra-abdominal drains [76]. In selected emergency and trauma settings, a single-stage procedure with primary anastomosis has demonstrated feasibility and outcomes comparable to stoma formation, even in minimally invasive surgery [77]. These decisions are guided by multiple intraoperative and patient-related factors, including haemodynamic stability, degree of contamination, extent of bowel injury, tissue quality, comorbidities, and overall physiological reserve, in addition to surgeon experience and available technology [78]. From a tool-centred perspective, mechanical anastomosis has been shown to be non-inferior to hand-sewn techniques [79]. Although it requires dedicated stapling devices and entails higher costs with a potential risk of device malfunction, it offers advantages such as faster execution, reduced technical demand, and shorter operative time, which may be particularly relevant in emergency settings [80, 81]. The choice between manual and mechanical anastomosis should therefore be individualized according to the specific clinical scenario [82]. Abdominal drains are intended to evacuate infected or inflammatory fluid, gas, or collections and to provide early indication of postoperative complications. However, drain placement is not without risk and may result in organ or vessel injury, tissue pressure damage, infection, or obstruction [83]. Drains may be classified as open passive, closed passive, or closed active systems, depending on their mechanism of action. Evidence from enhanced recovery pathways has increasingly questioned their routine use. The 2018 ERAS Society guidelines for elective colorectal surgery and the 2023 ERAS guidelines for emergency laparotomy report no clear benefit of routine drain placement in terms of anastomotic leak, mortality, wound infection, or reoperation rates, and therefore recommend avoiding drains whenever possible [84–87]. Accurate intraoperative assessment of gastrointestinal integrity is essential in emergency laparoscopy. The use of methylene blue dye, administered via a nasogastric tube or transanally, represents a simple and cost-effective method to detect gastrointestinal perforations or anastomotic leaks by directly visualizing dye extravasation, even in cases of diffuse peritonitis [88, 89]. Its diagnostic value may be reduced or contraindicated in the presence of significant gastrointestinal bleeding or obstruction [90]. Similarly, the air-leak test is a widely used adjunct for evaluating the integrity of bowel anastomoses and surgical repairs. Air insufflation into the gastrointestinal tract, followed by observation for bubble formation in a saline-filled operative field, allows prompt identification of leaks and immediate correction [91]. However, its reliability may be limited by factors such as bowel distension, adhesions, or active bleeding, and it does not provide quantitative information on leak size nor predict delayed or postoperative leakage [92, 93].

2.5 Limits and Safe Use of Technology in Emergency Settings

Patients undergoing surgical procedures in the emergency setting have been reported to experience significantly higher mortality compared with those undergoing the same procedures electively, with substantial associated healthcare costs [94]. In this context, the safe and appropriate use of surgical technology requires continuous intraoperative reassessment and a low threshold for strategy modification. Conditions such as extensive adhesions, bowel distension, diffuse inflammation or peritonitis with loss of normal anatomical planes, improper patient or trocar positioning, inadequate visualization, prolonged operative time without meaningful progress, iatrogenic organ injury, uncontrolled bleeding, or haemodynamic instability—particularly in the presence of the lethal triad of hypothermia, acidosis, and coagulopathy—represent clear warning signs that continuation of a minimally invasive approach may be unsafe and that conversion to laparotomy should be strongly considered [95]. Conversion to open surgery should not be regarded as a failure of minimally invasive techniques but rather as a timely and prudent decision aimed at safeguarding patient safety [96, 97]. Laparotomy provides direct access and comprehensive visualization of abdominal structures and facilitates more effective haemorrhage control. In patients with severe physiological derangement and diffuse contamination, where definitive repair exceeds the patient's remaining physiological reserve, a damage control strategy may be indicated to abbreviate operative time and allow prompt transfer to the intensive care unit for resuscitation and stabilization, thereby improving survival and outcomes [98, 99]. Nevertheless, open surgery is associated with relevant disadvantages, including increased morbidity, higher postoperative complication rates, greater postoperative pain, and prolonged recovery and hospital stay. It may also necessitate staged procedures, delay definitive treatment, and increase overall resource utilization [100]. These considerations underscore the importance of balancing the potential benefits of advanced surgical technologies with their limitations in emergency settings.

2.6 Conclusions and Future Perspectives

Emergency surgery increasingly relies on the appropriate integration of essential surgical tools and imaging technologies to support timely, safe, and effective decision-making. As outlined in this chapter, advances in energy devices, stapling systems, haemostatic tools, and intraoperative visualization have expanded the feasibility of minimally invasive approaches in selected emergency and trauma settings. At the same time, perioperative and intraoperative imaging modalities—including ultrasound, cross-sectional imaging, fluorescence-guided surgery, and targeted endoscopic techniques—provide critical anatomical and functional information that enhances surgical precision and situational awareness. However, the use of advanced technologies in emergency surgery must remain context-driven and patient-centred, with continuous reassessment of physiological status, anatomical conditions, and procedural progress. Awareness of the limits and risks associated with these tools is essential to avoid technology-driven persistence when conversion or alternative strategies better serve patient safety. Future perspectives in emergency surgery will likely focus on improved integration rather than mere technological expansion, emphasizing standardization, training, and evidence-based adoption. Emerging developments in real-time imaging, fluorescence guidance, and data-assisted intraoperative support may further enhance decision-making, provided that their implementation is guided by robust clinical validation, accessibility, and cost-effectiveness. Ultimately, technology should function as an adjunct to—not a substitute for—surgical judgement, experience, and responsibility in the management of critically ill emergency patients.

Conflicts of Interest All authors have no conflicts of interest to declare.

Funding This research received no external funding or financial support from any organization for the submitted work.

References

1. Ahmed K, Zygourakis C, Kalb S, Pennington Z, Molina C, Emerson T, Theodore N. Protocol for urgent and emergent cases at a large academic level 1 trauma center. Cureus. 2019;11(1):e3973. PMID: 30956925; PMCID: PMC6438689.
2. Kluger Y, Ben-Ishay O, Sartelli M, Ansaloni L, et al. World society of emergency surgery study group initiative on timing of acute care surgery classification (TACS). World J Emerg Surg. 2013;1:17. https://doi.org/10.1186/1749-7922-8-17. PMID: 23634 784; PMCID: PMC36 52724.
3. Weinbroum AA, Ekstein P, Ezri T. Efficiency of the operating room suite. Am J Surg. 2003;185:244–50.

4. De Simone B, Kluger Y, Moore EE, et al. The new timing in acute care surgery (new TACS) classification: a WSES Delphi consensus study. World J Emerg Surg. 2023;1:32. https://doi.org/10.1186/s13017-023-00499-3. PMID: 37118816; PMCID: PMC10147354.
5. Levtzion-Korach O, Murphy KG, Madden S, Dempsey C. For urgent and emergent cases, which one goes to the OR first? OR Manager. 2010;26(7):1, 11–3.
6. Leppäniemi A, Jousela I. A traffic-light coding system to organize emergency surgery across surgical disciplines. Br J Surg. 2014;101(1):e134–40. https://doi.org/10.1002/bjs.9325.
7. Haesler E, European Pressure Ulcer Advisory Panel, National Pressure Injury Advisory Panel, and Pan Pacific Pressure Injury Alliance. Prevention and treatment of pressure ulcers/injuries: clinical practice guideline. The International Guideline. EPUAP, NPIAP, PPPIA. 2019.
8. Guzman S, Allegretti AL, Kormos RL, Brienza DM. A comparison of air-cell and gel surgical table pads and an evaluation of the influence of pressure distribution and other factors on pressure injury prevention. J Tissue Viability. 2021;30(1):9–15. https://doi.org/10.1016/j.jtv.2020.12.006.
9. Gómez-Ríos MA, Abad-Gurumeta A, Casans-Francés R, Calvo-Vecino JM. Keys to optimizing operating room efficiency. Rev Esp Anestesiol Reanim (Engl Ed). 2019;66(2):104–12. https://doi.org/10.1016/j.redar.2018.08.002.
10. Benini B, Piagnerelli R. Cap 2. Strumentario per Chirurgia Laparoscopica. [book auth.] Bruno Benini. Manuale (Molto) Pratico di Chirurgia Laparoscopica. Info Stampa: Roma; 2008.
11. Shadduck PP, Paquentin EM, Carvalho GL, Redan JA. Mini-laparoscopy: instruments and economics. Surg Technol Int. 2015;27:59–64.
12. Warps A-LK, Zwanenburg ES, Dekker JWT, et al. Laparoscopic versus open colorectal surgery in the emergency setting: a systematic review and meta-analysis. Ann Surg Open. 2021;2:e097. https://doi.org/10.1097/AS9.0000000000000097.
13. Firat N, Mantoglu B, Akin E, Bas E, Altintoprak F. Why diagnostic laparoscopy. Pol Przegl Chir. 2021;93(3):15. https://doi.org/10.5604/01.3001.0014.8220.
14. Pau L, Navez J, Cawich SO, Dapri G. Laparoscopic management of blunt and penetrating abdominal trauma: a single-center experience and review of the literature. J Laparoendosc Adv Surg Tech A. 2021;31(11):1262–8. https://doi.org/10.1089/lap.2020.0552.
15. Boni L, Cassinotti E, Benevento A, et al. Principi di Tecnica Chirurgica. [book auth.] Cabitza P, Carcano G, et al. Dionigi R. Dionigi Chirurgia: Basi teoriche e Chirurgia Generale. Milano: Edra; 2017.
16. Benini B. Cap 11. Emostasi in Chirurgia Laparoscopica. [book auth.] R. Piagnerelli B. Benini. Manuale (Molto) Pratico di Chirurgia Laparoscopica. Roma: Info Stampa; 2008.
17. Applewhite MK, White MG, James BC, Abdulrasool L, Kaplan EL, Angelos P, Grogan RH. Ultrasonic, bipolar, and integrated energy devices: comparing heat spread in collateral tissues. J Surg Res. 2017;207:249–54. https://doi.org/10.1016/j.jss.2016.06.077.
18. Abi Antoun M, Etrusco A, Chiantera V, Laganà AS, Feghali E, Khazzaka A, Stabile G, Della Corte L, Dellino M, Sleiman Z. Outcomes of conventional and advanced energy devices in laparoscopic surgery: a systematic review. Minim Invasive Ther Allied Technol. 2024;33(1):1–12. https://doi.org/10.1080/13645706.2023.2274396.
19. McGinnis DE, Strup SE, Gomella LG. Management of hemorrhage during laparoscopy. J Endourol. 2000;14(10):915–20. https://doi.org/10.1089/end.2000.14.915.
20. Lattouf JB, Beri A, Klinger CH, Jeschke S, Janetschek G. Practical hints for hemostasis in laparoscopic surgery. Minim Invasive Ther Allied Technol. 2007;16(1): 45–51. https://doi.org/10.1080/13645700601157984.
21. Seehofer D, Mogl M, Boas-Knoop S, Unger J, Schirmeier A, Chopra S, Eurich D. Safety and efficacy of new integrated bipolar and ultrasonic scissors compared to conventional laparoscopic 5-mm sealing and cutting instruments. Surg Endosc. 2012;26(9):2541–9. https://doi.org/10.1007/s00464-012-2229-0. PMID: 22447285; PMCID: PMC3427482.
22. Chiara O, Cimbanassi S, Bellanova G, et al. A systematic review on the use of topical hemostats in trauma and emergency surgery. BMC Surg. 2018;18(1):68. https://doi.org/10.1186/s12893-018-0398-z. PMID: 30157821; PMCID: PMC6116382.

23. Vecchio R, Catalano R, Basile F, Spataro C, Caputo M, Intagliata E. Topical hemostasis in laparoscopic surgery. G Chir. 2016;37(6):266–70. https://doi.org/10.11138/gchir/2016.37.6.266. PMID: 28350974; PMCID: PMC5505485.
24. Koea JK, Baldwin P, Shen J, Patel B, Batiller J, Arnaud A, et al. Safety and hemostatic effectiveness of the fibrin pad for severe soft-tissue bleeding during abdominal retroperitoneal, pelvic, and thoracic (non-cardiac) surgery: a randomized, controlled, superiority trial. World J Surg. 2015;39:2663–9.
25. Klingler CH, Remzi M, Marberger M, Janetschek G. Haemostasis in laparoscopy. Eur Urol. 2006;50(5):948–56. https://doi.org/10.1016/j.eururo.2006.01.058.
26. Lewis KM, Spazierer D, Urban MD, Lin L, Redl H, Goppelt A. Comparison of regenerated and non-regenerated oxidized cellulose hemostatic agents. Eur Surg. 2013;45:213–20.
27. Dumville JC, Coulthard P, Worthington HV, Riley P, Patel N, Darcey J, et al. Tissue adhesives for closure of surgical incisions (review). Cochrane Database Syst Rev. 2014;11:CD004287.
28. Bulger EM, Snyder D, Schoelles K, Gotschall C, Dawson D, Lang E, et al. An evidence-based prehospital guideline for external hemorrhage control: American College of Surgeons Committee on trauma. Prehospital Emergency Care. 2014;18(2):163–73.
29. McGuire J, Wright IC, Leverment JN. Surgical staplers: a review. J R Coll Surg Edinb. 1997;42(1):1–9.
30. Burgio V, Bei J, Rodriguez Reinoso M, Civera M, Grimaldo Ruiz O, Surace C, Pugno NM. Mechanical stapling devices for soft tissue repair: a review of commercially available linear, linear cutting, and circular staplers. Appl Sci. 2024;14(6):2486.
31. Shivdekar S, Rojatkar P, Cummings JF, Clymer JW, Ricketts CD, Petraiuolo WJ. Comparison of circular staplers with adjustable staple height vs. fixed graduated staple height. World J Surg Surgical Res. 2021;4:1344.
32. Park SY, et al. Clinical and economic benefits associated with the use of powered and tissue-specific endoscopic staplers among the patients undergoing Thoracoscopic lobectomy for lung cancer. J Med Econ. 2019;22:1274–80.
33. Luo Y, Qiu YE, Mu YF, Qin SL, Qi Y, Zhong M, Yu MH, Ma LY. Plastic wound protectors decreased surgical site infections following laparoscopic-assisted colectomy for colorectal cancer: a retrospective cohort study. Medicine (Baltimore). 2017;96(37):e7752. https://doi.org/10.1097/MD.0000000000007752. PMID: 28906360; PMCID: PMC5604629.
34. Sajid MS, Rathore MA, Sains P, Singh KK. A systematic review of clinical effectiveness of wound edge protector devices in reducing surgical site infections in patients undergoing abdominal surgery. Updates Surg. 2017;69(1): 21–8. https://doi.org/10.1007/s13304-017-0415-2.
35. Web Appendix 18, Summary of a systematic review on wound protector devices. Global Guidelines for the Prevention of Surgical Site Infection. [Online] 2018. [Cited: 22 05 2024.] https://www.ncbi.nlm.nih.gov/books/NBK536418/.
36. Top 3 Global Video Endoscopy Companies. iData Research: Intelligence behind the Data. [Online] 28 05 2021. [Cited: 22 05 2024.] https://idataresearch.com/top-3-global-video-endoscopy-companies/.
37. Kokudo N, Sugawara Y. Intraoperative ultrasonography in liver surgery. J Hepato-Biliary-Pancreatic Sci. 2006;13(1):1–7.
38. Rizk N, Smith B. Intraoperative ultrasound in trauma surgery: a comprehensive guide. J Trauma Acute Care Surg. 2020;89(2): 352–61. https://doi.org/10.1097/TA.0000000000002694.
39. Petrov MS, Windsor JA. Current and future applications of intraoperative ultrasound in abdominal surgery. World J Surg. 2019;43(3): 658–69. https://doi.org/10.1007/s00268-018-4829-1.
40. Aucar JA, Webb T. Utility of intraoperative radiography in trauma surgery. J Trauma Acute Care Surg. 2019;86(5): 850–7. https://doi.org/10.1097/TA.0000000000002201.
41. Stawicki SP, Grossman MD. Intraoperative imaging techniques in trauma and emergency surgery. Int J Critic Illness Injury Sci. 2017;7(1):10–15. https://doi.org/10.4103/2229-5151.201939.
42. Long, B., & Koyfman, A. Radiographic imaging in trauma and emergency surgery: an overview. Emerg Med Clin N Am. 2018;36(1):1–25. https://doi.org/10.1016/j.emc.2017.09.002.

43. Singh R, Gupta S. Intraoperative imaging in orthopedic surgery. J Clin Orthopaedics Trauma. 2013;4(3):151–6.
44. Collins JA, Levy JH. Intraoperative imaging techniques in trauma surgery: CT and beyond. Am J Surg. 2019;217(2):341–9. https://doi.org/10.1016/j.amjsurg.2018.09.027.
45. Jansen JO, Morrison JJ. Intraoperative computed tomography in the management of trauma patients. Br J Surg. 2017;104(10):1313–20. https://doi.org/10.1002/bjs.10594.
46. Chiu WC, Dutton RP. Intraoperative CT imaging in trauma and emergency surgery: indications and outcomes. J Trauma Manage Outcomes. 2016;10(1):9–18. https://doi.org/10.1186/s13032-016-0039-4.
47. Gong RH, Hu J, Zhu J, Zhang Q. Clinical application of intraoperative angiography in vascular surgery. J Vasc Surg. 2019;69(3):759–5.
48. Miller PR, Meredith JW. Applications of intraoperative angiography in trauma surgery. Trauma Surg Acute Care Open. 2019;4(1):e000297. https://doi.org/10.1136/tsaco-2019-000297.
49. Friese RS, Hunt JL. The role of intraoperative angiography in managing abdominal vascular trauma. J Trauma Acute Care Surg. 2018;85(6):1043–50. https://doi.org/10.1097/TA.0000000000002037.
50. Feigl GC, Ulmer S, Klein J, Tronnier, V. M. Intraoperative imaging in neurosurgery: an overview. J Magn Reson Imaging. 2007;27(2):304–8.
51. Gervaise A, Chapiro J. Clinical applications of intraoperative MRI in abdominal trauma surgery. Abdomin Radiol. 2019;44(5): 1729–37. https://doi.org/10.1007/s00261-019-01965-2.
52. Benzel EC. Spine surgery: techniques, complication avoidance, and management. s.l.: Elsevier Health Sciences; 2011.
53. Spinoglio G, Bertani E, Borin S, Piccioli A, Petz W. Green indocyanine fluorescence in robotic abdominal surgery. Updates Surg. 2018;70(3):375–9, https://doi.org/10.1007/s13304-018-0585-6.
54. Fransvea P, Chiarello MM, Fico V, Cariati M, Brisinda G. Indocyanine green: the guide to safer and more effective surgery. World J Gastrointest Surg. 2024;16(3): 641–9. https://doi.org/10.4240/wjgs.v16.i3.641. PMID: 38577071; PMCID: PMC10989327.
55. Marshall MV, Rasmussen JC, Tan IC, Aldrich MB, Adams KE, Wang X, Fife CE, Maus EA, Smith LA, Sevick-Muraca EM. Near-infrared fluorescence imaging in humans with indocyanine green: a review and update. Open Surg Oncol J. 2010;2:12–25.
56. Mangano A, Gheza F, Chen LL, Minerva EM, Giulianotti PC. Indocyanine green (Icg)-enhanced fluorescence for intraoperative assessment of bowel microperfusion during laparoscopic and robotic colorectal surgery: the quest for evidence-based results. Surg Technol Int. 2018;32:101–4.
57. Manny TB, Hemal AK. Fluorescence-enhanced robotic radical cystectomy using unconjugated indocyanine green for pelvic lymphangiography, tumor marking, and mesenteric angiography: the initial clinical experience. Urology. 2014;83:824–9.
58. Cassinotti E, Al-Taher M, Antoniou SA, Arezzo A, et al. European Association for Endoscopic Surgery (EAES) consensus on Indocyanine Green (ICG) fluorescence-guided surgery. Surg Endosc. 2023;37(3): 1629–48. https://doi.org/10.1007/s00464-023-09928-5. PMID: 36781468; PMCID: PMC10017637.
59. Keller DS, Boulton R, Rodriguez-Justo M, Cohen R, Chand M. A novel application of Indocyanine green immunofluorescence in emergent colorectal surgery. J Fluoresc. 2018;28:487–90.
60. Osterkamp JTF, Patel MQ, Steyn E, Svendsen LB, Forgan T, Achiam MP. Usability of fluorescence angiography with indocyanine green in the surgical management of penetrating abdominal trauma. A case series. Int J Surg Open. 2021;30:100319.
61. Rizzo R, Vallicelli C, Ansaloni L, Coccolini F, Fugazzola P, Sartelli M, Agnoletti V, Luca Baiocchi G, Catena F. Usefulness of fluorescence imaging with indocyanine green for evaluation of bowel perfusion in the urgency setting: a systematic review and meta-analysis. Int J Surg. 2024; https://doi.org/10.1097/JS9.0000000000001529. Epub ahead of print.

62. Afifi I, Abdelrahman H, El-Faramawy A, Mahmood I, Khoschnau S, Al-Naimi N, El-Menyar A, Al-Thani H, Rizoli S. The use of Indocyanine green fluorescent in patients with abdominal trauma for better intraoperative decision-making and less bowel anastomosis leak: case series. J Surg Case Rep. 2021;rjab235
63. Machicado JD, Raijman I, Shah RJ. Future of Cholangioscopy. Gastrointest Endosc Clin N Am. 2022;32(3):583–96. https://doi.org/10.1016/j.giec.2022.03.002. Epub 2022 May 11.
64. Mauro A, Mazza S, Scalvini D, Lusetti F, Bardone M, Quaretti P, Cobianchi L, Anderloni A. The role of cholangioscopy in biliary diseases. Diagnostics (Basel). 2023;13(18):2933. https://doi.org/10.3390/diagnostics13182933. PMID: 37761300; PMCID: PMC10528268.
65. Fugazzola P, Bianchi CM, Calabretto F, Cicuttin E, et al. Intraoperative transcystic laparoscopic common bile duct stone clearance with SpyGlass™ discover during emergency and elective cholecystectomy: a single-center case series. World J Emerg Surg. 2024;19(1):8. https://doi.org/10.1186/s13017-023-00529-0. PMID: 38438899; PMCID: PMC10913229.
66. Becq A, Soualy A, Camus M. Cholangioscopy for biliary diseases. Curr Opin Gastroenterol. 2023;39(2):67–74. https://doi.org/10.1097/MOG.0000000000000907.
67. Lacy AM, Adelsdorfer C, Delgado S. Minimally invasive surgery for colorectal cancer: laparoscopy, robotics, and other emerging techniques. Surg Oncol Clin N Am. 2006;15(3):467–86.
68. Herron DM, Marohn M. SAGES-MIRA robotic surgery consensus group. A consensus document on robotic surgery. Surg Endosc. 2008;22:313.
69. Shah J, Vyas A, Vyas D. The history of robotics in surgical specialties. Am J Robot Surg. 2014;1(1):12–20.
70. Reza T, Bokhari SFH. Partnering with technology: advancing laparoscopy with artificial intelligence and machine learning. Cureus. 2024;16(3):e56076. https://doi.org/10.7759/cureus.56076. PMID: 38618354; PMCID: PMC11009890.
71. Tan A, Ashrafian H, Scott AJ, Mason SE, Harling L, Athanasiou T, Darzi A. Robotic surgery: disruptive innovation or unfulfilled promise? A systematic review and meta-analysis of the first 30 years. Surg Endosc. 2016;30(10):4330–52.
72. Murphy KP, Di Ruggiero M, Chadehumbe S. The future of robotic surgery: the human touch. J Robotic Surg. 2020;14(2):121–7.
73. Milone M, Anoldo P, de'Angelis N, Coccolini F, Khan J, Kluger Y, Sartelli M, Ansaloni L, Morelli L, Zanini N, Vallicelli C, Vigutto G, Moore EE, Biffl W, Catena F and Group, ROEM Collaborative. The role of RObotic surgery in EMergency setting (ROEM): protocol for a multicentre, observational, prospective international study on the use of robotic platform in emergency surgery. World J Emerg Surg. 2024;19(1):20. https://doi.org/10.1186/s13017-024-00542-x. PMID: 38835071; PMCID: PMC11149189.
74. Sermonesi G, Tian BWCA, Vallicelli C, et al. Cesena guidelines: WSES consensus statement on laparoscopic-first approach to general surgery emergencies and abdominal trauma. World J Emerg Surg. 2023;18(8):57.
75. De Angelis N, Khan J, Marchegiani F, et al. Robotic surgery in emergency setting: 2021 WSES position paper. World J Emeg Surg. 2022;17:4.
76. Skovsen AP, Korgaard Jensen T, Gögenur I, Tolstrup MB. Small bowel anastomosis in emergency surgery. World J Surg. 2024;48(2):341–9. https://doi.org/10.1002/wjs.12059.
77. Tantardini C, Godiris-Petit G, Noullet S, Raux M, Menegaux F, Chereau N. Management of the injured bowel: preserving bowel continuity as a gold standard. BMC Surg. 2021;21(1):339. https://doi.org/10.1186/s12893-021-01332. PMID: 34496803; PMCID: PMC8425099.
78. Howard AL, Stocchi L, Ashburn JH. Comparison of stapled and Hand-Sewn anastomoses in emergency surgery. J Gastrointest Surg. 2018;22(6):1124–30.
79. Khan A, Ullah K, Nabi, M. Mechanical vs. manual bowel anastomosis in emergency surgery: a randomized controlled trial. World J Emerg Surg. 2013;8(1):34.
80. King PM, Blazeby JM, Ewings P, Franks PJ, Longman RJ, Kipling RM. Randomized clinical trial comparing the effectiveness and quality of life in stapled versus Hand-Sewn bowel anastomoses. Br J Surg. 2006;93(8):851–7.
81. Cannon JW, Rabinovici R. Emergency laparoscopic intestinal resection and anastomosis: Hand-Sewn versus stapled techniques. Surg Endosc. 2017;31(4):1885–900.

82. McLean RC, St. Louis ER, Irani JL. Review of techniques and outcomes in emergency bowel anastomosis: manual vs. mechanical. Ann Surg. 2019;269(2):303–10.
83. McLatchie G, Borley N, Chikwe J. Principles of surgery. In: Oxford handbook of clinical surgery. Oxford: Oxford Medical Publications; 2013.
84. Gustafsson UO, Scott MJ, Hubner M, et al. Guidelines for perioperative care in elective colorectal surgery: Enhanced Recovery After Surgery (ERAS®) Society Recommendations: 2018. World J Surg. 2019;43(3):659–95. https://doi.org/10.1007/s00268-018-4844-y.
85. Jesus EC, Karliczek A, Matos D, et al. Prophylactic anastomotic drainage for colorectal surgery. Cochrane Database Syst Rev. 2004; https://doi.org/10.1002/14651858.CD002100.pub2.
86. Zhang HY, Zhao CL, Xie J, et al. To drain or not to drain in colorectal anastomosis: a meta-analysis. Int J Color Dis. 2016;31:951–60.
87. Scott MJ, Aggarwal G, Aitken RJ, et al. Consensus guidelines for perioperative care for emergency laparotomy Enhanced Recovery After Surgery (ERAS®) Society recommendations part 2-emergency laparotomy: intra- and postoperative care. World J Surg. 2023;47(8):1850–80. https://doi.org/10.1007/s00268-023-07020-6. PMID: 37277507; PMCID: PMC10241558.
88. Jones DB, Stefanidis D. Intraoperative use of methylene blue for leak detection in laparoscopic surgery. J Minim Invas Surg. 2019;23(4):202–8. https://doi.org/10.1016/j.jmis.2019.03.007.
89. Omnia MR. Evaluation of methylene blue in difficult laparoscopic cholecystectomy. Int J Surg Res. 2019;8(1):5–10. https://doi.org/10.5923/j.surgery.20190801.02.
90. Celik S, Almalı N, Aras A, Yılmaz Ö, Kızıltan R. Intraoperatively testing the anastomotic integrity of esophagojejunostomy using methylene blue. Scand J Surg. 2016;106(1):62–7. https://doi.org/10.1177/1457496916630652.
91. Bingham J, Kaufman J, Hata K, et al. A multicenter study of routine versus selective intraoperative leak testing for sleeve gastrectomy. Surg Obes Relat Dis. 2017;13(9):1469–75. ISSN 1550-7289. https://doi.org/10.1016/j.soard.2017.05.022.
92. Liu N, Cusack MC, Venkatesh M, et al. 30-day outcomes after intraoperative leak testing for bariatric surgery patients. J Surg Res. 2019;242:136–44. https://doi.org/10.1016/j.jss.2019.04.047. PMID: 31077945; PMCID: PMC6679992.
93. Rehman H, Ali M. Role of air leak test in preventing postoperative complications in laparoscopic gastrointestinal surgery. Int J Surg. 2019;64:40–5. https://doi.org/10.1016/j.ijsu.2019.02.014.
94. Havens JM, Peetz AB, Do WS, et al. The excess morbidity and mortality of emergency general surgery. J Trauma Acute Care Surg. 2015;78:306–11.
95. Pucher PH, Rahman SA, Mackenzie H, Tucker V, Mercer SJ. Feasibility of laparoscopy and factors associated with conversion to open in minimally invasive emergency major abdominal surgery: population database analysis. Surg Endosc. 2022;36(6): 4499–06. https://doi.org/10.1007/s00464-021-08803-5.
96. Yamamoto R, Cestero RF, Kameyama N, Sasaki J. Characteristics of laparoscopic surgery for trauma patients and risks of conversion to open laparotomy. World J Surg. 2022;46(11): 2616–24. https://doi.org/10.1007/s00268-022-06714-7.
97. Blikkendaal MD, Twijnstra AR, Stiggelbout AM, et al. Achieving consensus on the definition of conversion to laparotomy: a Delphi study among general surgeons, gynecologists, and urologists. Surg Endosc. 2013;27(12): 4631–9. https://doi.org/10.1007/s00464-013-3086-1.
98. Ball CG. Damage control surgery. Curr Opin Crit Care. 2015, 6:538–543. https://doi.org/10.1097/MCC.0000000000000252.
99. Roberts DJ, Leppäniemi A, Tolonen M, Mentula P, et al. The open abdomen in trauma, acute care, and vascular and endovascular surgery: comprehensive, expert, narrative review. BJS Open. 2023;7(5):zrad084. https://doi.org/10.1093/bjsopen/zrad084. PMID: 37882630; PMCID: PMC10601091.
100. Yamamoto R, Cestero RF, Kameyama N, Sasaki J. Characteristics of laparoscopic surgery for trauma patients and risks of conversion to open laparotomy. World J Surg. 2022;46(11):2616–24. https://doi.org/10.1007/s00268-022-06714-7.

3 Introduction to Precision Medicine and Personalized Treatment in Acute Care and Emergency Surgery

Vignesh Lakshmanan, Priyanka Bhattacharya, and Rajarshi Mukherjee

3.1 Introduction

The landscape of medicine and surgery is currently undergoing a transformation with the rapid development of precision medicine and personalized treatment. Historically, medical interventions in emergency settings have relied on standardized protocols designed to deliver emergent and effective care. While these approaches have saved countless lives, they often overlook the individual variability that can significantly impact treatment outcomes. Precision medicine focusses on tailoring medical care to the unique genetic, environmental, and lifestyle factors of each patient, promising to enhance the efficacy and safety of acute interventions [1].

The integration of personalized treatment strategies in emergency settings presents both opportunities and challenges. On one hand, Matchett et al. (2017) quite rightly outlined how the ability to rapidly analyse a patient's genetic profile can guide the selection of pharmacological agents, surgical techniques, and perioperative management tailored to their specific needs [2]. However crucially, Chude-Okonkwo et al. (2023) highlighted how the urgency and high-stakes nature of

V. Lakshmanan
Department of Emergency General & Major Trauma Surgery, Aintree University Hospital, NHS University Hospitals Liverpool Group, Liverpool, UK

P. Bhattacharya
Manchester Centre for Genomic Medicine, Manchester NHS Foundation Trust, Manchester, UK

R. Mukherjee (✉)
Department of Emergency General & Major Trauma Surgery, Liverpool University Hospitals NHS Foundation Trust, Aintree University Hospital, Liverpool, UK

Institute of Systems, Molecular and Integrative Biology, University of Liverpool, Liverpool, UK
e-mail: RAJARSHI.MUKHERJEE@liverpoolft.nhs.uk

B. De Simone et al. (eds.), *New Technologies, Precision Medicine, and AI in Emergency General Surgery*, Hot Topics in Acute Care Surgery and Trauma,
https://doi.org/10.1007/978-3-032-09357-8_3

emergency care require the seamless incorporation of precision tools into established workflows without compromising the speed of care delivery due to the time critical nature of acute care surgery [3].

In this chapter, we will first discuss the definition and principles of precision medicine, then consider it within the context of acute care and emergency surgery. How advancements in genomics, bioinformatics, and molecular diagnostics are enabling healthcare professionals to move beyond the one-size-fits-all paradigm in acute care surgery will then be outlined [4]. Finally a focus will be placed on application specifically to major trauma surgery, where the benefits from precision medicine are becoming increasingly evident.

3.2 Definition and Principles of Precision Medicine

Healthcare and patient management have progressively changed throughout the last hundred years, with an initial focus on treating disease now shifting towards a focus on ensuring health. Mukherjee (2023) emphasized that it is vital that surgeons of the present are aware of this change and those of the future fully engage with it [5, 6]. The catalyst to this progression has been the development of technology, allowing a move away from symptomatology and signology, relying on individual clinical excellence for maximal patient benefit in the past, to a system-based approach delivered in specialist units based on evidence-based medicine to guide patient management. Within this current landscape, the latest technologies exist centred on cellular-level interrogation of the genome with its upstream controllers and downstream effectors, alongside artificial intelligence to analyse the wealth of data produced. These innovations provide us with a sturdy platform looking to the future for an era of targeted treatments and personalized medicine (Fig. 3.1).

Although the principle of personalized treatment is not new [5], the invention of the term ‘Precision Medicine’ is believed to be from around the period of the late 90s from a small but impactful article in *The Wall Street Journal* entitled ‘New Era of Personalized Medicine: Targeting Drugs for Each Unique Genetic Profile’, and it has since been adapted by many. Recently it was adopted into mainstream global clinical research in 2015 when the National Institute of Health, USA, started the ‘Precision Medicine Initiative’ currently known as ‘All of Us’ [7]. Delpierre and Lefèvre (2023) reported that the term ‘Precision Medicine’ was interchangeably used with the term ‘Personalized Medicine’, at that stage; however, more recently ‘Precision Medicine’ is used more to avoid confusion following a conceptual argument that ‘Precision medicine’ can be defined as a healthcare model that relies on bioinformatics, analytics, and molecular information to focus on traits of population cohorts to improve therapeutic benefit or efficiency, and ‘Personalized Medicine’ is considered a practice of tailoring therapies to each patient uniquely based on their genetic makeup [8]. These concepts are now well established and summarized by the definition from the US National Human Genome Research Institute stating: ‘Precision medicine is an innovative approach that uses data about an individual’s

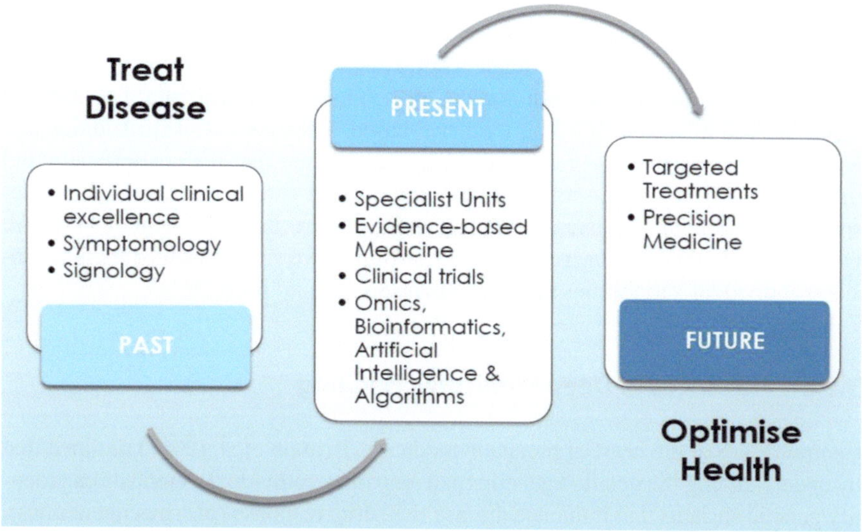

Fig. 3.1 Summary of key priorities in healthcare over time. Focus has shifted away from treating disease based predominantly on individual clinician excellence to our current systems of evidence-based healthcare delivered in specialist units, moving towards the future where the key focus will be optimizing health utilizing Precision Medicine approaches

genomic, environmental, and lifestyle information to guide decisions related to their medical management'. [9].

Precision Medicine is thus unique. Unlike traditional medicine, which often relies on generalized treatments based on the average patient and conventional quantitative and qualitative analytic research evidence, precision medicine seeks to understand and address the unique molecular profile and diversity of each patient.

3.2.1 Key Principles of Precision Medicine

The use of precision medicine in oncology and toxicology has been in use for years; however, their use in acute care and emergency medicine is still at an early stage [10, 11]. Precision medicine, with its emphasis on customized treatment plans based on lifestyle and genetic characteristics, may have the greatest impact in emergency surgery and acute care, where heterogeneity in terms of patient presentation and outcome is great and where prompt and efficient interventions are vital, if not potentially lifesaving [56].

Precision medicine aims to achieve its goals through the provision of personalized prevention and treatment strategies based on a patient's unique characteristics and their evolving health status. Kashoka et al. (2022) highlight that this approach involves detailed categorizing of individuals into subpopulations based on disease susceptibility, biology, prognosis, or response to treatments [12]. Precision medicine also emphasizes evidence-based clinical approaches and has garnered significant attention from healthcare providers [13].

In the realm of precision medicine, Ogino et al. (2022) and Handra et al. (2022) showed that applying epidemiological principles in clinical and translational research is vital for establishing evidence-based practices [14, 15]. Additionally, Kasztura et al. (2019) and Lee et al. (2021) concluded that the cost-efficient and timely integration of genomic medicine into clinical care is crucial for the widespread adoption of precision medicine and realizing its full potential [11, 16]. Overall, precision medicine represents a transformative shift in healthcare that considers individual variabilities in genes, environment, and lifestyle.

3.2.2 Advances in Deep Molecular Profiling

Genomics lies at the heart of precision medicine. Brittain et al. (2017) outlined that by understanding the detailed genetic road map of an individual, scientists can identify genetic variants that influence disease risk, drug response (pharmacogenomics), and health-related outcomes, leading to the treatment of diseases with accuracy and efficiency [17]. The pace of change in genetic technologies to allow such approaches has been rapid. In 2001, Lander et al. published 'The Human Genome Project' that took 13 years to sequence the first human genome and was completed in 2003 with costs of almost 2.7 billion US dollars [18]. Nowadays, the advancements in genomics and technology, such as next-generation sequencing (NGS), have made it possible to sequence a patient's genome within hours and for few hundred dollars or less (Fig. 3.2) [19].

McShane et al. (2013) in collaboration with US National Cancer Institute (NCI) derived a checklist for the use of omics-based predictors in medicine [20]. Tebani et al. (2016) reviewed the different omics technologies in clinical practice to achieve precision medicine along with the challenges that each faced [21]. Increasingly, over the last decade, other 'Omics' approaches, complementary to and enhancing genomic approaches that scientists use, have also been well developed and implemented:

- Proteomics—study of products of RNA.
- Metabolomics—study of metabolites.
- Transcriptomics—study of gene expression in a cell.
- Epigenomics—study of epigenetic changes (e.g. methylation, acetylation, etc.) in a cell.
- And other Omics such as metagenomics, inflamomics, lipidomics, and glycomics.

These various approaches and their relation to the cellular organelle that they focus on are summarized in Fig. 3.3.

Some of the most successful examples of precision medicine with the use of whole genome sequencing (WGS) along with the other 'Omics' technologies have been for the understanding, diagnosis, and management of familial

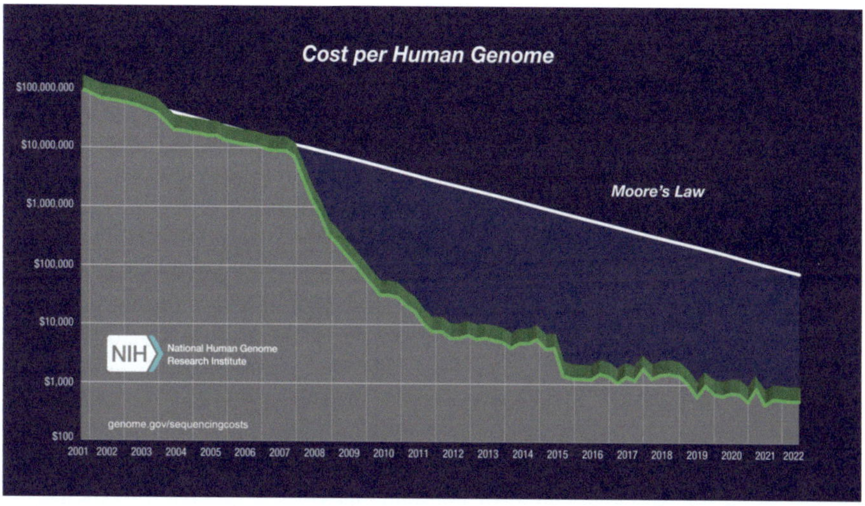

Fig. 3.2 Cost to sequence a single human genome over time. Graph reproduced from NIH data showing the cost to sequence a single human genome alongside hypothetical data representing Moore's Law, which demonstrates a trend in the computer hardware industry predicting a doubling of 'compute power' every 2 years. Technology improvements that 'keep up' with Moore's Law are widely regarded to be doing exceedingly well. Costs are represented on a logarithmic scale on the Y axis. The sudden and profound out-pacing of Moore's Law beginning in January 2008 is likely as a result of the implementation of next-generation DNA sequencing technologies. Wetterstrand KA. (DNA Sequencing Costs: Data from the NHGRI Genome Sequencing Program (GSP) Available at: www.genome.gov/sequencingcostsdata. Accessed [06/08/2024])

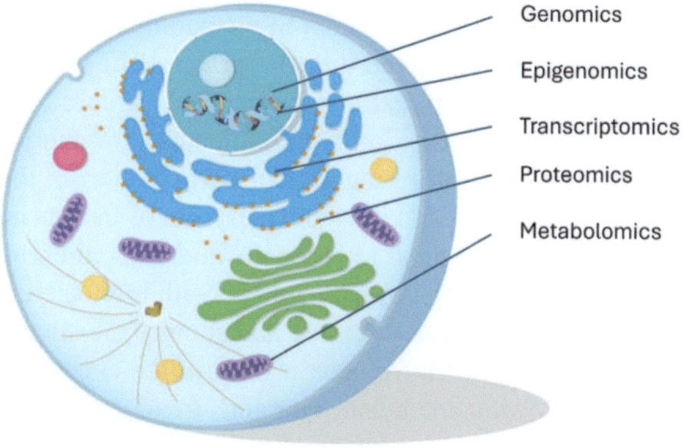

Fig. 3.3 Omics technologies based on sub-cellular organelle site. A variety of 'omics' approaches exist: Genomics (studying DNA held within the cellular nucleus), Epigenomics (profiling the mechanisms controlling the expression of DNA), Transcriptomics (assessing RNA within and outside the endoplasmic reticulum following DNA transcription), Proteomics (assessing protein once translated from RNA at the ribosome), Metabolomics (characterizing metabolites produced through the production of cellular energy predominantly orchestrated by the mitochondria). AI-generated base image created with OpenAI (2024), ChatGPT (version GPT-4) with original annotation

hypercholesterolemia (Ahangari et al. 2020), autosomal dominant polycystic kidney disease (Lanktree and Chapman 2017), epilepsy (Striano and Minnassian 2020), melanoma (Chapman et al. 2011), cystic fibrosis (Haq et al. 2022), and breast cancers (Subhan et al. 2023) [22–27].

3.2.3 Bioinformatics and Big Data Integration

Bioinformatics, a multidisciplinary field merging biology, computer science, and information technology, facilitates the analysis and interpretation of intricate biological data, such as genomic sequences and molecular pathways. Hulsen et al. (2019) and Yu et al. (2018) eloquently put the case forward that it is evident that through the utilization of bioinformatics tools, healthcare providers can pinpoint genetic variations, biomarkers, and molecular profiles that guide personalized treatment strategies tailored to individual patients [28, 29]. Qian et al. (2019) make the key point that the application of big data analytics in precision medicine for emergency surgery enables the processing and analysis of extensive amounts of clinical, genomic, and patient data to extract valuable insights and patterns [30]. This methodology is particularly advantageous in emergency surgery scenarios where prompt decision-making and personalized interventions are imperative. Thus, the integration of bioinformatics and big data analytics in precision medicine for emergency surgery harbours immense potential for revolutionizing patient care.

3.2.4 Personalized Diagnostics and Therapeutics

In 2015, a report of the European Parliament Symposium on Precision Medicine in allergy and airway diseases highlighted the core principle of precision medicine is to create diagnostic and therapeutic strategies precisely tailored to each patient's requirements by integrating information from molecular, immunologic, and functional genotyping of diseases; informing patient participation in therapeutic decisions; and considering predictive and preventive aspects of treatment [31]. It aimed to use genomic technologies, medical record data, and clinical knowledge to tailor treatments to individuals, reducing costs associated with ineffective therapies.

Zhang et al. (2023) reviewed the literature and showed advancements in cancer genomics and novel therapeutics have been pivotal in the emergence of personalized diagnostics and precision medicine, enabling treatments based on genomic profiling of tumours [32]. Similarly, McCrea et al. (2018) discussed precision medicine applications in prostate cancer that have been facilitated by developments in diagnostics and therapeutics, leading to customized treatments for the majority of individuals as a current standard of care [33]. Kannan et al. (2023) showed precision medicine has significantly enhanced the diagnosis, treatment, and management of chronic diseases like diabetes [34]. Furthermore, in transplantation, accurate diagnoses are essential for the success of precision medicine, emphasizing the widespread importance of precision diagnostics in healthcare [35]. This is particularly important considering the wide range of comorbidities that a patient might present with to an acute care surgeon.

3.3 Critical Areas of Acute Surgical Benefit from Personalised Medicine

Genomics and molecular profiling have revolutionized healthcare by enabling personalized patient care through precision medicine. Precision medicine tailors medical treatment to individual characteristics by analysing genetic makeup, DNA blueprint, lifestyle, and environment to optimize outcomes and minimize side effects and to improve efficiency. Artificial intelligence (AI) has emerged as a powerful tool in various medical fields, including emergency general surgery, by enhancing clinical decision-making and promoting precision medicine [36]. The integration of AI in emergency surgery settings has the potential to improve clinical practice, operating room management, and decision-making processes, ultimately leading to consistent, high-quality care [37].

In Emergency General Surgery (EGS), the use of AI has the potential to predict morbidity and mortality, particularly in the geriatric population, aiding in better risk assessment and patient management [38]. AI has been increasingly utilized, with innovative approaches applied in hand surgery, for example. Bodansky et al. (2023) studied the use of 3D modelling and printing for planning procedures and surgical templating, demonstrating the potential for AI to enhance surgical practices and outcomes [39]. In EGS the potential impact of precision approaches is diverse and far-reaching and is summarized in Fig. 3.4.

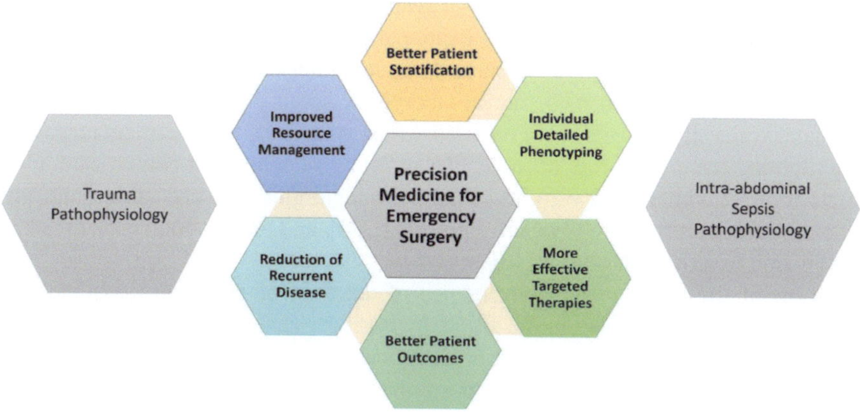

Fig. 3.4 Summary of potential benefits of precision medicine in Emergency General Surgery. By adopting approaches that help us better understand Trauma Pathophysiology and Intra-abdominal Sepsis Pathophysiology through precision medicine, we can develop better patient stratification, individual detailed phenotyping, more effective targeted therapies, better patient acute outcomes, reduce recurrence of disease, reduce potential morbidity and mortality, and better manage available resources

Lander et al. (2001) published the completion of the Human Genome Project, identifying the 3.2 billion base pairs that make up the human genome, often referred to as the 'Book of Life' [18]. The genome is composed of nucleotide sequences, with the bases adenine (A), cytosine (C), guanine (G), and thymine (T), which regulate the functioning of organisms through a variety of combinations or codes. This comprehensive analysis of the human genome, along with more recent larger projects such as 'Our Future Health' within the UK, is providing or has the potential to provide valuable insights into the genetic factors that influence health, disease, and responses to treatment [40]. The Human Genome Project marked a phenomenal leap in our ability to decode the human genome, laying the groundwork for modern genomics.

By exploring genetic variations and their implications for diseases, precision medicine aims to revolutionize healthcare by providing personalized and targeted solutions that consider the unique genetic makeup of each individual [41–43]. Identifying these variations helps in understanding the genetic predisposition to conditions like cancer, cardiovascular diseases, and neurodegenerative disorders. For instance, Subhan et al. (2023) showed that BRCA1 and BRCA2 mutations are well-known markers for increased breast and ovarian cancer risk, guiding preventive strategies and treatment choices [27].

Molecular profiling involves the comprehensive analysis of genomic, transcriptomic, and proteomic profiles, providing essential information for tailoring individualized treatment strategies. Precision medicine in emergency surgery has been significantly enhanced by the integration of molecular profiling techniques, reviewed by Alkhatib et al. (2024) who outlined the current and future genomic applications in surgery [44]. Tebani et al. (2016) showed by identifying biomarkers through omics data, precision medicine can predict outcomes related to disease susceptibility, diagnosis, prognosis, and treatment response [21]. Molecular and functional profiling plays a pivotal role in guiding clinical decision-making processes in emergency surgery, ensuring personalized and targeted interventions for optimal patient outcomes [45]. Precision medicine in emergency surgery relies on validated biomarkers to classify patients based on disease risk, prognosis, and treatment response, highlighting the critical role of molecular profiling in enhancing patient care. One such example comes from Watkins (2022) who highlighted the use and monitoring of antibiotics in relation to C-reactive protein (CRP) and procalcitonin (PCT) levels optimizing treatment strategies [46].

Some of the examples of convergence of the field of precision medicine and emergency surgery are seen in the article by Springer et al. (2016) who identified a panel of molecular markers that aid in classification and management of pancreatic cysts [47]. Popovtzer et al. (2011) demonstrated the possibility of computed tomography (CT) detection of molecular markers of cancers rather than conventional anatomical changes [48].

The integration of molecular profiling into emergency surgical practice represents a significant advancement, offering a personalized approach to patient management and treatment selection, ultimately improving outcomes in emergency surgical settings. Genomics and molecular profiling represent a paradigm shift in personalized patient care, offering many opportunities for disease prevention, diagnosis, and treatment. As technology advances, costs and efficiency reduce to make these technologies translatable into practical point-of-care tests, and as our understanding of the human genome deepens, personalized medicine will become increasingly integrated into routine clinical practice.

3.4 Biomarkers and Their Role in Early Diagnosis and Treatment Response Prediction

Slikker (2019) defines that biomarkers are measurable indicators of biological processes, pathogenic processes, or pharmacologic responses to therapeutic interventions [49]. Biomarkers have significantly impacted the field of medicine, providing crucial insights into early disease detection and prediction of treatment responses. In emergency surgery, biomarkers play a pivotal role in guiding clinical decisions promptly and effectively. Numerous studies have emphasized the importance of various biomarkers across a wide range of medical conditions, demonstrating their potential in improving patient care in critical surgical situations.

3.4.1 Early Diagnosis: Sooner Is Better

Early detection in acute care and emergency surgery is crucial for timely intervention and improved patient outcomes. Well-known use of biomarkers such as use of CRP in infection and inflammation and monitoring of postoperative patients is a good example (Watkins 2022). Screening of viral load blood borne viral infections, the screening for breast cancer with BRCA mutations, or the use of B-type natriuretic peptide (BNP) in cardiovascular diseases are all examples of other situations where biomarkers play a significant role. New advancements in the use of biomarkers in cancer (that may present as an emergency) and acute inflammatory emergency surgery conditions are discussed below.

In the realm of oncology, for instance, Ferreira et al. (2021) discussed the early detection of cancers such as non-small-cell lung cancer (NSCLC), through liquid biopsies that detect genetic alterations in genes like EGFR and ALK that have been studied and are becoming increasingly implemented [50]. Satam et al. (2023) reported that advancements in genetic engineering and bioinformatics have led to next-generation sequencing (NGS) methods, with genetic variant biomarkers enabling clinicians to identify actionable variants impacting a patient's management, guiding treatment decisions, and potentially improving surgical outcomes [51]. Similarly, Christodoulidis et al. (2024) showed that in oesophageal cancer, the application of exosomes as biomarkers has been explored for early detection and treatment, showcasing the evolving landscape of precision medicine in oncological emergencies [52]. Deulkar et al. (2024) tackled the challenges of endocrine illness in emergency settings and outlined the use of biomarkers, such as chromogranin A (CgA), cancer antigen (CA), beta-human chorionic gonadotropin (hCG), and alpha-fetoprotein (AFP), and thyroid-stimulating hormone (TSH), in early detection and treatment of endocrine disorders in critical care settings [53]. In the field of breast cancer, Davis and Hanash (2006) showed that plasma-based proteomics has emerged as a promising avenue for early detection and therapy, offering insights into disease progression and treatment response [54]. Furthermore, Hayes et al. (2018) argue that the development of point-of-care diagnostic technologies in healthcare and for cancer detection holds promise in emergency surgery settings, potentially changing the laboratory-based testing to on-site testing by medical staff or by patient themselves in real time, being cost-effective, simple to use, and function without excessive prior processing of samples [55].

In summary, developments have been significant, and continuing research and development in the use of biomarkers in early diagnosis through improved point-of-care devices can help clinicians streamline diagnostic process, reduce delays in treatment initiation, and ultimately enhance patient care in emergency surgical scenarios. A global survey showed it is crucial that future efforts are focussed on translation of significant progress from the oncology setting to acute care, identifying a wide gap between oncological, acute medical, and acute surgical trials and published outputs [56].

3.4.2 Treatment Response Prediction

By identifying novel biomarkers with diagnostic and prognostic value, clinicians can optimize treatment strategies and improve patient outcomes in emergency surgical scenarios.

For instance, Chen et al. (2019) reported the use of circulating tumour DNA (ctDNA) in the immediate postoperative period has been proposed to detect minimal residual disease (MRD) following surgery, providing valuable insights into treatment efficacy and the need for additional interventions [57]. Moreover, Berretta et al. (2017) reported the identification of biomarkers such as CA19-9 and CEA with diagnostic and prognostic implications in hepatocellular carcinoma and cholangiocarcinoma is crucial for guiding treatment decisions [58]. A common complication in emergency surgery like postoperative delirium has been studied by Saller et al. (2019) who reported biomarkers like tau and neurofilament proteins have shown promise in predicting and detecting delirium [59]. In HER2-positive metastatic breast cancer, Li et al. (2018) identified a serum microRNA signature as a predictive biomarker for trastuzumab benefit, offering insights into treatment sensitivity and prognosis, albeit in the field of oncology [60]. Stepanyan et al. (2023) investigated biopsy-based immune biomarkers as predictors of response to neoadjuvant therapy in rectal cancer patients [61]. Matshuoka and Yashira (2024) reported that great impact of bioinformatic analysis integrated with multi-omics platforms offers a promising tool for identifying prognostic and predictive biomarkers in gastric cancer [62]. Wang et al. (2021) reported the advancements of precision surgery treatment for gastric cancer with interventions such as targeted therapy or immunotherapy combined with molecular targets [63].

By incorporating biomarker-based predictive models into clinical practice, healthcare providers can enhance treatment prediction accuracy, improve patient care, and ultimately optimize outcomes for patients requiring urgent surgical interventions. Future focus is required on non-oncological acute inflammatory disorders presenting to the acute care surgeon that have been neglected until this stage. Significant advances have been made recently in gallstone disease following genome-wide association meta-analysis, yielding 20 loci associated with gallstone disease; however, this needs to be extended to other conditions [64].

3.5 Trauma Surgery in the Era of Precision Medicine and Artificial Intelligence

Trauma surgery is a critical field that deals with injuries caused by accidents, violence, or other physical impacts. The integration of precision medicine and artificial intelligence (AI) holds great promise to revolutionize clinical practice in this field, offering innovative approaches to patient care, treatment prediction, and surgical outcomes. This section explores the collaboration of precision medicine and AI in trauma surgery, highlighting key advancements and future directions in this rapidly evolving field.

Elhassan et al. (2024) reported that daily multidisciplinary (MDT) trauma meeting can significantly benefit patient care by holistic approach for patients, involving different teams to deal with speciality-specific injuries as traumas come unplanned, contrary to oncology [65]. Bach et al. (2017) also emphasized that the main focus of MDT trauma meetings lies in specialty synergies including surgical and non-surgical interventions along with rehabilitation course [66]. Overall, trauma surgery, being a multidisciplinary field, requires great collaboration amongst surgeons, emergency physicians, and other healthcare staff to deliver optimal care in medical centres. Precision medicine includes the use of modern molecular diagnostic technology, accurate molecular typing, and staging to develop precise and individualized surgical treatment plans. This approach emphasizes the importance of patient-specific care, where computer-based surgical planning and guidance play a crucial role in advancing therapy. By aligning interventions with the molecular drivers of disease, precision medicine in trauma care seeks to stratify risks, detect pathophysiological processes early, and personalize treatments accordingly [67, 68].

The use of genomic profiling, genomic susceptibility, and pharmacogenetics can predict susceptibility to infections and wound healing complications and response to drugs in acute settings. Davis et al. (2022) reported the significant potential of precision medicine in trauma following a thorough review of the literature, concluding that traumatic brain injury (TBI), trauma-induced coagulopathy, and infectious complications could benefit from applications of genomics and precision medicine [69]. Zhou et al. (2008) conducted a meta-analysis which showed the association between presence of apolipoprotein E4 (APOE4) allele and poor long-term prognosis following TBI [70]. Molecular analysis study of trauma intensive care patients by McDaniel et al. (2007) demonstrated a significant relation in cytokine expression profile with risk of developing sepsis, indicating low-producing genotype for IL-10 expressions had a two- to threefold lower risk of developing sepsis [71]. Tompkins (2015) published the article about 'The Glue Grant Experience—Genomics of Injury', which is a research collaborative that has led genomic and proteomics research in trauma since its inception in 2001 with support from the National Institutes of General Medical Sciences and has resulted in extensive knowledge and insights in metabolomics, proteomics, and genomics in trauma injuries. Thus, biomarkers play a vital role in identification and monitoring of illness in acute settings, and their utilization and implementation are gradually becoming more routine [72].

Surgeons and healthcare professionals are increasingly recognizing the potential of AI to revolutionize emergency and trauma surgery practices. Simone et al. (2022) have shown that trauma and acute care surgeons are not only open to but enthusiastic about incorporating AI into their clinical workflows, acknowledging its capacity to enhance patient care and outcomes. This positive attitude towards AI reflects a growing acceptance of technological advancements in the medical field and a willingness to embrace novel approaches to improve surgical interventions [37].

Bianchi et al. (2024) reviewed the different applications of AI and machine learning (ML) in diagnosing and management of acute appendicitis, a common presentation in general surgery [73]. Wu et al. (2023) proved that artificial intelligence image recognition systems could indeed assist orthopaedic surgeons in preventing the occurrence of wrong site left and right upper limb surgery [74]. In spine surgery, AI with augmented and virtual reality provides potential aids for surgeons to tackle anatomical challenges [75]. Thus, the application of AI extends from general surgery to trauma and orthopaedic surgery including specialized surgical specialties which have all demonstrated the ability to rapidly analyse vast amounts of clinical data enabling more informed decision-making. By leveraging AI capabilities, surgeons can navigate complex surgical procedures more efficiently and deliver personalized care that aligns with the unique needs of each patient. As AI continues to evolve, its impact on surgical education, decision support systems, and personalized care delivery is becoming increasingly evident. The future trajectory of AI in surgery is looking at significant growth, with machine learning playing a pivotal role in empowering medical teams to deliver superior care through accurate diagnosis and treatment.

3.6 Personalized Treatment Strategies for Trauma Patients

Trauma, with its complex presentation and varied individual responses, has long been a challenge for medical practitioners. However, the advancements in next-generation sequencing and the integration of diverse '-omics' data have opened new avenues for a more tailored and precise approach to trauma care. This paradigm shift from a 'one-size-fits-all' approach to a more targeted and individualized strategy has the potential to revolutionize the way trauma patients are managed [5, 76].

Several studies have demonstrated the potential benefits of precision medicine in trauma surgery. Lewy et al. (2023) have demonstrated feasibility of focused assessment with sonography in trauma (FAST) in improving patient care imaging interpretation with positivity and accuracy, positioning AI as a valuable tool for point-of-care clinical decision-making [77]. The applications of AI are evident in other areas of emergency general surgery, such as in improving care in acute appendicitis by ML prediction of appendicitis histopathological categorization using biomarkers and demographics (Kang et al. 2021) [78] and the prediction of postoperative outcomes using Random Forest (RF) plots, a well-studied accurate machine learning model (Eickhoff et al. 2022; Hseih et al. 2011) [79, 80]. Other applications such as ensuring procedural accuracy and improving patient safety in orthopaedic surgery (Wu et al. 2023) and enhancing surgical interventions in spinal surgery (Liawrungrueang et al. 2024) have all been demonstrated [74, 75].

In orthopaedic surgery, Lisacek-Kiosoglous et al. (2023) reported that AI has found practical applications in diagnostics, such as fracture recognition and tumour detection, predictive modelling of clinical outcomes, and real-time rehabilitation monitoring, contributing to personalized treatment approaches. The present status of robot-assisted surgery in trauma and orthopaedics in China highlights the direction of orthopaedic precision treatment technology in the twenty-first century, emphasizing the importance of technological advancements in personalized surgical interventions [76, 81]. Jayaraman et al. (2018) discussed the role of metabolomics and precision medicine in trauma care, emphasizing the importance of early interventions and close monitoring for successful outcomes [82].

In severe trauma cases, precision medicine plays a role in stratifying genetic risk factors rather than demographic factors. For instance, Rubin-Asher (2010) reported the failure of heparin therapy to prevent venous thromboembolism (VTE) in trauma patients with elevated factor VIII (FVIII), homocysteine (hcy) levels, and prothrombin carrier mutation [83]. Thus, routine testing for thrombophilia could assist and guide healthcare professionals to consider intense anticoagulation regimes. In trauma-related coagulopathies, viscoelastic tests such as thromboelastography (TEG) and rotational thromboelastometry (ROTEM) are excellent examples of real time, point-of-care diagnostic tests aiding surgeons and anaesthetists to correct patient's coagulation status and bleeding (Cappellini et al. 2023) [84].

In 2017, Kurowski et al. identified 33 genes related to recovery in traumatic brain injury (TBI) patients [85]. For instance, angiotensin-converting enzyme (ACE) genetic variations are associated with poor cognitive outcomes (Ariza et al. 2006) [86], interleukin-1 beta (IL-1β) gene polymorphisms are linked to prognosis in TBI patients; however, implementation into routine clinical practice is awaited.

3.7 Conclusion

The field of acute care and emergency surgery is poised to benefit significantly from the advancements in precision medicine and personalized treatment strategies that have gathered momentum over the course of the last few years. Concerted effort by multidisciplinary teams utilizing global networks is required to develop expertise and translate advancements identified in the laboratory to the patient bedside. This is likely to be achieved through improved point-of-care diagnostics, prognostication tools, and tailored treatment methods. In this way, surgeons will not only treat disease in the future, but also contribute more holistically to optimizing an individual's health.

References

1. Abdelhalim H, Berber A, Lodi M, Jain R, Nair A, Pappu A, Patel K, Venkat V, Venkatesan C, Wable R, Dinatale M, Fu A, Iyer V, Kalove I, Kleyman M, Koutsoutis J, Menna D, Paliwal M, Patel N, et al. Artificial intelligence, healthcare, clinical genomics, and pharmacogenomics approaches in precision medicine. Front Genet. 2022;13 https://doi.org/10.3389/fgene.2022.929736.
2. Matchett KB, Lynam-Lennon N, Watson RW, Brown JAL. Advances in precision medicine: tailoring individualized therapies. Cancers (Basel). 2017;9(11):Article 11. https://doi.org/10.3390/cancers9110146.
3. Chude-Okonkwo UK, Paul BS, Vasilakos AV. Enabling precision medicine via contemporary and future communication technologies: a survey. IEEE Access. 2023;11:21210–40. https://doi.org/10.1109/ACCESS.2022.3175573.
4. Hsiao WW-W, Lin J-C, Fan C-T, Chen SS-S. Precision health in Taiwan: a data-driven diagnostic platform for the future of disease prevention. Comput Struct Biotechnol J. 2022;20:1593–602. https://doi.org/10.1016/j.csbj.2022.03.026.
5. Mukherjee R. An acute need: precision medicine for acute care surgery. BJS Open. 2023;7(2):zrad003. https://doi.org/10.1093/bjsopen/zrad003.
6. Mukherjee R, Nunes Q, Huang W, Sutton R. Precision medicine for acute pancreatitis: current status and future opportunities. Precis Clin Med. 2019;2(2):81–6. https://doi.org/10.1093/pcmedi/pbz010.
7. https://allofus.nih.gov/.
8. Delpierre C, Lefèvre T. Precision and personalized medicine: what their current definition says and silences about the model of health they promote. Implication for the development of personalized health. Front Sociol. 2023;8:1112159. https://doi.org/10.3389/fsoc.2023.1112159.
9. Definition of precision medicine—NCI Dictionary of Cancer Terms—NCI (nciglobal,ncienterprise). (2011, February 2). [nciAppModulePage]. https://www.cancer.gov/publications/dictionaries/cancer-terms/def/precision-medicine.
10. Aslanidis T. Precision medicine in emergency medicine. Digital Med Healthcare Technol. 2022; https://doi.org/10.5772/dmht.01.
11. Lee S, Lam SH, Hernandes Rocha TA, Fleischman RJ, Staton CA, Taylor R, Limkakeng AT. Machine learning and precision medicine in emergency medicine: the basics. Cureus. 2021;13(9):e17636. https://doi.org/10.7759/cureus.17636.
12. Kahkoska AR, Freeman NLB, Hassmiller Lich K. Systems-aligned precision medicine—building an evidence base for individuals within complex systems. JAMA Health Forum. 2022;3(7):e222334. https://doi.org/10.1001/jamahealthforum.2022.2334.
13. Aron DC. Precision medicine and the challenges of human complexity. Psychother Psychosom. 2023;92(6):349–53. https://doi.org/10.1159/000534728.

14. Ogino S, Nowak JA, Hamada T, Phipps AI, Peters U, Milner DA, Giovannucci EL, Nishihara R, Giannakis M, Garrett WS, Song M. Integrative analysis of exogenous, endogenous, tumour and immune factors for precision medicine. Gut. 2018;67(6):1168–80. https://doi.org/10.1136/gutjnl-2017-315537.
15. Handra J, Elbert A, Gazzaz N, Moller-Hansen A, Hyunh S, Lee HK, Boerkoel P, Alderman E, Anderson E, Clarke L, Hamilton S, Hamman R, Hughes S, Ip S, Langlois S, Lee M, Li L, Mackenzie F, Patel MS, et al. The practice of genomic medicine: A delineation of the process and its governing principles. Front Med. 2023;9:1071348. https://doi.org/10.3389/fmed.2022.1071348.
16. Kasztura M, Richard A, Bempong N-E, Loncar D, Flahault A. Cost-effectiveness of precision medicine: a scoping review. Int J Public Health. 2019;64(9):1261–71. https://doi.org/10.1007/s00038-019-01298-x.
17. Brittain HK, Scott R, Thomas E. The rise of the genome and personalised medicine. Clin Med. 2017;17(6):545–51. https://doi.org/10.7861/clinmedicine.17-6-545.
18. Lander ES, Linton LM, Birren B, Nusbaum C, Zody MC, Baldwin J, Devon K, Dewar K, Doyle M, FitzHugh W, Funke R, Gage D, Harris K, Heaford A, Howland J, Kann L, Lehoczky J, LeVine R, McEwan P, et al. Initial sequencing and analysis of the human genome. Nature. 2001;409(6822):860–921. https://doi.org/10.1038/35057062.
19. Siegel V. The human genome project turns 20: here's how it altered the world. MIT Department of Biology; 2023. https://biology.mit.edu/the-human-genome-project-turns-20-heres-how-it-altered-the-world/.
20. McShane LM, Cavenagh MM, Lively TG, Eberhard DA, Bigbee WL, Williams PM, Mesirov JP, Polley M-YC, Kim KY, Tricoli JV, Taylor JMG, Shuman DJ, Simon RM, Doroshow JH, Conley BA. Criteria for the use of omics-based predictors in clinical trials. Nature. 2013;502(7471):317–20. https://doi.org/10.1038/nature12564.
21. Tebani A, Afonso C, Marret S, Bekri S. Omics-based strategies in precision medicine: toward a paradigm shift in inborn errors of metabolism investigations. Int J Mol Sci. 2016;17(9):Article 9. https://doi.org/10.3390/ijms17091555.
22. Ahangari N, Doosti M, Ghayour Mobarhan M, Sahebkar A, Ferns GA, Pasdar A. Personalised medicine in hypercholesterolaemia: the role of pharmacogenetics in statin therapy. Ann Med. 2020;52(8):462–70. https://doi.org/10.1080/07853890.2020.1800074.
23. Lanktree MB, Chapman AB. New treatment paradigms for ADPKD: moving towards precision medicine. Nat Rev Nephrol. 2017;13(12):750–68. https://doi.org/10.1038/nrneph.2017.127.
24. Striano P, Minassian BA. From genetic testing to precision medicine in epilepsy. Neurotherapeutics. 2020;17(2):609–15. https://doi.org/10.1007/s13311-020-00835-4.
25. Chapman PB, Hauschild A, Robert C, Haanen JB, Ascierto P, Larkin J, Dummer R, Garbe C, Testori A, Maio M, Hogg D, Lorigan P, Lebbe C, Jouary T, Schadendorf D, Ribas A, O'Day SJ, Sosman JA, Kirkwood JM, et al. Improved survival with vemurafenib in melanoma with BRAF V600E mutation. N Engl J Med. 2011;364(26):2507–16. https://doi.org/10.1056/NEJMoa1103782.
26. Haq I, Almulhem M, Soars S, Poulton D, Brodlie M. Precision medicine based on CFTR genotype for people with cystic fibrosis. Pharmacogenomics Pers Med. 2022;15:91–104. https://doi.org/10.2147/PGPM.S245603.
27. Subhan MA, Parveen F, Shah H, Yalamarty SSK, Ataide JA, Torchilin VP. Recent advances with precision medicine treatment for breast cancer including triple-negative sub-type. Cancer. 2023;15(8):2204. https://doi.org/10.3390/cancers15082204.
28. Hulsen T, Jamuar SS, Moody AR, Karnes JH, Varga O, Hedensted S, Spreafico R, Hafler DA, McKinney EF. From big data to precision medicine. Front Med. 2019;6:34. https://doi.org/10.3389/fmed.2019.00034.
29. Yu MK, Ma J, Fisher J, Kreisberg JF, Raphael BJ, Ideker T. Visible machine learning for biomedicine. Cell. 2018;173(7):1562–5. https://doi.org/10.1016/j.cell.2018.05.056.
30. Qian T, Zhu S, Hoshida Y. Use of big data in drug development for precision medicine: an update. Expert Rev Precis Med Drug Dev. 2019;4(3):189–200. https://doi.org/10.1080/23808993.2019.1617632.

31. Muraro A, Fokkens WJ, Pietikainen S, Borrelli D, Agache I, Bousquet J, Costigliola V, Joos G, Lund VJ, Poulsen LK, Price D, Rolland C, Zuberbier T, Hellings PW. European symposium on precision medicine in allergy and airways diseases: report of the European Union parliament symposium (October 14, 2015). Rhinol J. 2015;53(4):303–7. https://doi.org/10.4193/Rhino15.400.
32. Zhang Q, Fu Q, Bai X, Liang T. Molecular profiling–based precision medicine in cancer: a review of current evidence and challenges. Front Oncol. 2020;10:532403. https://doi.org/10.3389/fonc.2020.532403.
33. McCrea EM, Lee DK, Sissung TM, Figg WD. Precision medicine applications in prostate cancer. Ther Adv Med Oncol. 2018;10:1758835918776920. https://doi.org/10.1177/1758835918776920.
34. Kannan S, Chellappan DK, Kow CS, Ramachandram DS, Pandey M, Mayuren J, Dua K, Candasamy M. Transform diabetes care with precision medicine. Health Sci Rep. 2023;6(11):e1642. https://doi.org/10.1002/hsr2.1642.
35. Mengel M, Campbell P, Gebel H, Randhawa P, Rodriguez ER, Colvin R, Conway J, Hachem R, Halloran PF, Keshavjee S, Nickerson P, Murphey C, O'Leary J, Reeve J, Tinckam K, Reed EF. Precision diagnostics in transplantation: from bench to bedside. Am J Transplant. 2013;13(3):562–8. https://doi.org/10.1111/j.1600-6143.2012.04344.x.
36. Nicolas J, Pitaro NL, Vogel B, Mehran R. Artificial intelligence—advisory or adversary? 2023. https://www.icrjournal.com/articles/artificial-intelligence-advisory-or-adversary.
37. De Simone B, Chouillard E, Gumbs AA, Loftus TJ, Kaafarani H, Catena F. Artificial intelligence in surgery: the emergency surgeon's perspective (the ARIES project). Discov Health Sys. 2022;1(1):9. https://doi.org/10.1007/s44250-022-00014-6.
38. Elamin A, Tsoutsanis P, Sinan L, Tari SPH, Elamin W, Kurihara H. Emergency general surgery: predicting morbidity and mortality in the geriatric population. Surg J. 2022;08(3):e270–8. https://doi.org/10.1055/s-0042-1756461.
39. Bodansky DMS, Sandow MJ, Volk I, Luria S, Verstreken F, Horwitz MD. Insights and trends review: the role of three-dimensional technology in upper extremity surgery. J Hand Surg Eur. 2023;48(5):383–95. https://doi.org/10.1177/17531934221150498.
40. Our research mission. (n.d.). Our Future Health. Retrieved August 2, 2024, from https://ourfuturehealth.org.uk/our-research-mission/.
41. Anandakrishnan R, Carpenetti TL, Samuel P, Wasko B, Johnson C, Smith C, Kim J, Michalak P, Kang L, Kinney N, Santo A, Anstrom J, Garner HR, Varghese RT. DNA sequencing of anatomy lab cadavers to provide hands-on precision medicine introduction to medical students. BMC Med Educ. 2020;20(1):437. https://doi.org/10.1186/s12909-020-02366-0.
42. Tada H, Usui S, Sakata K, Takamura M, Kawashiri M. Challenges of precision medicine for atherosclerotic cardiovascular disease based on human genome information. J Atheroscler Thromb. 2021;28(4):305–13. https://doi.org/10.5551/jat.60087.
43. Hamazaki T, El Rouby N, Fredette NC, Santostefano KE, Terada N. Concise review: induced pluripotent stem cell research in the era of precision medicine. Stem Cells. 2017;35(3):545–50. https://doi.org/10.1002/stem.2570.
44. Alkhatib O, Miles T, Jones R, Mair R, Palmer R, Winter H, McDermott F. Current and future genomic applications for surgeons. Ann R College Surg Engl. 2024;106(4):321–8. https://doi.org/10.1308/rcsann.2024.0031.
45. Di Meo A, Bartlett J, Cheng Y, Pasic MD, Yousef GM. Liquid biopsy: a step forward towards precision medicine in urologic malignancies. Mol Cancer. 2017;16(1):80. https://doi.org/10.1186/s12943-017-0644-5.
46. Watkins RR. Antibiotic stewardship in the era of precision medicine. JAC Antimicrob Resist. 2022;4(3):dlac066. https://doi.org/10.1093/jacamr/dlac066.
47. Springer S, Wang Y, Molin MD, Masica DL, Jiao Y, Kinde I, Blackford A, Raman SP, Wolfgang CL, Tomita T, Niknafs N, Douville C, Ptak J, Dobbyn L, Allen PJ, Klimstra DS, Schattner MA, Schmidt CM, Yip-Schneider M, et al. A combination of molecular markers and clinical features improve the classification of pancreatic cysts. Gastroenterology. 2015;149(6):1501–10. https://doi.org/10.1053/j.gastro.2015.07.041.

48. Popovtzer R, Reuveni, Motiei, Romman, Popovtzer. Targeted gold nanoparticles enable molecular CT imaging of cancer: an in vivo study. Int J Nanomedicine. 2011;6:2859. https://doi.org/10.2147/IJN.S25446.
49. Slikker W. Biomarkers and their impact on precision medicine. Exp Biol Med. 2018;243(3):211–2. https://doi.org/10.1177/1535370217733426.
50. Ferreira D, Miranda J, Martins-Lopes P, Adega F, Chaves R. Future perspectives in detecting EGFR and ALK gene alterations in liquid biopsies of patients with NSCLC. Int J Mol Sci. 2021;22(8):Article 8. https://doi.org/10.3390/ijms22083815.
51. Satam H, Joshi K, Mangrolia U, Waghoo S, Zaidi G, Rawool S, Thakare RP, Banday S, Mishra AK, Das G, Malonia SK. Next-generation sequencing technology: current trends and advancements. Biology. 2023;12(7):997. https://doi.org/10.3390/biology12070997.
52. Christodoulidis G, Koumarelas KE, Kouliou MN. Pivotal role of exosomes in diagnosis and treatment of esophageal cancer in a new era of precision medicine. World J Methodol. 2024;14(1) https://doi.org/10.5662/wjm.v14.i1.90624.
53. Deulkar P, Singam A, Jain A, Sr, P. D., Singam A, Jain A. A comprehensive review of the role of biomarkers in the early detection of endocrine disorders in critical illnesses. Cureus. 2024;16(5) https://doi.org/10.7759/cureus.61409.
54. Davis MA, Hanash S. High-throughput genomic technology in research and clinical management of breast cancer. Plasma-based proteomics in early detection and therapy. Breast Cancer Res. 2006;8(6):217. https://doi.org/10.1186/bcr1619.
55. Hayes B, Murphy C, Crawley A, O'Kennedy R. Developments in point-of-care diagnostic technology for cancer detection. Diagnostics. 2018;8(2):39. https://doi.org/10.3390/diagnostics8020039.
56. Ng O-H, O'Connell E, Mukherjee R. A global survey of precision medicine in emergency general surgery. Br J Surg. 2023;110(Supplement_10):znad388.025. https://doi.org/10.1093/bjs/znad388.025.
57. Chen Q, Zhang Z-H, Wang S, Lang J-H. Circulating cell-free DNA or circulating tumor DNA in the management of ovarian and endometrial cancer. Onco Targets Ther. 2019;12:11517–30. https://doi.org/10.2147/OTT.S227156.
58. Berretta M, Cavaliere C, Alessandrini L, Stanzione B, Facchini G, Balestreri L, Perin T, Canzonieri V. Serum and tissue markers in hepatocellular carcinoma and cholangiocarcinoma: clinical and prognostic implications. Oncotarget. 2016;8(8):14192–220. https://doi.org/10.18632/oncotarget.13929.
59. Saller T, Petzold A, Zetterberg H, Kuhle J, Chappell D, von Dossow V, Klawitter F, Schürholz T, Hagl C, Reuter DA, Zwissler B, Ehler J. A case series on the value of tau and neurofilament protein levels to predict and detect delirium in cardiac surgery patients. Biomed Papers. 2019;163(3):241–6. https://doi.org/10.5507/bp.2019.043.
60. Li H, Liu J, Chen J, Wang H, Yang L, Chen F, Fan S, Wang J, Shao B, Yin D, Zeng M, Li M, Li J, Su F, Liu Q, Yao H, Su S, Song E. A serum microRNA signature predicts trastuzumab benefit in HER2-positive metastatic breast cancer patients. Nat Commun. 2018;9(1):1614. https://doi.org/10.1038/s41467-018-03537-w.
61. Stepanyan A, Fassan M, Spolverato G, Castagliuolo I, Scarpa M, Scarpa M, Group, the I. S. IMMUNOREACT 0: biopsy-based immune biomarkers as predictors of response to neoadjuvant therapy for rectal cancer—a systematic review and meta-analysis. Cancer Med. 2023;12(17):17878–90. https://doi.org/10.1002/cam4.6423.
62. Matsuoka T, Yashiro M. Bioinformatics analysis and validation of potential markers associated with prediction and prognosis of gastric cancer. Int J Mol Sci. 2024;25(11):Article 11. https://doi.org/10.3390/ijms25115880.
63. Wang Y, Zhang L, Yang Y, Lu S, Chen H. Progress of gastric cancer surgery in the era of precision medicine. Int J Biol Sci. 2021;17(4):1041–9. https://doi.org/10.7150/ijbs.56735.
64. Ferkingstad E, Oddsson A, Gretarsdottir S, Benonisdottir S, Thorleifsson G, Deaton AM, Jonsson S, Stefansson OA, Norddahl GL, Zink F, Arnadottir GA, Gunnarsson B, Halldorsson GH, Helgadottir A, Jensson BO, Kristjansson RP, Sveinbjornsson G, Sverrisson DA, Masson

G, Olafsson I, et al. Genome-wide association meta-analysis yields 20 loci associated with gallstone disease. Nat Commun. 2018;9(1):5101. https://doi.org/10.1038/s41467-018-07460-y.
65. Elhassan H, Bulliment KL, Blood C, Buxton T, Read M, Cowlam T, Race A, Anathasayanam A, Morris K, Qadri SSA, Tentzeris V, Cowen ME, Gooseman MR. The importance of a daily multi-disciplinary team meeting in the management of patients with thoracic trauma. Shanghai. Chest. 2024;8(0):Article 0. https://doi.org/10.21037/shc-23-31.
66. Bach JA, Leskovan JJ, Scharschmidt T, Boulger C, Papadimos TJ, Russell S, Bahner DP, Stawicki SPA. The right team at the right time—multidisciplinary approach to multi-trauma patient with orthopedic injuries. Int J Crit Illn Inj Sci. 2017;7(1):32. https://doi.org/10.4103/IJCIIS.IJCIIS_5_17.
67. Kassab GS, An G, Sander EA, Miga M, Guccione JM, Ji S, Vodovotz Y. Augmenting surgery via multi-scale modeling and translational systems biology in the era of precision medicine: a multidisciplinary perspective. Ann Biomed Eng. 2016;44(9):2611–25. https://doi.org/10.1007/s10439-016-1596-4.
68. Cholerton B, Larson EB, Quinn JF, Zabetian CP, Mata IF, Keene CD, Flanagan M, Crane PK, Grabowski TJ, Montine KS, Montine TJ. Precision medicine: clarity for the complexity of dementia. Am J Pathol. 2016;186(3):500–6. https://doi.org/10.1016/j.ajpath.2015.12.001.
69. Davis CS, Wilkinson KH, Lin E, Carpenter NJ, Georgeades C, Lomberk G, Urrutia R. Precision medicine in trauma: a transformational frontier in patient care, education, and research. Eur J Trauma Emerg Surg. 2022;48(4):2607–12. https://doi.org/10.1007/s00068-021-01817-7.
70. Zhou W, Xu D, Peng X, Zhang Q, Jia J, Crutcher KA. Meta-analysis of APOE4 allele and outcome after traumatic brain injury. J Neurotrauma. 2008;25(4):279–90. https://doi.org/10.1089/neu.2007.0489.
71. McDaniel DO, Hamilton J, Brock M, May W, Calcote L, Tee LY, Vick L, Newman DB, Vick K, Harrison S, Timberlake G, Toevs C. Molecular analysis of inflammatory markers in trauma patients at risk of postinjury complications. Journal of Trauma: Injury, Infection & Critical Care. 2007;63(1):147. https://doi.org/10.1097/TA.0b013e31806bf0ab.
72. Tompkins RG. Genomics of injury: the glue grant experience. J Trauma Acute Care Surg. 2015;78(4):671–86. https://doi.org/10.1097/TA.0000000000000568.
73. Bianchi V, Giambusso M, De Iacob A, Chiarello MM, Brisinda G. Artificial intelligence in the diagnosis and treatment of acute appendicitis: A narrative review. Updat Surg. 2024;76(3):783–92. https://doi.org/10.1007/s13304-024-01801-x.
74. Wu Y-C, Chang C-Y, Huang Y-T, Chen S-Y, Chen C-H, Kao H-K. Artificial intelligence image recognition system for preventing wrong-site upper limb surgery. Diagnostics. 2023;13(24):Article 24. https://doi.org/10.3390/diagnostics13243667.
75. Liawrungrueang W, Cho ST, Sarasombath P, Kim I, Kim JH. Current trends in artificial intelligence-assisted spine surgery: a systematic review. Asian Spine J. 2023;18(1):146–57. https://doi.org/10.31616/asj.2023.0410.
76. Xu D, Lou W, Li M, Xiao J, Wu H, Chen J. Current status of robot-assisted surgery in the clinical application of trauma orthopedics in China: A systematic review. Health Sci Rep. 2022;5(6):e930. https://doi.org/10.1002/hsr2.930.
77. Levy BE, Castle JT, Virodov A, Wilt WS, Bumgardner C, Brim T, McAtee E, Schellenberg M, Inaba K, Warriner ZD. Artificial intelligence evaluation of focused assessment with sonography in trauma. J Trauma Acute Care Surg. 2023;95(5):706. https://doi.org/10.1097/TA.0000000000004021.
78. Kang C-B, Li X-W, Hou S-Y, Chi X-Q, Shan H-F, Zhang Q-J, Li X-B, Zhang J, Liu T-J. Preoperatively predicting the pathological types of acute appendicitis using machine learning based on peripheral blood biomarkers and clinical features: A retrospective study. Annals of Transl Med. 2021;9(10):Article 10. https://doi.org/10.21037/atm-20-7883.
79. Eickhoff RM, Bulla A, Eickhoff SB, Heise D, Helmedag M, Kroh A, Schmitz SM, Klink CD, Neumann UP, Lambertz A. Machine learning prediction model for postoperative outcome after perforated appendicitis. Langenbeck's Arch Surg. 2022;407(2):789–95. https://doi.org/10.1007/s00423-022-02456-1.

80. Hsieh C-H, Lu R-H, Lee N-H, Chiu W-T, Hsu M-H, Li Y-C. Novel solutions for an old disease: diagnosis of acute appendicitis with random forest, support vector machines, and artificial neural networks. Surgery. 2011;149(1):87–93. https://doi.org/10.1016/j.surg.2010.03.023.
81. Lisacek-Kiosoglous AB, Powling AS, Fontalis A, Gabr A, Mazomenos E, Haddad FS. Artificial intelligence in orthopaedic surgery: exploring its applications, limitations, and future direction. Bone Joint Res. 2023;12(7):447–54. https://doi.org/10.1302/2046-3758.127.BJR-2023-0111.R1.
82. Jayaraman SP, Anand RJ, DeAntonio JH, Mangino M, Aboutanos MB, Kasirajan V, Ivatury RR, Valadka AB, Glushakova O, Hayes RL, Bachmann LM, Brophy GM, Contaifer D, Warncke UO, Brophy DF, Wijesinghe DS. Metabolomics and precision medicine in trauma: the state of the field. Shock. 2018;50(1):5. https://doi.org/10.1097/SHK.0000000000001093.
83. Rubin-Asher D, Zeilig G, Ratner A, Asher I, Zivelin A, Seligsohn U, Lubetsky A. Risk factors for failure of heparin thromboprophylaxis in patients with acute traumatic spinal cord injury. Thromb Res. 2010;125(6):501–4. https://doi.org/10.1016/j.thromres.2009.09.012.
84. Cappellini I, Lai F, Magazzini S, Consales G. Precision medicine in hemostasis: a review of prothrombin complex concentrates and the role of viscoelastic tests in tailoring therapy. Emerg Care J. 2023;19(4):Article 4. https://doi.org/10.4081/ecj.2023.11500.
85. Kurowski BG, Treble-Barna A, Pitzer AJ, Wade SL, Martin LJ, Chima RS, Jegga A. Applying systems biology methodology to identify genetic factors possibly associated with recovery after traumatic brain injury. J Neurotrauma. 2017;34(14):2280–90. https://doi.org/10.1089/neu.2016.4856.
86. Ariza M, Matarin MD, Junqué C, Mataró M, Clemente I, Moral P, Antonia Poca M, Garnacho A, Sahuquillo J. Influence of angiotensin-converting enzyme polymorphism on neuropsychological subacute performance in moderate and severe traumatic brain injury. J Neuropsychiatry Clin Neurosci. 2006;18(1):39–44. https://doi.org/10.1176/jnp.18.1.39.

Part II

Artificial Intelligence and Surgical Decision-Making Support

4 Basics of AI in Surgical Practice and the Role of AI in Decision-Making for Risk Assessment and Clinical Decision Support

Francesca Dal Mas, Justyna Fijalkowska, Justyna Rdzanek, and Lorenzo Cobianchi

4.1 Introduction to AI in Surgical Practice

Artificial intelligence (AI) can be defined as the development of algorithms that enable machines to behave with human-like rationality in complex tasks, such as problem-solving and decision-making [1, 2]. AI has emerged as a transformative Industry 4.0 technology in various industries [3], and healthcare is no exception [4–7]. AI-based advanced techniques have the power to disrupt and revolutionize the way healthcare professionals approach patient care.

Currently, AI is predominantly employed to enhance the speed and precision of healthcare. AI algorithms are particularly valuable in analyzing medical imaging data, including X-rays, Magnetic Resonance Imaging (MRI), and computed tomography (CT) scans, to aid healthcare professionals in rapidly and accurately diagnosing patients [8–11]. Digital pathology represents one more relevant application, as

F. Dal Mas (✉)
Department of Management, Ca Foscari University of Venice, Venice, Italy

Collegium Medicum, SAN University, Łodz, Poland
e-mail: francesca.dalmas@unive.it

J. Fijalkowska
Department of Management, SAN University, Łodz, Poland

J. Rdzanek
Collegium Medicum, SAN University, Łodz, Poland

L. Cobianchi
Collegium Medicum, SAN University, Łodz, Poland

Department of Clinical, Surgical, Diagnostic, and Pediatric Sciences, University of Pavia, Pavia, Italy

General Surgery Department and Pancreas Unit Directorship, IRCCS Foundation San Matteo, Pavia, Italy

B. De Simone et al. (eds.), *New Technologies, Precision Medicine, and AI in Emergency General Surgery*, Hot Topics in Acute Care Surgery and Trauma,
https://doi.org/10.1007/978-3-032-09357-8_4

it empowers pathologists to deliver more accurate diagnoses and improve clinical decision-making in patients with cancer or other diseases [12, 13]. AI is also applied in surgical practice. By harnessing the power of AI, surgeons can now make more informed decisions, enhance risk assessment, and provide better clinical outcomes for their patients [5, 14].

The ability to accurately assess risks and make informed clinical decisions is paramount in the dynamic and high-stakes surgery world. Traditional methods of risk assessment and decision-making, while valuable, can be limited by human biases, cognitive constraints, and the sheer volume of data that surgeons must process [15]. AI can provide surgeons with a valid aid to these challenges, offering powerful tools to enhance their decision-making capabilities and improve patient outcomes.

4.2 Applications of AI in Surgical Practice

AI algorithms can analyze vast amounts of patient data, including medical histories, imaging scans, and surgical records, to identify patterns and predict potential risks. By leveraging these technologies, surgeons can gain a more comprehensive understanding of a patient's unique risk profile, allowing them to make more informed decisions about the appropriate course of treatment [16, 17]. Therefore, AI may offer the opportunity to combine traditional clinical data-based prediction algorithms with quantified surgeon intuition [16].

Numerous examples of successful applications of AI in surgical practice have emerged in recent years, and they involve the preoperative, intraoperative, and postoperative phases.

Concerning the preoperative phase, AI can assist in the planning of complex surgical procedures. AI-empowered systems can support the early detection of surgical complications and risks, including potential postoperative bleeding or infections [18–20] and the need for early access to intensive care units [21]. By continuously monitoring patient data, these systems can provide timely alerts, enabling surgeons to intervene promptly and mitigate risks, also supporting a virtual hospital model of care [22]. AI can also support surgical planning and simulation by generating detailed 3D models of a patient's anatomy, allowing surgeons to rehearse complex procedures and optimize their surgical approach before the actual operation. This level of precision and preparation can lead to improved outcomes and reduced operating times [23, 24]. This information can then be used to tailor the surgical plan, optimize patient preparation, and implement targeted preventive measures, ultimately enhancing patient safety and improving surgical outcomes [25].

Concerning the intraoperative phase, AI has been instrumental in the development of robotic-assisted surgical systems [26, 27], which leverage these technologies to enhance the precision, stability, and dexterity of surgical interventions. By integrating AI algorithms, these systems can provide real-time guidance and decision support to the operating surgeon, enhancing the overall quality of care. Still, according to the recent literature, there is no available summary of the current stage of development and the degree of autonomy of this technology [26, 27].

AI can then support the postoperative phases, including the monitoring of postoperative complications [28], pain management [29], and rehabilitation through specific algorithms [30]. Moreover, the analysis of surgical data can benchmark the quality of surgical care by employing nonlinear methods for more comprehensive evaluation to understand areas of excellence versus suboptimal care [31].

AI can also represent a new subject as well as a methodology for innovative surgical education [32], including performance assessment using virtual simulators.

4.3 The Role of AI in Clinical Decision Support for Surgeons

In addition to risk assessment, AI applications play a crucial role in clinical decision support for surgeons [33, 34]. The importance of competent clinical judgment is widely recognized, as it is necessary to integrate evidence-based medicine into clinical practice appropriately. In daily practice, junior surgeons seek counsel from their more experienced colleagues, patients inquire about the surgeon's opinion when navigating treatment options, and physicians frequently rely on their gestalt to make clinical decisions [16].

AI technologies can analyze a vast array of medical data, including research studies, clinical guidelines, and patient-specific information, to provide personalized recommendations and insights. For instance, AI-powered systems can suggest the most appropriate surgical approach based on the patient's unique characteristics, the complexity of the procedure, and the surgeon's expertise. By considering a multitude of factors, these systems can help surgeons make more informed decisions, reducing the risk of complications and improving the overall quality of care. Still, to positively impact surgical care, decision-support models must surpass the current reporting guideline requirements by performing external and real-time validation, enrolling sufficient sample sizes, reporting model precision, assessing performance across vulnerable populations, and achieving clinical implementation. A recent literature review highlighted how the extent to which published models meet these criteria is unknown [33].

Clinical decision-making can be extremely challenging, especially in the context of trauma and emergency surgery [35], when clinicians need to act fast despite several aspects that could be uncertain, including the patient's identity and care preferences, existing conditions or ongoing treatments, and the trauma's causes. Therefore, in such contexts, high cognitive demands and time constraints imposed by the vast amounts of information necessitate the use of cognitive shortcuts, which can result in preventable patient injury and errors [36].

In recent years, the literature has devoted significant attention to decision-support systems that are founded on AI algorithms [5]. Still, AI systems in routine trauma and emergency surgical care remain a critical opportunity that seems largely unfulfilled [14, 37, 38].

The World Society of Emergency Surgery (WSES), one of the major scientific societies in the field of trauma and emergency surgery, has endorsed a number of clinical and organizational studies in the field of AI.

For instance, the artificial intelligence in emergency and trauma surgery (ARIES) survey [39] assessed the knowledge, attitude, and practices of international acute care and emergency surgeons in the application of AI in the emergency setting. The investigation demonstrated that the implementation of AI in the emergency and trauma setting is eagerly anticipated, despite the fact that it is still in the early stages, and that trauma and emergency surgeons are ebullient about participating [39, 40].

The WSES team dynamics study on clinical decision-making [41–44] assessed, through an online survey filled in by 650 surgeons from 71 distinct countries, the knowledge, perspectives, facilitators, and barriers in the use of AI-based applications to support clinical decision-making in complex settings.

Concerning knowledge, participating surgeons were questioned regarding their familiarity with the term "AI." Interestingly, almost 70% of participants declared that they were acquainted with the term, while the remaining 30% acknowledged that they were not. Still, such declarations were questioned, as they were required to include a written explanation of the application of AI to surgery. A manual analysis made by the principal investigators revealed that only 17% of participants submitted a definition that met the criteria, namely, emphasizing the machine's ability to replicate human intelligence. Almost 30% of participants provided a definition that revealed only a partial understanding of the phenomenon. More than half of the participants (55% of the sample) provided responses that did not align with the concept of AI, its objectives, or its potential. Moreover, the majority of these participants declared that they were unaware of the potential implications of AI in surgical practice [41].

Concerning facilitators in medical decision-making, clinicians underscored the significance of clinical guidelines, training, and multidisciplinary committees and meetings [41]. Interestingly enough, tools that are now at the center of the academic and practice debate, namely, risk stratification by additive scores using static variable thresholds, AI, regression modeling tools, and calculations, received the lowest scores, with AI recording the highest standard deviation in responses, showing a divide in the surgical community between technology enthusiasts and those who are more skeptical. To dig deeper into the matter, the sample was divided using descriptive statistics, analyzing the responses concerning the potential use of AI by type of institution (academic vs. non-academic), the position held by the respondent, and the work country. Intriguingly, there was no discernible distinction between the role and the institution (academic or non-academic). The analysis of the countries revealed significant differences, with some exhibiting a high mean and a low standard deviation, such as Argentina, and others demonstrating a very low mean and a high standard deviation, such as Switzerland [41]. Additionally, the responses were analyzed simultaneously with respect to the institution, position, and country. Despite the reduction in numbers, some intriguing discoveries emerged. For example, the senior consultants of Malaysian academic institutions were unanimous in their support of AI, scoring the item at 5/5 on the Likert scale, in contrast to the division commanders in the United States, who rated it at 2.5 with a standard deviation of 1.05. Residents and younger surgeons do not occupy the highest positions despite their status as digital natives [41].

Concerning the barriers, the WSES study results emphasize the perceived misalignment between the actual clinical scenario and the independent assessment, the absence of complete data availability, the risk of anticipating specific outcomes based on inaccurate data, the presence of bias derived from the most recent experiences, and the potential for making mistakes throughout the clinical journey. The potential support provided by new technologies such as AI was rated as the lowest item by surgeons [41].

The results of the WSES Team Dynamics survey are consistent with the ARIES one [39]. Trauma and emergency surgeons demonstrate an interest in AI, but they continue to harbor numerous doubts and apprehensions regarding its actual applicability and potential as a decision-making tool. Still, they rely more on the support of their multidisciplinary staff and colleagues, clinical guidelines, and training. Geographical disparities appear intriguing as well, and more aspects may be worth investigating, namely, the areas of cultural perspective, the training opportunities in place, the availability of technology or technology partners, and the presence of technological surgical leaders or ambassadors.

4.4 Challenges and Limitations of AI in Surgery

As AI continues to evolve, the potential for its application in surgical practice is expected to grow exponentially. Advancements in areas such as natural language processing (NLP), computer vision, and predictive analytics will enable even more sophisticated risk assessment, clinical decision support, and surgical planning capabilities. Additionally, the integration of AI with other emerging technologies, such as augmented reality (AR), virtual reality (VR), and wearable devices, will likely lead to the development of innovative surgical tools and techniques [3]. These advancements will empower surgeons to make more informed decisions, enhance patient safety, and improve overall surgical outcomes.

While the potential benefits of AI-based tools in surgical practice are substantial, it is essential to acknowledge the challenges and limitations associated with these technologies. Ethical considerations, data privacy concerns, and the need for robust validation and regulatory oversight are critical factors that must be addressed [40, 45, 46]. Ensuring the transparency and interpretability of AI models is crucial, as surgeons and patients must understand the reasoning behind the recommendations and decisions [45]. Surgeons and healthcare institutions must work closely with ethicists, policymakers, and the broader community to develop robust guidelines and frameworks for the responsible use of AI in surgical settings. This includes ensuring that patient consent is obtained, that data is securely stored and protected, and that the decision-making process of these technologies is transparent and accountable.

Additionally, the integration of these technologies into existing workflows, the design of new organizational models, the understanding of the new technical and non-technical skills, and the need for comprehensive training and support for healthcare professionals can present significant implementation hurdles [47].

Moreover, while surgeons emphasize the necessity of reliable decision aids when analyzing the dynamics of the decision-making process, especially in challenging scenarios like trauma and emergency [39, 41], they still seem skeptical about the value of using AI tools to support their medical decisions. The degree of technology acceptance seems low [48], and this topic is worth investigating, leading to research and practice implications that require a multidisciplinary approach to competencies, including information technology, computer sciences, management, statistics, and psychology.

4.5 Implementing AI in Surgical Settings: What Should We Expect?

The successful implementation of AI in surgical practice requires a multifaceted approach that addresses technological, organizational, and cultural factors [41]. Healthcare institutions must invest in the necessary infrastructure, including secure data storage, high-performance computing resources, and specialized AI expertise.

Furthermore, the integration of these technologies must be accompanied by competency alignment and comprehensive training and support for surgeons and other healthcare professionals [47]. This ensures that they can effectively leverage the capabilities of AI, interpret the results, and make informed decisions that prioritize patient safety and well-being. A profound revision of medical schools' curricula or residents' training plans may also be necessary to align the required skills with the teaching contents and methods [41].

As the adoption of AI-based solutions in surgical practice continues to grow, it is essential that healthcare institutions, surgeons, and the broader healthcare community and ecosystem work together to address the challenges and ethical considerations associated with these technologies. By doing so, the transformative power of AI can be harnessed to the fullest extent, ultimately improving patients' lives and advancing the field of surgical practice [40, 45].

References

1. Secinaro S, Calandra D, Secinaro A, Muthurangu V, Biancone P. The role of artificial intelligence in healthcare: a structured literature review. BMC Med Inform Decis Mak [Internet]. 2021;21(1):1–23. Available from: https://doi.org/10.1186/s12911-021-01488-9.
2. Wehde M. Healthcare 4.0. IEEE Eng Manag Rev. 2019;47(3):24–8.
3. Bagnoli C, Albarelli A, Biazzo S, Biotto G, Marseglia GR, Massaro M, et al. Digital business models for industry 4.0. Cham: Springer; 2022.
4. Kemppainen L, Pikkarainen M, Hurmelinna-Laukkanen P, Reponen J. Connected health innovation: data access challenges in the Interface of AI companies and hospitals [Internet]. Vol. 9,

Technology Innovation Management Review. Ottawa: Talent First Network; 2019. Available from: http://timreview.ca/article/1291.

5. Loftus TJ, Tighe PJ, Filiberto AC, Efron PA, Brakenridge SC, Mohr AM, et al. Artificial intelligence and surgical decision-making. JAMA Surg. 2020;155(2):148–58.
6. Hashimoto DA, Rosman G, Rus D, Meireles OR. Artificial intelligence in surgery: promises and perils. Ann Surg [Internet]. 2018;268(1). Available from: https://journals.lww.com/annalsofsurgery/fulltext/2018/07000/artificial_intelligence_in_surgery__promises_and.13.aspx.
7. Birkmeyer JD. The future of artificial intelligence in surgical care. Ann Surg [Internet]. 2020;272(3). Available from: https://journals.lww.com/annalsofsurgery/fulltext/2020/09000/the_future_of_artificial_intelligence_in_surgical.32.aspx.
8. Calisto FM, Nunes N, Nascimento JC. Modeling adoption of intelligent agents in medical imaging. Int J Hum Comput Stud [Internet]. 2022;168:102922. Available from: https://www.sciencedirect.com/science/article/pii/S1071581922001422.
9. Dicuonzo G, Donofrio F, Fusco A, Shini M. Healthcare system: moving forward with artificial intelligence. Technovation. 2022:102510.
10. Dal Mas F, Massaro M, Rippa P, Secundo G. The challenges of digital transformation in healthcare: an interdisciplinary literature review, framework, and future research agenda. Technovation [Internet]. 2023;123:102716. Available from: https://www.sciencedirect.com/science/article/pii/S0166497223000275.
11. Wein W, Brunke S, Khamene A, Callstrom MR, Navab N. Automatic CT-ultrasound registration for diagnostic imaging and image-guided intervention. Med Image Anal [Internet]. 2008;12(5):577–85. Available from: https://www.sciencedirect.com/science/article/pii/S1361841508000637.
12. Hijazi A, Bifulco C, Baldin P, Galon J. Digital pathology for better clinical practice. Cancers (Basel). 2024;16(9)
13. Sulaieva O, Dudin O, Koshyk O, Panko M, Kobyliak N. Digital pathology implementation in cancer diagnostics: towards informed decision-making. Front Digit Heal. 2024;6:1358305.
14. Loftus TJ, Upchurch GR, Bihorac A. Building an artificial intelligence–competent surgical workforce. JAMA Surg. 2021;156(6):511.
15. O'sullivan ED, Schofield SJ. Cognitive bias clinical medicine. J R Coll Physicians Edinb. 2018;48(3):225–32.
16. Berrigan MT, Beaulieu-Jones BR, Marwaha J, Fladger A, Katlic MR, Brat GA. Integrating human intuition into prediction algorithms for improved surgical risk stratification. Ann Surg [Internet]. 2024;279(1). Available from: https://journals.lww.com/annalsofsurgery/fulltext/2024/01000/integrating_human_intuition_into_prediction.4.aspx.
17. El Hechi M, Gebran A, Bouardi HT, Maurer LR, El Moheb M, Zhuo D, et al. Validation of the artificial intelligence-based trauma outcomes predictor (TOP) in patients 65 years and older. Surgery. 2022;171(6):1687–94.
18. Loftus TJ, Vlaar APJ, Hung AJ, Bihorac A, Dennis BM, Juillard C, et al. Executive summary of the artificial intelligence in surgery series. Surgery. 2022;171(5):1435–9.
19. Byerly S, Maurer LR, Mantero A, Naar L, An G, Kaafarani HMA. Machine learning and artificial intelligence for surgical decision making. Surg Infect (Larchmt) [Internet]. 2021;22(6):626–34. Available from: https://doi.org/10.1089/sur.2021.007.
20. Maurer LR, Bertsimas D, Bouardi HT, El Hechi M, El Moheb M, Giannoutsou K, et al. Trauma outcome predictor: an artificial intelligence interactive smartphone tool to predict outcomes in trauma patients. J Trauma Acute Care Surg [Internet]. 2021;91(1). Available from: https://journals.lww.com/jtrauma/Fulltext/2021/07000/Trauma_outcome_predictor__An_artificial.15.aspx.
21. Gebran A, Vapsi A, Maurer LR, El Moheb M, Naar L, Thakur SS, et al. POTTER-ICU: an artificial intelligence smartphone-accessible tool to predict the need for intensive care after emergency surgery. Surgery. 2022;172(1):470–5.
22. Bidoli C, Pegoraro V, Dal Mas F, Bagnoli C, Bert F, Bonin M, et al. Virtual hospitals: the future of the healthcare system? An expert consensus. J Telemed Telecare. 2023:1–13.

23. Chen-Yoshikawa TF. Evolution of three-dimensional computed tomography imaging in thoracic surgery. Cancers. 2024;16.
24. Dal Mas F, Piccolo D, Edvinsson L, Skrap M, D'Auria S. Strategy innovation, intellectual capital management and the future of healthcare. The case of Kiron by nucleode. In: Matos F, Vairinhos V, Salavisa I, Edvinsson L, Massaro M, editors. Knowledge, people, and digital transformation: approaches for a sustainable future. Cham: Springer; 2020. p. 119–31.
25. Nederpelt CJ, Mokhtari AK, Alser O, Tsiligkaridis T, Roberts J, Cha M, et al. Development of a field artificial intelligence triage tool: confidence in the prediction of shock, transfusion, and definitive surgical therapy in patients with truncal gunshot wounds. J Trauma Acute Care Surg. 2021;90(6):1054–60.
26. Vasey B, Lippert KAN, Khan DZ, Ibrahim M, Koh CH, Layard Horsfall H, et al. Intraoperative applications of artificial intelligence in robotic surgery: a scoping review of current development stages and levels of autonomy. Ann Surg [Internet]. 2023;278(6). Available from: https://journals.lww.com/annalsofsurgery/fulltext/2023/12000/intraoperative_applications_of_artificial.10.aspx.
27. Panesar S, Cagle Y, Chander D, Morey J, Fernandez-Miranda J, Kliot M. Artificial intelligence and the future of surgical robotics. Ann Surg [Internet]. 2019;270(2). Available from: https://journals.lww.com/annalsofsurgery/fulltext/2019/08000/artificial_intelligence_and_the_future_of_surgical.7.aspx.
28. Tseng P-Y, Chen Y-T, Wang C-H, Chiu K-M, Peng Y-S, Hsu S-P, et al. Prediction of the development of acute kidney injury following cardiac surgery by machine learning. Crit Care [Internet]. 2020;24(1):478. Available from: https://doi.org/10.1186/s13054-020-03179-9.
29. Wang R, Wang S, Duan N, Wang Q. From patient-controlled analgesia to artificial intelligence-assisted patient-controlled analgesia: practices and perspectives. Front Med [Internet]. 2020;7. Available from: https://www.frontiersin.org/journals/medicine/articles/10.3389/fmed.2020.00145.
30. Bongiorno G, Sisti G, Tsiotas G, Biancuzzi H, Dal Mas F, Miceli L. Artificial intelligence as a potential teaching tool for athletes: when the skate and the smartphone run together. J Sports Med Phys Fitness Italy. 2023;63:974–6.
31. Dorken-Gallastegi A, El Hechi M, Amram M, Naar L, Maurer LR, Gebran A, et al. Use of artificial intelligence for nonlinear benchmarking of surgical care. Surgery. 2023;174(6):1302–8.
32. Winkler-Schwartz A, Bissonnette V, Mirchi N, Ponnudurai N, Yilmaz R, Ledwos N, et al. Artificial intelligence in medical education: best practices using machine learning to assess surgical expertise in virtual reality simulation. J Surg Educ [Internet]. 2019;76(6):1681–90. Available from: https://www.sciencedirect.com/science/article/pii/S1931720419301060.
33. Loftus TJ, Altieri MS, Balch JA, Abbott KL, Choi J, Marwaha JS, et al. Artificial intelligence–enabled decision support in surgery: state-of-the-art and future directions. Ann Surg [Internet]. 2023:278(1). Available from: https://journals.lww.com/annalsofsurgery/fulltext/2023/07000/artificial_intelligence_enabled_decision_support.9.aspx.
34. Cobianchi L, Dal Mas F, Ansaloni L. Editorial: new frontiers for artificial intelligence in surgical decision making and its organizational impacts. Front Surg [Internet]. 2022;9(933673). Available from: https://www.frontiersin.org/article/10.3389/fsurg.2022.933673.
35. Cobianchi L, Dal Mas F, Massaro M, Fugazzola P, Coccolini F, Kluger Y, et al. Team dynamics in emergency surgery teams: results from a first international survey. World J Emerg Surg. 2021;16:47.
36. Litvin A, Korenev S, Rumovskaya S, Sartelli M, Baiocchi G, Biffl WL, et al. WSES project on decision support systems based on artificial neural networks in emergency surgery. World J Emerg Surg. 2021;16(1):50.
37. Balch J, Upchurch GR, Bihorac A, Loftus TJ. Bridging the artificial intelligence valley of death in surgical decision-making. Surgery. 2021;169(4):746–8.
38. Loftus TJ, Shickel B, Ruppert MM, Balch JA, Ozrazgat-Baslanti T, Tighe PJ, et al. Uncertainty-aware deep learning in healthcare: a scoping review. Lai Y, editor. PLOS Digit Heal. 2022;1(8):e0000085.

39. De Simone B, Abu-Zidan FM, Gumbs AA, Chouillard E, Di Saverio S, Sartelli M, et al. Knowledge, attitude, and practice of artificial intelligence in emergency and trauma surgery, the ARIES project: an international web-based survey. World J Emerg Surg. 2022;17(1):10.
40. De Simone B, Di Saverio S. Invited commentary: artificial intelligence in surgical care: we must overcome ethical boundaries. J Am Coll Surg [Internet]. 2022;235(2). Available from: https://journals.lww.com/journalacs/fulltext/2022/08000/invited_commentary__artificial_intelligence_in.18.aspx.
41. Cobianchi L, Piccolo D, Dal Mas F, Agnoletti V, Ansaloni L, Balch J, et al. Surgeons' perspectives on artificial intelligence to support clinical decision – making in trauma and emergency contexts: results from an international survey. World J Emerg Surg. 2023;18:1–17.
42. Cobianchi L, Dal Mas F, Agnoletti V, Ansaloni A, Biffl V, Butturini G, et al. Time for a paradigm shift in shared decision-making in trauma and emergency surgery? Results from an international survey. World J Emerg Surg. 2023.
43. Dal Mas F, Massaro M, Woltz S, Ruta F, Catena F, Fugazzola P, et al. Shared decision-making in trauma and emergency surgery settings. A literature review. In: Cerchione R, Centobelli P, editors. Proceedings of the 23rd European Conference on Knowledge Management – ECKM. Naples: Academic Conferences & Publishing International Ltd.; 2022. p. 278–88.
44. Cobianchi L, Dal Mas F, Catena F, Ansaloni A. Artificial intelligence and clinical decision-making in emergency surgery. A research protocol. In: Sousa MJ, Kumar PS, Dal Mas F, Sousa S, editors. Advancements in artificial intelligence in the service sector. London: Routledge; 2023.
45. Cobianchi L, Verde JM, Loftus TJ, Piccolo D, Dal Mas F, Mascagni P, et al. Artificial intelligence and surgery: ethical dilemmas and open issues. J Am Coll Surg [Internet]. 2022;235(2):268–275. Available from: https://journals.lww.com/journalacs/Fulltext/9900/Artificial_Intelligence_and_Surgery__Ethical.215.aspx.
46. O'Sullivan S, Nevejans N, Allen C, Blyth A, Leonard S, Pagallo U, et al. Legal, regulatory, and ethical frameworks for development of standards in artificial intelligence (AI) and autonomous robotic surgery. Int J Med Robot Comput Assist Surg. 2019;15(1):1–12.
47. Sousa MJ, Dal Mas F, Pesqueira A, Lemos C, Verde JM, Cobianchi L. The potential of AI in health higher education to increase the students' learning outcomes. TEM J. 2021;10(2):488–97.
48. Biancone P, Secinaro S, Marseglia R, Calandra D. E-health for the future. Managerial perspectives using a multiple case study approach. Technovation [Internet]. 2021:102406. Available from: https://www.sciencedirect.com/science/article/pii/S0166497221001875.

5 Application of AI in Acute Care and Emergency Surgery for the Management of Surgical Patients

Lydia R. Maurer and Haytham M. A. Kaafarani

5.1 Introduction

Emergency general surgery (EGS) patients have been shown to have significantly higher mortality and complications compared with elective surgery patients undergoing similar procedures. Additionally, this population of patients can have incredibly diverse disease presentations and constellations of underlying conditions, making clinical decision-making particularly complex. To assist with surgical decision-making, a number of risk prediction tools have been adapted from other situations and applied to the emergency surgery realm, and more recently, some tools have been developed and validated for EGS specifically. In this chapter, we will discuss the growth in artificial intelligence (AI)-based methodology that has allowed for the development of risk calculators that adapt to and reflect the complexity of the EGS population and can provide support for surgeons and families making critical surgical decisions.

5.2 Linear Versus Nonlinear Risk Calculators in Emergency Surgery

A number of surgical risk prediction tools have been developed over the last several decades and applied to the EGS population. Two of the most common are the American Society of Anesthesiologists (ASA) classification system and the American College of Surgeons National Surgical Quality Improvement Program (ACS-NSQIP) calculator [1, 2]. More recently, a calculator was specifically developed for this population called the Emergency Surgery Score (ESS), which has

L. R. Maurer (✉) · H. M. A. Kaafarani
Department of Surgery, Massachusetts General Hospital, Harvard University, Boston, MA, USA
e-mail: lrmaurer@mgb.org; hkaafarani@mgh.harvard.edu

B. De Simone et al. (eds.), *New Technologies, Precision Medicine, and AI in Emergency General Surgery*, Hot Topics in Acute Care Surgery and Trauma,
https://doi.org/10.1007/978-3-032-09357-8_5

since been validated in a multicenter context [3, 4]. These traditional (non-AI-based) risk calculators all have one thing in common—they can be considered "linear"—with the same data points included for every patient, every time. In each case, these data points carry the same weight and have the same relationship in the risk calculation algorithm. In contrast, AI-based risk calculators have the potential to reflect nonlinear relationships between patient characteristics in a way that can be more reflective of clinical reality. In a prior explanation of linear versus nonlinear risk, El Hechi et al. offer the hypothetical example of an elderly gentleman who needs a Graham patch for a perforated duodenal ulcer [5]. Depending on the presence or absence of individual comorbidities, the role of other patient factors may vary as to their importance in predicting mortality and complications. For example, if this older patient comes in well nourished, the most important contributors to his or her outcome may be underlying lung or cardiac disease. Conversely, if he or she comes in malnourished, poor nutrition status may predominate in contributing to a poor outcome and supersede the other underlying comorbidities. "Linear" prediction models do not allow for this degree of model adaptation based on individual patient factors.

5.3 AI-Based Risk Calculation in Emergency Surgery

In contrast to linear calculators, risk calculators developed with AI methodology are inherently nonlinear. For example, the Predictive OpTimal Trees in Emergency Surgery Risk (POTTER) Calculator was developed in 2018 and is an interpretable, AI-based calculator available as a smartphone application that can be used at the bedside [6, 7]. The interpretable AI methodology is called optimal classification trees (OCTs), and it has since been used to generate predictive algorithms in multiple clinical contexts, including trauma [5, 8], intensive care [9], surgical oncology [10], cardiac surgery [11], and pediatric surgery [12], among others. With regard to the OCT methodology, this algorithm was derived and tested on patients from the ACS-NSQIP database, generating a tree-like architecture of patient variables (in the appearance of a decision tree) that creates outcome prediction for patients with various combinations of these characteristics (Fig. 5.1). The model itself iterates numerous versions of the overall OCT, and in doing so optimizes the performance of the entire model. A benefit of this particular AI-based methodology is that it is interpretable, meaning that the individual patient variables contributing to a particular outcome prediction can be seen by the clinician using the data. Not only did this model have the benefit of interpretability, but it also outperformed other commonly used risk calculators, including the ASA classification system and the ACS-NSQIP Surgical Risk Calculator.

Another set of AI-based models was recently developed to predict postoperative mortality, pneumonia, surgical site infection, thrombosis, and mechanical ventilation in EGS patients [13]. The authors tested multiple machine-learning-based methodologies (random forest [14], XGBoost [15], etc.) to find the best-performing model for each outcome and have an available web-based application. They also

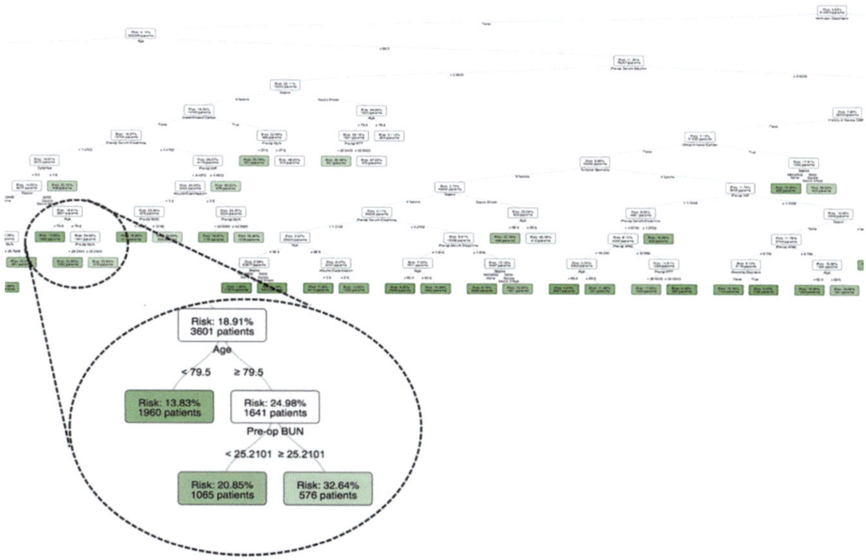

Fig. 5.1 *Optimal Classification Tree (OCT) example.* This model was developed using an iterative machine-learning-based methodology called OCTs. The tree-like structure illustrates how patient variables are sequentially used to predict clinical outcomes. Each node's split is internally generated by the model (for example, age, which here diverges at 79.5 years) to optimize the overall performance of the model as a whole. After following patient-specific splits to the terminal nodes, a final risk prediction is given

compared their algorithm for mortality to the ESS, APACHE II, and ASA and found their ML-based algorithm to have better discrimination performance with an AUROC of 0.89. The highest-performing methodology was ultimately the random forest, which is a "black box" methodology, meaning that after inputting a series of patient variables, the relationship of those variables and the calculations that yield an ultimate prediction are invisible to the end user. A benefit of these "black box" methodologies is that they can be quite powerful and perform very well to discriminate between outcomes. However, a downside is that these methods are not interpretable, and it is not clear to the clinician user which patient factors led to a particular outcome prediction [16]. Additionally, bias can be inadvertently introduced and propagated without the user realizing it [17].

Beyond the initial development of these algorithms, it is important to test them in patient populations that mimic clinical practice. For instance, while a particular clinical algorithm may have excellent performance in a large population of EGS patients, there may be certain groups in which it performs better than in others. Looking specifically at the POTTER calculator in geriatric patients, for instance, the calculator performed well up to the age of 85, but in the oldest patients, the model did not perform as well [18]. Ultimately, the performance of these AI-based models is integrally tied to the availability of the data used to create them. For instance, a calculator developed from patient data with a very limited geriatric sample should not necessarily be applied to a population of older adults unless it is validated and found to be high-performing for that specific group. This applies to any unique population or environment, and it is important for the clinician to look in detail at the data source of the original calculator and whether any validation studies have been performed in particular populations before applying the outcomes to clinical practice for an individual patient.

5.4 AI Versus Surgeon Gestalt in Clinical Practice

The potential for risk calculators to predict surgical outcomes has been studied in many arenas, but there is a paucity of research comparing AI or non-AI-based risk calculators to decision-making by the surgeon, often referred to as a surgeon's "gestalt." A recent study used clinical vignettes based on real-life EGS scenarios to compare a surgeon's outcome prediction without access to a risk calculator versus their prediction of the patient's outcome with the POTTER prediction available to them [19]. These were both compared to the prediction of POTTER alone. In this study, all groups performed quite well—POTTER had the best discrimination performance, followed by surgeons + POTTER, and then the surgeons alone. There was some variation in the relative performance of the groups for individual complications, but overall, surgeons with the POTTER prediction available to them came up with predictions that were more in line with clinical reality than those who did not.

In another study examining the potential impact of risk calculators in surgical decision-making and patient counseling, researchers found that when risk calculator predictions were available to surgeons (in this case, the ACS-NSQIP risk calculator), there was less variability in their assessment of operative risk regarding mortality and complications, but no difference in whether they would advocate for an operation [20]. This study is interesting in that it examines the potential role of a risk calculator not just for outcome prediction and patient counseling but also for surgical decision-making. Outside of clinical vignettes, more studies are needed to better understand the optimal way to incorporate risk calculators into day-to-day clinical reality.

5.5 Avoiding Bias in AI-Based Risk Calculators

As AI has become increasingly widespread in both general society and within healthcare, there have been a number of warning signs as to the potential risks of perpetuating bias for sensitive groups in areas as widespread as criminal recidivism [20], facial recognition [21], skin cancer detection [22], and others. At numerous stages in clinical algorithm development, bias can be introduced—from the data source itself and any discriminatory practices embedded in the care of patients in that original source data to data processing and outcome analysis. The potential risk for bias encoding and propagation in AI methodologies is well-established. To combat this, interpretable methodologies can be valuable in revealing areas of bias in algorithms [17]. Additionally, when evidence of bias is exposed within an algorithm, studies have shown that mathematical fairness adjustment can process a biased dataset in an attempt to reduce the bias of a final outcome prediction [23, 24]. Conversely, simply removing race (or another sensitive attribute) as a variable has not been shown to be as effective [24]. In healthcare, as in other fields, it is imperative that we continue to investigate and take active efforts to reduce bias in AI-based algorithms.

5.6 Conclusion

AI-based technology has expanded the potential for risk calculators in emergency surgery. Still, a number of areas remain to be studied, particularly when it comes to understanding how best to implement these calculators into clinical practice. While there are some isolated examples in the literature of incorporating risk predictors into the electronic medical record, there has not yet been widespread implementation and evaluation at a health system or multicenter level. AI has the potential to process massive amounts of data and continue to iterate and "learn," and we have not yet fully realized this potential. As AI becomes increasingly widespread in healthcare, continued evaluation of outcomes, optimal implementation, and investigations of potential bias are critical to ensure appropriate use of this technology.

References

1. Wolters U, Wolf T, Stützer H, Schröder T. ASA classification and perioperative variables as predictors of postoperative outcome. Br J Anaesth. 1996;77(2):217–22. https://doi.org/10.1093/BJA/77.2.217.
2. Bilimoria KY, Liu Y, Paruch JL, et al. Development and evaluation of the universal ACS NSQIP surgical risk calculator: a decision aid and informed consent tool for patients and surgeons. J Am Coll Surg. 2013;217(5):833. https://doi.org/10.1016/J.JAMCOLLSURG.2013.07.385.
3. Kaafarani HMA, Kongkaewpaisan N, Aicher BO, et al. Prospective validation of the emergency surgery score in emergency general surgery: an eastern Association for the Surgery of trauma multicenter study. J Trauma Acute Care Surg. 2020;89(1):118–24. https://doi.org/10.1097/TA.0000000000002658.
4. Nandan AR, Bohnen JD, Sangji NF, et al. The Emergency Surgery Score (ESS) accurately predicts the occurrence of postoperative complications in emergency surgery patients. J Trauma Acute Care Surg. 2017;83(1):84–9. https://doi.org/10.1097/TA.0000000000001500.
5. El Hechi M, Gebran A, Bouardi HT, et al. Validation of the artificial intelligence–based trauma outcomes predictor (TOP) in patients 65 years and older. Surgery. 2022;171(6):1687–94. https://doi.org/10.1016/J.SURG.2021.11.016.
6. Bertsimas D, Dunn J, Velmahos GC, Kaafarani HMA. Surgical risk is not linear: derivation and validation of a novel, user-friendly, and machine-learning-based Predictive OpTimal Trees in Emergency Surgery Risk (POTTER) calculator. Ann Surg. 2018;268(4):574–83. https://doi.org/10.1097/SLA.0000000000002956.
7. Bertsimas D, Dunn J. Optimal classification trees. Mach Learn. 2017;106(7):1039–82. https://doi.org/10.1007/S10994-017-5633-9.

8. Maurer LR, Bertsimas D, Bouardi HT, et al. Trauma outcome predictor: an artificial intelligence interactive smartphone tool to predict outcomes in trauma patients. J Trauma Acute Care Surg. 2021;91(1):93–9. https://doi.org/10.1097/TA.0000000000003158.
9. Gebran A, Vapsi A, Maurer LR, et al. POTTER-ICU: an artificial intelligence smartphone-accessible tool to predict the need for intensive care after emergency surgery. Surgery. 2022;172(1):470–5. https://doi.org/10.1016/J.SURG.2022.03.023.
10. Bertsimas D, Margonis GA, Tang S, et al. An interpretable AI model for recurrence prediction after surgery in gastrointestinal stromal tumour: an observational cohort study. EClinicalMedicine. 2023;64:102200. https://doi.org/10.1016/j.eclinm.2023.102200.
11. Orfanoudaki A, Giannoutsou A, Hashim S, Bertsimas D, Hagberg RC. Machine learning models for mitral valve replacement: a comparative analysis with the Society of Thoracic Surgeons risk score. J Card Surg. 2022;37(1):18–28. https://doi.org/10.1111/JOCS.16072.
12. Bertsimas D, Masiakos PT, Mylonas KS, Wiberg H. Prediction of cervical spine injury in young pediatric patients: an optimal trees artificial intelligence approach. J Pediatr Surg. 2019;54(11):2353–7. https://doi.org/10.1016/J.JPEDSURG.2019.03.007.
13. Chen B, Sheng W, Wu Z, et al. Machine learning based peri-surgical risk calculator for abdominal related emergency general surgery: a multicenter retrospective study. Int J Surg. Published online March 15, 2024. https://doi.org/10.1097/JS9.0000000000001276.
14. Breiman L. Random forests. Mach Learn. 2001;45(1):5–32. https://doi.org/10.1023/A:1010933404324.
15. Chen T, Guestrin C. XGBoost: a scalable tree boosting system. Proceedings of the ACM SIGKDD international conference on knowledge discovery and data mining. 2016;13–17-August-2016:785–94. https://doi.org/10.1145/2939672.2939785.
16. Rudin C. Stop explaining black box machine learning models for high stakes decisions and use interpretable models instead. Nat Mach Intell. 2019;1(5):206–15. https://doi.org/10.1038/S42256-019-0048-X.
17. Maurer LR, Bertsimas D, Kaafarani HMA. Machine learning reimagined: the promise of interpretability to combat bias. Ann Surg. 2022;275(6):E738–9. https://doi.org/10.1097/SLA.0000000000005396.
18. Maurer LR, Chetlur P, Zhuo D, et al. Validation of the AI-based Predictive OpTimal Trees in Emergency Surgery Risk (POTTER) calculator in patients 65 years and older. Ann Surg. 2023;277(1):E8–E15. https://doi.org/10.1097/SLA.0000000000004714.
19. El Moheb M, Gebran A, Maurer LR, et al. Artificial intelligence versus surgeon gestalt in predicting risk of emergency general surgery. J Trauma Acute Care Surg. 2023;95(4):565–72. https://doi.org/10.1097/TA.0000000000004030.
20. Sacks GD, Dawes AJ, Ettner SL, et al. Impact of a risk calculator on risk perception and surgical decision making: a randomized trial. Ann Surg. 2016;264(6):889–95. https://doi.org/10.1097/SLA.0000000000001750.
21. Perkowitz S. The Bias in the Machine: Facial Recognition Technology and Racial Disparities. MIT Case Studies in Social and Ethical Responsibilities of Computing; 2021. https://doi.org/10.21428/2C646DE5.62272586.
22. Guo LN, Lee MS, Kassamali B, Mita C, Nambudiri VE. Bias in, bias out: underreporting and underrepresentation of diverse skin types in machine learning research for skin cancer detection—a scoping review. J Am Acad Dermatol. 2022;87(1):157–9. https://doi.org/10.1016/j.jaad.2021.06.884.
23. Gebran A, Thakur SS, Maurer LR, et al. Development of a machine learning-based prescriptive tool to address racial disparities in access to care after penetrating trauma. JAMA Surg. 2023;158(10):1088–95. https://doi.org/10.1001/JAMASURG.2023.2293.
24. Park Y, Hu J, Singh M, et al. Comparison of methods to reduce bias from clinical prediction models of postpartum depression. JAMA Netw Open. 2021;4(4):e213909. https://doi.org/10.1001/JAMANETWORKOPEN.2021.3909.

6 AI-Driven Prediction Models, Image Analysis, and Computer-Assisted Diagnosis in Acute Care Surgery

Elisa Reitano, Stefano Piero Bernardo Cioffi, and Stefano Granieri

6.1 Introduction

Artificial intelligence (AI) refers to the development of algorithms that can lead a machine to think, learn, and perform just as a human mind would [1].

Machine learning (ML) represents a subset of AI, which involves training algorithms on large datasets to learn patterns and make predictions or decisions without being explicitly programmed [2].

Computer vision (CV) represents the application of algorithms to analyze and interpret visual data [3].

AI models have enormous potential to improve clinical care across many specialties, including surgery, becoming a fundamental technology to study the intraoperative phase of care with the objectives of augmenting surgeons' decision-making processes, supporting a safer surgery, and expanding access to surgical care [4].

Currently, AI is supporting surgical practice using technological advances in imaging, patient management, and navigation, as well as the development of new technologies [4].

E. Reitano (✉)
Department of General, Digestive, and Endocrine Surgery, University Hospital of Strasbourg, IRCAD France, Strasbourg, France

Institute of Image-Guided Surgery, IHU-Strasbourg, Strasbourg, France
e-mail: elisa.reitano@ircad.fr

S. P. B. Cioffi
General Surgery and Trauma Team, ASST GOM Niguarda, Milano, Milan, Italy

Department of Surgical Sciences, Sapienza University of Rome, Rome, Italy
e-mail: stefanopiero.cioffi@ospedaleniguarda.it

S. Granieri
General Surgery and Trauma Team, ASST GOM Niguarda, Milano, Milan, Italy

B. De Simone et al. (eds.), *New Technologies, Precision Medicine, and AI in Emergency General Surgery*, Hot Topics in Acute Care Surgery and Trauma,
https://doi.org/10.1007/978-3-032-09357-8_6

AI in medicine has evolved dramatically over the past 5 decades, improving diagnostic accuracy, improving efficiency in provider workflow and clinical operations, facilitating better disease and therapeutic monitoring, and improving procedure accuracy and overall patient outcomes.

Nowadays, AI is applied in different branches of medicine and surgery. In neurology, AI can help to predict the progression of Alzheimer's disease by analyzing amyloid imaging data and the responses to drug therapy [5]. In endoscopy, AI can characterize either neoplastic or non-neoplastic polyps or the degree of dysplasia for Barrett's disease [6].

In the last year, different researchers focused on the role of AI in acute care surgery, where the analysis of complex data and rapid decision-making are critical [7, 8]. AI analysis could be a valuable support for healthcare decisions in preoperative, intraoperative, and postoperative periods, potentially leading to reduced morbidity and mortality rates in emergency surgery [3].

Although some authors reported their concern about the complete automation of medical decisions using artificial intelligence, the shift toward computer-guided surgery is inevitable and will modify the surgical approach from before to after surgery.

6.2 Applications of AI in Preoperative Planning

Surgeons make complex, high-stakes decisions under time constraints and uncertainty, with significant effects on patient outcomes. Surgical decision-making is dominated by hypothetical deductive reasoning and individual judgment, education, and resources, which are highly variable [9, 10]. Timely interventions require an early and accurate identification of patients who may benefit from them [11]. Consequently, the use of AI to perform diagnostic decisions in the emergency setting has been the focus of many AI-based studies. Farahmand et al. used the development of a software application to triage patients with abdominal pain referred to the emergency department, which subsequently contributed to potentially reducing the time before surgery [12].

Reismann et al. focused their study on the diagnosis of acute appendicitis using a supervised learning algorithm based on predicting biomarkers, reaching the conclusion that two-thirds of the sample had been prevented from unnecessary anesthesiology and surgery [13].

Other studies recommended the use of AI in acute care surgery for imaging recognition. Cheng PM et al. investigated the use of AI in the diagnosis of small bowel obstruction (SBO), reporting a sensitivity of 91.4% and a specificity of 91.9% [14].

Cheng et al. investigated the performance of ultrasound detection of abdominal free fluid in the hepatorenal fossa, also known as Morison's pouch, after abdominal trauma, using a deep learning algorithm, reporting a model sensitivity of 0.985 and a specificity of 0.913 [14]. The AI system for ultrasound detection of free fluids may be helpful for inexperienced sonographers and paramedics in their interpretation of the Focused Assessment with Sonography for Trauma (FAST) assessment [15].

Although many AI solutions are mainly developed for elective minimally invasive surgery procedures, the imaging analysis may also be critical in emergency settings.

Different studies developed algorithms for the automatic recognition of retained surgical bodies, such as sponges, needles, or misplaced enteric tubes [16].

In a preoperative setting, AI may also be used to create personalized learning experiences for surgical trainees [17]. Simulation-based training aims to recreate the gestures of standard procedures with the AI interface and to decrease the learning curve for a specific procedure [18]. Nowadays, simulation tools are often available on the main robotic platforms. Simulation-based programs are also currently available for endoscopic or laparoscopic procedures, allowing for practice without any risks for patients [19].

In an era in which emergency surgery increasingly takes advantage of new technologies, surgical simulation becomes of paramount importance for training in acute care surgery [7, 19, 20].

Additionally, for educational purposes, AI may also be used to provide remote training for surgical trainees, allowing telemonitoring and democratizing surgery despite geographical considerations [7]. The importance of AI in the acute setting was also underlined by the Artificial Intelligence in Emergency and Trauma Surgery (ARIES) project survey [7], showing that most surgeons believe that AI in emergency surgery can be useful to support perioperative decision-making and to improve surgical vision, surgical practice, training, and education.

6.3 Application of AI in the Operating Room (OR)

Over the last few years, different studies have underlined the increasing role of minimally invasive surgery and new technologies in the field of acute care surgery.

Robotic surgery (RS) was shown to reduce the in-hospital length of stay and improve patient outcomes [21].

Lunardi et al. conducted the first propensity score-matched cohorts for emergency procedures, showing that RS had a lower risk of conversion to open surgery than laparoscopy and was associated with an expedited postoperative course [22]. RS in emergency settings may only be applied in selected clinically stable patients [23]. In addition, RS is highly dependent on the surgeon's experience and should only be performed in an appropriately equipped operating room with trained nursing staff [23]. The greater limitation to the use of RS in emergency settings seems to be the availability of the robotic platforms, as well as the presence of an equipped staff in emergency situations [23].

AI can help the surgeons to recognize the anatomy, to automatically assess anatomical structures, and to obtain the critical view of safety (CVS) [24]. Automatic anatomical recognition increases patient safety, and it could be useful in educational settings, especially in the first part of the learning curve [25]. For educational purposes, Jin et al. showed that automatically inferred information about tool use patterns, range of motion, and cost effectiveness correlated with the performance assessed by surgeons using validated evaluation metrics [26]. Lavanchy et al. proposed a regression model to predict surgical skills and to distinguish good versus poor technical performance [27].

The real-time workflow analysis could be used to improve communication, situational awareness, and the readiness of the entire surgical team [28].

Analysis of surgical videos, detection models, and algorithms to estimate the remaining surgical time can help to track the progress of the operation and assist operating room staff and anesthesia in planning the current and next case [28].

6.4 Postoperative Care and Monitoring with AI

6.4.1 Predictive Analytics for Postoperative Complications

Recent research studies have extensively explored the use of AI in predictive analytics for postoperative complications in acute care surgery. AI algorithms, such as the Predictive Optimal Trees in Emergency Surgery Risk (POTTER) calculator, have demonstrated excellent performance in predicting postoperative complications and mortality among emergency surgery patients. Studies have reported a high accuracy in predicting outcomes such as mortality, morbidity, and specific complications, with area under the receiver operating characteristic curve (AUROC) values ranging from 0.77 to 0.93 [29–33].

The MySurgeryRisk AI system, using automated electronic health record (EHR) data inputs and machine learning algorithms, has shown stable predictive performance in forecasting postoperative complications. This system provides automated outputs directly to the mobile devices of surgeons, matching the predictive accuracy of the surgeons themselves [29]. AI algorithms such as XGBoost, random forest, and neural networks have proven effective in analyzing large datasets, identifying patterns, and making accurate predictions about patient outcomes. This reduces surgical errors and postoperative complications [34].

The feasibility of providing automated outputs directly to surgeons' mobile devices has been demonstrated, enhancing real-time predictions and clinical workflows [33]. The role of AI in predictive analytics for postoperative complications in acute care surgery showed a significant potential for improving prediction accuracy, resource utilization, and patient outcomes. However, challenges such as data access, privacy concerns, and ethical considerations must be addressed, and the performance of AI algorithms should be rigorously evaluated using key metrics such as AUROC values and precision.

6.4.2 Remote Patient Monitoring and Telemedicine

AI has the potential to significantly impact all phases of perioperative care, including accurate risk prediction, operating room organization, and perioperative decision-making, leading to increased cost-effective care quality and better outcomes [3]. AI may enhance patient safety and satisfaction while reducing rising healthcare costs, particularly in postoperative care through telemedicine and remote patient monitoring [35]. The use of AI in telemedicine can provide advanced methods of coordination, improve patient outcomes through patient monitoring, and aid in early prevention and detection, ultimately enhancing patient safety and satisfaction [36].

Challenges associated with implementing AI in telemedicine include technical adaptation, loss of managerial control, data privacy, and accountability [37]. Ethical considerations such as algorithmic bias, lack of transparency, data privacy issues, and the potential for AI to deskill healthcare professionals and erode humanistic values in patient care are also crucial challenges to address [38]. AI may assist physicians in decision-making strategies, improve healthcare delivery, and automate administrative tasks, ultimately enhancing the efficiency and accuracy of telemedicine in acute care surgery [38].

The use of AI in remote patient monitoring and telemedicine in acute care surgery bears great promise in improving patient outcomes, enhancing healthcare delivery, and addressing various challenges. However, ethical considerations and implementation challenges need to be carefully addressed to ensure the successful integration of AI in acute care surgery.

6.4.3 Personalized Follow-Up Care

The use of AI to implement follow-up care in patients with acute traumatic and non-traumatic surgical diseases poses unique challenges based on ethical considerations. These include the reliability of robotic and AI systems, respect for privacy and sensitive data, transparency and uncertainties in AI, fairness, and the potential for exacerbating inequalities in access to healthcare [25].

Other ethical concerns involve algorithmic bias, lack of transparency, data privacy issues, and the potential for AI to deskill healthcare professionals and erode humanistic values in patient care [39].

AI can ensure the early identification of patients at a higher risk of developing postoperative complications, thereby personalizing postoperative follow-up care. Computer vision (CV) and artificial intelligence (AI) are emerging as key players in transforming patient care, with the potential to enhance surgical procedures, increase accuracy and safety, and enable real-time patient data and proactive interventions [40]. AI and computer vision may be used to intraoperatively support the identification of instruments, anatomical structures, or activities in real time and to postoperatively support the analysis and understanding of surgical processes [3].

AI and machine learning (ML) techniques may facilitate shared decision-making and improve patient outcomes by accurately predicting patient-reported outcomes (PROs) following surgery [39]. AI technologies may aid in preoperative patient risk stratification, intraoperative anesthesia maintenance, and prevention of postoperative complications, thereby enhancing patient safety and improving health outcomes [41].

AI-assisted follow-up conversational agents have been developed to simulate a human voice and select appropriate follow-up times for patient follow-up, showing potential cost effectiveness and comprehensive feedback collection [42]. Key AI-based tools to enhance postoperative follow-up in surgical patients include telemedicine, remote patient monitoring, computer vision, AI and ML techniques for predicting patients' reporting outcomes (PROs), and AI-assisted follow-up conversational agents. Such technologies have the potential to improve patient safety, satisfaction, and outcomes while reducing healthcare costs. However, it is crucial to address challenges and limitations, such as ethical use, potential biases in AI algorithms, and resistance from medical professionals and patients [39, 40, 42].

6.5 Future Direction and Challenges

6.5.1 Advances in AI Technologies

AI has gained a pivotal role in the field of intraoperative imaging. The integration of AI algorithms in the Picture Archiving and Communication System (PACS), mainly based on deep learning (DL) models, allowed a clearer and facilitated visualization of anatomical structures and pathological entities during surgery.

The AI-driven generation of three-dimensional (3D) models that could be exploited to better understand the anatomy and the spatial relationship between a pathologic entity and neighboring structures represents another major progress. A growing body of evidence has highlighted how such 3D models may be helpful in the preoperative planning of complex hepatobiliary resections with vascular involvement [43–46].

A further evolution of this concept is represented by real-time image segmentation and augmentation. The possibility to promptly generate images and models, which can be used intraoperatively to give the surgeon supplementary information (such as the demarcation of safe surgical margins), assumes a critical role, especially in emergency procedures. In this context, the combination of hyperspectral imaging (HSI) and machine learning (ML) has been recently proposed to identify characteristic tissue signatures, enabling automatic tissue recognition intraoperatively. In the EX-MACHYNA prospective trial, RGB images obtained through hyperspectral gathering were annotated with different organ labels, and data were analyzed using convolutional neural networks (CNNs). The results of the study underlined that in vivo, real time, anatomical tissue recognition using HSI and deep learning (DL) is feasible. However, model performances are heavily dependent upon the source of data, and the generalization of results remains to be demonstrated [47].

Another example is provided by the so-called phase recognition. Automating the identification of a specific step or phase of a surgical procedure may offer the potential to reduce operative errors, maximizing surgical training [48]. Such applications are even more evident in minimally invasive and robotic surgery. The possibility of real-time overlaying AI-generated 3D images and dynamic models onto the surgical field of view can contribute to minimizing surgical trauma and boosting the recovery process [49–51].

6.5.2 Integration with Electronic Health Records and Healthcare Systems

AI is revolutionizing the healthcare landscape by seamlessly merging with electronic health records (EHR) and broader healthcare systems. This integration enhances the capacity to collect, organize, and interpret vast amounts of patient data, ultimately driving better clinical outcomes. By integrating such vast and intricate datasets, AI facilitates a more holistic view of patient health, improving the accuracy of surgical planning and outcomes. The integration of AI with EHRs and healthcare systems also streamlines workflow efficiency and reduces administrative burdens. For instance, automated data entry minimizes the risk of human error and frees up healthcare professionals to focus more on patient care [1]. Additionally, AI may facilitate continuous learning and improvement within surgical teams by analyzing outcomes and providing feedback on performance. This iterative process fosters a culture of excellence and innovation, where surgical practices are constantly refined based on the latest data-driven insights.

6.5.3 Addressing Barriers to Adoption and Implementation

Despite the advances in AI development systems, several issues still need to be overcome.

The non-negligible costs required to guarantee and maintain the widespread use of such technology are way too high to be affordable on a large scale.

As the artificial intelligence in emergency and trauma surgery (ARIES) survey pointed out, the limited availability and accessibility of high-technology tools merged with AI in the emergency and trauma surgery setting contribute to hindering its diffusion [7].

A huge amount of input data is necessary to develop and validate machine learning models. However, even in large datasets, elements such as the representativeness of the included populations, missing data, and outliers may impact generalizability across subgroups. In this context, the quality and the reliability of medical information are of the utmost importance. To overcome such an issue, it is critical to regularly update and upload new data to the algorithms in order to produce appropriate responses.

Despite all such efforts, some AI algorithms may "misinterpret" input data, providing forecasts without an actual cause-and-effect relationship [36]. This concept underscores the need for external supervision by healthcare professionals, along with AI experts, to verify the validity of AI algorithm outputs and their applicability.

Further drawbacks arise from the security of data storage. As already mentioned, AI systems often require access to large datasets to function effectively. In healthcare, this involves sensitive patient information, which must be protected to comply with privacy regulations such as the Health Insurance Portability and Accountability Act (HIPAA) in the United States or the General Data Protection Regulation (GDPR) in Europe. Ensuring that data is anonymized or encrypted before it is used by AI systems is essential to prevent unauthorized access and potential data breaches. In this context, implementing robust cybersecurity measures, such as advanced encryption methods, multi-factor authentication, and regular security audits, is crucial to protect data storage systems from attacks [50].

The diffusion of AI in healthcare has also led to ethical concerns. For instance, in the case of biased data, the AI algorithm's prediction will also be biased. This can lead to unfair treatment of certain groups of people. Ensuring that training datasets are representative and implementing algorithms to detect and mitigate bias are necessary steps to promote fairness. AI systems, especially those based on complex neural networks, can often be "black boxes" in which the decision-making process is not transparent. It is essential to develop AI systems that can provide explanations for the decisions made, which is key to building trust and accountability. In addition, individuals should have control over their personal data and over the ways such data is used by AI systems. Obtaining informed consent before collecting and using personal data is an ethical imperative [52, 53].

Balancing the benefits of AI innovation with the need for security and ethical responsibility is a complex yet essential task. Ensuring that AI systems are designed, developed, and deployed with security and ethical considerations in mind will help to maximize their positive impact while minimizing potential risks and harms. This requires collaboration between technologists, ethicists, policymakers, and the general public to create frameworks and guidelines that support responsible AI development and use.

References

1. Hashimoto DA, Rosman G, Rus D, Meireles OR. Artificial intelligence in surgery: promises and perils. Ann Surg. 2018;268(1):70–6.
2. Satapathy P, Pradhan KB, Rustagi S, Suresh V, Al-Qaim ZH, Padhi BK, et al. Application of machine learning in surgery research: current uses and future directions-editorial. Int J Surg. 2023;109:1550–1.
3. Mascagni P, Alapatt D, Sestini L, Altieri MS, Madani A, Watanabe Y, et al. Computer vision in surgery: from potential to clinical value. Npj Digit Med. 2022;5:1–9.
4. Kitaguchi D, Takeshita N, Hasegawa H, Ito M. Artificial intelligence-based computer vision in surgery: recent advances and future perspectives. Ann Gastroenterol Surg. 2022;6:29–36.
5. Dabbaghi KG, Khosravirad Z, Jamalnia S, GhorbaniNia R, Mahmoudikohani F, Zakeri H, et al. The use of artificial intelligence in the management ofNeurodegenerative disorders; focus on Alzheimer's disease. Galen Med J. 2023;12:1.
6. Tsai MC, Yen HH, Tsai HY, Huang YK, Luo YS, Kornelius E, et al. Artificial intelligence system for the detection of Barrett's esophagus. World J Gastroenterol. 2023;29:6198–207.

7. De Simone B, Chouillard E, Gumbs AA, Loftus TJ, Kaafarani H, Catena F. Artificial intelligence in surgery: the emergency surgeon's perspective (the ARIES project). Discov Heal Syst. 2022;1(1):9.
8. Cheng K, Li Z, Guo Q, Sun Z, Wu H, Li C. Emergency surgery in the era of artificial intelligence: ChatGPT could be the doctor's right-hand man. Int J Surg. 2023;109(6):1816–8.
9. Carenzo L, Mercalli C, Reitano E, Tartaglione M, Ceolin M, Cimbanassi S, et al. State of the art of trauma teams in Italy: a nationwide study. Injury. 2024 May;55(5):111388.
10. Cobianchi L, Dal Mas F, Agnoletti V, Ansaloni L, Biffl W, Butturini G, et al. Team dynamics study group. Time for a paradigm shift in shared decision-making in trauma and emergency surgery? Results from an international survey. World J Emerg Surg. 2023;18(1):14.
11. Reitano E, Bini R, Difino M, Chiara O, Cimbanassi S. Nine year in-hospital mortality trends in a high-flow level one trauma center in Italy. Updates Surg. 2022;74:1445–51.
12. Farahmand S, Shabestari O, Pakrah M, Hossein-Nejad H, Arbab M, Bagheri-Hariri S. Artificial intelligence-based triage for patients with acute abdominal pain in emergency department; a diagnostic accuracy study. Adv J Emerg Med. 2017;1:5.
13. Reismann J, Romualdi A, Kiss N, Minderjahn MI, Kallarackal J, Schadid M, et al. Diagnosis and classification of pediatric acute appendicitis by artificial intelligence methods: an investigator-independent approach. PLoS One. 2019;14(9):e0222030.
14. Yang Y, Li Y-X, Yao R-Q, Du X-H, Ren C. Artificial intelligence in small intestinal diseases: application and prospects conflict-of-interest statement: open-access. World J Gastroenterol. 2021;27:3734–47.
15. Cheng CY, Chiu IM, Hsu MY, Pan HY, Tsai CM, Lin CHR. Deep learning assisted detection of abdominal free fluid in Morison's pouch during focused assessment with sonography in trauma. Front Med. 2021;8:1–7.
16. Eibschutz L, Lu MY, Abbassi MT, Gholamrezanezhad A. Artificial intelligence in the detection of non-biological materials. Emerg Radiol. 2024;31:391–403.
17. Khan R, Plahouras J, Johnston BC, Scaffidi MA, Grover SC, Walsh CM. Virtual reality simulation training in endoscopy: a Cochrane review and meta-analysis. Endoscopy. 2019;51:653–64.
18. Satapathy P, Hermis AH, Rustagi S, Pradhan KB, Padhi BK, Sah R. Artificial intelligence in surgical education and training: opportunities, challenges, and ethical considerations-correspondence. Int J Surg. 2023;109:1543–4.
19. Kleebayoon A, Wiwanitkit V. Artificial intelligence in surgical education. Cleft Palate Craniofac J. 2023:86–97.
20. Reitano E, Famularo S, Dallemagne B, Mishima K, Perretta S, Riva P, et al. Educational scoring system in laparoscopic cholecystectomy: is it the right time to standardize? Medicina (Kaunas). 2023;59(3):446.
21. Fairag M, Almahdi RH, Siddiqi AA, Alharthi FK, Alqurashi BS, Alzahrani NG, et al. Robotic revolution in surgery: diverse applications across specialties and future prospects review article. Cureus. 2024;16:1–10.
22. Lunardi N, Abou-Zamzam A, Florecki KL, Chidambaram S, Shih IF, Kent AJ, et al. Robotic Technology in Emergency General Surgery Cases in the era of minimally invasive surgery. JAMA Surg. 2024;159:493–9.
23. de'Angelis N, Khan J, Marchegiani F, Bianchi G, Aisoni F, Alberti D, et al. Robotic surgery in emergency setting: 2021 WSES position paper. World J Emerg Surg. 2022;17:1–12.
24. Mascagni P, Fiorillo C, Urade T, Emre T, Yu T, Wakabayashi T, et al. Formalizing video documentation of the critical view of safety in laparoscopic cholecystectomy: a step towards artificial intelligence assistance to improve surgical safety. Surg Endosc. 2019;34:2709–14.
25. Ward TM, Mascagni P, Madani A, Padoy N, Perretta S, Hashimoto DA. Surgical data science and artificial intelligence for surgical education. J Surg Oncol. 2021;124:221–30.
26. Jin A, Yeung S, Jopling J, Krause J, Azagury D, Milstein A, et al. Tool detection and operative skill assessment in surgical videos using region-based convolutional neural networks. Proc – 2018 IEEE Winter Conf Appl Comput Vision, WACV 2018. 2018;691–9.

27. Lavanchy JL, Zindel J, Kirtac K, Twick I, Hosgor E, Candinas D, et al. Automation of surgical skill assessment using a three-stage machine learning algorithm. Sci Rep. 2021;11(1):8933.
28. Twinanda AP, Yengera G, Mutter D, Marescaux J, Padoy N. RSDNet: learning to predict remaining surgery duration from laparoscopic videos without manual annotations. IEEE Trans Med Imaging. 2019;38:1069–78.
29. Stam WT, Goedknegt LK, Ingwersen EW, Schoonmade LJ, Bruns ERJ, Daams F. The prediction of surgical complications using artificial intelligence in patients undergoing major abdominal surgery: a systematic review. Surg (United States). 2022;171:1014–21.
30. El Hechi MW, Maurer LR, Levine J, Zhuo D, El Moheb M, Velmahos GC, et al. Validation of the artificial intelligence-based predictive optimal trees in emergency surgery risk (POTTER) calculator in emergency general surgery and emergency laparotomy patients. J Am Coll Surg 2021;232:912–919.e1.
31. Junior MAFR, Smaniotto R, Gebran A, Zamudio JP, Mohseni S, da Silva Rodrigues JM, et al. The use of POTTER (predictive optimal trees in emergency surgery risk) calculator to predict mortality and complications in patients submitted to emergency surgery. Rev Col Bras Cir. 2023;50:e20233624.
32. Gebran A, Vapsi A, Maurer LR, El Moheb M, Naar L, Thakur SS, et al. POTTER-ICU: an artificial intelligence smartphone-accessible tool to predict the need for intensive care after emergency surgery. Surg (United States). 2022;172:470–5.
33. Hassan AM, Rajesh A, Asaad M, Nelson JA, Coert JH, Mehrara BJ, et al. Artificial intelligence and machine learning in prediction of surgical complications: current state, applications, and implications. Am Surg. 2023;89:25.
34. Loftus TJ, Altieri MS, Balch JA, Abbott KL, Choi J, Marwaha JS, et al. Artificial intelligence-enabled decision support in surgery: state-of-the-art and future directions. Ann Surg. 2023;278:51–8.
35. Sonawane A, Shah S, Pote S, He M. The application of artificial intelligence: perceptions from healthcare professionals. Health Technol (Berl). 2023;13:861–7.
36. Elhassan BT, Arabi AA. Ethical forethoughts on the use of artificial intelligence in medicine. Int J Ethics Syst. 2024; https://doi.org/10.1108/IJOES-08-2023-0190.
37. Meskó B, Görög M. A short guide for medical professionals in the era of artificial intelligence. Npj Digit Med. 2020:3.
38. Sharma S, Rawal R, Shah D. Addressing the challenges of AI-based telemedicine: best practices and lessons learned. J Educ Health Promot. 2023:12.
39. Chadebecq F, Vasconcelos F, Mazomenos E, Stoyanov D. Computer vision in the surgical operating room. Visc Med. 2020;36:456.
40. Hassan AM, Biaggi-Ondina A, Rajesh A, Asaad M, Nelson JA, Coert JH, et al. Predicting patient-reported outcomes following surgery using machine learning. Am Surg. 2023;89:31–5.
41. Bian Y, Xiang Y, Tong B, Feng B, Weng X. Artificial intelligence–assisted system in postoperative follow-up of orthopedic patients: exploratory quantitative and qualitative study. J Med Internet Res. 2020:22.
42. Shafik W, Hidayatullah AF, Kalinaki K, Aslam MM. Artificial intelligence (AI)-assisted computer vision (CV) in healthcare systems. Comput Vis AI-Integrated IoT Technol Med Ecosyst 2024:17–36.
43. Famularo S, Bannone E, Collins T, Reitano E, Okamoto N, Mishima K, et al. Partial hepatic vein occlusion and venous congestion in liver exploration using a hyperspectral camera: a proposal for monitoring intraoperative liver perfusion. Cancers (Basel). 2023;15:1–14.
44. Ruzzenente A, Alaimo L, Conci S, De Bellis M, Marchese A, Ciangherotti A, et al. Hyper accuracy three-dimensional (HA3D™) technology for planning complex liver resections: a preliminary single center experience. Updat Surg. 2023;75:105.
45. Cotsoglou C, Granieri S, Bassetto S, Bagnardi V, Pugliese R, Grazi GL, et al. Dynamic surgical anatomy using 3D reconstruction technology in complex hepato-biliary surgery with vascular involvement. Results from an international multicentric survey. HPB (Oxford). 2024 Jan;26(1):83–90.

46. Granieri S, Bassetto S, Bonomi A, Germini A, Bruno F, Chierici A, et al. Three-dimensional reconstruction technology in the preoperative workup of complex hepatic resections. Our experience on 11 consecutive cases. Updat Surg. 2024;76:2221.
47. Bannone E, Collins T, Esposito A, Cinelli L, De Pastena M, Pessaux P, et al. Surgical optomics: hyperspectral imaging and deep learning towards precision intraoperative automatic tissue recognition—results from the EX-MACHYNA trial. Surg Endosc. 2024:1–15.
48. Garrow CR, Kowalewski KF, Li L, Wagner M, Schmidt MW, Engelhardt S, et al. Machine learning for surgical phase recognition: a systematic review. Ann Surg. 2021;273:684–93.
49. Mascagni P, Alapatt D, Urade T, Vardazaryan A, Mutter D, Marescaux J, et al. A computer vision platform to automatically locate critical events in surgical videos: documenting safety in laparoscopic cholecystectomy. Ann Surg. 2021;274:E93–5.
50. Kitaguchi D, Takeshita N, Matsuzaki H, Oda T, Watanabe M, Mori K, et al. Automated laparoscopic colorectal surgery workflow recognition using artificial intelligence: experimental research. Int J Surg. 2020;79:88–94.
51. Hashimoto DA, Rosman G, Witkowski ER, Stafford C, Navarette-Welton AJ, Rattner DW, et al. Computer vision analysis of intraoperative video: automated recognition of operative steps in laparoscopic sleeve gastrectomy. Ann Surg. 2019;270:414–21.
52. Kruse CS, Frederick B, Jacobson T, Kyle D. Cybersecurity in healthcare: a systematic review of modern threats and trends. Technol Heal Care. 2017;25:1–10.
53. Mittelstadt BD, Allo P, Taddeo M, Wachter S, Floridi L. The ethics of algorithms: Mapping the debate. Big Data Soc. 2016:3.

7 Artificial Intelligent Assistants in Support of Trauma Surgery

Juan Wachs, Yupeng Zhuo, and Andrew W. Kirkpatrick

7.1 Introduction

In-person training is the classic educational method of learning surgical and resuscitative techniques, and has been shown to be an effective method of such. Traditionally acquiring these complex psychomotor surgical skills and especially the background knowledge regarding when and how to perform these skills has taken many years of intense apprenticeship in a Residency Training Program. To augment and refresh such formal training, shorter condensed hand-on courses have also been developed such as the Advanced Trauma Life Support Course (ATLS), The Advanced Surgical Skills for Exposure in Trauma (ASSET) [1], and the Definitive Surgical Trauma Care course (DSTC), among many other courses have improved outcomes in the management of polytrauma patients [2]. Such courses typically are based on one or two (students)-to-one (faculty) mentoring model [3] where an expert teaches and challenges learners to perform complex procedures such as thoracostomies, tracheostomies, and fasciotomies on cadavers and simulators.

J. Wachs (✉)
Industrial Engineering, Purdue University, West Lafayette, IN, USA

School of Medicine, Indiana University, Indianapolis, IN, USA
e-mail: jpwachs@purdue.edu

Y. Zhuo
Industrial Engineering, Purdue University, West Lafayette, IN, USA

A. W. Kirkpatrick
Trauma Services, Calgary, AB, Canada

Telementord Ultrasound Supported Medical Interventions (TMUSMI) Research Group, Calgary, AB, Canada

University of Calgary, Calgary, AB, Canada

B. De Simone et al. (eds.), *New Technologies, Precision Medicine, and AI in Emergency General Surgery*, Hot Topics in Acute Care Surgery and Trauma,
https://doi.org/10.1007/978-3-032-09357-8_7

While such courses are becoming part of the surgical training curricula as well as in maintenance of competence programs, in-person training is often not possible because trauma procedures require immediate readiness, and the experts may not be physically available when required [4]. In addition, for most community surgeons, it is impossible or undesirable to leave their surgical practices to complete training due to their continual need to provide care to their communities [5]. Instead, knowledge must come from another method that still allows for "hands-on" training but avoids long travel and absences for those surgeons from their current practices.

Remote instruction has been proposed as a possible solution to this problem [6], and yet telemedicine is not yet "out there" and commonly accessible at many rural hospitals. Infrastructure constraints due to austere conditions (e.g., poor telecommunications, lacking infrastructure, uncontrolled remote environments, and other "stressors") are significant barriers to the introduction of this technology in the civilian domain. In the military domain, while telemedicine has tremendous theoretical appeal in far forward and especially prolonged field care situations [7], military drone technology has rapidly rewritten the rules of modern conflict, and the use of a telemedical technique may allow electronic targeting of the user. The term Disconnected, Denied, Intermittent, and/or with Limited bandwidth (DDIL) environment has been used to describe contested spaces where communications are contested, denied, or precluded to secrecy requirements [8]. As discussed further in our accompanying chapter in this textbook, the term still applies to many non-military situations where communications are not available, such as during disasters when communication failures may be expected, or simply when a suitable remote mentor is unavailable [9].

Artificial intelligence-based solutions (AIBS) hold the promise to be completely autonomous and self-contained [10], and thus we believe AIBS may hold great promise in disconnected environments anywhere on earth, as well as above the earth in long-duration space exploration [11, 12]. Therefore, AIBS could be deployed in resource-limited environments even when network connectivity is unavailable. From the pedagogical perspective, the Joint Program Committee-1 (JPC-1) Medical Simulation and Information Sciences Research Program (MSISRP) and the Office of Naval Research (ONR) invested in skills decay research, providing the foundation for future research efforts to explore augmented reality (AR) medical simulation training interfaces [13, 14]. AR-based learning technologies focused on the learner can allow for the performance of routine and complex skills where virtual instruments can be mapped to and projected over a mannequin and/or human [15]. Consequently, AR systems can be leveraged to provide real-time, embedded feedback via the on-board computer vision systems of the AR hardware, haptics, and the actual visual environment [16]. The computer vision component is necessary in such cases in order to produce models from images which can allow for the understanding of fundamental concepts captured by the images, such as anatomical structures. Such models generated are then used to provide feedback mechanisms to provide the learner with positive or negative feedback [17]. These AR-based learning capabilities can have straightforward applications in airway management skills, such as cricothyroidotomy and endotracheal intubation, and hemorrhage control involving such advanced concepts as resuscitative endovascular balloon occlusion of the aorta placement [18], to name a few. Therefore, these procedural applications often are seen as near-term targets for experimentation with AI, with copilots and virtual assistants with AR support for display of instructions when telemedicine support is not available. While AI assistance can offer support for prehospital care providers (civilian and military), students and residents in training are an important goal, moving these capabilities to the austere setting and rural regions would require major developments [19].

Thus, there is a necessary focus on providing effective prehospital intervention tools and training to support first responders to utilize AI agents closer to point of injury, to allow heroic LSIs where it is so critically needed. In such environments it will also be critical to utilize AI to guide less experienced providers to know not only "how" to perform such an intervention, but "whether" the severity is such that the risks justify the benefits. In addition, there is significant knowledge to be gained from developing AI-based technologies for trainers and mentors. Such knowledge can be key building blocks and support significant improvements in surgical education at all levels, as technological and scientific advances in training and simulation, cognitive models, augmented reality, natural language processing, and human-computer interaction and will easily carryover to mentoring in other knowledge domains (e.g., artificial intelligence [AI] in diagnostic expert systems, equipment maintenance, and navigation vehicles).

7.2 State of the Art and Its Limitations in AI Mentorship and Trainers

Personal assistants, AI copilots, and AR/VR trainers struggle to understand and infer the user needs unless those needs are clearly communicated to them. Market acceptance has been a barrier because "human behavioral" models have been dramatically simplified to the extent that the models are not usable in practical settings (e.g., equipment maintenance, home assistance, delivering first-aid). In these simplifications, the user is a static, unidimensional entity who responds in a predictable manner. Calisto proposed to use AI/AR to assist an operator in a breast image diagnosis task [20]. While Calisto's approach was presented as human-centric AI, it lacks attentional modeling. Research by Shen, Nama, and Jin developed an AI assistant for Eco-Skills through user demonstration and instruction [21]. Differences in skill or style were not considered, however, and only the sequence of actions was relevant. User cognition was recently considered through an augmented reality cognitive assistant for the blind [22]. The assistant can provide navigation assistance while modeling the user's spatial memory, but the model is too generic to be useful. An AR virtual assistant for cooking activities was proposed to help users with cognitive impairments [23]. Physiological and optical sensors were used to assess task state (and not user state) in the kitchen procedural task. Likewise, Miyawaki and Sano [24] proposed a virtual agent using AI/VR for cooking support but without including the user state, style, expertise, or needs. In the self-aware and active-guiding training assistant for intelligent manufacturing [25], the user current state was inferred and used for quantifying and assessing the worker performance with the goal of adapting the guidance style. However, the user model was limited to only user intent. Similar approaches [26] have been adopted to develop AR instructional systems for mechanical assembly, where the user intention determines the type of assistance.

In the field of medicine, AI-MEDIC [27–30] proposed to support a special operations medic with lifesaving skills. While multiple sources of knowledge have been included for task guidance, AI-MEDIC had no implicit user modeling to adapt the user's guidance. Recent work using AI copilots has shown significant assistance and impact in diagnostic reasoning [31], yet there is no action recognition integrated as part of that system. To summarize, state-of-the-art personal assistants, copilots, and AR/VR AI trainers have the following limitations:

1. *Lack of mutual grounding*: People use different modal perceptual representations to understand and manipulate the environment. While such metaphors require mutual grounding between the user perception and the agent, current agents rely on unimodal representations of the actions, objects, and tasks that do not align well with abstractions that people commonly use.
2. *Poor knowledge transfer*: Most agents rely on curated datasets with the knowledge sources expressed through visual, text, and acoustic forms. While parsing between knowledge sources into different modalities is not a trivial problem, without a mentor, it is not clear in what form (including metaphors) the necessary instructions should be presented to the user.
3. *Attention models*: Most AI agents aim to maximize situational awareness by adding more camera and sensors and increasing bandwidth and big data computing capabilities. Yet, humans are very effective at decision-making based on only salient factors that go beyond object recognition and link to user intention and goals and how physiological vision and hearing work.
4. *Emotion and state*: When guiding a medic during a lifesaving procedure, experts often provide reassurance and a sense of companionship that reduce stressors effecting cognitive load and, therefore, task performance. To mimic mentor support that modulates according to operator stress level, confusion, and decisiveness, some AI/VR agents collect physiological signals from highly intrusive wearable sensors but do not assess user state through gestures, pose, and proxemics.

7.3 Requirements and Needs in Surgical AI Copilots, Mentorship, and Trainers

AI mentors, copilots, and assistants could potentially surpass the current state of the art in telementoring by "amplifying" individual performer capabilities to address new tasks without the associated learning curve, costs, time, and reallocation. The expectation is that systems such as *CoPiSMs* will bridge the perception, reasoning, and action gaps by taking an egocentric approach of sensemaking and instruction. User models could innovatively address the four challenges of *perceptual grounding, perceptual attention, knowledge transfer, and user modeling* (a meta-model):

Perceptual grounding innovation will draw on the role of commonsense and intuition in how people solve problems [32]. New techniques can generate *multitask graphs with multiple levels* (Fig. 7.1) to adapt to user proficiency levels and find alternative pathways to solutions [33]. A user can be "rewarded" by finding effective solutions instead of being forced to follow one single sequence of actions. Such a *user-focused* approach allows alterations from the documented source, as seen, for example, in the creative and divergent thinking as well as protocol following of Captain Chesley "Sully" Sullenberger in his emergency landing of U.S. Airways Flight 1549 onto the Hudson River [34]. AI mentors will have the ability to adapt procedural knowledge to parallel and potentially ambiguous sources to discover new solutions.

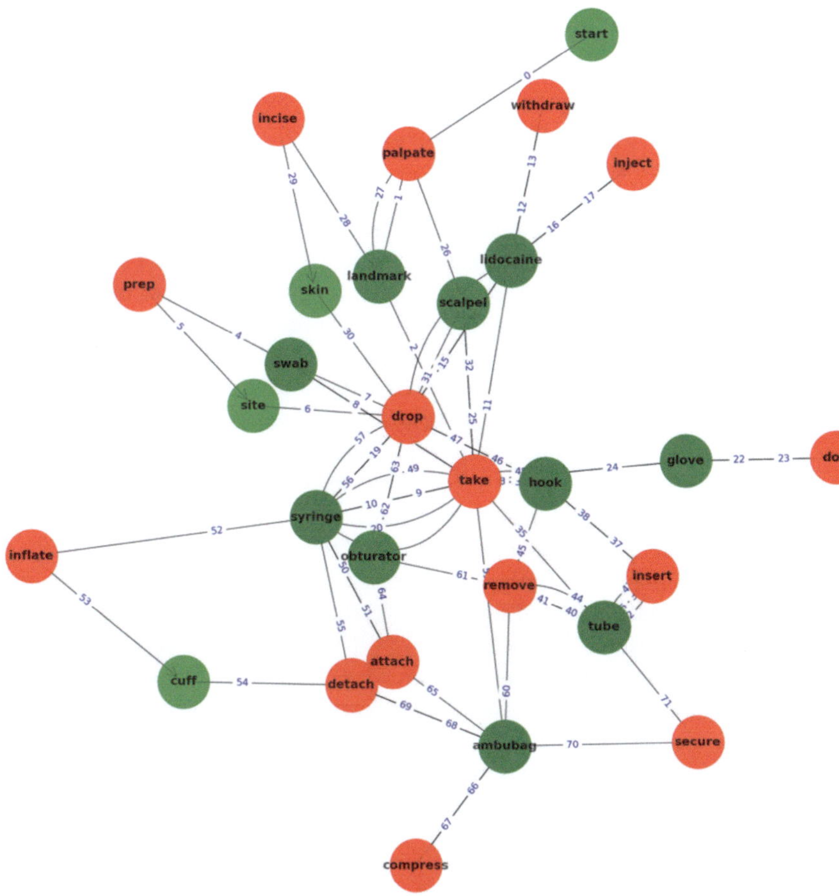

Fig. 7.1 Multitask graph of a cricothyrotomy procedure

Attention modeling innovation varies from traditional attentional techniques that model either the top-down or bottom-up and instead combines both in a biomimetic approach. Attentional models gained interest during the surge of deep convolutional neural networks (DCNN) [35] as a mechanism to understand what makes artificial neural networks "see" differences in massive datasets of objects and activities. This type of *saliency* is referred as bottom-up [36], pushed by characteristics of the objects regardless of what the user makes of them. Top-down is the attention motivated by users' personal goals and intentions. The human motor system is a formidable proxy for top-down attention as human gaze and gestures both indicate intent [37]. A key component of AI assistance is the proper selection of events and objects through a combination of bottom-up and top-down mechanisms that engage the sensorimotor aspects of user behavior. Hand maneuvers and gaze direction are predictors of hotspots of attention. *Contextual saliency through relevancy* is based on the role of the object/action in the task context. This unique approach on selective attention may offload unnecessary items from short-term memory and thus reduce the cognitive load. The importance of cognitive load and the capacity of humans to function in catastrophic situations is a poorly studied area, but one with immense implications for the psychological health of first responders [38]. Telemedicine, AI, AR, and decision support may be one tool to protect the psychological health of first responders but much more research is required [38].

Knowledge transfer innovation addresses the system underperformance due to sample selection bias [39] when adapting learned models of procedural instruction to new domains [40] in what becomes a "domain gap" problem [41, 42]. While current adaptation, at best, deals with sensor acquisition, passing of time [43], location change (new environments), and short-term and long-term temporal offsets [44], future algorithms could *simultaneously learn objects, actions, and tasks* using data augmentation with minimum retraining using different representations. Optical transformations and semantic representations will go well beyond the traditional paradigm of image-text mapping to address *a compound domain gap* [45]. With very little data of the new domain (few shots, one or even zero shot) and in real-time, one generalizes a model to a new hyperspace [46]. Likewise, additional domain variance from neighbor semantics using free text forms linked to ontologies, such as ConceptNet, can be incorporated [47].

User modeling innovation further addresses the domain gap by focusing on user changes during the task [48] and involves awareness of the user state in terms of proficiency, style, attention, and preferences [49]. Our egocentric approach for the first time *integrates usability studies* to learn what "cannot" be learned in an unsupervised manner. For example, instead of re-learning and re-annotating all task-completion observations in the EPIC Kitchen [50] or TA2 dataset [51], micro-studies need to be conducted that can be propagated and scaled up based on key features detected through user-dialogue timing of the interaction.

AI Copilots The use of AI-powered applications to support surgeons [52], first responders, and medics is a viable direction for future development [53]. Simplistically, we consider this paradigm the provision to a less experienced care provider of an extremely capable assistant who can navigate, communicate, and even actually "fly the plane" if the first responder is overwhelmed or uncomfortable. Copilots are applications developed using AI-based algorithms which display human-like traits and are designed to work alongside individuals, providing personalized support and guidance, in order to achieve a cognitive task [54]. The straightforward application is the use for content generation, question answering, and documentation [55]. Fundamentally, the main aspects of generating, understanding, and responding to natural verbal and written language, are basic reuquirements in AI copilots. In addition, AI copilots can be used to personalize treatment and to diagnose faster and more accurately between different conditions that could be difficult for the bare human eye to see and understand. Furthermore, with the advent of self-driving labs (SDL) [56], it is not difficult to envision copilots than could design a battery of clinical tests, run the tests through automation, conduct the data analysis, and ultimately deliver the most likely diagnosis with best potential treatments.

7.4 Lessons from the Trauma THOMPSON Challenge

In order to assess the potential of using AI for supporting frontline healthcare providers, the Trauma THOMPSON Challenge (Fig. 7.2) was recently conducted. This was a research competition at the 26th International Conference on Medical Image Computing and Computer-Assisted Intervention, MICCAI 2023, held in Vancouver, Canada, in October 2023. The goal of the challenge was to submit machine learning algorithms capable of recognizing first responders' surgical activities and anticipate events in uncontrolled and unscripted settings [57]. The end goal of creating such algorithms was to allow their use in real-time, to provide autonomous medical instructions to untrained individuals performing life-saving procedures in austere environments. Such settings include infrastructures with poor network connectivity and limited resources, as might be expected on a remote battlefield or remote resource-limited setting. The challenge provided a diverse dataset of first-person view video footage of medics and surgeons conducting LSIs such as tourniquet application, needle thoracostomy, and cricothyroidotomy [58, 59]. In these initial studies, the recognition accuracies for the best performers were all well below 25%.

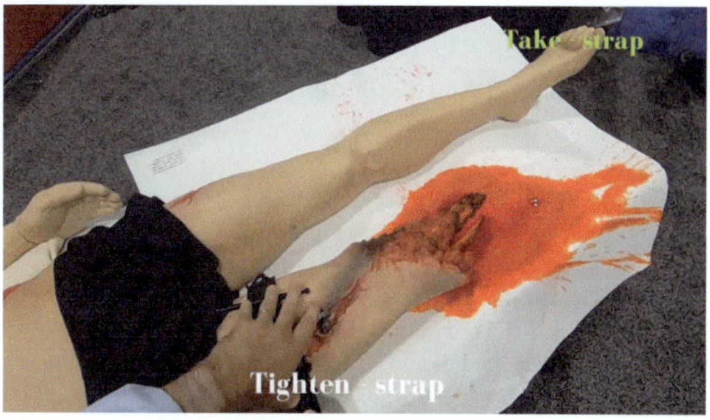

Fig. 7.2 Action recognition (green caption) and action anticipation (white caption) on the Trauma THOMPSON dataset

Therefore these results are strong indicators that, in spite of the progress in AI and machine learning, it is difficult to generalize surgical activities in new environments, especially when there is no prior information about the number and type of procedures to be recognized. This type of problems is referred as Open Set Problems [60], and represents the difficulties to be expected in the creation of such a real-time copilot for austere and field medicine. However, in environments with no other realistic options, and a clinical need to save lives, further development and research efforts are strongly encouraged.

7.5 Conclusions

The vision of an artificial intelligent mentor that can assist a user in the completion of a task that involves both cognitive and physical challenges such as special ops medic, equipment maintenance, or pilot assistance is an endeavor that computer scientists, engineers, and clinicians have been focusing on for the last several years. This vision depicts a mentor (or copilot) that is an agent with a defined set of skills (e.g., airway management), but also capable of learning new skills (e.g., hemorrhage control) presented in a variety of modalities (speech, videos, written instructions, such as checklists in Tactical Combat Casualty Care [TCCC]) and use dialogue and visual annotations augmented in the visual field to guide a mentee (user) through the LSI task completion, such as cricothyrotomy. While this surrogate mentor is embodied, it does not interfere with task performance. It only intervenes when guidance is needed by being situational aware of the task performance, environment, and user states. Such systems are transferable. That is, they can be validated with cooking or driving surrogate tasks, such as the Epic Kitchen Dataset. The main "feature" of such copilot, referred as the *Copilots Surgical Mentors (CoPiSMs)* is that they have (and can enable) complete situation awareness. That is, user, task, and context are modeled in a joint framework that evolves. This is necessary because complex decision-making relies on a disparate amount of information that humans are very good at perceiving, processing, and acting but machines in most cases operate with a limited "glimpse" of the world, thus lacking critical situation awareness. Creating models that can jointly address complete situation awareness, such as *Copilots Surgical Mentors (CoPiSMs)*, is an essential part to achieve robust intelligence of such personal assistants, especially when the tasks demand major physical, cognitive, and emotional requirements, as often found in medicine.

Disclosures *Andrew W Kirkpatrick* serves as the PI of the COOL trial, which previously was partially supported by the 3M/Acelity Corporation until August 2022. AW Kirkpatrick has consulted for the 3M/Acelity Corporation, Zoll Medical, Innovative Trauma Care, and CSL Behring. He is the Director of the TeleMentored Ultrasound Supported Medical Interventions (TMUSMI) Research group.

Juan P Wachs serves as the CEO of AI-MEDIC, a company that aims to provide AI-based solutions to medical, clinical, and surgical challenges using AI-based decision-making.

References

1. Bowyer MW, Kuhls DA, Haskin D, Sallee RA, Henry SM, Garcia GD, Luchette FA. Advanced surgical skills for exposure in trauma (ASSET): the first 25 courses. J Surg Res. 2013; https://doi.org/10.1016/j.jss.2013.02.005.
2. Wild H, Marfo C, Mock C, Gaarder T, Gyedu A, Wallis L, Makasa E, Hagander L, Reynolds T, Hardcastle T, Jewell T, Stewart B. Operative trauma courses: a scoping review to inform the development of a trauma surgery course for low-resource settings. World J Surg. 2023;47:1662.
3. Ali J, Sorvari A, Henry S, Kortbeek J, Tremblay L. The advanced trauma operative management course-a two student to one faculty model. J Surg Res. 2013; https://doi.org/10.1016/j.jss.2013.03.019.
4. Rosser JC, Young SM, Klonsky J. Telementoring: an application whose time has come. Surg Endosc Other Interv Tech. 2007; https://doi.org/10.1007/s00464-007-9263-3.
5. Sebajang H, Trudeau P, Dougall A, Hegge S, McKinley C, Anvari M. The role of telementoring and telerobotic assistance in the provision of laparoscopic colorectal surgery in rural areas. Surg Endosc Other Interv Tech. 2006;20(9):1389–93. https://doi.org/10.1007/s00464-005-0260-0.
6. Sebajang H, Trudeau P, Dougall A, Hegge S, McKinley C, Anvari M. Telementoring: an important enabling tool for the community surgeon. Surg Innov. 2005;12(4):327–31. https://doi.org/10.1177/155335060501200407.
7. Vasios WN, Pamplin JC, Powell D, Loos PE, Riesberg JC, Keenan S. Teleconsultation in prolonged field care position paper. J Spec Oper Med. 2017;17(3):141–4. https://doi.org/10.55460/MGJ0-L27W.
8. Scott K, Refaei T, Trivedi N, Trinh J, Macker JP. Robust communications for disconnected, intermittent, low-bandwidth (DIL) environments. In: 2011 – MILCOM 2011 military communications conference. IEEE; 2011. p. 1009–14.
9. Kirkpatrick AW, McKee JL, Tomlinson C, Donley N, Ball CG, Wachs J. A randomized controlled pilot trial of video-modelling versus telementoring for improved hemorrhage control wound packing. Am J Surg. 2022; https://doi.org/10.1016/j.amjsurg.2022.02.039.
10. Wachs JP, Kirkpatrick AW, Tisherman SA. Procedural telementoring in rural, underdeveloped, and austere settings: origins, present challenges, and future perspectives. Annu Rev Biomed Eng. 2021;23(1):115–39. https://doi.org/10.1146/annurev-bioeng-083120-023315.
11. Kirkpatrick AW, Campbell MR, Novinkov OL, Goncharov IB, Kovachevich IV. Blunt trauma and operative care in microgravity: a review of microgravity physiology and surgical investigations with implications for critical care and operative treatment in space. J Am Coll Surg. 1997;184(5):441–53.
12. Kirkpatrick AW, Ball CG, Campbell M, Williams DR, Parazynski SE, Mattox KL, Broderick TJ. Severe traumatic injury during long duration spaceflight: light years beyond ATLS. J Trauma Manag Outcomes. 2009;3(1):4. https://doi.org/10.1186/1752-2897-3-4.
13. Linde AS, Caridha J, Kunkler KJ. Skills decay in military medical training: a meta-synthesis of research outcomes. Mil Med. 2017;183(1–2):e40–4.
14. Sotomayor TM, Mazzeo MV, Maraj CS, Page AJ. Saving female lives using simulation: elevating the training experience. J Cyber Secur Inf Syst. 2018;6(4):28–37.
15. Rojas-Muñoz E, Cabrera ME, Andersen D, Popescu V, Marley S, Mullis B, Zarzaur B, Wachs J. Surgical telementoring without encumbrance: a comparative study of see-through augmented reality-based approaches. Ann Surg. 2019;270(2):384–9. https://doi.org/10.1097/SLA.0000000000002764.
16. Sekhar LN, Juric-Sekhar G, Qazi Z, Patel A, McGrath LB, Pridgeon J, Kalavakonda N, Hannaford B. The future of skull base surgery: a view through tinted glasses. World Neurosurg. 2020;142:29.
17. Linde AS, Miller GT. Applications of future technologies to detect skill decay and improve procedural performance. Mil Med. 2019;184:72.

18. Ribeiro J, Marcelo AF, de Oliveira AM, Junior G, Reva V, Fajer S. Vascular damage control surgery in limited resource environments: a narrative review. Panam J Trauma Crit Care Emerg Surg. 2024;13(2):88–95. https://doi.org/10.5005/jp-journals-10030-1458.
19. Shrestha AB, Taha AM, Siddiq A, Shrestha S, Thakur P, Chapagain S, Sharma S, Halder A, Rajak K, Shah V. Virtual and augmented reality in cardiovascular care in low and middle income country. Curr Probl Cardiol. 2024;49(3):102380. https://doi.org/10.1016/j.cpcardiol.2024.102380.
20. Calisto FM, Santiago C, Nunes N, Nascimento JC. Introduction of human-centric AI assistant to aid radiologists for multimodal breast image classification. Int J Hum-Comput Stud. 2021; https://doi.org/10.1016/j.ijhcs.2021.102607.
21. Shen Y, Nama S, Jin H. Teach once and use everywhere -- building AI assistant eco-skills via user instruction and demonstration (poster). In: Proceedings of the 17th annual international conference on mobile systems, applications, and services. New York: ACM; 2019. p. 606–7.
22. Liu Y, Stiles NRB, Meister M. Augmented reality powers a cognitive assistant for the blind. elife. 2018;7 https://doi.org/10.7554/eLife.37841.
23. Dagostini J, Bonetti L, Salee A, Passerini L, Fiacco G, Lavanda P, Motti E, Stocco M, Gashay KT, Abebe EG, Alemu SM, Haghani R, Voltolini A, Strobbe C, Covre N, Santolini G, Armellini M, Sacchi T, Ronchese D, Furlan C, Facchinato F, Maule L, Tomasin P, Fornaser A, De Cecco M. An augmented reality virtual assistant to help mild cognitive impaired users in cooking a system able to recognize the user status and personalize the support. In: 2018 workshop on Metrology for Industry 4.0 and IoT, MetroInd 4.0 and IoT 2018 – Proceedings; 2018.
24. Yoshimitsu K, Miyawaki F, Sadahiro T, Ohnuma K, Fukui Y, Hashimoto D, Masamune K. Development and evaluation of the second version of scrub nurse robot (SNR) for endoscopic and laparoscopic surgery. In: 2007 IEEE/RSJ international conference on intelligent robots and systems. IEEE; 2007. p. 2288–94.
25. Tao W, Lai ZH, Leu MC, Yin Z, Qin R. A self-aware and active-guiding training & assistant system for worker-centered intelligent manufacturing. Manuf Lett. 2019; https://doi.org/10.1016/j.mfglet.2019.08.003.
26. Lai ZH, Tao W, Leu MC, Yin Z. Smart augmented reality instructional system for mechanical assembly towards worker-centered intelligent manufacturing. J Manuf Syst. 2020; https://doi.org/10.1016/j.jmsy.2020.02.010.
27. Rojas-Muñoz E, Couperus K, Wachs J. The AI-Medic: an artificial intelligent mentor for trauma surgery. In: 14th Augmented Environments for Computer Assisted Interventions Workshop (AE-CAI), part of 23rd International Conference on Medical Image Computing & Computer Assisted Intervention (MICCAI '20); 2020a.
28. Rojas-Munoz E, Couperus K, Wachs JP. The AI-medic: an artificial intelligent mentor for trauma surgery. In: Computer methods in biomechanics and biomedical engineering: imaging & visualization; 2021.
29. Rojas-Muñoz E, Couperus K, Wachs J. DAISI: database for AI surgical instruction. 2020b.
30. Rojas-Muñoz E, Couperus K, Wachs JP. The AI-medic: a multimodal artificial intelligent mentor for trauma surgery. In: Proceedings of the 2020 international conference on multimodal interaction. New York: ACM; 2020c. p. 766–7.
31. Goh E, Gallo R, Hom J, Strong E, Weng Y, Kerman H, Cool JA, Kanjee Z, Parsons AS, Ahuja N, Horvitz E, Yang D, Milstein A, Olson APJ, Rodman A, Chen JH. Large language model influence on diagnostic reasoning. JAMA Netw Open. 2024;7(10):e2440969. https://doi.org/10.1001/jamanetworkopen.2024.40969.
32. Fischbein E. Intuition and proof. For Learn Math. 1982;3(2):9–24.
33. Zhuo Y, Jiang N, Kirkpatrick AW, Couperus K, Tran O, Beck J, DeVane DA, Candelore R, McKee J, Gorbatkin C, Birch E, Colombo C, Duerstock B, Wachs J. TON-ViT: a neurosymbolic AI based on task oriented network with a vision transformer. In: Annual conference on medical image understanding and analysis; 2024. p. 157–70.
34. Northouse PG. Leadership-theory and practice. 5th ed. London; 2010.

35. Mehrjardi S, Mansour AT, Zaïane OR. Self-attentional models application in task-oriented dialogue generation systems. In: Proceedings – natural language processing in a deep learning world. Shoumen: Incoma Ltd; 2019. p. 1031–40.
36. Rutishauser U, Walther D, Koch C, Perona P. Is bottom-up attention useful for object recognition? In: Proceedings of the 2004 IEEE computer society conference on computer vision and pattern recognition, 2004. CVPR 2004, vol. 2. IEEE; 2004. p. 37–44.
37. Huang CM, Andrist S, Sauppé A, Mutlu B. Using gaze patterns to predict task intent in collaboration. Front Psychol. 2015; https://doi.org/10.3389/fpsyg.2015.01049.
38. Kirkpatrick AW, McKee JL, Barrett R, Couperus K, Wachs J. Considering human cognitive architecture in stressful medical prehospital interventions might benefit care providers. Can J Surg. 2023;66(6):E532–4. https://doi.org/10.1503/cjs.015422.
39. Heckman JJ. Sample selection bias as a specification error. Econometrica. 1979;47(1):153. https://doi.org/10.2307/1912352.
40. Damen D, Doughty H, Farinella GM, Furnari A, Kazakos E, Ma J, Moltisanti D, Munro J, Perrett T, Price W, Wray M. Rescaling egocentric vision. ArXiv. 2020b; https://doi.org/10.5523/bris.2g1n6qdydwa9u22shpxqzp0t8m.
41. Chang D, Sain A, Ma Z, Song Y-Z, Guo J. Mind the gap: enlarging the domain gap in open set domain adaptation. ArXiv. 2020.
42. Ueberla JP. Domain adaptation with clustered language models. In: ICASSP, IEEE international conference on acoustics, speech and signal processing – proceedings; 1997.
43. Sattler T, Maddern W, Toft C, Torii A, Hammarstrand L, Stenborg E, Safari D, Okutomi M, Pollefeys M, Sivic J, Kahl F, Pajdla T. Benchmarking 6DOF outdoor visual localization in changing conditions. In: Proceedings of the IEEE computer society conference on computer vision and pattern recognition; 2018.
44. Wulfmeier M, Bewley A, Posner I. Incremental adversarial domain adaptation for continually changing environments. In: Proceedings – IEEE international conference on robotics and automation; 2018.
45. Liu Z, Miao Z, Pan X, Zhan X, Lin D, Yu SX, Gong B. Open compound domain adaptation. In: Proceedings of the IEEE computer society conference on computer vision and pattern recognition; 2019. https://doi.org/10.1109/CVPR42600.2020.01242.
46. Kadam S, Vaidya V. Review and analysis of zero, one and few shot learning approaches. In: Advances in intelligent systems and computing; 2020.
47. Speer R, Chin J, Havasi C. ConceptNet 5.5: an open multilingual graph of general knowledge. In: Proceedings of the AAAI conference on artificial intelligence; 2017. https://doi.org/10.1609/aaai.v31i1.11164.
48. Liu J, Belkin NJ, Zhang X, Yuan X. Examining users' knowledge change in the task completion process. Inf Process Manag. 2013;49(5):1058–74. https://doi.org/10.1016/j.ipm.2012.08.006.
49. Krätzig GP, Arbuthnott KD. Perceptual learning style and learning proficiency: a test of the hypothesis. J Educ Psychol. 2006;98(1):238–46. https://doi.org/10.1037/0022-0663.98.1.238.
50. Damen D, Doughty H, Farinella GM, Fidler S, Furnari A, Kazakos E, Moltisanti D, Munro J, Perrett T, Price W, Wray M. The EPIC-KITCHENS dataset: collection, challenges and baselines. ArXiv. 2020a.
51. Duffner S, Motlicek P, Korchagin D. The TA2 database – a multi-modal database from homeentertainment. Int J Electr Comput Eng. 2012; https://doi.org/10.7763/ijcee.2012.v4.581.
52. Birch E, Couperus K, Gorbatkin C, Kirkpatrick AW, Wachs J, Candelore R, Jiang N, Tran O, Beck J, Couperus C, McKee J, Curlett T, DeVane DA, Colombo C. Trauma THOMPSON: clinical decision support for the frontline medic. Mil Med. 2023;188(Supplement_6):208–14. https://doi.org/10.1093/milmed/usad087.
53. Rakauskas TR, Da Costa A, Moriconi C, Gill G, Kwong JW, Lee N. Evaluation of chat generative pre-trained transformer and microsoft copilot performance on the American Society of Surgery of the hand self-assessment examinations. J Hand Surg Glob Online. 2024; https://doi.org/10.1016/j.jhsg.2024.10.001.

54. Coyle J, Jeske S. The rise of AI copilots: how LLMs turn data into actions, advance the business intelligence industry and make data accessible company-wide. Appl Mark Anal. 2023; https://doi.org/10.69554/sjei6374.
55. Lu MY, Chen B, Williamson DFK, Chen RJ, Zhao M, Chow AK, Ikemura K, Kim A, Pouli D, Patel A, Soliman A, Chen C, Ding T, Wang JJ, Gerber G, Liang I, Le LP, Parwani AV, Weishaupt LL, Mahmood F. A multimodal generative AI copilot for human pathology. Nature. 2024;634(8033):466–73. https://doi.org/10.1038/s41586-024-07618-3.
56. Abolhasani M, Kumacheva E. The rise of self-driving labs in chemical and materials sciences. Nat Synth. 2023;*2:483*.
57. Bao R, Grant E, Kirkpatrick A, Wachs J, Ou Y. AI for brain lesion detection and trauma video action recognition, vol. 14567. Cham: Springer Nature Switzerland; 2025.
58. Zhuo Y, Kirkpatrick AW, Couperus K, Tran O, Beck J, DeVane D, Candelore R, McKee J, Colombo C, Gorbatkin C, Birch E, Duerstock B, Wachs J. Overview of the trauma THOMPSON challenge at MICCAI 2023. 2025a. p. 47–60.
59. Zhuo Y, Kirkpatrick AW, Couperus K, Tran O, Wachs J. The trauma THOMPSON challenge report MICCAI 2023. 2025b. p. 61–71.
60. Boudiaf M, Bennequin E, Tami M, Toubhans A, Piantanida P, Hudelot C, Ayed IB. Open-set likelihood maximization for few-shot learning. 2023.

Clinical Decision Support for Extreme Prehospital Emergencies

8

Andrew W. Kirkpatrick, Kyle Couperus, John Van Eaton, Jason R. Bingham, Jessica L. McKee, Christopher J. Colombo, and Juan Wachs

8.1 Introduction

Human health is often taken for granted but can be rapidly impacted by acute medical, surgical, and traumatic emergencies. The most promising opportunities to impact potentially preventable deaths are in the prehospital phase of care, where early decisive decision-making is critical. However, this phase of care may be the most challenging, as providers must deal with unknown or uncertain clinical information,

A. W. Kirkpatrick (✉)
Departments of Critical Care Medicine and Surgery, University of Calgary, Calgary, AB, Canada

TeleMentored Ultrasound Supported Medical Interventions Research Group, Calgary, AB, Canada

Canadian Forces Medical Services (Retired), Calgary, AB, Canada
e-mail: Andrew.kirkpatrick@albertahealthservices.ca

K. Couperus
Madigan Army Medical Centre, Department of Emergency Medicine, Tacoma, WA, USA

J. Van Eaton
Madian Army Medical Center, Tacoma, WA, USA

J. R. Bingham
Department of General Surgery, Madigan Army Medical Center, Tacoma, WA, USA

J. L. McKee
TeleMentored Ultrasound Supported Medical Interventions Research Group, Calgary, AB, Canada

C. J. Colombo
Uniformed Services University of Health Sciences, Bethesda, MD, USA
e-mail: ccolombo@genevausa.org

J. Wachs
Industrial Engineering, Purdue University, West Lafayettte, IN, USA

B. De Simone et al. (eds.), *New Technologies, Precision Medicine, and AI in Emergency General Surgery*, Hot Topics in Acute Care Surgery and Trauma,
https://doi.org/10.1007/978-3-032-09357-8_8

potentially dangerous or hostile physical environments to work within, and balancing transport with treatment, among a host of other challenges. Acute medical, surgical, and traumatic emergencies dramatically bring to light the fragility of the human operator within this paradigm. Thus, most health care systems have developed clinical algorithms and treatment guidelines to attempt to optimize the care delivered while decreasing the variability introduced when providers provide care under immense pressure. In evaluations of hospital-based care, however, compliance with guidelines is poor, and unwarranted variance in clinical management predominates [1, 2].

With the rapid advancement of technology, there is hope that despite the ever-changing clinical scenarios the system is faced with, there will be a framework to bolster the health care system's ability to take on any acute challenge. Human history has entered the information age, where immense data are readily available almost anywhere anytime due to ubiquitous internet and connected devices such as the tablet or smartphone. These advances have also been termed mobile-health (mHealth), where portable communication technologies provide a range of potential health benefits, including remote clinical management support [3, 4]. These technologies have enabled a revolution in clinical decision support systems (CDSS) which are processes or computing systems that provide clinicians with information to enhance health care. Ideally, CDSS should provide information at the point of care, in the right place and format, at the right time, and in the right context [3, 5] and can be easily accessed by less experienced providers using mHealth technologies.

While unlimited information and communication can be potentially available to prehospital providers, there is an unanswered question "will it be helpful?" Pinsky recently postulated that the intensive care unit presents the most challenging environment to consider the potential of CDSS and machine learning (ML)-based artificial intelligence (AI) techniques [6]. However, the TeleMentored Ultrasound Supported Medical Interventions (TMUSMI) Research group counter postulates that prehospital care is actually a more challenging environment with even more potential for these technologies using an expanded conceptual appreciation of clinical decision support (CDS).

8.2 The Expanded (and Practical) Concept of What Constitutes Clinical Decision Support

Given the immense cognitive and technical challenges non-physician caregivers experience in attending to devastating injuries in the field, it is a logical starting point to integrate cognitive aid or decision support. Assessment, initial care, and triage in prehospital settings ideally occur in a systematic and often concurrent system that gathers the necessary information and guides the provider to treat the most likely injury to kill the patient first. A calamitous polytrauma can overwhelm even the most experienced trauma surgeon with sheer amount of information delivered in the trauma bay. Experience, however, allows one to filter information so that only the most necessary data points are used to make the right decisions and save the patient. CDSS tools are able to bring this experience and knowledge to the point of injury and can extend the

Table 8.1 Types of augmented clinical decision support systems

Computer-based	Standalone	Database
	Standalone	Artificial Intelligence
	Fused	
Human based	Telementored	
	Video modeled	
	Action Recognition	
	Autonomous	
	Rich Immersive Video	
	Modeled Autonomous	

See text for details

spectrum of clinical capabilities of pre-hospital providers. Despite its benefits, a CDSS can also be a double-edged sword. Unwanted, misguided, or unnecessary prehospital decision support may be counterproductive and build barriers and resentment between prehospital providers and remote experts who might potentially have been helpful otherwise [7, 8]. CDSS is most frequently conceptualized as being computer-based. However, a CDS is a much broader concept that encompasses any paradigm or technology that enhances or supports the prehospital or hospital care provider that provides better clinical care, off-loads cognitive load, or ideally both. This expanded domain of CDSS can include advanced computer-based options that leverage machine learning (ML) and artificial intelligence (AI). Often these systems will involve human-based paradigms leveraging human experience and problem solving, such as remote telementoring (RTM), just-in-time video modeling, or combinations and permutations of all best embraced under augmented intelligence (Table 8.1).

8.3 The Challenge: Prehospital Decision Making in Life Threatening Emergencies

Most of the potentially preventable deaths from acute life-threatening emergencies occur before a victim can ever be transported to a hospital. This means that diagnoses and interventions required to save lives will need to be delivered by first responders either at the scene or en route to higher levels of care. As Paliokaite and colleagues have well described, prehospital providers are expected to "rapidly recognize and manage a wide variety of conditions, determine the acuity level, and make appropriate decisions regarding transportation to further treatment facilities [9]." Further, they highlighted that "prehospital decision-making is challenging and depends on system influences, environmental factors, patient characteristics, available resources, and provider experience and knowledge" [9]. Whenever prehospital caregivers respond to a patient, the caregivers must conduct a diagnostic analytical decision-making process in addition to continuously assessing the patients' ongoing needs based on their health status (stable, improving, or deteriorating) [10]. TMUSMI and others have long sought to enable remote advanced diagnoses and interventions performed by less experienced non-physician care providers remotely guided by distant experts utilizing communication informatics. TMUSMI has also attempted to learn more about how first responders think when required to perform life-saving resuscitations on critically injured/ill patients that may require performing beyond the boundaries of personal comfort and/or competence [11]. A much greater understanding of the magnitude and direction of the effect on first responders such remote support creates on stress and cognitive load is required. Post-traumatic stress disorder is associated with reduced working memory, and neuronal resources that should be allocated to cognition are partially diverted to emotion-related brain areas [12]. In addition to the well-understood exposure to traumatic life-threatening events, further aggravating factors for first responders include self-criticism regarding performance and retrospective rumination over critical but prior decision making. Therefore, as health systems attempt to improve and potentially expand the scope and expectations placed on prehospital care, the human thought processes related to critical prehospital decision-making require deeper consideration.

To ideally support the prehospital care providers' cognitive capacity to function under stress and uncertainty, human cognitive processing should be understood [11]. Current theory holds that human cognitive architecture in relation to clinical reasoning frameworks can be modeled by dual-process reasoning, which postulates two distinct systems of reasoning: System 1, representing intuition or automatic thinking; and System 2, representing analytic or deductive thinking [4]. Caregivers need to utilize both intuition and analytical thinking to make critical decisions quickly and accurately, as they are often, if not usually, operating with uncertain and limited information. Both systems are critical; neither is better, although using only one exclusively would be detrimental. For example, when a care provider, with clinical experience and confident pattern recognition, is operating with System 1 thinking, further and/or deeper analysis with System 2 thinking would result in unnecessarily slow responses and could potentially be harmful when immediate responses are required. However, when this same care provider is faced with confusing clinical findings or unforeseen complications, System 2 analytical reasoning is absolutely critical. Thus, efficient toggling between both systems is critical and relates to the concept of cognitive load (CL) [11]. TMUSMI postulates that expanded CDS should preserve System 1 intuition while enabling a "turbo-charged" System 2 resource always in the background ready to interact when appropriate. Again, for example, System 1 is a faster intuitive system, so when a first provider sees external bleeding, they are trained to intuitively find the source and provide pressure. However, System 2 requires a slower, deeper process. This means collecting aggregate data, separating signal from noise in this data set, and finding the pattern within it to come to a conclusion or best next steps when faced with internal torso bleeding that has no immediate solution on a battlefield.

8.4 Human Cognitive Load and Cognitive Load Theory

Cognitive load theory (CLT) refers to the cognitive resources required by the working memory of a care provider to make critical decisions or perform complex tasks. If the CL is excessive, it may overwhelm the working memory, leading to increased stress as well as errors [6, 13]. CLT recognizes three resources; sensory memory and long term memory which are considered to have an infinite capacity; and working memory which, while critical to task performance and recalling stored information, has a fixed finite capacity [14]. The functional strain on working memory is comprised of 3 categories of CL: intrinsic load, extrinsic load, and germane load. Intrinsic load relates to the details of the task at hand (diagnostic or procedural), and is associated with both the complexity of the task and the providers skills, as well as, familiarity with that task [13]. Extrinsic load relates to the cognitive processing required extraneous to the task. Simply put, extrinsic load is the stimuli a provider will face that may not be directly related to the patient but still must be filtered into decision-making. In the prehospital care, extrinsic load may be especially overwhelming, especially if there is a hostile environment, a mass casualty event, strained resources, uncertainty of transport, and innumerable other potential stressors. Germane load relates to potentially useful information that may be incorporated into a future framework for long term memory [14]. Inexperienced providers are assumed at greater risk of cognitive overload as their cognitive resources for knowledge transfer are usually less honed compared to experienced caregivers [13].

Using such frameworks of cognitive architecture allows speculation as to how CDSS might address cognitive load capacities to preserve working memory, improve patient care, and potentially decrease negative long-term effects on caregivers performing such stressful tasks. Remotely guided decision-making can decrease performance and increase the stress on first responders [8], so assumptions are dangerous. Therefore, how and when to provide remote guidance and CDSS to first responders should be more formally studied to understand how these techniques might either greatly benefit or alternatively exacerbate CL with potential positive or adverse results in first responders. Well-designed CDSS should improve situational awareness and decrease CL in care providers [6].

While the front end of the challenge is to improve prehospital care for the dying patient, a parallel but absolutely vital goal should be to improve the psychological well being for caregivers to prevent the development of secondary victims of trauma [11, 15]. Potential targets for stress mitigation and CDS are illustrated in Table 8.2. Given the toll psychological stress places upon first responders, study is urgently required to understand how providing potentially life-saving care seems to exacerbate and exponentiate the psychological trauma experienced in witnessing traumatic injuries in others.

Table 8.2 Potential attributes and pitfalls of CDSS

CDSS Potential Benefits
Better patient care
Reduced provider stress
CDSS Potential Downsides
Slower time-critical patient care
Increased provider stress

8.5 Decision Support Systems and Clinical Decision Support Systems

Decision support systems have been defined as information systems that support business or organizational decision-making activities. They can be either fully computerized or human-powered, or a combination of both [16]. A traditional CDSS is intended to improve healthcare delivery by enhancing medical decisions with targeted clinical knowledge and patient information [17, 18]. In hospitals, they are typically comprised of software designed to aid clinical decision-making, in which patient characteristics are matched to computerized clinical knowledge bases and specific assessments or recommendations are thereafter presented to the responsible clinician [17, 18]. CDSS can be classified by whether they have active or passive delivery, as well as whether they are knowledge-based, involving a database, or non-knowledge-based, meaning that the system leverages artificial intelligence [17]. Non-knowledge-based CDSS are associated with concerns regarding the understanding of the logic used to produce recommendations and problems with data availability and the inherent "black box" nature of many predictive algorithms [6, 17]; nonetheless, they have immense future potential and are considered to be "here to stay," and thus they must be studied properly and integrated [6]. No matter what the architecture, CDSS may potentially be utilized to support patient safety, clinical management, cost containment, administrative functions, diagnostic support, patient decision support, documentation optimization, and workflow improvements [17]. This chapter will hereafter focus on clinical management, diagnostics support, and workflow improvements focused on the prehospital environment, perhaps the least studied domain of practice, but arguably the most in need of such study.

There is a general consensus that readily available guidelines, protocols, and other decision support tools should be made available in prehospital care [9]. Strategies to improve human performance and mitigate human limitations in safety-critical endeavors include the provision and use of cognitive aids and tools that include algorithms, checklists, and decision aids [19]. Recent meta-analysis confirms the ability of checklists and cognitive aids to aid in accurately following checklists and improving teamwork on clinical emergencies [19]. Greig and colleagues concluded that cognitive aids significantly reduced the incidence of missed care steps with the quality of evidence rated as moderate. Further, the use of cognitive aids decreased the incidence of errors, increased the rate of correctly performed steps and improved clinical teamwork, non-technical skills scores, subjective conflict resolution, and globally improved team performance [19]. These authors did reflect on the aviation industry and commented on the continuous tension between practical usability, which promotes simplicity, and the attractiveness of adding clinical detail [19], which may augment education. A further fundamental paradigm tension is whether CDS algorithms should consist of "read then do" steps, where an algorithm is strictly followed, or a "do-confirm" approach, where steps are completed and then confirmed to be correct or warranted [19].

8.6 Computer-Based Clinical Decision Support Systems to Improve Prehospital Care

CDSS may be represented by interactive computer systems for situational decision-making and can improve decision efficiency and safety of care [10]. They are an analytical tool that converts raw clinical data into useful information to inform better decision-making. Bashiri and colleagues recently reviewed the role of CDSS systems in enhancing prehospital care. They concluded that there were four key factors related to the ability of CDS to improve decision making, reduce error, and improve safety. They considered these factors to be computer-based platforms, offering support as a natural part of the workflow, providing support in the same time and space as decision-making, and simply offering practical advice [10]. Bashiri and colleagues also nicely summarized CDSS as being [10];

> These systems use data, models, and algorithms to make recommendations in the form of warnings, color codes, or picture messages to solve diagnostic, therapeutic, and organizational problems. Although these systems are not designed to replace humans, they can improve quality of care. Humans will inevitably make errors, and these systems are designed to help healthcare providers remember relevant diagnostic and treatment options, offer easy-to-follow instructions, reduce diagnostic and therapeutic errors, and change incorrect behaviors.

CDSS still require robust examination to determine their functionality and usefulness. Vicente showed that a prehospital CDS developed for 11 medical conditions could safely direct geriatric patients to the most appropriate care facility with greater accuracy and safety [20]. Hagiwara performed a systemic review of randomized trials concerning prehospital CDS in 2011 and noted that their use might decrease "time to definitive care" and improve diagnostic accuracy among prehospital personnel. However, their final conclusions at that time were that the amount of data was too small to be able to draw any reliable conclusions about the impact of the CDSS in prehospital care [21]. They subsequently carried out another randomized controlled simulation study utilizing or not a CDS tool to manage a critical case with ambulance nurses participating. They found that the CDS tool increased provider compliance with regional guidelines but at the cost of an increased scene time [22].

Paliokaite theorized that standardized interactive field protocols with evidence-based diagnostic and management steps for prehospital providers integrated with access to patient care records could allow for an expedited and critical review of the necessary steps and interventions for the anticipated emergency to be encountered, especially enroute to the patient [9]. These Lithuanian investigators thus developed a series of electronic field protocol modules as cognitive aids to first responders. There were 12 resuscitation scenarios involving the most common life-threatening emergencies prehospital care responders must deal with. Experienced prehospital personnel (paramedics, community nurses, and emergency care nurses) were thereafter randomized to spend 15 minutes cognitively planning for their expected resuscitation sequence after receiving an initial synopsis simulating a 911 dispatcher call-out. They were randomized to either reflect on their own memories and experience or to formally review the specific electronic field protocol module that applied to the scenario in question [9]. The most remarkable result was that the study revealed that being able to review the online cognitive aid resources compared to memory alone significantly improved performance in 10 out of 12 simulation scenarios, with adherence to standardized checklists increasing from 65% to 85% ($p < 0.001$) [9]. Previous studies in both prehospital and hospital settings have shown improvements in provider performance and adherence to guidelines using CDS and cognitive assistance [22, 23], although success has not been universal [21, 22, 24, 25].

Paliokaite and others thus concluded that a well-designed cognitive aid should offer clear and goal-specific guidance to help providers prioritize actions, recall treatment steps, consider relevant diagnoses, and deliver evidence-based care [9, 26]. However, despite the theoretical advantages in delivering CDSS capabilities to first responders, Greig and colleagues [19] have realistically noted that "it is not yet clear if the utilization of cognitive aids in medicine is universally beneficial [27], and some evidence suggests that they may result in minimal advantage or can even worsen team performance [22]. CDSS can disrupt workflow if designed without attention to efficient human information processing or cognitive processing [17].

8.7 A Realistic Appraisal of Cognitive Aids and Their Potential Adverse Effects on Real-Time Resuscitative Care

Greig and colleagues noted in their systematic review of cognitive aid utilization during clinical emergencies that there were possible "drawbacks" that included prolonged times to complete definitive management of life-threatening problems [19, 28]. At the current time it is unknown whether such concerns regarding the usefulness relate to a limitation in the overall concept or in the practical logistics of delivering CDSS to prehospital providers. Pinsky recently concluded that CDSSs could not replace bedside clinicians in acute and critical care environments due to immature situational awareness, technical barriers to timely and valid data, and limitations in data display useful for clinical workflows [6]. If these limitations exist in the intensive care unit, these challenges will only be greatly increased in the prehospital arena. Nevertheless, efforts to overcome the inherent challenges will be discussed. Pinsky also noted a wide gap between artificial intelligence (AI)-based clinical decision support systems (AI-CDSS) in theory and practice, a phenomenon termed the AI chasm [6, 29, 30].

In an effort to "fill" the AI Chasm, in June 2018, the American Medical Association adopted policy, H-480.940, "Augmented Intelligence in Health Care," to provide a framework for the incorporation of AI into health care with the goal of ensuring that AI realizes the benefits to all stakeholders that it promises [31]. This paradigm rebrands the vision of human-machine cooperation as "augmented intelligence" as opposed to artificial intelligence, as humans will remain central as opposed to being excluded in care delivery [6]. Augmented intelligence is an alternative conceptualization that focuses on AI's assistive role, emphasizing a design approach and implementation that enhances human intelligence rather than replaces it [31]. Further, these healthcare leaders emphasized two fundamental concepts regarding the appropriate integration of AI into health care. These are that AI should be recognized as being simply a tool to augment professional clinical judgment and not as a technology to replace or override it. Second, that the development of AI technology should attend specifically to individual applications, with deep concern for patient privacy, and fundamentally reflect thoughtful clinical implementation [31].

8.8 Real-Time Clinical Decision Support When Connectivity Supports On-Line Mentorship

A practical and current means of augmenting provider intelligence is through the utilization of real-time remote expert guidance. The world is increasingly connected with internet availability as standard networks expand, satellite internet develops, and even drone-delivered connectivity solutions proliferate [32]. If there is connectivity, TMUSMI and others suggest that involving an expert human to provide CDS and cognitive aid (particularly for System 2 cognition) is another possibly superior paradigm to support cognitively overwhelmed prehospital providers in a potentially more advanced form of CDSS delivery. TMUSMI is a voluntary international collaboration of academic, government, industry, and military collaborators dedicated to the study of the Science of Telementoring and Teleintervention to improve healthcare, especially focused on vulnerable populations, recognizing populations may be vulnerable through many varied circumstances ranging from geography to hostile environments to socioeconomic conditions [33]. Chronologically, TMUSMI has been a logical evolution from the Damage Control Surgery In Austere Environments Research Group [34, 35], which was itself a logical and iterative evolution from Tele-Ultrasound work performed over the last two decades and derived from Space Medicine [36–48].

We categorize and conceptualize remote telementoring as an expert human-based form of CDSS in which the human factors become essential to successful implementation and for which the true potential of this paradigm has not yet been fully scientifically evaluated [49]. Subjectively, we propose there is a huge potential for this paradigm, which is the least technically complex of all the other paradigms, as remote telementoring simply requires an expert to communicate with, reassure, and direct a novice to perform beyond their perceived limitations and self-imposed boundaries. A remarkable range of diagnoses and interventions have been shown to be feasible in controlled studies [50]. In both clinical [41] and laboratory [50] scenarios, such remote support is reassuring to first responders. A simulation study of remotely mentored damage control packing of exsanguinating intra-abdominal hemorrhage demonstrated significantly increased self-assessed non-surgeon procedural confidence and improved heart rate variability compared to unmentored non-surgeons

[50]. Overall, remote mentor-to-first responder communication may either be considered helpful and reassuring [8, 41, 50], or it may be counterproductive and engender unnecessary delay [8]. Thus, further studies are required to elucidate the efficacy of these techniques in prehospital care as well as in global health and determine the factors predicting efficacy or interference. TMUSMI does believe, though, that the potential is nearly unlimited for most healthcare when internet connectivity is not impeded such that "remote digital medicine" or mHealth will soon become a specialty unto itself, but one for which the entire scope of practice and especially human factors aspects require urgent and meticulous establishment [33, 51].

8.9 Disconnected, Denied, Intermittent, and/or with Limited Bandwidth (DDIL) and Clinical Decision Support for Prehospital Resuscitation

The term Disconnected, Denied, Intermittent and/or with Limited bandwidth (DDIL) environment has been used to describe contested spaces where communications are contested, denied, or precluded due to secrecy requirements [52]. However, the term still applies to many non-military situations where communications are not available, such as during disasters when communication failures may be expected, or simply when a suitable remote mentor is unavailable [53]. Thus, solutions to provide clinical decision support in DDIL environments should be independent from connectivity requirements and ideally autonomous/semi-autonomous. Such solutions would also be required for Space Medicine if humans are to safely travel to Mars, with distances that preclude real-time communication and guidance [54, 55].

8.10 Video Modeling

Video modeling constitutes a form of behavior modeling that involves the demonstration of desired behaviors, outcomes, and attitudes through active visual representations [14] and can be as simple as trying to recreate something depicted on a YouTube video. While ubiquitous in everyday life, little has been explored in empowering life-saving medical interventions with this technique, which is surprising given its potential. Potential limitations include the critical time pressures associated with providing heroic life-saving interventions (LSIs), knowing what content the novice users will require education on, and the near-infinite variety of human anatomy and physiology related to even standard categories of wounds. Considering the potential, however, TMUSMI did conduct the first randomized trials comparing the utility of remote telementoring (RTM) versus video-modeled review prior to undertaking simulated life-saving interventions by first responders. The overall results were mixed, noting that both techniques were complementary [53, 56]. RTM provides an engaged human mentor who may provide real-time guidance and corrective troubleshooting during the performance of an unfamiliar and likely stressful intervention. A previous RCT involving tube thoracostomy insertion was associated with increased success and improved confidence in those remotely supported [56]. A remote expert may also provide real-time corrective guidance to avoid both iatrogenic injury and procedure failure and thus might be applicable to more complex "out-of-scope" tasks. When communications permit, RTM is thus a technique that both reassures first responders and may be quicker if there is no information or opportunity to review techniques prior to arrival on scene [53, 56].

8.11 Autonomous Disconnected CDSS

Research is actively underway to attempt to harness the potential of AI coupled to action recognition software to enable autonomous diagnosis and interventions for far-forward resuscitation. The TeleHelper for Operational Medical Procedure Support and Offline Network (Trauma-THOMPSON) Project is such an example, which explores an autonomous approach to providing real-time guidance for non-medical personnel to perform LSIs, independent of both connectivity and mentors [57]. Trauma THOMPSON is a user interface platform designed to be used as a clinical decision tool for point-of-care and PCC settings powered by an AI engine. As a mobile-based application, Trauma THOMPSON will provide a repository of videos, downloadable and available offline, to serve as a reference when performing specific critical care procedures [57]. Trauma-THOMPSON is a virtual artificial intelligence mentor that analyzes the previous steps of an invasive procedure to guide the next step autonomously. The intent of the Trauma THOMPSON is multifactorial, intending to develop voice-controlled mobile applications with video references for procedural guidance, audio narration of video procedures with mentoring scripts, and most disruptive and potentially powerful, creating an AI-guided autonomous intervention system using AR overlay and voice command to create immersive video modeling [57, 58]. Trauma THOMPSON represents efforts to provide an augmented reality (AR)/virtual reality-guided intervention system that could facilitate life-saving interventions performed by inexperienced users (when absolutely required) using natural language. To do this, the system interprets the procedure in real time and guides the user through the procedure by identifying actions and anticipating the next steps through both AR overlay and voice command [57]. At the present time the system performs more than 154 times better than random prediction [57], but it is ever improving with experience and data input.

8.12 Rich Immersive Video-Modeling (RIVM) of Life Saving Interventions

As discussed, video-modeling (VM) is a medically underappreciated approach to just-in-time learning that teaches through active visual representation with immediate repetition. Augmenting the standard VM with the Trauma-THOMPSON Deep learning capability may potentially create a new paradigm designated as rich immersive video-modeling (RIVM) that is independent of connectivity, remote mentors, and the need for a prepared library of procedures, as action-recognition software could recognize and guide procedures autonomously. With ML and advanced AI, just-in-time videos demonstrating what steps should occur could be created real time with the conduct of necessary life-saving intervention such that a novice just needs to replicate the content of what is being created for them by the autonomous resuscitation guide. At the present such technology does not yet exist, but given the explosive advance in AI and decision support, it may provide health care solutions that ill require serious clinical evaluation. There is hope with the use of technologies like Trauma-THOMPSON. The more global use of Trauma-THOMPSON, the greater its accuracy and versatility. RIVM thus provides a potential just-in-time paradigm to save lives in remote or disadvantaged areas of the globe as well as in deep space.

8.13 Conclusions

Saving lives in chaotic, confusing, and potentially dangerous situations is an extremely stressful human undertaking. Those people who accept and undertake this challenge should not only be thanked but also supported. Thankfully there now exist multiple technological solutions to remotely or autonomously support clinical point-of-care decisions to both save more lives and to cognitively protect the caregivers. At the present nothing is definitively proven, and nothing can be assumed. However, the potential seems unlimited to improve prehospital care with information delivered and received by many different technologies. Therefore, there is an urgent need for well-designed research to discern how to incorporate augmented intelligence into prehospital care for all of humanity.

Disclosures *Andrew W Kirkpatrick* serves as the PI of the COOL trial, which previously was partially supported by the 3 M/Acelity Corporation until Aug 2022. AW Kirkpatrick is also a member of the Canadian Forces Medical Services and has consulted for the 3 m/Acelity Corporation, Zoll Medical, Innovative Trauma Care, and CSL Behring. He is the Director of the TeleMentored Ultrasound Supported Medical Interventions (TMUSMI) Research group and serves in the Canadian Forces Medical Services. He has previously disclosed a personal relationship with Jessica L McKee.

Kyle Couperus reported no disclosures.
Jason R Bingham reported no disclosures.
Jessica L McKee reported no disclosures.
Jan Van Eaton reported no disclosures.
Christopher J. Colombo reported no disclosures.
Juan Wachs reported no disclosures.

References

1. Albrecht V, Schafer N, Sturmer EK, Driessen A, Betsche L, Schenk M, et al. Practice management of acute trauma haemorrhage and haemostatic disorders across German trauma centres. Eur J Trauma Emerg Surg. 2017;43(2):201–14.

2. Hamada SR, Gauss T, Pann J, Dunser M, Leone M, Duranteau J. European trauma guideline compliance assessment: the ETRAUSS study. Crit Care. 2015;19:423.
3. Nishimwe A, Ibisomi L, Nyssen M, Conco DN. The effect of a decision-support mHealth application on maternal and neonatal outcomes in two district hospitals in Rwanda: pre – post intervention study. BMC Pregnancy Childbirth. 2022;22(1):52.
4. Free C, Phillips G, Watson L, Galli L, Felix L, Edwards P, et al. The effectiveness of mobile-health technologies to improve health care service delivery processes: a systematic review and meta-analysis. PLoS Med. 2013;10(1):e1001363.
5. Optimizing strategies for clinical decision support: summary of a meeting series. Washington, D. C.: National Academy of Medicine; 2017.
6. Pinsky MR, Bedoya A, Bihorac A, Celi L, Churpek M, Economou-Zavlanos NJ, et al. Use of artificial intelligence in critical care: opportunities and obstacles. Crit Care. 2024;28(1):113.
7. Netzer I, Kirkpatrick AW, Nissan M, McKee JL, McBeth P, Dobron A, et al. Rubrum Coelis: the contribution of real-time telementoring in acute trauma scenarios-a randomized controlled trial. Telemed J E Health. 2019;25(11):1108–14.
8. Kirkpatrick AW, McKee JL, Netzer I, McKee IA, McBeth P, Wachs JP, et al. A randomized trial of mentored vs nonmentored military medics compared in the application of a wound clamp without prior training: when to shut up and just watch! Mil Med. 2020;185(Suppl 1):67–72.
9. Paliokaite I, Dambrauskas Z, Dobozinskas P, Pukenyte E, Mankute-Use A, Vaitkaitis D. Electronic field protocols for prehospital care quality improvement in Lithuania: a randomized simulation-based study. Scand J Trauma Resusc Emerg Med. 2023;31(1):83.
10. Bashiri A, Alizadeh Savareh B, Ghazisaeedi M. Promotion of prehospital emergency care through clinical decision support systems: opportunities and challenges. Clin Exp Emerg Med. 2019;6(4):288–96.
11. Kirkpatrick AW, McKee JL, Barrett R, Couperus K, Wachs J. Considering human cognitive architecture in stressful medical prehospital interventions might benefit care providers. Can J Surg. 2023;66(6):E522–E34.
12. Shim M, Hwang HJ, Lee SH. Impaired functional cortical networks in the theta frequency band of patients with post-traumatic stress disorder during auditory-cognitive processing. Front Psych. 2022;13:811766.
13. Vella KM, Hall AK, van Merrienboer JJG, Hopman WM, Szulewski A. An exploratory investigation of the measurement of cognitive load on shift: application of cognitive load theory in emergency medicine. AEM Educ Train. 2021;5(4):e10634.
14. Harris E, Santhosh L. Dual process theory and cognitive load: how intensivists make diagnoses. Crit Care Clin. 2022;38(1):27–36.
15. Joseph B, Pandit V, Hadeed G, Kulvatunyou N, Zangbar B, Tang A, et al. Unveiling posttraumatic stress disorder in trauma surgeons: a national survey. J Trauma Acute Care Surg. 2014;77(1):148–54; discussion 54.
16. Wikepedia. Decision support system: Wikepedia; [updated 28 March 2024; cited 2024 April 14 2024]. Available from: https://en.wikipedia.org/wiki/Decision_support_system.
17. Sutton RT, Pincock D, Baumgart DC, Sadowski DC, Fedorak RN, Kroeker KI. An overview of clinical decision support systems: benefits, risks, and strategies for success. NPJ Digit Med. 2020;3:17.
18. Sim I, Gorman P, Greenes RA, Haynes RB, Kaplan B, Lehmann H, et al. Clinical decision support systems for the practice of evidence-based medicine. J Am Med Inform Assoc. 2001;8(6):527–34.
19. Greig PR, Zolger D, Onwochei DN, Thurley N, Higham H, Desai N. Cognitive aids in the management of clinical emergencies: a systematic review. Anaesthesia. 2023;78(3):343–55.
20. Vicente V, Sjostrand F, Sundstrom BW, Svensson L, Castren M. Developing a decision support system for geriatric patients in prehospital care. Eur J Emerg Med. 2013;20(4):240–7.
21. Hagiwara M, Henricson M, Jonsson A, Suserud BO. Decision-support tool in prehospital care: a systematic review of randomized trials. Prehosp Disaster Med. 2011;26(5):319–29.

22. Hagiwara MA, Sjoqvist BA, Lundberg L, Suserud BO, Henricson M, Jonsson A. Decision support system in prehospital care: a randomized controlled simulation study. Am J Emerg Med. 2013;31(1):145–53.
23. Peran D, Kodet J, Pekara J, Mala L, Truhlar A, Cmorej PC, et al. ABCDE cognitive aid tool in patient assessment – development and validation in a multicenter pilot simulation study. BMC Emerg Med. 2020;20(1):95.
24. Nelson McMillan K, Rosen MA, Shilkofski NA, Bradshaw JH, Saliski M, Hunt EA. Cognitive aids do not prompt initiation of cardiopulmonary resuscitation in simulated pediatric cardiopulmonary arrests. Simul Healthc. 2018;13(1):41–6.
25. Porter A, Dale J, Foster T, Logan P, Wells B, Snooks H. Implementation and use of computerised clinical decision support (CCDS) in emergency pre-hospital care: a qualitative study of paramedic views and experience using strong structuration theory. Implement Sci. 2018;13(1):91.
26. Abir G, Austin N, Seligman KM, Burian BK, Goldhaber-Fiebert SN. Cognitive aids in obstetric units: design, implementation, and use. Anesth Analg. 2020;130(5):1341–50.
27. Writing Group for the C-ICUI, the Brazilian Research in Intensive Care N, Cavalcanti AB, Bozza FA, Machado FR, Salluh JI, et al. Effect of a quality improvement intervention with daily round checklists, goal setting, and clinician prompting on mortality of critically Ill patients: a randomized clinical trial. JAMA. 2016;315(14):1480–90.
28. Forristal C, Hayman K, Smith N, Mal S, Columbus M, Farooki N, et al. Does utilization of an intubation safety checklist reduce omissions during simulated resuscitation scenarios: a multicenter randomized controlled trial. CJEM. 2021;23(1):45–53.
29. Heavan WD. Hundreds of AI tools have been built to catch covid. None of them helped: MIT Technology Review; 2021 [cited 2024. Available from: https://www.technologyreview.com/2021/07/30/1030329/machine-learning-ai-failed-covid-hospital-diagnosis-pandemic/.
30. Vasey B, Nagendran M, Campbell B, Clifton DA, Collins GS, Denaxas S, et al. Reporting guideline for the early-stage clinical evaluation of decision support systems driven by artificial intelligence: DECIDE-AI. Nat Med. 2022;28(5):924–33.
31. Crigger E, Khoury C. Making policy on augmented intelligence in health care. AMA J Ethics. 2019;21(2):E188–91.
32. Cabrera-Castellanos DF, Aragon-Zavala A, Castanon-Avila G. Closing connectivity gap: an overview of mobile coverage solutions for not-spots in rural zones. Sensors (Basel). 2021;21(23):8037.
33. Kirkpatrick AW. Point-of-care resuscitation research: from extreme to mainstream: trauma Association of Canada Fraser Gurd Lecture 2019. J Trauma Acute Care Surg. 2019;87(3):571–81.
34. Kirkpatrick AW, McKee JL, McBeth PB, Ball CG, LaPorta A, Broderick T, et al. The Damage Control Surgery in Austere Environments Research Group (DCSAERG): a dynamic program to facilitate real-time telementoring/telediagnosis to address exsanguination in extreme and austere environments. J Trauma Acute Care Surg. 2017;83(1 Suppl 1):S156–S63.
35. Kirkpatrick AW, McKee JL, Tien CH, LaPorta AJ, Lavell K, Leslie T, et al. Abbreviated closure for remote damage control laparotomy in extreme environments: a randomized trial of sutures versus wound clamps comparing terrestrial and weightless conditions. Am J Surg. 2017;213(5):862–9.
36. Sargsyan AE, Hamilton DR, Jones JA, Melton S, Whitson PA, Kirkpatrick AW, et al. FAST at MACH 20: clinical ultrasound aboard the International Space Station. J Trauma. 2005;58(1):35–9.
37. Kirkpatrick AW, Jones JA, Sargsyan A, Hamilton DR, Melton S, Beck G, et al. Trauma sonography for use in microgravity. Aviat Space Environ Med. 2007;78(4 Suppl):A38–42.
38. Kirkpatrick AW, Hamilton DR, Nicolaou S, Sargsyan AE, Campbell MR, Feiveson A, et al. Focused assessment with sonography for trauma in weightlessness: a feasibility study. J Am Coll Surg. 2003;196(6):833–44.

39. Kirkpatrick AW, Nicolaou S, Campbell MR, Sargsyan AE, Dulchavsky SA, Melton S, et al. Percutaneous aspiration of fluid for management of peritonitis in space. Aviat Space Environ Med. 2002;73(9):925–30.
40. Dyer D, Cusden J, Turner C, Boyd J, Hall R, Lautner D, et al. The clinical and technical evaluation of a remote telementored telesonography system during the acute resuscitation and transfer of the injured patient. J Trauma. 2008;65(6):1209–16.
41. Al-Kadi A, Dyer D, Ball CG, McBeth PB, Hall R, Lan S, et al. User's perceptions of remote trauma telesonography. J Telemed Telecare. 2009;15(5):251–4.
42. Crawford I, McBeth PB, Mitchelson M, Tiruta C, Ferguson J, Kirkpatrick AW. Telementorable "just-in-time" lung ultrasound on an iPhone. J Emerg Trauma Shock. 2011;4(4):526–7.
43. Crawford I, Tiruta C, Kirkpatrick AW, Mitchelson M, Ferguson J. Big brother could actually help quite easily: telementored "just-in-time" telesonography of the FAST over a smartphone. Ann Emerg Med. 2011;58(3):312–4.
44. Crawford I, McBeth PB, Mitchelson m, Fergusen J, Tiruta C, Kirkpatrick AW. How to set up a low-cost tele-ultrasound capable video-conferencing system with wide applicability. Crit Ultrasound J. 2012;4(13)
45. Biegler N, McBeth PB, Tevez-Molina M, McMillan JR, Crawford I, Hamilton DR, et al. Just-in-time cost-effective off-the-shelf remote telementoring of paramedical personnel in bed-side lung sonography – a technical case study. Telemed J E Health. 2012;18(10):807–9.
46. Biegler N, McBeth PB, Tiruta C, Hamilton DR, Xiao Z, Crawford I, et al. The feasibility of nurse practitioner-performed, telementored lung telesonography with remote physician guidance – 'a remote virtual mentor'. Crit Ultrasound J. 2013;5(1):5.
47. McBeth P, Crawford I, Tiruta C, Xiao Z, Zhu GQ, Shuster M, et al. Help is in your pocket: the potential accuracy of smartphone- and laptop-based remotely guided resuscitative telesonography. Telemed J E Health. 2013;19(12):924–30.
48. McBeth PB, Crawford I, Blaivas M, Hamilton T, Musselwhite K, Panebianco N, et al. Simple, almost anywhere, with almost anyone: remote low-cost telementored resuscitative lung ultrasound. J Trauma. 2011;71(6):1528–35.
49. Wachs JP, Kirkpatrick AW, Tisherman SA. Procedural telementoring in rural, underdeveloped, and austere settings: origins, present challenges, and future perspectives. Annu Rev Biomed Eng. 2021;23:115–39.
50. Kirkpatrick AW, Tien H, LaPorta AT, Lavell K, Keillor J, Wright Beatty HE, et al. The marriage of surgical simulation and telementoring for damage-control surgical training of operational first responders: a pilot study. J Trauma Acute Care Surg. 2015;79(5):741–7.
51. Kirkpatrick AW, LaPorta A, Brien S, Leslie T, Glassberg E, McKee J, et al. Technical innovations that may facilitate real-time telementoring of damage control surgery in austere environments: a proof of concept comparative evaluation of the importance of surgical experience, telepresence, gravity and mentoring in the conduct of damage control laparotomies. Can J Surg. 2015;58(3 Suppl 3):S88–90.
52. Scott K, Refaei T, Trivedi N, Trinh J. Robust communications for disconnected, intermittent, low-bandwidth (DIL) environments. The 2011 military communications conference – track 2 – network protocols and performance; 7–10 Nov 2011.
53. Kirkpatrick AW, McKee JL, Tomlinson C, Donley N, Ball CG, Wachs J. A randomized controlled pilot trial of video-modelling versus telementoring for improved hemorrhage control wound packing. Am J Surg. 2022;224(2):769–74.
54. Kirkpatrick AW, Campbell MR, Novinkov OL, Goncharov IB, Kovachevich IV. Blunt trauma and operative care in microgravity: a review of microgravity physiology and surgical investigations with implications for critical care and operative treatment in space. J Am Coll Surg. 1997;184:441–53.
55. Kirkpatrick AW, Ball CG, Campbell M, Williams DR, Parazynski SE, Mattox KL, et al. Severe traumatic injury during long duration spaceflight: light years beyond ATLS. J Trauma Manag Outcomes. 2009;3:4.

56. Kirkpatrick AW, Tomlinson C, Donley N, McKee JL, Ball CG, Wachs JP. To watch before or listen while doing? A randomized pilot of video-modelling versus telementored tube thoracostomy. Prehosp Disaster Med. 2022;37(1):71–7.
57. Birch E, Couperus K, Gorbatkin C, Kirkpatrick AW, Wachs J, Candelore R, et al. Trauma THOMPSON: clinical decision support for the frontline medic. Mil Med. 2023;188(Suppl 6):208–14.
58. Wachs J, Jiang N, Zhuo Y, Couperus K, Colombo C, Birch E, et al. The Trauma THOMPSON Challenge Proposal. International Conference on Medical Image Computing and Computer Assisted Intervention (MICCAI) 2023 (MICCAI 2023); Vancouver: International Conference on Medical Image Computing and Computer Assisted Intervention 2023.

AI in the Trauma Bay

9

Zain Khalpey and Joseph F. Sucher

9.1 Introduction

The intensive care unit (ICU) is a nexus of complexity and uncertainty, where clinicians work under immense pressure to decode a cacophony of data streams—vital signs, laboratory results, imaging studies, ventilator parameters, fluid inputs and outputs, and pharmacological regimens. The overarching objective is to stabilize critically ill patients, identify subtle signs of decompensation, and implement interventions swiftly enough to alter the disease trajectory. Yet, despite decades of technological progress in monitoring hardware and data acquisition platforms, the capacity to synthesize and interpret this avalanche of information in real time has remained constrained by human cognitive limits and fragmented information systems.

The ascendancy of artificial intelligence, particularly machine learning (ML) and deep neural networks, promises a paradigm shift in ICU monitoring and care delivery. These tools excel at pattern recognition, predictive modeling, and adaptive learning—capabilities that map seamlessly onto the demands of acute care. Such advancements become even more critical when considering the dual challenges of increased cognitive workload (CW) that clinicians face, thus negatively impacting situational awareness (SA). AI systems designed with principles from human factors and cognitive engineering have demonstrated significant potential to mitigate these challenges. AI tools can reduce cognitive burden, enhance situational awareness, and ensure that critical decisions are informed by the most salient data, intelligently organized and displayed.

A definition of cognitive workload (CW), also referred to as "cognitive load," is subjective. There is no universally accepted definition. There is a consensus that

Z. Khalpey (✉) · J. F. Sucher (✉)
HonorHealth Deer Valley Medical Center, Phoenix, AZ, USA
e-mail: zain@khalpey.ai; jsuche@honorhealth.com

B. De Simone et al. (eds.), *New Technologies, Precision Medicine, and AI in Emergency General Surgery*, Hot Topics in Acute Care Surgery and Trauma,
https://doi.org/10.1007/978-3-032-09357-8_9

defines CW as the cognitive "cost" of a task to the operator. Humans have limited resources for cognition, and CW refers to the subjective experiences associated with the demands on these resources, especially working memory.

Factors that contribute to the experience of CW are influenced by many dimensions that are unique to the individual in the situation. More simply stated, what is "hard" for one person may be "easy" for another. The factors that result in what is hard for one and easy for another are multidimensional and include mental demand, temporal demand, physical demand, performance, effort, and frustration level. Hart and Staveland examined the dimensions that comprise CW in a scientifically rigorous and replicable way over a 3-year period and produced a validated and reliable instrument for measuring a person's CW: The NASA-TLX (Task Load Index)(XX2).

The current generation of electronic medical records, along with computerized provider order entry systems, has failed to provide an adequate solution(XX1). One reason for this failure is that many health information technology (HIT) systems have not leveraged human factors and cognitive engineering design methodologies. This has led to failed or suboptimal implementation of HIT, which either has not improved clinical decision support (CDS) or, worse, may have decreased our ability to identify problems(XX3). The current HIT implementations are largely passive, serving only to provide the clinician with the ability to query the clinical database. Instead, we require HIT systems that leverage AI to present salient information (synthesized data) to the provider at the point of care (Fig. 9.1). This is an active process that seeks to aid the expert clinician by decreasing CW and improving situation awareness (SA).

Situation awareness is the area of study that examines the knowledge and comprehension of the environment that is essential to those who make decisions in complex domains such as critical care medicine. Optimizing SA by providing clinicians with information that has been intelligently organized can reduce the CW. Having complete, accurate, and up-to-the-minute SA is considered to be vital in any area where the effects of technological and situational complexity on decision-makers are of concern. The SICU is one such domain.

A definition of situation awareness (SA) general enough to account for everything and anything runs the risk of being too broad to be useful. A definition that is overly specific often prevents transferring issues, concepts, and results from one domain to another. Much of the literature regarding SA is in the realm of aerospace engineering. Aviation and high-intensity clinical environments (e.g., trauma bays, intensive care units, and operating rooms) share many core features: They are all complex and dynamic with high volumes of data and high CW. Endsley proposes this definition of SA:

> "the perception of elements in the environment within a volume of time and space, the comprehension of their meaning, and the projection of their status into the near future."—Endsley MR (1988) Design and evaluation for situation awareness enhancement. Proceedings of the Human Factors Society 32nd Annual Meeting (Vol. 1, pp. 97). Santa Monica, CA: Human Factors Society.

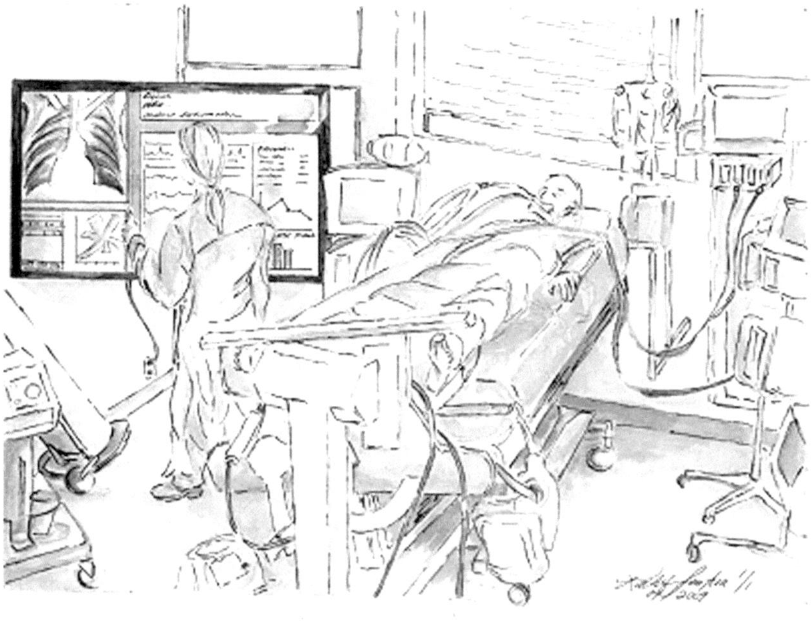

Fig. 9.1 Concept rendering of an intelligent video display. Salient patient-specific information provided in an organized, intelligent fashion at the bedside of each complex, critically ill patient

This definition forms the basis of a model of SA that seems applicable in the SICU (see Fig. 9.2).

Level 1 SA entails the perception of cues in the environment that are pertinent to the current situation. Without perception of important information relevant to the situation, the odds of forming an incorrect decision increase. Jones et al. found that 76% of errors in pilots could be linked to problems with the perception of essential information(XX5).

Level 2 SA is a measure of the relevance of each fact, which facts are more salient, and the ability to make accurate judgments about the situation. Jones and Endsley found that 20% of pilot errors were linked to problems with Level 2 SA(XX5).

Level 3 SA involves the ability of the person to project and forecast events and dynamics of the situation into the immediate future. This level of SA has marked implications for timely decision-making. Skilled experts in a domain demonstrate a high level 3 SA(XX5).

This hierarchical model of SA has direct applicability to the dynamic and complex environments found in the SICU. Singh et al. (XX6) used the following mapping of this model from aviation to health care:

Level 1 SA: What are the relevant facts in this case?
Level 2 SA: What is the story?
Level 3 SA: What is most likely to happen if?

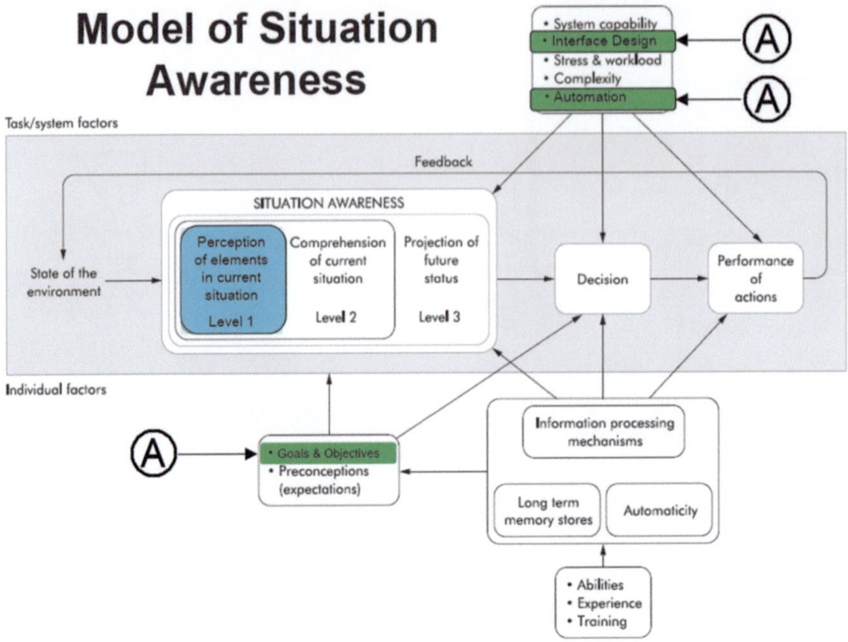

Fig. 9.2 Model of Situation Awareness. Factors marked by (A) indicate areas where human factors, cognitive engineering, and systems design intersect to optimize SA. (Figure adapted from Endsley [16] (XX4))

This framework provides targets for measuring and studying SA. Situation awareness (SA) has been demonstrated to be a factor in decision-making in complex environments(XX7).

In the trauma bay, for example, AI can stratify risk and prioritize life-saving interventions within seconds, enhancing SA at each decision point. Postoperatively, AI-driven systems predict arrhythmias before they strike, optimize fluid balance, and deliver timely alerts, allowing clinicians to address potential crises before they manifest overtly. By synthesizing fragmented data streams into a coherent and actionable format, AI systems enable clinicians to focus on higher-order problem-solving rather than routine data management.

This chapter dissects the emergence of AI in ICU monitoring, from conceptual frameworks to robust clinical applications. With a focus on trauma admission, intraoperative decision support, postoperative predictive analytics, fluid management, and arrhythmia surveillance, we highlight the synergy of domain knowledge and computational sophistication. We provide real-world scenarios, drawn from early adopter institutions, to illuminate how these technological innovations reshape the ICU landscape. We also examine data stewardship, ethics, bias mitigation, and regulatory considerations, delineating best practices for sustainable implementation. Ultimately, this chapter offers a roadmap for clinicians, administrators, and policymakers eager to embrace AI's potential to revolutionize critical care medicine.

9.2 The Trauma Bay and AI-Driven Efficiency

The trauma bay is a uniquely challenging microcosm of the hospital, where seconds can separate survival from mortality. Current trauma protocols, such as ATLS, have standardized the approach to acute injuries, yet integrating dynamic, multimodal data under intense time pressure remains daunting. AI can shoulder some of the cognitive load, enabling trauma teams to focus on clinical acumen while data-driven tools orchestrate the recognition of patterns and priorities.

9.2.1 Rapid Diagnostics and Triage

Trauma patients often present with complex, polytraumatic injuries that defy quick classification. Machine learning algorithms, trained on extensive trauma registries and enriched by continuous physiological monitoring, can rapidly identify the probability of major hemorrhage, organ laceration, or traumatic brain injury. Within seconds of patient arrival, AI tools may integrate portable imaging findings, such as fast-acquired CT scans or even point-of-care ultrasound images, to generate probability scores. This can guide clinicians to target interventions—e.g., deciding whether to rush the patient to the operating suite, consider a massive transfusion protocol, or activate interventional radiology services for potential embolization.

9.2.2 Workflow Integration and Communication

The trauma bay thrives on coordination. Voice recognition and NLP systems can convert spoken commands into actionable orders, while dashboards highlight patient allergies, prior surgeries, and home medications pulled automatically from the EHR. These elements can all be re-presented to the entire team in a context-sensitive format to minimize CW and enhance SA. For instance, an AI-driven display might show relevant home medications such as beta blockers and anticoagulants while calculating the shock index, which can help prompt clinical decisions for earlier interventions of blood transfusions or anticoagulation reversal.

Interfaces utilizing NLP can improve efficiencies by triggering the necessary blood bank notifications, nursing tasks, and medication orders when the attending surgeon verbalizes "Massive transfusion protocol now." Additionally, AI can also analyze the timing and sequence of interventions, recommending subtle process improvements that streamline care and minimize delays.

9.2.3 Three Examples in the Trauma Bay

Example 1: A 27-year-old patient arrives after a fall from a height. AI algorithms integrate the patient's oxygen saturation, heart rate variability, and initial portable chest X-ray, flagging a potential tension pneumothorax. The care team receives an immediate alert, prompting a rapid needle decompression before hemodynamic collapse ensues.

Example 2: A motor vehicle collision victim presents with unstable pelvic fractures. The AI system correlates pre-hospital vital signs, pelvic imaging, and known pelvic injury patterns, predicting significant hemorrhage risk. The trauma surgeon initiates a massive transfusion protocol, and interventional radiology is preemptively mobilized.

Example 3: A patient with blunt abdominal trauma arrives hypotensive. The AI model, referencing thousands of similar cases, quickly identifies a high likelihood of intra-abdominal hemorrhage. The team expedites a focused assessment with sonography for trauma (FAST) exam, confirms a hemoperitoneum, and moves directly to the operating room for emergent laparotomy.

9.3 Intraoperative AI: Real-Time Monitoring and Decision Support

In the operating room, surgeons and anesthesiologists navigate a labyrinth of continuous data streams. Conventional monitors display heart rate, blood pressure, oxygenation, and end-tidal CO2, but integration and prediction remain limited without advanced analytics. AI augments this scenario by distilling data into actionable foresight, reducing unforeseen complications, and improving surgical precision.

9.3.1 Integrating Continuous Data Streams

Deep learning models can detect hemodynamic signatures of impending instability. For example, subtle deviations in arterial waveform morphology may forecast hypotension minutes in advance. By providing early warnings, the anesthesiologist can titrate vasopressors or fluids before the patient's blood pressure plummets. Similarly, integration of neuromonitoring signals with ventilator parameters can help anticipate changes in intracranial pressure or cerebral perfusion, which is critical in neurosurgical procedures.

9.3.2 Image Recognition and Guidance

Advanced computer vision tools analyze intraoperative imaging—be it laparoscopic feeds during abdominal surgery or fluoroscopic images in vascular interventions. By identifying anatomical landmarks, highlighting critical structures such as coronary arteries or vascular grafts, and even suggesting optimal suture angles, these AI tools function as a digital surgical assistant. For intricate cardiac surgeries, real-time AI guidance may mean fewer intraoperative complications and more precise reconstructions.

9.3.3 Three Intraoperative Examples

Example 1: During a complex CABG, AI-driven predictive models detect early signals of declining cardiac output. An alert prompts the anesthesiologist to adjust inotropes and fluid balance, stabilizing the patient before a full hemodynamic crash.

Example 2: In a laparoscopic cholecystectomy, computer vision identifies the cystic duct and artery clearly, reducing the risk of accidental bile duct injury. The surgical resident, guided by these image overlays, performs the dissection more confidently and safely.

Example 3: For a spinal tumor resection, ML-based algorithms process intraoperative neuromonitoring data (somatosensory and motor-evoked potentials) to detect early signs of cord ischemia. The surgical team modifies their approach mid-procedure, preserving neurological function.

9.4 Postoperative Monitoring, Arrhythmia Prediction, and Fluid Management

The postoperative period is a critical juncture. Patients, though stabilized surgically, remain vulnerable to silent complications such as arrhythmias, fluid overload, acute kidney injury, and respiratory failure. AI-driven predictive analytics excel in this setting, transforming raw telemetry, laboratory, and imaging data into early warning systems.

9.4.1 Arrhythmia Surveillance and Prediction

Arrhythmias like atrial fibrillation (AF) can emerge unpredictably post-cardiac or major vascular surgery, posing risks of hemodynamic compromise and stroke. ML models can analyze continuous ECG telemetry, applying pattern recognition techniques to detect atrial ectopy patterns, changes in P-wave morphology, or RR interval variability that precede AF onset by hours. By alerting clinicians early, the ICU team can optimize electrolytes, initiate rate or rhythm control strategies, and prevent full-blown arrhythmic events.

9.4.2 Chest X-ray Analysis and Fluid Management

Chest radiographs are standard postoperative studies, especially after cardiac or thoracic interventions. AI-based image recognition quantifies pulmonary edema, identifies pleural effusions, and tracks subtle vascular redistribution. Integrating these imaging findings with hemodynamic data and fluid balance charts allows AI tools to optimize the presentation of this information to the clinician and recommend precise fluid titration and diuretic regimens, providing a reduction in CW and optimizing SA. The result is a more finely tuned fluid management strategy that minimizes the risk of acute kidney injury and respiratory compromise.

9.4.3 Three Postoperative Examples

Example 1: A patient recovering from valve replacement surgery shows subtle ECG changes and rising ventilator pressures. The AI platform correlates these findings, suggesting that early AF or fluid overload may be developing. Intervening early with beta blockers and diuretics prevents deterioration.

Example 2: In a post-liver transplant patient, AI-driven chest X-ray analysis detects incremental vascular congestion over 24 hours. By adjusting IV fluid rates and diuretics, the team averts acute respiratory distress.

Example 3: A patient with complex orthopedic trauma surgery remains sedated and ventilated. Continuous predictive modeling identifies a likelihood of impending atrial arrhythmias, guiding a prophylactic electrolyte correction and medication adjustment that stabilizes the patient's cardiac rhythm.

9.5 Data Integration, Storage, and Security in AI-Driven ICUs

The backbone of any AI implementation is data—continuous, reliable, and secure. Handling massive data streams from multiple devices and integrating them into a unified platform is nontrivial. Ensuring data quality, interoperability, and privacy is paramount.

9.5.1 Structured Data Pipelines

Effective pipelines begin with real-time data capture from bedside monitors, ventilators, infusion pumps, imaging systems, and laboratory information systems. Data cleaning, normalization, and preprocessing are essential before AI algorithms can interpret these signals. Adopting standards like FHIR enhances interoperability across EHR systems. Advanced data engineering tools ensure resiliency against missing data and noise, which are common in critical care environments.

9.5.2 Ethics, Bias, and Equity

AI systems risk embedding historical biases if their training datasets are not representative. For instance, arrhythmia prediction models must be validated on diverse populations to ensure equitable performance. Ethical frameworks and institutional review boards should oversee algorithm development, focusing on fairness and explainability. Continuous performance monitoring and recalibration against bias are essential, as inaccurate predictions in underrepresented groups can have dire consequences.

9.5.3 Three Examples of Robust Data Management

Example 1: A hospital implements a secure, cloud-based repository for high-frequency waveforms. With end-to-end encryption, role-based access controls, and regular audits, clinicians trust the integrity and confidentiality of patient data.

Example 2: An ICU in a large academic center employs a federated learning model. Instead of centralizing all patient data, the algorithm trains locally at each institution and aggregates learned parameters, preserving patient privacy while improving model generalizability.

Example 3: A rural trauma center invests in bias detection tools. Their arrhythmia prediction model is tested against demographic subsets, ensuring similar predictive accuracy for patients of different ages, ethnic backgrounds, and comorbidity profiles, thus maintaining equitable care standards.

9.6 Clinical Validation and Regulatory Considerations

No AI intervention should reach mainstream ICU practice without rigorous clinical validation and regulatory oversight. Clinical trials, prospective cohort studies, and real-world evidence generation ensure that the tools truly improve patient outcomes.

Simulated environments should be maximized in testing before, during, and even after implementation into the clinical environment. The NASA-TLX framework provides a quantifiable measure of CW by evaluating mental demand, temporal demand, and frustration levels, among other factors. Endsley's hierarchical SA model, encompassing the perception, comprehension, and projection of environmental elements, offers a robust lens for understanding the cognitive processes that underpin decision-making in high-stakes settings like the trauma bay or ICU.

9.6.1 Performance Metrics and Validation Studies

Performance must be judged against established benchmarks: sensitivity, specificity, positive predictive value, and net clinical benefit. Controlled trials can compare AI-assisted care against standard physician-led management, highlighting incremental improvements. Meta-analyses and systematic reviews provide a higher-level synthesis of evidence, guiding policymakers and hospital administrators in adopting proven solutions.

Hogan et al. leveraged SAGAT, as described by Endsley, to measure SA in a human patient simulated environment for trauma skills training and assessment(XX8). They found the SAGAT method to be valid and reliable in this scenario. SAGAT queries allow for detailed information about a subject's SA to be collected on an element-by-element basis that can be evaluated against reality, thus providing a more objective measure of operator SA. This is a direct measure of SA since it relies upon objective assessment of the operator's perception and understanding rather than upon observations and inferences of subject behavior. It does not require subjects or observers to make judgments or inferences about situation knowledge on a foundation of incomplete information, which subjective assessments often do. The SAGAT technique is suited for simulated environments since it relies upon multiple randomly spaced snapshots of operator SA across the full spectrum of operator SA. This method helps address potential problems with subject attention bias in that subjects cannot prepare for the queries in advance.

For SAGAT to provide relevant information regarding the operators SA, a detailed analysis of the situation scenarios must be performed in advance. This process is necessary to glean relevant queries for each situation. This requires the application of human factors goals and user analysis techniques to obtain insight into each subject's goals for any particular scenario (e.g., "Identify source of infection," or "Keep MAP above 65 mm Hg"). Queries are derived for each goal and subgoal that address projection (Level 3 SA), comprehension (Level 2 SA), and data (Level 1 SA). This process defines what is needed to effectively make decisions in the context of the operator's goals and subgoals. It is important to note that this analytical process is preferred over simple task analysis because goals, rather than tasks, form the basis of decision-making in complex and dynamic environments such as the SICU. The process seeks to identify what the operator would ideally need to know to arrive at the best decision. It is also important to note that the results of this type of analysis are technology independent and can be used to evaluate different tools (e.g., different displays derived from other groups' efforts) for their effect on SA in similar clinical scenarios.

Analysis of the SAGAT results obtained in the simulation lab can be used to validate AI tools that are most effective at optimizing SA.

9.6.2 The Regulatory Landscape

The U.S. FDA, European Medicines Agency (EMA), and other global regulatory bodies have begun establishing frameworks for AI-based Software as a Medical Device (SaMD). Requirements often include rigorous testing, transparency, documentation of training data, and post-market surveillance. Maintaining a feedback loop with regulatory agencies encourages iterative refinement and can accelerate market authorization.

9.6.3 Three Examples of Validation

Example 1: A multicenter randomized controlled trial tests an arrhythmia prediction tool in postoperative cardiac surgery patients. The tool reduces time-to-intervention by 30% and lowers severe arrhythmic event rates by 15%, satisfying FDA criteria for approval.

Example 2: A European consortium evaluates an AI model for trauma risk stratification across five countries. Consistent performance across diverse healthcare settings convinces the EMA of its robustness, paving the way for continental adoption.

Example 3: A hospital system implements continuous quality improvement cycles, where performance metrics are re-evaluated monthly. Adjustments to the model are documented and submitted to regulators, ensuring ongoing compliance and maintaining public trust.

9.7 Beyond Monitoring: Emerging Applications of AI in the ICU

While the current AI focus largely remains on monitoring, prediction, and decision support, the horizon extends far beyond these domains. Emerging applications include antimicrobial stewardship, sedation management, and even psychosocial interventions guided by AI insights.

9.7.1 Antimicrobial Stewardship and Infection Control

Predictive analytics can identify patients at high risk of sepsis or nosocomial infections earlier, prompting timely antibiotic administration or isolation measures. Similarly, AI can aid in antibiotic de-escalation when clinical and laboratory trends suggest resolution of infection. By balancing aggressive treatment with antibiotic stewardship, the ICU can curb the rise of multidrug-resistant organisms.

9.7.2 Sedation and Pain Management

Optimizing sedation to maintain patient comfort and safety is a delicate task. ML algorithms integrate patient vitals, ventilator settings, sedation scores, and EEG-based brain monitoring data to recommend precise dosing. Over-sedation risks delirium and prolonged ventilation, while under-sedation causes distress and agitation. AI-based sedation management can thus strike the optimal balance, improving both immediate comfort and long-term neurological outcomes.

9.7.3 Nutritional and Metabolic Guidance

Patients in the ICU often experience metabolic derangements. Integrating metabolomic profiles, glucose trends, and caloric intake data, AI tools can personalize nutritional plans. For example, a postoperative patient at risk of hyperglycemia and insulin resistance may benefit from algorithmically optimized feeding strategies, improving wound healing and recovery.

9.7.4 Three Emerging Examples

Example 1: A sepsis prediction model flags patients at risk hours before standard criteria are met. Prompt antibiotic and fluid resuscitation guided by AI reduces septic shock incidence and improves survival.

Example 2: A sedation management algorithm integrates EEG bispectral index (BIS) monitors with hemodynamic data, suggesting subtle dosage reductions of propofol. The patient awakens more alert and without agitation, facilitating timely extubation.

Example 3: Nutritional guidance algorithms incorporate metabolomic fingerprints and continuously updated insulin requirements. The patient recovers with better glycemic control, fewer complications, and improved muscle mass retention.

9.8 Future Directions: Continuous Learning and Personalization

As data lakes grow and computational techniques mature, AI models in the ICU will become adaptive, continuously learning from each patient encounter. Such systems transcend static protocols, evolving with changes in clinical practice, emerging pathogens, and patient demographics.

9.8.1 Continuous Learning Health Systems

Future AI-driven ICUs may leverage reinforcement learning, where algorithms learn from their own performance and user feedback. For instance, if an arrhythmia prediction tool repeatedly notes that certain electrolyte correction protocols yield better outcomes, it can self-calibrate, improving predictive accuracy over time. This dynamic adaptation nurtures a virtuous cycle of optimization.

9.8.2 Personalized, Precision Medicine

Integrating genomics, metabolomics, proteomics, and even microbiome data into AI models can tailor interventions at the molecular level. For a patient with a predisposition to malignant hyperthermia or drug hypersensitivities, personalized medicine guided by AI could suggest safer anesthetic regimens or prophylactic measures. Over time, these personalized predictions will refine risk stratification, therapeutic targeting, and long-term prognostication.

9.8.3 Three Examples of the Future ICU

Example 1: A hybrid cloud platform integrates global data on ICU patients with rare genetic conditions. The AI model learns from these cases, improving its ability to predict unique complications and tailor therapies.

Example 2: As an infectious disease evolves (e.g., a novel coronavirus), the ICU's AI system updates its sepsis and ventilation strategies based on early data from other centers. Continuous learning ensures the hospital remains agile in its response.

Example 3: Longitudinal patient monitoring, stretching beyond the ICU stay, provides feedback loops. Post-discharge outcomes inform the AI's recommendations for future similar patients, closing the gap between critical and post-acute care.

Highlights/Take-Home Messages for Readers

Rapid Triage and Intervention: AI streamlines trauma bay diagnostics, ensuring earlier recognition of critical injuries and timely activation of life-saving interventions.

Intraoperative Synergy: Real-time AI guidance in the OR anticipates hemodynamic instability, refines surgical navigation, and improves anesthetic management.

Predictive Postoperative Surveillance: Arrhythmia prediction and fluid management algorithms preempt destabilization, optimizing patient recovery and ICU throughput.

Robust Data and Ethical Foundations: Secure data pipelines, bias mitigation strategies, and adherence to regulatory standards form the ethical bedrock of AI implementations.

Expanding Horizons: From antimicrobial stewardship to sedation management and personalized care, the future AI-driven ICU continuously learns, adapts, and refines clinical decision-making.

References

1. Lynn LA. Artificial intelligence systems for complex decision-making in acute care medicine: a review. Patient Saf Surg. 2019;13:6.
2. Topol EJ. High-performance medicine: the convergence of human and artificial intelligence. Nat Med. 2019;25(1):44–56.
3. Esteva A, Robicquet A, Ramsundar B, Kuleshov V, DePristo M, Chou K, et al. A guide to deep learning in healthcare. Nat Med. 2019;25(1):24–9.
4. Johnson AEW, Ghassemi MM, Nemati S, Niehaus KE, Clifton DA, Clifford GD. Machine learning and decision support in critical care. Proc IEEE. 2020;108(1):83–102.
5. Sendak M, D'Arcy J, Kashyap S, Gao M, Nichols M, Corey KM, et al. A path for translation of machine learning products into healthcare delivery. EMJ Innov. 2020;4(1):78–84.
6. Kim H, Goo JM, Lee KH. Artificial intelligence in medical imaging: lung and chest. Korean J Radiol. 2020;21(7):837–47.
7. Komorowski M. Artificial intelligence in intensive care: are we there yet? Intensive Care Med. 2019;45(9):1298–300.
8. Ercole A, Standley T, Zaffuto M, Parker R, Menon DK, Harrison DA. Predicting trauma patient outcomes using automated machine learning methods. BMC Med Inform Decis Mak. 2021;21:142.
9. Gulshan V, Peng L, Coram M, Stumpe MC, Wu D, Narayanaswamy A, et al. Development and validation of a deep learning algorithm for detection of diabetic retinopathy in retinal fundus photographs. JAMA. 2016;316(22):2402–10.
10. U.S. Food and Drug Administration. Artificial Intelligence/Machine Learning (AI/ML)-Based Software as a Medical Device (SaMD) Action Plan. 2021. Available at: https://www.fda.gov/media/145022/download.
11. Churpek MM, Yuen TC, Park SY, Gibbons R, Edelson DP. Using electronic health record data to develop and validate a prediction model for adverse outcomes in the wards. Crit Care Med. 2014;42(4):841–8.
12. Belle A, Thiagarajan R, Soroushmehr SMR, Samarabandu J, LaRocca G, Najarian K. Big data analytics in healthcare. Biomed Res Int. 2015;2015:370194.
13. Stead WW, Lin HS, editors. Computational technology for effective health care: immediate steps and strategic directions. Washington, DC: The National Academies Press; 2009.
14. Hart SG, Staveland LE. Development of NASA-TLX (Task Load Index): results of empirical and theoretical research. In: Hancock PA, Meshkati N, editors. Advances in psychology, Vol. 52: human mental workload. North-Holland: Elsevier Science Publishers; 1988. p. 139–83.
15. Koppel R, Metlay JP, Cohen A, Abaluck B, Localio AR, Kimmel SE, Strom BL. Role of computerized physician order entry systems in facilitating medication errors. JAMA. 2005;293(10):1197–203.
16. Endsley MR. Toward a theory of situation awareness in dynamic systems. Hum Factors. 1995;37(1):32–64.
17. Jones DG, Endsley MR. Sources of situation awareness errors in aviation. Aviat Space Environ Med. 1996;67(6):507–12.
18. Singh H, Petersen LA, Thomas EJ. Understanding diagnostic errors in medicine: a lesson from aviation. Qual Saf Health Care. 2006;15(3):159–64.
19. Adams MJ, Tenney YJ, Pew RW. Situation awareness and the cognitive management of complex systems. Hum Factors. 1995;37(1):85–104.
20. Hogan MP, Pace DE, Hapgood J, Boone DC. Use of human patient simulation and the situation awareness global assessment technique in practical trauma skills assessment. J Trauma. 2006;61(5):1047–52.

10 Introduction to Telemedicine/Teleconsultation/Teletriage and Its Impact on Acute Care, Trauma, and Emergency Surgery (Challenges, Regulatory Considerations, and Future Directions)

Evika Karamagioli, Anastasia Pikouli,
Ioanna Antonopoulou, and Eleni Chatzi

10.1 The Evolution and Expanding Role of Telemedicine in Modern Healthcare

Telemedicine (TM), a term first introduced in the 1970s, refers to the remote provision of healthcare services utilizing information and communication technologies (ICT) [27]. It encompasses a wide array of methodologies, including store-and-forward consultations, home-based monitoring with direct patient interaction, and interprofessional communication for specialized medical advice. The evolution of telemedicine is intricately linked to its integration into the multidisciplinary domain of healthcare, which leverages ICTs to facilitate remote diagnosis, treatment, prevention, and education [263]. Although telemedicine has been in practice for over six decades, its widespread adoption experienced a notable acceleration during the COVID-19 pandemic. This surge in adoption was largely due to the ability of telemedicine to alleviate travel burdens and reduce the risk of interpersonal exposure [99]. The pandemic served as a pivotal moment, prompting an extensive body of literature that highlights the rapid expansion of telehealth services [241].

E. Karamagioli (✉) · E. Chatzi
Disaster Medicine, Medical School, National and Kapodistrian University of Athens, Athens, Greece

A. Pikouli
3rd Department of Surgery, University Hospital "Attikon", National and Kapodistrian University of Athens, Athens, Greece

I. Antonopoulou
National and Kapodistrian University of Athens, Athens, Greece

B. De Simone et al. (eds.), *New Technologies, Precision Medicine, and AI in Emergency General Surgery*, Hot Topics in Acute Care Surgery and Trauma,
https://doi.org/10.1007/978-3-032-09357-8_10

Telemedicine and telehealth have long demonstrated effectiveness in various aspects of healthcare, including routine medical and surgical care, primary healthcare, and specialized consultations. Their utility extends beyond conventional medical settings, playing a crucial role in critical scenarios such as disasters, remote regions, and resource-limited environments [136]. Despite their well-documented advantages, widespread acceptance of telemedicine among healthcare professionals has been a challenge. However, the COVID-19 pandemic significantly accelerated telemedicine's adoption, focusing on its indispensable role in modern healthcare. Recent studies have emphasized telemedicine's role in overcoming geographical and logistical barriers, particularly in acute care settings where timely intervention is essential for patient outcomes. The adoption of telemedicine in trauma, emergency care, and surgery has shown substantial growth in recent years, representing considerable progress in healthcare provision [64].

The modern era of telemedicine began with remote physiological monitoring for NASA's Mercury Space Program in the late 1950s [63], with video technology later being used for psychiatric consultations between the Norfolk State Hospital and the Nebraska Psychiatric Institute [32]. Interest in telemedicine grew rapidly in the context of disaster management [181] and battlefield medicine [54]. One of the major transformations brought about by telemedicine is the increased accessibility of healthcare services, especially in overcoming geographical barriers. Initiatives like telehealth vans, which provide consultations, diagnostics, and teletherapy services, shift healthcare delivery from traditional brick-and-mortar structures to more equitable and inclusive models [4, 67]. Over the years, telemedicine's scope has expanded beyond remote consultations to include telediagnostics, telemonitoring, and teletherapy [27, 72, 271].

Technological advancements have since expanded telemedicine's applications across various specialties, where it has primarily been studied for feasibility and resource utilization [262]. Telemedicine techniques have been employed in psychiatry [214], neurology [211], primary care [42], radiology [163], and emergency medicine [265]. Additionally, telemedicine's capabilities have expanded with the rise of technologies such as wearable devices, digital health records, and mobile health applications, broadening its reach in modern healthcare delivery [179]. The integration of Artificial Intelligence (AI) into telemedicine marks a significant shift in healthcare, offering improvements in diagnostic precision, treatment planning, and overall system efficiency. Machine learning algorithms, a core component of AI, are increasingly being used to analyze extensive datasets, enabling early disease detection and personalized treatment strategies [237].

Rural and remote populations face significant challenges in accessing specialized medical services, which contributes to poorer patient outcomes, higher mortality rates, and a greater incidence of preventable deaths [261]. This disparity in healthcare access between rural and urban populations stresses the critical equity and accessibility issues, particularly in areas such as emergency care and obstetrics [48, 159]. For instance, rural populations experience a threefold greater risk of mortality within the emergency department [92]. Telemedicine has emerged as a potential solution to bridge this gap by offering remote consultations and monitoring services, especially for rural and underserved populations, which often face barriers such as limited healthcare facilities, socioeconomic challenges, and mobility issues. Virtual consultations, by reducing travel distances and associated costs, can alleviate these difficulties [28]. Furthermore, telemedicine has been shown to decrease hospital readmissions, prevent unnecessary emergency department visits, and increase the availability of critical care beds. By providing regular monitoring and consultations, telemedicine enhances accessibility to healthcare for vulnerable groups, such as the elderly and those with chronic conditions, helping to address healthcare inequalities and improve health outcomes [57].

The integration of telemedicine and AI into emergency medicine, for example, can significantly improve clinical decision-making and extend the reach of healthcare professionals to underserved regions [51]. The incorporation of virtual reality (VR) and augmented reality (AR) into telemedicine has transformed both medical training and patient care. VR immerses healthcare professionals in simulated clinical environments, allowing for realistic training in surgical procedures, emergency interventions, and medical decision-making without exposing patients to risk [233]. AR, in contrast, overlays digital information onto real-world settings, assisting healthcare providers during medical procedures by highlighting anatomical structures and displaying real-time patient data [120].

Telemedicine's transformation aligns with the principles of patient-centered care by tailoring healthcare solutions to individual needs. Culturally competent telehealth services ensure that healthcare delivery is accessible and adapted to diverse population preferences, making telemedicine an effective tool for reducing healthcare disparities [4]. Telemedicine empowers patients by placing them at the center of their care, enabling virtual consultations where individuals can actively engage in their healthcare journey, discuss symptoms, ask questions, and participate in decision-making. This collaborative approach improves patient satisfaction and health outcomes [29]. By considering individual preferences and values, telemedicine also promotes patient education and self-management. Through remote monitoring, educational materials, and guidance on lifestyle modifications, patients gain a better understanding of their health conditions and are encouraged to adhere to treatment plans [189]. Enhanced communication between patients and healthcare providers, facilitated by secure messaging platforms and virtual consultations, reduces communication barriers, ensuring timely feedback and continuous supportive healthcare relationships.

Telemedicine is defined as the use of information and communication technologies to deliver healthcare remotely, aligning with the World Health Organization's (WHO) characterization [179]. While the terms telemedicine and telehealth are often used interchangeably, it is important to differentiate between them. Telehealth refers to a broader range of remote health-related activities and services facilitated through ICT, aimed at dismantling barriers and improving public health outcomes [9]. Telemedicine, as a subset of telehealth, focuses specifically on the remote delivery of health services by professionals for promotion, prevention, diagnosis, treatment, and rehabilitation, ultimately improving accessibility and timeliness of care [9].

Telemedicine has become an essential tool in emergency response, offering numerous advantages such as improved quality of treatment, increased efficiency, and enhanced access to care [39]. The adoption of telemedicine in emergency settings has accelerated due to advancements in digital health technologies and the increasing demand for scalable healthcare solutions. Survey studies have pointed out benefits such as reduced patient wait times and improved coordination between healthcare providers [107]. This paper reviews telemedicine practices in acute care, trauma, and emergency services.

10.1.1 Teletrauma: Bridging the Gap in Trauma Care Between Rural and Urban Settings

The effective management of trauma patients necessitates prompt, coordinated care, appropriate access to resources, and specialized expertise [160]. In trauma scenarios, rapid action is critical to achieving positive patient outcomes. Unfortunately, trauma centers are often concentrated in urban areas, leaving rural populations underserved [145]. Injuries impose a substantial healthcare burden on a global scale, with trauma being responsible for a significant part of fatalities. Inequities in the availability of specialized trauma care are present, especially in rural regions, where the scarcity of experience and resources impedes prompt responses [137]. Telemedicine has been shown to improve the quality and timeliness of emergency care, particularly in rural areas, by reducing the time to essential procedures like electrocardiograms and fibrinolysis for myocardial infarction patients [55].

A growing body of literature supports telemedicine's role in evaluating and managing acutely injured patients [142, 254, 259]. Telemedicine, particularly the practice of "teletrauma," provides a solution by linking rural hospitals with trauma specialists at prominent centers, enabling expert assessment and enhancing the delivery of care. This concept shows potential in connecting rural and urban trauma care, guaranteeing prompt access to sophisticated resources and knowledge [80, 135]. The term "teletrauma" refers to the use of telehealth technologies in trauma care and management. However, only a few studies have used the term "teletrauma" to describe a telehealth system specifically designed for trauma care. Instead, many studies have labeled their telehealth services based on the technology used, such as tele-ultrasound, teleradiology, and telesonography. While these systems serve similar functions, they are named according to their diagnostic or technological focus. Despite the lack of a clear definition, any telehealth technology used during the management of traumatic injuries can be broadly classified as "teletrauma," regardless of its specific focus, such as sonography, basic consultations, or airway management. In conclusion, the inconsistency in terminology related to teletrauma may hinder the synthesis of knowledge in this area [268].

Trauma is considered a surgical subspecialty, frequently managed at high-level designated trauma centers with trained trauma experts and requiring multiple subspecialty resources. For example, MacKenzie et al. [146] reported a reduction in mortality among moderate to severely injured patients receiving care at designated

Level 1 trauma centers compared to non-trauma centers. Yet, severe injuries occur broadly, with patients often presenting initially to rural or outlying hospitals for evaluation and stabilization, where they are managed by clinicians with varying degrees of trauma training (including nurse practitioners, family physicians, or emergency medicine physicians). Secondary transfers to higher-level trauma centers introduce additional risks and resource burdens. Numerous opportunities exist to compromise trauma resuscitation through errors of omission, commission, and misprioritization, which can be life-threatening.

Similarly, Duchesne et al. [66] demonstrated that telemedicine reduced transfer rates while increasing injury severity scores and reducing emergency department stays, with no difference in mortality. Aucar et al. [22] demonstrated high concordance in trauma assessments, supporting the potential for telemedicine to improve trauma management. Ricci et al. [200] found that telemedicine reduced discrepancies in trauma care, while Rogers et al. [207] reported that telemedicine consultations improved early trauma care in rural settings. Alser et al. [12] examined WhatsApp-based telemedicine used to support surgical teams at Nasser Medical Complex in Gaza amid ongoing military assaults. Between January 28 and February 12, 2024, 12 patient cases were analyzed, with 92% sustaining penetrating injuries and 33% being children. A global network of over 1000 specialists provided remote guidance, enhancing clinical decision-making despite extreme resource limitations.

Remote evaluation of trauma resuscitation began with the use of video recordings as a teaching tool [104] and later as a quality assurance tool using an ATLS-based protocol [21]. Despite its potential, the use of telemedicine in trauma care has received relatively little scientific scrutiny. A recent white paper from the American College of Surgeons states that telemedicine can be instrumental for rapid expert consultations in emergent situations, potentially guiding on-site staff in urgent surgical interventions and improving patient outcomes [118]. However, applying telemedicine to acute trauma care presents challenges due to its broader scope and lack of predetermined diagnoses; while proponents emphasize its benefits, including improved diagnostic efficiency, better-informed therapeutic decisions, and optimized transfer processes, there are concerns that remote evaluation may lead to overdiagnosis, missed injuries, inappropriate interventions, increased diagnostic costs, or unnecessary transfers. Resolving these conflicting viewpoints will require well-structured quantitative studies [118].

Kamine et al. [113] evaluated the feasibility of a teletrauma surgery consultation service between Level I trauma centers (LITC) and rural and community hospitals (RCH). Over 5 months, TACS surgeons provided remote consultations for 21 trauma patients, reducing unnecessary transfers. Six patients were discharged, four were admitted locally, and nine were directly admitted to LITC. There were no missed injuries, complications, or deaths, and only one 30-day readmission. Both RCH providers and TACS surgeons reported high levels of satisfaction. The study demonstrated that teletrauma consultations can effectively reduce resource use while maintaining quality care.

The study by Wood et al. [268] explored user perspectives on the factors influencing the use of teletrauma in rural areas, specifically focusing on northern British Columbia. The analysis of 14 qualitative interviews revealed four key themes: the context of teletrauma in rural settings, factors that facilitate its use, its role in team-based care, and the interconnectedness of the healthcare system. Key facilitators for teletrauma adoption included user-friendly technology, the flexibility of teletrauma systems, and strong interprofessional relationships. However, barriers such as technological complexity, lack of familiarity with the system, and workflow disruptions at consulting sites were also identified. While the study discussed the potential of teletrauma to improve care in remote areas, it emphasized that these challenges must be addressed for successful integration into clinical practice.

10.1.2 Teletriage Systems in Emergency Healthcare

Major accidents, such as rail accidents, and major disasters, such as hurricanes and typhoons, have caused injuries to many patients [206]. In these cases, triage provides an easy-to-use, scalable, and durable information collection infrastructure. Telemedicine facilitates real-time communication between on-site responders and off-site specialists, aiding in timely decision-making and enhancing patient care during emergencies [8]. Similarly, mHealth apps support efficient triage, patient tracking, and resource management, which are crucial for effective disaster response [2]. Portable diagnostic tools, such as point-of-care ultrasound, enable rapid injury assessment and improved treatment decisions in the field [46].

The triage process helps rapidly evaluate patients affected by disasters, identify response capabilities required, and manage assets when they arrive on the scene [206]. Patient prioritization is carried out to provide each patient with healthcare services at the right time. Based on the severity of the condition and vital signs of patients, rescuers determine the treatment and transportation priorities during the first phase of operation. In this phase, immediate life-saving treatments are administered to the most affected victims; patients are then identified, labeled, and followed up [270].

Patients in critical conditions in local and emergency department (ED) queues are prioritized [125]. The automation of this process can significantly improve the quality of care and hospitalization of patients, ultimately saving lives. Emergency departments (EDs) are frequently overcrowded, and trained staff utilize triage systems to ensure timely treatment for patients with the most urgent needs [168]. This technology enables physicians to conduct triage remotely, helping to prioritize rescue operations by tending to the most critical patients [273].

Teletriage primarily addresses how medical data, such as vital signs (heart rate, temperature, etc.), are prioritized and transmitted through telecommunication networks in healthcare settings. Since medical data can vary significantly in urgency and importance, proper prioritization (or triaging) is essential to ensure that critical information is transmitted first, especially in emergencies or high-congestion situations [170]. Quality of service (QoS) is crucial for prioritizing data flows based on urgency. QoS mechanisms ensure reliable transmission of critical data, particularly in telemedicine applications like telecardiology, where real-time communication is necessary [73].

One potential goal of remote triage centers is to achieve case resolution during the initial contact. Studies have shown that local, practice-based telephone triage services tend to achieve a higher percentage of case resolution compared to regional or national systems [52, 202]. The impact of telephone triage on healthcare service utilization, particularly in primary care (PC) services and emergency department (ED) visits, has been widely studied. A systematic review by Boggan et al. [33] revealed that only one study [166], a controlled before-and-after study with a high risk of bias (ROB), showed a reduction in PC service utilization due to the telephone triage system. In contrast, four other studies [41, 155, 245, 201] reported statistically significant increases in PC utilization when telephone triage was used. Interestingly, no significant difference was found in ED visits between telephone triage and in-person consultations, suggesting that telephone triage does not increase ED utilization [52, 203]. On the other hand, a study by Langabeer et al. [133] found that a telehealth-enabled emergency medical services (EMS) program led to a 6.7% reduction in unnecessary ambulance transports to urban EDs, while improving EMS efficiency by allowing paramedic units to return to service an average of 44 min faster.

Distant patient consultation, mobile triage technology, remote diagnostics, and other mobile technology services significantly reduce the burden on healthcare providers by enabling more efficient care delivery. These technologies, such as portable emergency telemedicine systems that utilize wireless networks, facilitate real-time data exchange, allowing physicians to monitor patients remotely [38]. For instance, Hong et al. [103] developed a portable emergency telemedicine system over wireless networks, using personal digital assistants (PDAs) for video, biosignal, message, and triage data exchange. This system allowed reliable patient monitoring and data sharing, improving the efficiency of remote care. The research by Clark et al. [49] demonstrates how teletriage systems can enhance resource utilization, especially in burn care, by ensuring that inpatient care is directed toward patients with more severe burns, resulting in a 17% reduction in short-stay admissions. Similarly, Tuetken et al. [243] applied a teletriage protocol in an emergency department setting, which improved triage consistency, reduced patient wait times, and led to fewer patients leaving without being seen (LWBS). This protocol contributed to improved workflow and patient outcomes despite occasional staffing shortages. Moreover, Meer [157] explored the use of a symptom checker using a computerized neural network on a tablet PC, which recommended appropriate triage levels based on patients' self-assessments. This system showed no hazardous undertriage instances, aligning with the reliability of technology-driven triage approaches.

However, while these advancements show promise, the conclusion of Lake et al.'s [130] review is that telephone triage and advice services (TTAS) have yet to provide conclusive evidence on certain aspects, such as service access, costs, and clinical outcomes. The review emphasizes that factors like healthcare context, demographics, and system integration significantly impact the effectiveness of TTAS.

Studies have also examined the effects of telemedicine consultations on children in the highest triage category, as these patients are most likely to receive treatment below current standards. The impact of telemedicine critical care consultations on the quality of care for acutely ill and injured children in rural areas has been investigated [62]. During disasters, hospitals can be overwhelmed, and pediatric specialists, who care for injured children, are often insufficient. Telemedicine has played a crucial role in pediatric emergency treatment by assisting in efficient triage and decreasing needless transfers to referral institutions [246, 247]. The additive effects of a telemedicine program and a hospital system on pediatric patients have been evaluated in a community hospital [129]. Researchers assumed that implementing a telemedicine program for pediatric consultation and a hospital program for pediatric hospital care in a community hospital would improve the identification of patients requiring continuous intensive care. As a result, the rate of transfer to higher levels of care was reduced. A study by Sarria Guerrero et al. [216] found that pediatric telephone triage and televisits significantly influenced emergency department (ED) utilization, with 46% of parents changing their initial decision to visit the ED after consultation. High compliance (76%) with recommendations and a satisfaction rating of 4.8 out of 5 highlighted the effectiveness of this approach. While telephone triage successfully directed patients to appropriate care, moderate concordance existed between phone-assigned and ED-confirmed severity levels. Overtriage often occurred when primary care services were unavailable, while undertriage was linked to communication difficulties and symptom misinterpretation.

Remote acute clinical triage centers are becoming increasingly common, particularly in larger healthcare organizations. These centers use varied contact methods and staffing models, aiming to improve access while reducing barriers such as distance, cost, and time for both patients and providers. Such centers also serve as an effective approach to prevent costly ED and urgent care visits by providing timely primary care (PC) advice [33]. A portable emergency telemedicine system over wireless networks has been developed, enabling video, biosignal, message, and triage data exchange with reliable patient information [103]. Additionally, web-based triage has been identified as an innovative and cost-saving system for patient empowerment, maintaining or improving treatment quality while minimizing unnecessary doctor visits and reducing healthcare costs [175]. A non-invasive radio frequency (RF) device can be used for heart rate (HR) and HR variability (HRV) monitoring, helping confirm individual identities prior to rescue efforts [94]. Furthermore, emergency department (ED) physician telemedical triage has been shown to improve operational metrics such as length of stay and time to physician evaluation [239] . Another study developed a computer-assisted self-triage instrument from a pen-and-paper version, validated for use in the ophthalmic emergency department [71]. A secure web-based computer imaging program, compliant with the Health Insurance Portability and Accountability Act (HIPAA), can help reduce unnecessary patient transfers and promote timely decision-making [164]. This system allows neurosurgeons to examine digital brain and spine images when a referring doctor applies for consultation or patient transfer. ECG transmission data and routine checkup results are collected and referred for primary percutaneous coronary intervention. For early diagnosis, decision-makers should receive an ECG diagnosis for patients with acute coronary syndromes, ensuring ideal reperfusion triage initiation for patients with ST-elevation myocardial infarction. This emergency triage can also extend to cardiology diagnoses, especially non-ST-elevation cases [50].

Wearable health monitoring devices have been explored to alleviate the burden on primary care, using simulation models to assess vital signs and consultation times [194]. Real-time HR signals and sensor data fusion, including temperature and blood pressure, are processed via Xbee modules for RF transmission [83]. A web server enables healthcare providers to access patient data, send daily heartbeat files, and support long-term monitoring and atrial fibrillation detection. A multi-priority queue model efficiently manages high- and low-priority data [255]. ECG data is prioritized using wavelet packet decomposition, optimizing bandwidth in wireless networks [119]. The Ad hoc On-Demand Distance Vector (AODV) routing protocol prioritizes critical data transmission, considering energy constraints in wireless body area networks (WBANs) [167]. Telemedicine transmission over wireless cellular networks has gained importance due to its ability to carry critical patient information. High priority is given to multimedia telemedicine traffic, particularly ECG data, which is encoded with priorities based on cardiac activities of interest [193]. A protocol for traffic control was developed, prioritizing ECG data using algorithms that define minimum priority levels for each area [100]. This protocol, integrated into middleware, manages burst traffic effects and uses cellular network location information to control transmission from a home broker to the patient. Data is triaged into non-real-time (normal health status) and soft-real-time (critical conditions) categories, with case studies on ad hoc sensor networks proposed for patient monitoring [226]. The performance of a multi-sensor remote monitoring system was evaluated using real-time operating systems (RTOS) versus general-purpose operating systems (GPOS), with RTOS providing better prioritization of high-priority tasks ([205], as cited in [23]). Internet of Things (IoT) systems also monitor patients at home using personal healthcare devices (PHDs), allowing medical staff to track emergency conditions [184]. EMPaD, a method for increasing track diversity while reducing traffic, was proposed to manage emergency messages in triage scenes, though node increases can lead to delays due to traffic [236].

From an organizational perspective, Boggan et al. [33] concluded that the organization of triage systems, including general practitioner (GP)-led after-hours care, deputizing services, and off-site triage, does not appear to have a significant impact on primary care utilization or emergency department visits. Comparative studies of different triage models, such as NHS Direct and GP cooperative telephone triage, indicate that there are minimal differences in patient outcomes and service utilization. Comparisons between centralized and decentralized triage systems, such as NHS Direct versus local GP services, reveal no substantial differences in patient referral rates or case resolution, indicating that both approaches can be effective [52, 166, 203].

The integration of telemedicine with triage processes has been emphasized for its cost-effectiveness, speed, and ease of operation, making it a valuable tool in emergency surgical settings [37]. In addition, web-based triage has emerged as an innovative and cost-saving system that empowers patients, maintains or improves treatment quality, minimizes unnecessary doctor visits, and reduces healthcare costs [170]. A telemedicine program involving emergency department physicians in triage has proven responsive and cost-effective, yielding positive results for both doctors and patients [235]. The rapid delivery of patient measurements is crucial for providing reliable data in emergency care [86].

10.1.3 Teleconsultation in Acute Care

Telemedicine has played a crucial role in trauma and emergency management, delivering effective care through telehealth consultations across various disciplines [242]. Teleconsultation refers to the use of information and communication technologies to facilitate either real-time or delayed consultations, aiming to overcome geographical and functional barriers in healthcare. It enables diagnostics and treatment exchanges between healthcare providers—such as physicians and nurses—or between providers and patients [36]. The broader term "remote consultation," as defined in Medical Subject Headings (MeSH), describes a consultation that occurs via telecommunications, typically for diagnosing or treating a patient who is located far from their primary healthcare provider [171]. Wang et al. [256] analyzed 11,987 telemedicine consultations in China and found that telemedicine frequently led to changes in diagnosis, treatment, and additional diagnostic work.

A review of the literature indicates that "teleconsultation" is frequently used in three primary contexts. The first is provider-to-provider communication, which occurs when both participants are healthcare professionals. This includes physician-to-physician consultations, often sought for second opinions [6, 75, 221], and physician-to-primary care provider (PCP) interactions, including communications with nurses [128]. The second context is provider-to-patient communication, where one party is a healthcare provider, and the other is a patient. This includes direct physician-patient consultations for telemonitoring or remote visits [198] and PCP-patient interactions, which involve virtual care provided by nurses or other primary care professionals [238]. The third context is tripartite communication, which involves a physician, a PCP, and a patient all being involved in the consultation process [238].

Studies have shown that teleconsulting systems can significantly reduce the number of patients requiring physical specialist consultations before surgical procedures, streamlining the process and improving efficiency [257]. The study by Accorsi [3] examined the use of direct-to-consumer telemedicine for managing acute respiratory tract infections (RTIs) during the COVID-19 pandemic in Brazil. It showed that telemedicine consultations, supported by digital tablets and HIPAA-compliant platforms, were as effective as face-to-face evaluations in the emergency department. Telemedicine consultations had similar diagnostic accuracy and test ordering rates, with the added benefit of fewer antibiotic prescriptions and shorter emergency department stays. Latifi et al. [138] reported that 77% of trauma patients receiving telemedicine consultations were transferred, with some undergoing surgery and others receiving non-operative care, with certain interventions considered life-saving. Mohr et al. [161] indicated that telemedicine consultations led to a 30% reduction in emergency department length of stay for transferred trauma patients. Waran et al. [258] and Ashkenazi et al. [20] used mobile phone image transfer and teleradiology for neurosurgical consultations, respectively, showing that telemedicine can aid remote diagnosis and treatment. Villa [251] examined the use of teledermatology through a store-and-forward method, where emergency physicians captured and transmitted images of skin lesions to dermatologists for remote evaluation. The study found complete agreement between telemedicine-based and in-person diagnoses, reinforcing telemedicine's diagnostic reliability.

Surgeons have increasingly embraced telemedicine for postoperative follow-up, showcasing its feasibility and acceptance among patients [172]. Furthermore, telemedicine has been instrumental in broadening access to vascular surgery care during the pandemic [44]. During the COVID-19 pandemic, teleconsultation played a critical role in maintaining essential surgical services while minimizing the risk of infection. Many healthcare facilities resorted to teleconsultations to manage oncological emergencies and prioritize high-priority surgeries, ensuring continuity of care amidst challenging circumstances [162]. This shift toward telemedicine has been a transformative change in healthcare delivery, emphasizing the importance of remote consultations to safeguard both patients and healthcare providers [145].

In rural areas, such as much of the United States [97], as well as in regions of Australia, Europe, Canada, and Africa with sparse populations [140], distances between healthcare facilities can limit access to care. Video consultation (VC) can alleviate the need for travel, thus improving access to essential healthcare. Video consultation (VC) is a form of telehealth that enables real-time visual and audio communication [123], offering a means to provide medical support to underserved regions. As a result, many healthcare responsibilities, especially in rural areas, have shifted from hospitals to primary care settings [264]. However, the potential role of VC in reducing healthcare disparities and whether it may inadvertently exacerbate them remains an open question that requires urgent exploration [58, 150].

Systematic reviews examining patient satisfaction with telehealth, including VC, generally show a positive effect [127, 180]. However, some studies indicate that both patients and healthcare professionals prefer face-to-face consultations over VC, if given the choice [248]. When comparing the content and quality of VC consultations to telephone consultations in primary care, the outcomes are generally comparable, although VC may offer advantages, such as enhanced rapport building [96]. Increasing evidence showcases the importance of patient involvement in healthcare improvements [224], and there is a recognized gap in understanding patient perspectives in the study of telemedicine effectiveness [72].

The increasing availability of technology, such as video-conferencing equipment, has transformed the nature of patient-provider interactions. Despite this, there remains limited insight into patients' views on this emerging mode of care [154]. Given the rising use of VC, particularly in rural settings, further research is needed to better understand this communication solution. Clear and consistent communication between healthcare professionals and patients is essential for patient engagement in emergency care visits [78]. In rural primary healthcare settings, patient experiences with specialist care via VC have shown that effective communication is critical for ensuring a sense of safety during consultations [111]. However, rural healthcare providers often lack adequate training or experience relevant to rural practice [1], while a systematic review by Sharifi Kia et al. [223] analyzing telemedicine in emergency departments found that while real-time video conferencing is preferred, technical and infrastructural challenges persist. The relationship between patients and healthcare providers, particularly with local registered nurses (RNs), is also a crucial factor in rural eHealth contexts [144].

In the literature, the most prevalent VC application in emergency care is the connection between rural hospitals and urban emergency departments for consultations between physicians [165]. The use of VC in emergency care has been studied for various acute conditions, such as psychiatric emergencies [240] and acute stroke [117, 232], though there are few studies focusing on VC in emergency care within rural primary care settings [65, 158]. In northern rural Sweden, residents have access to primary care through small community hospitals and emergency care with general practitioners via VC, although its effectiveness has not yet been evaluated [65].

Janssen et al. [110] conducted a study to evaluate the use of telemedicine, specifically audiovisual consultation (AVC), in providing on-call backup services within a general neurology department of an acute care hospital. The study aimed to address the increasing need for specialist support, especially during nighttime hours when hospital specialists may be in short supply. The findings demonstrated that AVC was valuable in enhancing the quality and safety of care, particularly in emergency situations. It led to a change in diagnosis in more than half of the cases when compared to traditional telephone consultations. Additionally, AVC was found to improve diagnostic accuracy, especially for stroke cases. Despite the positive outcomes, the study also pointed out that directly talking to patients and reviewing their history was as important as performing a clinical examination in many instances. McCormick et al. [152] examined the impact of a teleneurology (TN) program on hospital performance, focusing on the time it took to complete consultations, inpatient length of stay (LOS), and transfer rates to tertiary care. They found that after implementing the TN program, the time from consult request to completion significantly decreased, and the median length of stay for patients was reduced by about 28%. Despite these improvements, there was no notable change in the percentage of patients discharged home or transferred to other hospitals for specialized care. The study concluded that TN consultations helped speed up the process of care and reduced the length of hospital stays, making it a valuable tool for improving hospital efficiency. Libreros-Peña et al. [143] conducted a study that explored the implementation and clinical outcomes of telemedicine consultations in an emergency department at a high-complexity university hospital in Latin America. The study found that telemedicine significantly enhanced access to emergency care, reduced patient waiting times, and alleviated pressure on emergency departments, particularly during the COVID-19 pandemic.

Ärlebrant et al. [17] examined patient experiences with video consultations (VC) for emergency care in rural Sweden, reporting both positive and negative feedback. Patients appreciated the sense of teamwork with the local registered nurse (RN) and general practitioner (GP), especially when the RN was competent in facilitating the consultation. However, some patients found VC inadequate, particularly when remote assessments were not sufficient, leading to additional travel for in-person care. The rural context added complexity, as long travel distances and logistical challenges were common. While many valued the convenience of VC, others expressed dissatisfaction due to the lack of direct interaction with the GP. Moreover, telemedicine has been effectively utilized for teleconsults in neurological emergencies, such as traumatic brain injuries, and in telestroke scenarios, where it aids in assessing the risks and benefits of local thrombolytic therapy administration [185]. Telemedicine has proven particularly beneficial in scenarios such as orthopedic emergencies requiring urgent interventions like decompressive fasciotomy. Studies have also demonstrated the acceptability of teleconsultation among patients and clinicians in various surgical specialties, including oral and maxillofacial surgery, featuring its potential as a viable alternative to traditional face-to-face assessments [267].

Dharmar et al. [62] and Nadar et al. [169] both demonstrate the potential of telemedicine in enhancing clinical outcomes in pediatric acute care settings, but they approach the topic from different angles. Dharmar et al. [62] focused on rural emergency departments, where telemedicine consultations led to significant improvements in care quality, diagnosis accuracy, and therapeutic interventions. Their study found that telemedicine consultations led to more frequent changes in diagnosis and treatment compared to telephone consultations, with improved parental satisfaction. However, it lacked long-term outcome measures and did not explore the reasons behind the differences observed between telemedicine and telephone consultations. On the other hand, Nadar et al. [169] conducted a systematic review evaluating synchronous telemedicine in pediatric ICUs, neonatal ICUs, and emergency departments. Their findings indicated that telemedicine improved care quality, reduced transfer rates, shortened length of stay, and decreased complications and illness severity.

10.1.4 Telemonitoring

Remote patient monitoring (RPM), also referred to as telemonitoring, involves recording and transmitting patient biometrics, vital signs, or disease-related data to healthcare providers using information and communication technologies. The data collected is typically disease-specific and commonly includes measures such as blood pressure, weight, heart rate, respiration rate, pulse oximetry, spirometry, temperature, blood glucose levels, or specific symptoms [147]. RPM data can be collected automatically (e.g., by implanted or wearable devices) or manually (e.g., by patients using peripheral devices and a transmission hub). RPM interventions for cardiovascular disease (CVD) can be either invasive or non-invasive. Remote patient monitoring (RPM) has also gained prominence with the widespread adoption of wearable devices and biosensors, enabling continuous tracking of vital signs and other health metrics [234]. RPM plays a crucial role in chronic disease management, allowing for ongoing assessment of patients without necessitating frequent hospital visits [177].

Invasive RPM interventions involve direct measurement of biometric data, such as heart rate and pulmonary artery pressures, typically from implanted devices. These devices, including pacemakers and implantable cardioverter defibrillators (ICDs), transmit data to healthcare providers [186]. Non-invasive interventions involve the transmission of data like body weight, blood pressure, or pulse oximetry [249], commonly used in patients requiring long-term self-management support (e.g., heart failure patients) [108]. Wearable technologies, such as smartwatches and fitness trackers, provide real-time data that can be transmitted to healthcare providers, facilitating timely interventions and personalized care strategies. The integration of biosensors into these devices enhances their utility, particularly in monitoring chronic conditions like diabetes, cardiovascular diseases, and respiratory disorders [187].

RPM data can be reviewed either actively (when healthcare providers regularly monitor data) or passively (when healthcare providers are only alerted if data readings exceed a clinical threshold). Interventions resulting from abnormal readings may include telephone support, video consultations, or home visits. Chronic diseases are often associated with high rates of unplanned hospital use, especially when comorbid conditions are present [101]. This incurs substantial costs to the healthcare system. For example, in Australia, nearly half of all potentially avoidable hospitalizations are due to chronic conditions like congestive cardiac failure, diabetes complications, COPD, and angina [24]. Early detection and proactive management of chronic disease exacerbations may reduce costly acute hospital admissions [132].

Research has shown that RPM can alert healthcare teams to declines in patients' conditions, allowing for issues to be resolved outside of hospitals, thus reducing the need for urgent hospital admissions [222]. Existing studies have shown that for RPM to be cost-effective, it must reduce acute hospital use. Many disease-specific reviews (e.g., heart failure and COPD) have demonstrated the impact of RPM on hospital use, though these are often secondary outcomes [108]. Additionally, there is a gap in research related to newer technologies like implanted devices and other diseases, and more frequent literature reviews are warranted [234]. A 2024 study in France found that 90% of citizens had used telemedicine services, with 70% actively engaging with the telemedicine platform. Among these users, 74% recognized its positive impact on integrated care and telemonitoring French Ministry of Health, as cited in [115].

The largest study on RPM to date found that it was associated with reduced all-cause hospitalizations, particularly for patients with cardiac resynchronization therapy, suggesting greater benefits for those with more severe conditions [188]. The continuous biometric data collection provided by invasive RPM technologies tends to offer greater effectiveness than non-invasive methods, which provide only intermittent measurements. RPM also enhances the safety of implanted devices [10]. Notably, no study reviewed reported adverse events related to patient safety.

Additionally, significant variability exists in how RPM services are implemented, and this variability may influence outcomes. For instance, patients using smartphone applications for RPM demonstrated higher adherence compared to those using web-based services [219]. The severity of illness also plays a role in determining RPM's effectiveness in reducing acute care utilization [102].

Beyond emergency interventions, telemedicine plays a crucial role in remote patient monitoring and long-term care management. In countries with a low doctor-to-patient ratio, telemedicine ensures continuous patient tracking and data exchange, allowing physicians to oversee patients from a distance [103, 112]. Wireless health monitoring is particularly critical for elderly patients in remote areas, where limited healthcare access contributes to higher morbidity and mortality rates [236]. The concept of "connected healthcare" has evolved with advancements in network technologies, enabling real-time remote monitoring and improved chronic disease management [25, 192]. Additionally, structured telemedicine follow-ups have been shown to improve patient adherence and reduce re-consultations. A study by Soltane [230] found that patients receiving telemedicine follow-up calls had fewer re-consultations (14%) compared to the control group (26.5%), along with better treatment adherence (97.5% vs. 92%) and significantly higher patient satisfaction rates (90% vs. 37.5%). Such findings endorse telemedicine's potential not only in acute emergency settings but also in long-term patient engagement and healthcare optimization.

To ensure the success of RPM, a patient-centric approach is crucial. This approach should foster engagement, health literacy, and self-management skills. While some participants may become dependent on RPM systems and telemonitoring nurses, reducing their self-management skills, a comprehensive model involving various healthcare professionals has been shown to yield positive results [34]. Studies have demonstrated that RPM enhances quality of life, improves early detection of conditions like atrial fibrillation, and strengthens communication between patients and healthcare providers [108, 124].

10.2 Procedural Telementoring in Acute/Trauma Resuscitation/Surgery

In the context of emergencies, telemedicine has been instrumental in expanding access to specialized care, particularly in underserved and rural areas [61]. Telementoring has evolved from telemedicine, which initially focused on using communication technology to transfer medical information into a more complex and interactive field [253]. El-Sabawi and Magee [74] offer a detailed review of the origins of telementoring and identify two main applications: (a) remotely educating and supervising learners in simulated or real complex environments and (b) providing real-time corrective supervision and guidance during actual medical interventions. The core concept of telementoring involves an expert, such as a surgeon (the mentor), using telecommunications systems to instruct and guide another healthcare provider (the mentee) interactively during procedures [43]. Telementoring serves two primary purposes: it functions as a virtual classroom designed to help adult learners gain competency, and it acts as a safety net in critical situations where failure to act could result in preventable harm [151].

Telementoring has proven successful in developing surgeons' skills when experienced mentors are not available on-site [229] and in reducing delays caused by the transportation of medical equipment and personnel [87]. The mentor, an expert providing surgical knowledge, works with the mentee, the clinician performing the procedure. The mentee interacts with the patient by performing various actions, such as surgical maneuvers, handling tools, and interacting with tissues. The patient's condition is monitored using feedback, which includes vital signs, visual data, and alerts. This information is sent to the mentor to guide the next steps in the process. The mentor delivers instructions through voice, visual annotations, and gestures. The mentee receives these instructions and makes decisions on the next steps to take. Ultimately, the success of the mentorship is measured through patient-related outcomes [253].

Telementoring has been effective in disseminating surgical knowledge to remote regions and resource-constrained environments, thereby enhancing local surgical capabilities and reducing the need for costly hospital transfers [61]. Live telementoring has proven life-saving in managing critically ill trauma patients, as demonstrated by a study by Latifi et al. [138], where telementoring via teletrauma consults was potentially life-saving for six trauma cases and allowed 17 patients (29%) to be retained in rural hospitals, preventing unnecessary transfers.

Studies have highlighted the benefits of synchronous telementoring in various surgical contexts. For example, it has been shown to improve outcomes in open surgery [195] and help reduce discrepancies in rural trauma care [200]. In laparoscopic surgery, telementoring typically involves real-time video sharing, allowing mentors to view both the laparoscopic video and the operating room setup simultaneously. This dual perspective enhances remote procedural guidance, as demonstrated by studies on laparoscopic telementoring [77, 220].

Emergency surgery encompasses a range of priorities, with the most critical being those that are life-threatening. These include conditions such as hemodynamic instability and intracranial hematoma, where immediate intervention is essential to preserve life. Additionally, surgeries addressing limb- or organ-threatening injuries, such as vascular injuries or penetrating eye injuries, are prioritized to prevent irreversible damage. Other urgent surgical priorities involve conditions like peritonitis, open fractures, and the debridement of infected wounds or amputations, all of which require prompt intervention to minimize complications and improve outcomes [145].

Dawe et al. [59] showed that secure video-conferencing applications for remote guiding can be used to telementor non-surgeon medical officers during real tissue training exercises. Rojas-Munoz et al. [208] developed the system for telementoring with augmented reality (STAR) platform, a portable and self-contained telementoring platform for critical surgeries such as cricothyrotomies in disaster/conflict settings. For damage-control surgery telementored training, Kirkpatrick et al. [121] used realistic surgical training mannequins and Skype-enabled communication to provide real-time visual and auditory feedback. Dulou et al. [68] described a mobile neurosurgery unit that supports rural medicosurgical units, demonstrating its importance in delivering specialist help to underserved areas.

Beyond surgical applications, telementoring has also been explored in emergency airway management. A pilot study by Cho et al. [45] examined the Tele-Airway Management System (TAMS) for remote guidance during emergency intubation. This system, which includes two video cameras, a video laryngoscope, and a patient monitor, enables emergency physicians to supervise intubation procedures remotely. The study compared TAMS to traditional on-scene directed (OSD) intubation and found no significant differences in intubation time, success rate, or complications. These findings suggest that remote guidance via TAMS can serve as a viable alternative in emergency airway management, particularly in situations where immediate on-site supervision is unavailable. Furthermore, telemonitoring has been widely used in neurological emergencies, such as traumatic brain injuries and telestroke scenarios, where it aids in assessing the risks and benefits of local thrombolytic therapy [185].

A review evaluating the trade-offs between on-site mentoring and telementoring technologies revealed that each approach has its own challenges (e.g., travel and time costs versus equipment cost and network issues) [106], but more recently, several forms of telementoring have been adopted for surgical practice, with the cost of such equipment significantly reduced. For example, 40% of the US News Best Hospitals currently use the InTouch telemedicine system, an integrated telepresence system for the operating room that relies on multiple cameras pointing at the patient and mentee, designed to facilitate surgical telementoring through remote collaboration in the operating room [253].

Telemedicine and telesurgical support, often involving surgical guidance via telephone or messaging, help alleviate the pressure experienced by isolated and typically young surgeons, provided that sufficient computer infrastructure is in place—a factor that continues to improve in quality and reliability [68]. One emerging advancement in surgical telementoring is telestration, which allows mentors to draw annotations over live images or videos. Available in both 2D and 3D formats, 2D telestration is more commonly adopted due to its simplicity [228]. However, it presents occlusion challenges that can hinder depth perception and spatial awareness in 3D tasks. In contrast, 3D telestration eliminates these issues, enhancing performance in surgical procedures. Notably, Ali et al. [11] demonstrated its feasibility in a robotic surgical system, underscoring its ability to improve telementoring efficacy without negatively affecting user performance. Beyond telestration, AI-driven systems are advancing the field by generating step-by-step surgical instructions, bringing AI-based virtual mentors closer to reality, and supporting clinicians when human experts are unavailable [208]. Augmented reality (AR) also holds significant promise in surgical telementoring, as it can overlay critical information—such as anatomical structures or mentor instructions—onto the real-world environment, thereby improving both procedural safety and comprehension. For example, Chou et al. [47] implemented an AR-based preoperative planning system in remote robot-assisted neurosurgery, while Shenai et al. [227] integrated digital renderings of a surgical site with MRI data to provide enhanced visual context. Furthermore, telementoring has been acknowledged as a method to standardize the utilization of robotics in surgery, offering the potential for safe and efficient surgical practices, even in low-volume centers [82]. While the feasibility of using telementoring and telerobotics for open surgery has been demonstrated [30, 77], this initial work must be expanded further to ensure its widespread application. Despite the adoption of telementoring within fixed hospital settings for planned and scheduled surgical activities, the situation is different for urgent, just-in-time emergency care, which is a capability gap of health care systems worldwide. Simulation studies, however, suggest the promise of relatively low-tech audio and video approaches to telementoring. The Retention and Assessment of Surgical Performance Group at the University of Maryland has been studying the effectiveness and skill retention of the Advanced Surgical Skills for Exposure in Trauma (ASSET) course of the American College of Surgeons. This group has demonstrated that a telementor, using audio and three camera connections, significantly improved the ability of surgeons who had completed ASSET at least 6 months before to successfully complete upper- and lower-extremity fasciotomies on cadavers without colocated assistants [253]. Of note, a brief video tool also improved performance, but not as well as the telementor. Given the fundamental challenges in telementoring, several techniques and technologies have been developed to specifically ease the two-way transfer of information between the mentee and mentor and to enhance the understanding and appreciation of the task being performed, although no technological solution will satisfy all the requirements for procedural telementoring support. The environment in which procedural telementoring is performed dictates the practical solutions required. For instance, a fully immersive virtual reality (VR) environment with a holographic, lifelike, teleported mentor may be ideal for training surgical residents in a scheduled operating room in the continental United States. However, such a technology might prove a lethal liability for guiding a resuscitative life-saving intervention (LSI) performed by special forces medics in tactical situations, in which a dual focus must be maintained regarding performing the LSI and maintaining situational awareness to avoid becoming a secondary casualty. Thus, a practical theme for all advanced telementoring solutions will be to evaluate the relative attributes of far-forward and austere care versus scheduled in-hospital care. Borrowing from the military medicine lexicon, solutions may potentially support in-garrison care or far-forward operational needs [253].

10.2.1 Opportunities for Surgical Telementoring in Low-Income Countries, Rural Areas, and Austere Settings

There is a substantial need to enhance the delivery of surgical interventions globally. One promising solution is telementoring, which allows surgeons in developed nations to expand their capabilities by aiding local providers through teaching or real-time guidance in procedures. Following the limitations on international travel post-COVID-19, this need is now more critical than ever. Notable examples of international telementoring include the work of Lee et al. [141], where a high-bandwidth telecommunications line facilitated one-way video transfer from the laparoscope or external cameras, two-way voice communication, telestration, pan/tilt control of the laparoscopic camera, and electrocautery instruments. In this instance, telementoring was conducted internationally from Johns Hopkins Hospital (United States) to Bangkok (Thailand) and Innsbruck (Austria) [141]. Another application of telementoring supported an endoscopic laser-assisted dacryocystorhinostomy through a fast internet line (Integrated Service Digital Network line), enabling real-time communication between Honolulu, Hawaii, and Manila, Philippines [40]. Rosser et al. [209] also demonstrated telementoring's potential by remotely overseeing a laparoscopic cholecystectomy in rural Ecuador, utilizing low-bandwidth telemedical techniques in an area with minimal resources. Furthermore, Aguilera et al. [7] highlighted telementoring's potential in low- and middle-income countries, particularly in resource-constrained settings, and its integration with trauma mass casualty centers.

Rural areas in developed nations face unique challenges in accessing subspecialist care. In the United States, 25% of the population resides in rural areas, yet fewer than 15% of physicians practice there, a number that continues to decline [244]. General surgery residencies often do not prepare trainees adequately for the broad skillset required for rural practice, where generalists manage a wide array of pathologies [131]. This limitation becomes more pronounced as surgical education increasingly emphasizes sub-specialization [35]. Even when surgeons are exposed to skills outside their subspecialty during training, such skills are often lost due to their infrequent use in highly specialized practice [212]. In pediatric surgery, for example, certain procedures may occur only once every few years, leading to difficulties for even experienced surgeons [210]. The rapid learning curve for innovative technologies is another barrier to their adoption [266]. While in-person mentoring is effective for teaching new surgical techniques [76], it is not always feasible for trauma or emergency procedures that demand immediate attention, as experts may not be available on-site. Additionally, most surgeons in rural settings cannot afford to leave their practice for extended periods to receive training, creating a need for alternative methods of learning that do not disrupt their practice [16].

Operational medicine, which is practiced in environments where resources and caregivers are at risk, and austere medicine, which occurs in resource-poor settings, are areas where telementoring can be particularly valuable. The military medical systems of developed nations, such as the United States, have demonstrated success in delivering medical care comparable to civilian trauma systems under logistical and resource constraints [218]. However, future military engagements may involve operations where access to advanced medical care is even more limited [173]. In such cases, telementoring could prove essential in pushing advanced medical capabilities to frontline providers. Pamplin et al. [182] emphasize that care will need to be provided at the point of need, particularly as traditional echelons of care may become compressed in future conflicts. Similarly, military medical efforts have shown that preventing traumatic deaths relies heavily on rapid intervention to manage hemorrhage, often before the patient reaches definitive care [70]. To improve resuscitation in austere environments, concepts like remote damage-control resuscitation (RDCR) have emerged, focusing on hemorrhage control and minimizing the use of fluids [88]. While telemedicine was a vital component of RDCR, field implementation has been limited by technical and logistical challenges. However, studies such as the EM-ANGEL study [89] demonstrate that remote telementoring during trauma resuscitation can improve accuracy and efficiency. The TeleMentored Ultrasound Supported Medical Interventions (TMUSMI) group at the University of Calgary has also contributed to advancing telementoring in point-of-care settings, enabling providers to perform advanced interventions using simple, lightweight technologies. Although some studies have shown that not all telementoring interventions are perceived as useful [122], the field continues to evolve alongside technological advancements.

10.3 Future Directions in Telemedicine: AI, VR, AR, and Telementoring in Healthcare

In telemedicine triage, ensuring that high-priority data, such as emergency medical information, receives sufficient bandwidth is crucial. This can be achieved by implementing algorithms that dynamically adjust bandwidth based on data importance, preventing delays in life-critical information due to insufficient network resources. Media Access Control (MAC) protocols are essential for managing data transmission in wireless networks, particularly for WBANs. These protocols prioritize medical traffic by allocating specific slots or channels for high-priority data, such as emergency medical information, ensuring timely transmission. For example, protocols can distinguish between emergency, normal medical, and non-medical traffic, with emergency data receiving the highest priority [85, 199]. A new MAC protocol for WBANs integrates dual-band physical layer technology, utilizing both UWB transmission and narrowband receiving, to enhance performance. It employs a narrowband feedback path to reduce UWB receiver complexity and uses a guaranteed delivery mechanism for high priority data. The protocol also incorporates priority packet transmission techniques to meet the varying QoS needs of different sensors. Additionally, its balance control algorithm for the contention access period (CAP) and contention-free period (CFP) optimizes the transmission of medical data while improving non-medical traffic efficiency. By allocating specific CFP slots to non-medical data, the protocol reduces delays for non-medical packages and increases overall throughput. Adaptive resource allocation further boosts the data rate for sensor nodes by adjusting transmission intervals based on channel conditions, mitigating the effects of deep fading in WBANs. In the context of disaster response, the protocol facilitates the creation of regional telemedicine hubs that connect local healthcare infrastructures with external expertise, enabling efficient care during surges in casualties and overwhelming demands for medical attention [170]. A healthy traffic control mechanism has been proposed in modern heterogeneous wireless networks to prevent congestion and ensure the reliability of quality of service (QoS) and service responsiveness. Each health terminal device or router employs a proportionate allocation control strategy to regulate data flow, aligning the rate of transmission with the priority of the information. Priority is often linked to the bandwidth required for the reliable transmission of vital signals, as well as the level of urgency in specific clinical, acute care, and disaster situations. For instance, Koutsakis [126] suggests an easy-to-implement token-based and self-policing scheduling scheme combined with a mechanism to mitigate congestion. In this approach, telemedicine video applications over wireless LAN are assigned guaranteed bandwidth (QoS) for connection requests, ensuring smooth video transmission even in congested environments [191]. Additionally, Manfredi [149] emphasizes the importance of controlling congestion in emerging heterogeneous wireless body area networks to guarantee differentiated healthcare service delivery, thus supporting both reliability and responsiveness in telemedicine applications.

The role of informatics and AI in telemedicine is pivotal in enhancing its capabilities, particularly in the fields of acute care, emergency surgery, and trauma. Informatics systems provide the foundation for telemedicine platforms, enabling real-time access to crucial patient data, including electronic health records (EHRs), imaging, and laboratory results, which are essential for timely medical decision-making. AI further strengthens telemedicine by offering powerful tools for data analysis, predictive modeling, and clinical decision support. AI-powered algorithms, for instance, can assist healthcare providers in remotely diagnosing life-threatening conditions such as sepsis or myocardial infarction by analyzing patient data in real time, ensuring prompt and informed decision-making [51]. Additionally, AI can analyze vast datasets from remote patient monitoring devices, EHRs, and telehealth interactions to identify patterns indicative of potential health risks, allowing healthcare providers to intervene proactively [196]. This predictive capacity shifts the focus from reactive care to preventive health maintenance, offering personalized health recommendations, preventive screenings, and lifestyle interventions, which can significantly improve patient outcomes [237]. Moreover, AI-driven predictive models can contribute to population health management by identifying trends and risk factors on a broader scale, transforming telemedicine into a more anticipatory, data-driven, and preventive healthcare paradigm. In radiology, AI enhances image interpretation by automating the identification of abnormalities, thus optimizing diagnostic workflows [79]. Additionally, natural language processing (NLP) techniques facilitate the extraction of meaningful insights from unstructured clinical data, thereby improving the comprehensiveness of patient records [90]. AI algorithms can analyze genetic data, biomarkers, and patient-specific health information to generate personalized treatment plans [178], which telemedicine platforms can deliver through remote consultations. This integration not only enhances the effectiveness of treatments but also reduces the risk of adverse reactions and unnecessary interventions, benefiting patients regardless of their geographical location [237].

Beyond diagnostics, AI-driven virtual health assistants provide tailored health information, medication reminders, and lifestyle recommendations, contributing to improved patient engagement and adherence to treatment regimens [237].

AI-powered decision-support systems further aid healthcare professionals by analyzing patient-specific data—including genetic profiles, lifestyle habits, and previous treatment responses—to generate customized therapeutic interventions [237]. This level of personalization aligns with the principles of precision medicine, paving the way for individualized patient care and reducing the likelihood of misdiagnoses [79].

Advancements in virtual reality (VR) and augmented reality (AR) are transforming telemedicine, particularly in remote surgical interventions. VR platforms create immersive environments that enhance spatial awareness and precision during remote procedures [233], while AR overlays critical information onto the surgeon's field of view, offering real-time guidance during surgeries conducted at a distance [120]. VR, when used as an interface, allows more intuitive interactions with information, while as an environment, it creates a heightened sense of presence for both the mentor and mentee during the session [204, 217]. AR enhances the real-world visual scene with computer-generated elements, while VR immerses users entirely in a virtual world Studies by Huang et al. [105] suggest that VR provides a stronger sense of psychological immersion, whereas AR is more effective for visual and auditory communication. These technologies are particularly valuable for minimally invasive surgeries, robotic procedures, and other precision-based interventions, enabling expert surgeons to collaborate with local teams globally, overcoming geographical barriers and ensuring specialized care for patients [120].

The system for telementoring with augmented reality (STAR), developed by Purdue and Indiana University School of Medicine, enables field medics to receive guidance from surgeons via AR headsets and drone views [208]. Another innovative system, ARTEMIS, combines AR and VR, with VR creating an avatar of the expert surgeon and AR projecting 3D annotations onto the patient's body [260].

A key area of focus is haptics, which facilitates the transmission of tactile feedback between the mentor and mentee, thereby enhancing the remote mentoring experience. Two main methods are used: non-intrusive techniques, which provide force feedback through multimodal displays, alarms, or acoustic signals, and intrusive methods that involve wearable sensors, allowing the mentee to feel the pressure applied to their hands or arms. These tactile sensations are replicated at the mentor's side using virtual and augmented reality (VR/AR) systems, including cybergloves and exosuits, which help ensure that both the mentor and mentee can engage in seamless and synchronized interactions [225]. Another significant advancement is in assistive exoskeletons, which are being designed using lightweight, soft materials to enhance mobility without restricting joint function. These exosuits are particularly useful in rehabilitation, with pneumatic actuators and fluid-driven devices optimizing comfort and power transfer [18, 19, 190].

Beyond surgical applications, VR and AR are revolutionizing patient education and engagement. VR allows patients to explore 3D models of their conditions, treatment plans, and potential outcomes, fostering informed decision-making [250]. Similarly, AR enhances teleconsultations by visually demonstrating diagnoses, procedures, and medication instructions, strengthening provider-patient communication [237]. The integration of these technologies marks a shift toward patient-centered care, prioritizing education, transparency, and shared decision-making.

VR and AR are also redefining medical education and training. VR simulations offer immersive, hands-on experiences, allowing medical students and healthcare professionals to refine their skills and enhance decision-making abilities [233]. AR-powered overlays and holographic displays create interactive learning environments, enabling remote students to participate in virtual dissections, surgical simulations, and case discussions. These advancements democratize medical education, making high-quality training more accessible worldwide [250]. Moreover, cognitive collaborations in telementoring are transforming traditional mentor-mentee dynamics by enabling multi-expert teams to guide mentees during complex procedures. For example, the Rubrum Coelis Project [174] demonstrated how trauma surgeons, medics, and translators could collaborate remotely to mentor military medics. Although effective, further research is needed to optimize these multidisciplinary setups. Additionally, innovations in remote knobology control are allowing mentors to adjust ultrasound settings remotely, freeing up the mentee to focus on more critical aspects of patient care [109]. Finally, the future of telementoring is poised to benefit from the development of virtual teleportation, where 5D VR systems create a sense of co-presence between mentor and mentee, overcoming spatial barriers in teaching complex procedures [225, 253].

10.4 Ethical, Technical, and Quality-of-Care Challenges in Telemedicine

One of the central ethical concerns in telemedicine is patient privacy, particularly regarding the transmission and storage of sensitive health data in virtual environments. The security of patient information is a primary concern, as telemedicine systems must adhere to strict encryption protocols and secure communication channels to prevent unauthorized access and data breaches [4]. Striking a balance between accessibility for healthcare providers and safeguarding patient privacy is a nuanced challenge that requires ongoing collaboration among policymakers, technology developers, and healthcare professionals. Additionally, the use of remote monitoring devices and wearables in telemedicine introduces further privacy considerations. Continuous data collection from these devices necessitates clear and transparent communication about data usage, ownership, and implications of sharing such information with healthcare providers [4].

Vulnerable populations, such as those with lower socioeconomic status, may face barriers in accessing telehealth services due to limited digital literacy, lack of technology, or unreliable internet connectivity [27]. Without initiatives to enhance digital literacy, promote affordable internet access, and provide support for individuals encountering technological barriers, certain groups may be left behind. Ethical considerations in telemedicine extend beyond technology to include social determinants of health, ensuring that the benefits of telehealth are accessible to all individuals, regardless of socioeconomic status [272].

Telemedicine relies heavily on stable internet connectivity, which can present significant barriers in rural and remote areas that lack high-speed internet access [95]. Connectivity issues—such as bandwidth limitations, network reliability, and speed—hinder widespread adoption and equitable access to telehealth services. To address these challenges, collaborations between telecommunication providers, policymakers, and healthcare institutions are essential to improve infrastructure and expand broadband access in underserved regions [4]. Additionally, the digital divide, which includes disparities in access to smartphones, tablets, or computers, further exacerbates access challenges, particularly for individuals in low-resource settings. A 2023 study on integrated telemedicine care for cancer patients revealed that most respondents (91.7%) agreed that telehealth enhances access to early integrated palliative care, and 79.2% believed it simplifies the process for patients. However, elderly patients, particularly those in rural areas and from lower-income backgrounds, faced significant challenges in accessing telemedicine services [213]. Bridging this divide requires a comprehensive approach that incorporates both infrastructure improvements and educational initiatives to empower individuals to navigate virtual healthcare platforms [64].

Another critical technical challenge lies in the integration of telemedicine with existing healthcare systems, particularly in ensuring interoperability with electronic health record (EHR) systems. Many healthcare institutions operate on diverse EHR platforms, and ensuring compatibility with telehealth platforms is vital for the efficient flow of patient data [153]. Standardized protocols, such as Fast Healthcare Interoperability Resources (FHIR), facilitate data exchange between telemedicine applications and EHR systems [148]. However, as the use of digital platforms increases, cybersecurity risks also heighten. Rigorous cybersecurity measures are essential to protect patient data and maintain the integrity of healthcare systems, requiring collaborative efforts between healthcare IT professionals, cybersecurity experts, and policymakers (Henderson et al. 2021, as cited in Adeghe 2024).

The convergence of telemedicine and the Internet of Things (IoT) has further revolutionized healthcare by enabling seamless communication between interconnected medical devices, sensors, and data analytics platforms [134]. IoT-powered telemedicine allows healthcare providers to access comprehensive patient data, including vital signs and environmental factors, fostering a more holistic and proactive healthcare approach. Smart medical devices such as blood pressure monitors, glucose meters, and ECG trackers transmit real-time patient information securely, enhancing the efficiency of remote consultations [98]. However, as reliance on IoT increases, addressing data security and privacy concerns remains critical. Given the expanded risk of cyber threats, robust security measures such as encryption, secure authentication protocols, and routine software updates are necessary to protect patient data [4]. Additionally, compliance with regulations like the General Data Protection Regulation (GDPR) and the Health Insurance Portability and Accountability Act (HIPAA) ensures ethical and legal adherence while safeguarding patient privacy [4].

While telemedicine offers a range of healthcare services, certain diagnostic procedures are inherently limited in virtual settings. Physical examinations and certain imaging studies may be challenging to replicate remotely [116]. Healthcare providers must adapt to these limitations by leveraging available technologies, collaborating with on-site healthcare professionals, and establishing clear guidelines for when in-person assessments are necessary. The interpretation of subtle clinical cues, which are often observed during in-person visits, may also be challenging in telemedicine. Therefore, healthcare providers must rely on effective communication, patient history, and available data to make informed decisions [28]. Also, in areas with poor infrastructure, AI could serve as a fallback mechanism, providing support in the absence of human mentors [60]. Ongoing advancements in telehealth technologies, including high-fidelity imaging devices for home use, aim to address these limitations and improve diagnostic accuracy.

Teaching and providing care at a distance inherently pose significant challenges, as telementoring relies solely on telecommunications technologies. One of the primary weaknesses of telementoring in care delivery is the absence of the mentor's physical presence. From an educational standpoint, the lack of direct physical interaction can make learning less intuitive, and adjuncts aimed at enhancing personal engagement are often necessary. In procedural telementoring, the risks are even greater, as mentors cannot intervene physically or demonstrate techniques when an operating surgeon encounters difficulties [16]. This limitation has driven research into telepresence and telerobotic surgery. However, current commercial telerobotic systems are impractical for remote regions and community hospitals due to their large size, weight, complex setup, and high initial and maintenance costs [16].

Additionally, telementoring is heavily dependent on telecommunications infrastructure, making the reliability of these systems crucial to both the mentoring process and surgical outcomes [15]. Unfortunately, very few platforms are equipped with vigorous fail-safe mechanisms to address connectivity disruptions [14]. Effective verbal communication is also critical in telementoring, yet noise in the operating room can significantly interfere with the mentor's instructions. While headsets provide a partial solution, they can be cumbersome and may hinder the operating surgeon's interaction with the surgical team, particularly in high-stakes environments such as far-forward tactical interventions [210].

Another major limitation of current telementoring platforms is their restricted perceptual and physical access to the operative field. This gap makes it difficult for mentors to develop an accurate mental model of the surgical environment, forcing mentees to focus more on managing the technology rather than the patient. This contradicts the "come-as-you-are" usability principle in human-computer interaction, which emphasizes intuitive and seamless engagement with technology [252]. Furthermore, excessive or unnecessary mentoring can slow down critical procedures, particularly when the mentee is already proficient in certain tasks [174]. Research on human factors in telementoring remains underdeveloped and must address issues related to technique, technology, and communication to optimize remote mentoring effectiveness. In particular, understanding how virtual mentors can support learners in high-stress, complex environments is a key priority for future advancements in telementoring [174].

Building and maintaining trust in telemedicine is essential for effective healthcare delivery. The absence of physical presence in virtual consultations can create a sense of impersonality, leading to patient concerns [93]. To overcome these challenges, healthcare providers must prioritize clear, empathetic communication and work to foster strong therapeutic alliances with patients. Ensuring high-quality audio and video communication through telehealth platforms, along with training healthcare professionals in virtual communication skills, contributes to strengthening trust in telemedicine relationships [116].

10.5 Regulatory and Policy Implications of Telemedicine

The integration of telemedicine into healthcare delivery brings forth substantial regulatory and policy implications. As the legal framework evolves, it addresses the unique challenges and opportunities that telemedicine presents. Regulatory bodies are working to ensure the safety, privacy, and effectiveness of telehealth services, while simultaneously fostering innovation [114]. Key considerations such as licensing requirements, provider reimbursement, and liability issues are central to shaping telemedicine's legal framework [13]. Since telehealth policies vary between regions and nations, ongoing efforts aim to develop standardized guidelines to ensure the consistent quality of telemedicine services [114]. The expansion of telemedicine faces challenges tied to licensing and reimbursement. Healthcare has traditionally been governed by state-specific licensing rules, raising questions about jurisdictional boundaries for telemedicine practitioners [5]. Efforts to create interstate licensing agreements and reciprocity are helping resolve these issues and promote smooth telehealth delivery. Reimbursement is a critical factor in the broad adoption of telemedicine, with payers, including government and private insurers, reconsidering their reimbursement models to align with the value and efficiency of telehealth services [5].

Policy interventions play a key role in developing equitable reimbursement structures that sustain telemedicine initiatives while maintaining affordability and patient access. The rapid rise of digital health is driven by advances in data, computational power, and widespread internet access, positioning digital health at the forefront of global innovation [26]. The World Health Organization's Global Strategy on Digital Health 2020–2025 emphasizes principles such as transparency, accessibility, scalability, interoperability, security, and confidentiality [269]. This strategy is aligned with the United Nations' Sustainable Development Goals, calling for universal access to high-quality health services [81].

Standardization in telemedicine includes protocols, data security practices, and quality assurance measures to protect patient care and maintain ethical standards. Developing standardized guidelines requires collaboration between healthcare professionals, technology developers, and regulatory authorities. These guidelines should address licensure, reimbursement, and the integration of telemedicine within existing healthcare systems [5]. A universal framework can encourage the responsible expansion of telemedicine, minimize risks, and ensure high-quality care delivery. Since telemedicine can transcend geographic boundaries, international cooperation is vital to create comprehensive telehealth standards. Such global collaboration can lead to interoperable systems that allow seamless telemedicine across the globe [28].

Standardizing telemedicine practices worldwide also facilitates cross-border consultations, enabling patients to access specialized care from international experts. Additionally, international collaboration allows for the exchange of best practices, research, and lessons learned from telemedicine implementation. Regulatory bodies can benefit from the insights of their international counterparts, fostering a collective approach to solving challenges and driving telehealth innovation [5]. As telemedicine continues to evolve, a harmonized set of international standards ensures that its benefits are accessible to diverse populations.

Reimbursement models for telemedicine are also shifting toward value-based models, which prioritize care quality and outcomes over service volume. This aligns with the goals of telemedicine by encouraging healthcare providers to focus on patient outcomes, preventive care, and overall health improvement [114]. By focusing on value, reimbursement policies can promote efficient, patient-centered telehealth services. Implementing value-based models requires collaboration between providers, payers, and regulatory bodies to define quality indicators for telemedicine services [5]. These indicators include patient satisfaction, health outcomes, and cost-effectiveness, ensuring telemedicine contributes positively to healthcare delivery.

Telemedicine parity laws are crucial for ensuring equal compensation for telehealth services compared to in-person visits. Policymakers need to address reimbursement rates, coverage, and conditions for telemedicine consultations to eliminate barriers for healthcare providers [28]. Achieving telemedicine parity requires ongoing communication between healthcare stakeholders, insurers, and regulatory bodies to establish fair reimbursement structures. Furthermore, as new technologies and modalities emerge, reimbursement policies must evolve to cover a wide range of telehealth practices while maintaining parity with in-person services [5].

Finding the right balance in telemedicine reimbursement is vital for ensuring sustainability, affordability, and accessibility for both providers and patients. The ethical aspects of telemedicine require clear frameworks that guide healthcare professionals, technology developers, and policymakers. Ethical guidelines for telemedicine cover issues like patient autonomy, informed consent, confidentiality, and the responsible use of technology [114]. Telemedicine practitioners must adhere to ethical standards that respect patients' rights, privacy, and dignity. Developing these frameworks involves collaboration among healthcare institutions, professional organizations, and regulatory bodies and should remain flexible to adapt to technological advancements and evolving patient expectations [5].

Given that telemedicine relies on transmitting and storing sensitive health information, safeguarding patient privacy is essential. Policymakers and regulatory bodies must enforce strong privacy regulations that address the unique challenges of virtual healthcare interactions [28]. Telehealth platforms should implement encryption, secure communication channels, and data protection measures to prevent unauthorized access. Transparent patient consent mechanisms must also be in place to ensure patients understand how their health information will be used and shared in telehealth settings [5]. Ongoing evaluations of privacy practices, along with technologies like blockchain for secure health data exchange, will help maintain patient trust in virtual healthcare systems.

Telemedicine's regulatory considerations and policy implications encompass standardization, reimbursement, and ethics. As telehealth continues to reshape healthcare, regulatory bodies must adapt to ensure its responsible, ethical, and equitable integration into healthcare systems.

Telemedicine services are becoming increasingly accessible in both developed and developing nations, with reliable technological infrastructure supporting cost-effective services. Telemedicine eliminates the need for patients to travel to specialists, allowing specialized care to be delivered directly to patients. However, these advancements present new legal, ethical, and regulatory challenges that shape policymaking [91]. International ehealth laws are influenced not only by individual countries but also by global entities like the World Trade Organization (WTO), as well as agreements in trade, telecommunications, and healthcare services [197]. Despite its potential, telemedicine regulation and licensing are still underdeveloped in many nations, with challenges such as professional licensing, unapproved health practices, fraud, and jurisdictional conflicts continuing to pose obstacles

Telemedicine in the USA has been regulated since its initial stages. By 1992, five states had implemented telemedicine laws, and this number grew to 15 by 1995. Today, all 50 states have laws governing telemedicine, but these regulations vary by state and are complemented by federal and facility-based guidelines. This creates a complex regulatory landscape for providers, especially in specialized areas like sleep telemedicine. Providers must navigate regulations not only for the distant site but also for the patient's state of residence (originating site). Rules vary widely, including requirements for informed consent and in-person consultations before follow-up visits. To avoid legal and professional issues, providers must stay informed about the specific regulations in each state [84].

A report by Aizenberg [9] maps the differing progress of telemedicine regulation across Latin America and the Caribbean (LAC). While countries like Uruguay, Panama, and Peru have made strides by enacting telemedicine laws, many others remain in the early stages of regulatory development. Around 34.61% of countries are at Level 1 (basic), and 46.15% are at Level 2 (development phase). These countries face issues like limited integration of digital health into healthcare systems and inadequate coordination across sectors. While personal data protection laws are widespread, ensuring patient rights and expanding access to healthcare via telemedicine continue to be major challenges. Additionally, the Pan American Health Organization has urged countries in the Americas to adopt the Eight Guiding Principles for Digital Transformation of Health, ensuring no one is left behind [183].

In countries like Korea, telemedicine's legal foundation dates to 2002, and a supportive legal framework was established by 2013. However, telemedicine remained limited until 2015, when it was introduced in underserved regions [56].

In Malaysia, the nationwide telemedicine network links 37 service points to major hospitals, supported by the Telemedicine Act of 1997 [231]. In the US, telemedicine offers an affordable way to diagnose and treat conditions, especially for uninsured and low-income populations [176]. However, Europe still struggles with fragmented regulation regarding telemedicine and medical liability [197].

Malaysia's Telemedicine Act of 1997 regulates medical practices involving audio, visual, and data communications. While not yet fully enforced, the act complements the Malaysian Medical Act of 1971 and the Malaysian Medical Council's Code of Professional Ethics. Virtual consultations are permitted only for ongoing care, and telemedicine platforms must comply with the Personal Data Protection Act (PDPA) of 2010 [215]. Similarly, Argentina's Ministry of Health issued guidelines in 2019 for telehealth, establishing protocols for real-time consultations. By 2020, private insurers were required to offer teleconsultations while safeguarding patient data [215]. Other countries like Austria, Mexico, and Russia have also implemented their own telemedicine regulations to ensure safe, secure, and effective telehealth services aligned with international standards [215].

10.6 Conclusion

The COVID-19 pandemic significantly accelerated the adoption of telemedicine, spurring a surge in research and literature that examined the rapid expansion of telehealth services across various healthcare domains. This shift also drew attention to the critical role of telemedicine in emergency and acute trauma care, emphasizing its potential to enhance patient outcomes and bridge access gaps for timely medical interventions. Telemedicine, including teletrauma and remote patient monitoring (RPM), is revolutionizing healthcare by enhancing access to specialists, improving patient outcomes, and reducing unnecessary transfers, particularly in rural and underserved areas. Advances in teleconsultation, teletriage, and telementoring allow for real-time guidance and support in emergency care and surgical procedures, overcoming geographical and resource limitations. The integration of AI for predictive analytics, along with VR and AR for remote surgical interventions and medical education, will further enhance the expanding field. Despite its promise, telemedicine faces challenges such as ethical concerns, technical limitations, and access disparities, all of which must be addressed alongside regulatory hurdles to ensure its continued growth and successful integration into mainstream healthcare systems. Establishing universal guidelines and addressing reimbursement policies will be crucial for telemedicine's expansion, ensuring responsible and equitable development. The future of telemedicine holds immense promise in reshaping healthcare delivery, making it more efficient, personalized, and accessible. As we continue to navigate these technological advancements, a patient-centric approach—focused on fostering engagement, health literacy, and self-management—will be key to realizing the full potential of telemedicine.

References

1. Abelsen B, Strasser R, Heaney D, Berggren P, Sigurðsson S, Brandstorp H, et al. Plan, recruit, retain: a framework for local healthcare organizations to achieve a stable remote rural workforce. Hum Resour Health. 2020;18(1):63. https://doi.org/10.1186/s12960-020-00502-x.
2. Abualenain J. Use of technology in disaster medicine. Eur J Emerg Med. 2024;23(3):155–8. https://doi.org/10.4274/eajem.galenos.2024.45452.
3. Accorsi TA, Moreira FT, Pedrotti CH, et al. Telemedicine diagnosis of acute respiratory tract infection patients is not inferior to face-to-face consultation: a randomized trial. Einstein (Sao Paulo). 2022;20:eAO6800. https://doi.org/10.31744/einstein_journal/2022AO6800.
4. Adeghe EP, Okolo CA, Ojeyinka OT. A review of emerging trends in telemedicine: healthcare delivery transformations. Int J Life Sci Res Arch. 2024;6(1):137–47. https://doi.org/10.53771/ijlsra.2024.6.1.0040.
5. Adler-Milstein J, Kvedar J, Bates DW. Telehealth among US hospitals: several factors, including state reimbursement and licensure policies, influence adoption. Health Aff. 2014;33(2):207–15. https://doi.org/10.1377/hlthaff.2013.1054.
6. Agarwal S, Day DJ, Sibson L, Barry PJ, Collas D, Metcalf K, et al. Thrombolysis delivery by a regional telestroke network—experience from the U.K. National Health Service. J Am Heart Assoc. 2014;3(1):e000408. https://doi.org/10.1161/JAHA.113.000408.
7. Aguilera S, Quintana L, Khan T, Garcia R, Shoman H, Caddell L, Latifi R, Park KB, Garcia P, Dempsey R, Rosenfeld JV, Scurlock C, Crisp N, Samad L, Smith M, Lippa L, Jooma R, Andrews RJ. Global health, global surgery and mass casualties: II. Mass casualty Centre resources, equipment and implementation. BMJ Glob Health. 2020;5(1):e001945. https://doi.org/10.1136/bmjgh-2019-001945.
8. Ahmed AA, Mojiri ME, Daghriri AA, Hakami OA, Alruwaili RF, Khan RA, Madkhali HA, Almania MM, Hakami ZT, Mashraqi KO, Adawi KA, Alqattan SA, Alharbi AN, Albahlol MA, Moafa AI. The role of telemedicine in emergency department triage and patient care: A systematic review. Cureus. 2024;16(12):e75505. https://doi.org/10.7759/cureus.75505.
9. Aizenberg M. Regulatory framework for telemedicine: current status and next steps. 2022; https://doi.org/10.18235/0004176
10. Akar JG, Bao H, Jones PW, Wang Y, Varosy PD, Masoudi FA, Stein KM, Saxon LA, Normand SL, Curtis JP. Use of remote monitoring is associated with lower risk of adverse outcomes among patients with implanted cardiac defibrillators. Circ Arrhythm Electrophysiol. 2015;8(5):1173–80. https://doi.org/10.1161/CIRCEP.114.003030.
11. Ali MR, Loggins JP, Fuller WD, Miller BE, Hasser CJ, Yellowlees P, Vidovszky TJ, Rasmussen JJ, Pierce J. 3-D telestration: a teaching tool for robotic surgery. J Laparoendosc Adv Surg Tech A. 2008;18(1):107–12. https://doi.org/10.1089/lap.2007.0051.
12. Alser K, Mallah SI, El-Oun YRA, Ghayada M, Sammour AA, Gilbert M, Fitzgerald S, Shaikh Z, Alser O. Trauma care supported through a global telemedicine initiative during the 2023–24 military assault on the Gaza strip, Occupied Palestinian Territory: a case series. Lancet. 2024;404(10455):874–86. https://doi.org/10.1016/S0140-6736(24)01170-X.
13. American Medical Association. Licensure & telehealth. Chicago (IL): American Medical Association; 2022. Available from: https://www.ama-assn.org/system/files/issue-brief-licensure-telehealth.pdf.
14. Andersen DS, Cabrera ME, Rojas-Muñoz EJ, Popescu VS, Gonzalez GT, Mullis B, Marley S, Zarzaur BL, Wachs JP. Augmented reality future step visualization for robust surgical telementoring. Simul Healthc. 2019;14(1):59–66. https://doi.org/10.1097/SIH.0000000000000334.
15. Antoniou SA, Antoniou GA, Franzen J, Bollmann S, Koch OO, et al. A comprehensive review of telementoring applications in laparoscopic general surgery. Surg Endosc. 2012;26(8):2111–6. https://doi.org/10.1007/s00464-012-2175-x.
16. Anvari M. Telesurgery: remote knowledge translation in clinical surgery. World J Surg. 2007;31(8):1545–50. https://doi.org/10.1007/s00268-007-9076-5.

17. Ärlebrant L, Dubois H, Creutzfeldt J, Edin-Liljegren A. Emergency care via video consultation: interviews on patient experiences from rural community hospitals in northern Sweden. Int J Emerg Med. 2024;6:24. https://doi.org/10.1186/s12245-024-00703-4.
18. Asbeck AT, Dyer RJ, Larusson AF, Walsh CJ. Biologically-inspired soft exosuit. In: 2013 IEEE international conference on rehabilitation robotics (ICORR) (Paper No. 6650455). IEEE; 2013. https://doi.org/10.1109/ICORR.2013.6650455.
19. Asbeck AT, De Rossi SM, Holt KG, Walsh C. A biologically inspired soft exosuit for walking assistance. Int J Robot Res. 2015;34(6):744–62. https://doi.org/10.1177/0278364914562476.
20. Ashkenazi I, Haspel J, Alfici R, Kessel B, Khashan T, Oren M. Effect of teleradiology upon pattern of transfer of head injured patients from a rural general hospital to a neurosurgical referral centre. Emerg Med J. 2007;24(8):550–2. https://doi.org/10.1136/emj.2006.044461.
21. Aucar JA, Villavicencio RT, Wall MJ Jr, et al. Evaluation of clinical data by remote observation in trauma. In: Proceedings of the AMIA annual fall symposium. National Institutes of Health; 1997. p. 408–12. https://www.ncbi.nlm.nih.gov/pmc/articles/PMC2233260/.
22. Aucar JA, Granchi T, Liscum K, Wall M, Mattox K. Is regionalization of trauma care using telemedicine feasible and desirable? Am J Surg. 2000;180(6):535–9. https://doi.org/10.1016/s0002-9610(00)00516-x.
23. Auccahuasi W, Meza S, Porras E, Reyes M, Linares O, Rojas K, Inciso-Roja M, Pando-Ezcurra T, Aiquipa G, Nicolas-Roja Y, Auccahuasi A. Application of real-time operating systems in the design of medical devices. CEUR Workshop Proc. 2022;3445:44–50. https://ceur-ws.org/Vol-3445/PAPER_05.pdf
24. Australian Institute of Health and Welfare. Potentially preventable hospitalizations in Australia by small geographic areas. 2019. https://www.aihw.gov.au/reports/primary-health-care/potentially-preventable-hospitalisations/contents/oveview
25. Baig MM, Gholamhosseini H. Smart health monitoring systems: An overview of design and modeling. J Med Syst. 2013;37:9898. https://doi.org/10.1007/s10916-012-9898-z.
26. Basco AI, Beliz G, Coatz D, Garnero P. Industria 4.0: Fabricando el Futuro. 2018. https://doi.org/10.18235/0001229.
27. Bashshur R, Shannon G, Krupinski E, Grigsby J. The taxonomy of telemedicine. Telemed e-Health. 2011;17(6):484–94. https://doi.org/10.1089/tmj.2011.0103.
28. Bashshur RL, Howell JD, Krupinski EA, Harms KM, Bashshur N, Doarn CR. The empirical foundations of telemedicine interventions in primary care. Telemed e-Health. 2016;22(5):342–75. https://doi.org/10.1089/tmj.2016.0045.
29. Bergmo TS. How to measure costs and benefits of eHealth interventions: An overview of methods and frameworks. J Med Internet Res. 2015;17(11):e254. https://doi.org/10.1111/ijs.12032.
30. Bhatia PD, Bottoni DA, Malthaner RA. Telesurgical evaluation of stable thoracic trauma patients: a feasibility study. Eur J Trauma Emerg Surg. 2011;37(3):297–303. https://doi.org/10.1007/s00068-011-0094-5.
31. Bilgic E, Turkdogan S, Watanabe Y, Madani A, Landry R, et al. Role of telementoring in global health: telemedicine applications for underserved populations. Surg Innov. 2017;24(4):321–6. https://doi.org/10.1177/1553350617708725.
32. Board on Health Care Services; Institute of Medicine. The role of telehealth in an evolving health care environment: workshop summary. National Academies Press; n.d. Retrieved from https://www.ncbi.nlm.nih.gov/books/NBK207141/.
33. Boggan JC, Shoup JP, Whited JD, et al. Effectiveness of acute care remote triage systems: a systematic review. J Gen Intern Med. 2020;35(8):2136–45. https://doi.org/10.1007/s11606-019-05585-4.
34. Bohingamu Mudiyanselage S, Stevens J, Watts JJ, Toscano J, Kotowicz MA, Steinfort CL, Bell J, Byrnes J, Bruce S, Carter S, Hunter C, Barrand C, Hayles R. Personalised telehealth intervention for chronic disease management: a pilot randomised controlled trial. J Telemed Telecare. 2019;25(6):343–52. https://doi.org/10.1177/1357633X18775850.

35. Borman KR, Vick LR, Biester TW, Mitchell ME. Changing demographics of residents choosing fellowships: longterm data from the American Board of Surgery. J Am Coll Surg. 2008;206(5):782–8. https://doi.org/10.1016/j.jamcollsurg.2007.12.012.
36. Bove AA, Homko CJ, Santamore WP, Kashem M, Kerper M, Elliott DJ. Managing hypertension in urban underserved subjects using telemedicine—a clinical trial. Am Heart J. 2013;165(4):615–21. https://doi.org/10.1016/j.ahj.2013.01.004.
37. Brova M, Boggs KM, Zachrison KS, Freid RD, Sullivan AF, Espinola JA, Boyle TP, Camargo CA Jr. Pediatric telemedicine use in United States emergency departments. Acad Emerg Med. 2018;25(12):1427–32. https://doi.org/10.1111/acem.13629.
38. Brown S, Rudahinduka K. Use of mobile devices for medical services in resource-limited settings: case study in Rwanda. Telemed eHealth. 2014;20(5):389–96. https://doi.org/10.1049/cp.2014.0766.
39. Buvik A, Bugge E, Knutsen G, Småbrekke A, Wilsgaard T. Quality of care for remote orthopaedic consultations using telemedicine: a randomised controlled trial. BMC Health Serv Res. 2016;16(1) https://doi.org/10.1186/s12913-016-1717-7.
40. Camara JG, Rodriguez RE. Real-time telementoring in ophthalmology. Telemed J. 1998;4(4):375–7. https://doi.org/10.1089/tmj.1.1998.4.375.
41. Campbell JL, Fletcher E, Britten N, Green C, Holt TA, Lattimer V, Richards DA, Richards SH, Salisbury C, Calitri R, Bowyer V, Chaplin K, Kandiyali R, Murdoch J, Roscoe J, Varley A, Warren FC, Taylor RS. Telephone triage for management of same-day consultation requests in general practice (the ESTEEM trial): A cluster-randomised controlled trial and cost-consequence analysis. Lancet. 2014;384(9957):1859–68. https://doi.org/10.1016/S0140-6736(14)61058-8.
42. Carrillo de Albornoz S, Sia KL, Harris A. The effectiveness of teleconsultations in primary care: systematic review. Fam Pract. 2022;39(1):168–82. https://doi.org/10.1093/fampra/cmab077.
43. Challacombe B, Kavoussi L, Stoianovici D. Remote percutaneous renal access using a telesurgical robotic system. In: Kumon H, Murai M, Baba S, editors. Endourooncology. Springer-Verlag; 2006. p. 63–73.
44. Chen AJ, Yeh SL, Delfin D, Hoal G, Barron N, Riedinger T, Kashanijou N, Lieland J, Bickel K, O'Connell JB, Ulloa JG. Telemedicine and vascular surgery: expanding access and providing care through the COVID-19 pandemic. Am Surg. 2022;88(10):2561–4. https://doi.org/10.1177/00031348221109464.
45. Cho J, Chung HS, Choa M, Yoo SK, Kim J. A pilot study of the tele-airway management system in a hospital emergency department. J Telemed Telecare. 2011;17(1):49–53. https://doi.org/10.1258/jtt.2010.100202.
46. Choi W, Cho YS, Ha YR, Oh JH, Lee H, Kang BS, Kim YW, Koh CY, Lee JH, Jung E, Sohn Y, Kim HB, Kim SJ, Kim H, Suh D, Lee DH, Hong JY, Lee WW, Society Emergency and Critical Care Imaging (SECCI). Role of point-of-care ultrasound in critical care and emergency medicine: update and future perspective. Clin Exp Emerg Med. 2023;10(4):363–81. https://doi.org/10.15441/ceem.23.101.
47. Chou W, Wang T, Zhang Y. Augmented reality based preoperative planning for robot assisted tele-neurosurgery. In: Proceedings of the 2004 IEEE international conference on systems, man and cybernetics, vol. 3. IEEE; 2004. p. 2901–6. https://doi.org/10.1109/ICSMC.2004.1400773.
48. Chu C, Cram P, Pang A, Stamenova V, Tadrous M, Bhatia R. Rural telemedicine use before and during the covid-19 pandemic: repeated cross-sectional study. J Med Internet Res. 2021;23(4):e26960. https://doi.org/10.2196/26960.
49. Clark NM, Agoubi LL, Gibbs S, Stewart BT, De Grauw X, Vavilala MS, Rivara FP, Arbabi S, Pham TN. Impact of tele-triage pathways on short-stay admission after transfer to a regional burn center for acute burn injury. J Am Coll Surg. 2023;237(6):799–807. https://doi.org/10.1097/XCS.0000000000000854.

50. Clemmensen P, Loumann-Nielsen S, Sejersten M. Telemedicine fighting acute coronary syndromes. J Electrocardiol. 2010;43(6):615–8. https://doi.org/10.1016/j.jelectrocard.2010.06.012.
51. Conforti R. Informatics in emergency medicine: a literature review. Emerg Care Med. 2025;2(1):2. https://doi.org/10.3390/ecm2010002.
52. Cragg DK, McKinley RK, Roland MO, et al. Comparison of out-of-hours care provided by patients' own general practitioners and commercial deputizing services: A randomized controlled trial. I: the process of care. BMJ. 1997;314(7075):187–9. https://doi.org/10.1136/bmj.314.7075.187.
53. Cronin AJ, Lopez JTJ, Pabla R. Evaluation of remote OMFS assessments in the era of pandemic COVID-19 control measures. Br J Oral Maxillofac Surg. 2020;58(8):1023–8. https://doi.org/10.1016/j.bjoms.2020.07.010.
54. Crowther JB, Poropatich R. Telemedicine in the U.S. Army: case reports from Somalia and Croatia. Telemed J. 1995;1(1):73–80. https://doi.org/10.1089/tmj.1.1995.1.73.
55. Cruz MJ, Nieblas-Bedolla E, Young CC, Feroze AH, Williams JR, Ellenbogen RG, Levitt MR. United States medicolegal progress and innovation in telemedicine in the age of COVID-19: A primer for neurosurgeons. Neurosurgery. 2021;89(3):364–71. https://doi.org/10.1093/neuros/nyab185.
56. Damayanti FN, Absori A, Wardiono K, Rejeki S. Ethical and legal issues in the use of online-based health services (E-health). SOEPRA. 2020;6(1):15–23.
57. Darkins A, Cary MA. Telemedicine and telehealth: principles, policies, performance, and pitfalls. Springer; 2000.
58. Davidson SK, Sanci L, de Nicolás IC, Watson CJ, Baltag V, Sawyer SM. Best practice during teleconsultations with adolescents: A scoping review. J Adolesc Health. 2022;70(5):714–28. https://doi.org/10.1016/j.jadohealth.2021.11.012.
59. Dawe P, Kirkpatrick A, Talbot M, Beckett A, Garraway N, Wong H, Hameed SM. Telementored damage-control and emergency trauma surgery: A feasibility study using live-tissue models. Am J Surg. 2018;215(5):927–9. https://doi.org/10.1016/j.amjsurg.2018.01.016.
60. de Araújo Novaes M, Basu A. Disruptive technologies: present and future. In: Fundamentals of telemedicine and telehealth. Academic; 2020. p. 305–30.
61. De Biase G, Freeman WD, Bydon M, Smith N, Jerreld D, Pascual J, Casler J, Hasse C, Quiñones-Hinojosa A, Abode-Iyamah K. Telemedicine utilization in neurosurgery during the COVID-19 pandemic: a glimpse into the future? Mayo Clin Proc Innov Qual Outcomes. 2020;4(6):736–44. https://doi.org/10.1016/j.mayocpiqo.2020.07.013.
62. Dharmar M, Romano PS, Kuppermann N, Nesbitt TS, Cole SL, Andrada ER, Vance C, Harvey DJ, Marcin JP. Impact of critical care telemedicine consultations on children in rural emergency departments. Crit Care Med. 2013;41(10):2388–95. https://doi.org/10.1097/CCM.0b013e31828e9824.
63. Doarn CR. Development of telemedicine and NASA'S contribution. Aerosp Med Hum Perform. 2015;86(5):504–5. https://doi.org/10.3357/AMHP.4324.2015.
64. Doarn CR, Latifi R. Telementoring and teleproctoring in trauma and emergency care. Curr Trauma Rep. 2016;2(3):138–43. https://doi.org/10.1007/s40719-016-0055-x.
65. Dubois H, Bergenmar M, Härgestam M, Creutzfeldt J. Patient participation in tele-emergencies – experiences from healthcare professionals in northern rural Sweden. Rural Remote Health. 2022;22:7404. Retrieved from https://www.rrh.org.au/journal/article/7404/
66. Duchesne JC, Kyle A, Simmons J, Islam S, Schmieg RE, Olivier J, McSwain NE. Impact of telemedicine upon rural trauma care. J Trauma Injury Infect Crit Care. 2008;64(1):92–8. https://doi.org/10.1097/TA.0b013e31815dd4c4.
67. Dullet NW, Geraghty EM, Kaufman T, Kissee JL, King J, Dharmar M, Smith AC, Marcin JP. Impact of a university-based outpatient telemedicine program on time savings, travel costs, and environmental pollutants. Value Health. 2017;20(4):542–6. https://doi.org/10.1016/j.jval.2017.01.014.

68. Dulou R, Dagain A, Delmas JM, Lambert E, Blondet E, Goasguen O, Pouit B, Dutertre G, de Soultrait F, Pernot P. The French mobile neurosurgical unit. Neurosurg Focus. 2010;28(5):E13. https://doi.org/10.3171/2010.2.FOCUS1016.
69. Eadie L, Mulhern J, Regan L, Mort A, Shannon H, Macaden A, et al. Remotely supported prehospital ultrasound: a feasibility study of real-time image transmission and expert guidance to aid diagnosis in remote and rural communities. J Telemed Telecare. 2017;24(9):616–22. https://doi.org/10.1177/1357633x17731444.
70. Eastridge BJ, Mabry RL, Seguin P, Cantrell J, Tops T, et al. Death on the battlefield (2001–2011): implications for the future of combat casualty care. J Trauma Acute Care Surg. 2012;73(6 Suppl):431–7. https://doi.org/10.1097/TA.0b013e3182755dcc.
71. Eijk ES, Bettink-Remeijer MW, Timman R, Busschbach JJ. From pen-and-paper questionnaire to a computer-assisted instrument for self-triage in the ophthalmic emergency department: process and validation. Comput Biol Med. 2015;66:258–62.
72. Ekeland AG, Bowes A, Flottorp S. Effectiveness of telemedicine: a systematic review of reviews. Int J Med Inform. 2010;79(11):736–71. https://doi.org/10.1016/j.ijmedinf.2010.08.006.
73. El Kalam AA, Ferreira A, Kratz F. Bilateral teleoperation system using QoS and secure communication networks for telemedicine applications. IEEE Syst J. 2016;10(2):709–20. https://doi.org/10.1109/JSYST.2015.2422992.
74. El-Sabawi B, Magee W III. The evolution of surgical telementoring: current applications and future directions. Ann Transl Med. 2016;4(20):Article 391. https://doi.org/10.21037/atm.2016.10.04.
75. Engle X, Aird J, Tho L, Bintcliffe F, Monsell F, Gollogly J. Combining continuing education with expert consultation via telemedicine in Cambodia. Trop Dr. 2014;44(2):62–8. https://doi.org/10.1177/0049475513515654.
76. Entezami P, Franzblau LE, Chung KC. Mentorship in surgical training: a systematic review. Hand. 2012;7(1):30–6. https://doi.org/10.1007/s11552-011-9379-8.
77. Ereso AQ, Garcia P, Tseng E, Gauger G, Kim H, Dua MM, Victorino GP, Guy TS. Live transference of surgical subspecialty skills using telerobotic proctoring to remote general surgeons. J Am Coll Surg. 2010;211(3):400–11. https://doi.org/10.1016/j.jamcollsurg.2010.05.014.
78. Eriksson-Liebon M, Roos S, Hellström I. Patients' expectations and experiences of being involved in their own care in the emergency department: a qualitative interview study. J Clin Nurs. 2021;30(13–14):1942–52. https://doi.org/10.1111/jocn.15746.
79. Esteva A, Kuprel B, Novoa RA, Ko J, Swetter SM, Blau HM, Thrun S. Dermatologist-level classification of skin cancer with deep neural networks. Nature. 2017;542(7639):115–8. https://doi.org/10.1038/nature21056.
80. Evans CR, Medina MG, Dwyer AM. Telemedicine and telerobotics: from science fiction to reality. Updat Surg. 2018;70(3):357–62. https://doi.org/10.1007/s13304-018-0574-9.
81. Fatehi F, Samadbeik M, Kazemi A. What is digital health? Review of definitions. Stud Health Technol Inform. 2020;275:67–71. https://doi.org/10.3233/SHTI200696.
82. Fawaz HI, Forestier G, Weber J, Petitjean F, Idoumghar L, Muller P-A. Automatic alignment of surgical videos using kinematic data. arXiv. 2019; https://doi.org/10.48550/arXiv.1904.07302.
83. Fezari M, Rasras R, El Emary IM. Ambulatory health monitoring system using wireless sensors node. Proc Comput Sci. 2015;65:86–94. https://doi.org/10.1016/j.procs.2015.09.082.
84. Fields BG. Regulatory, legal, and ethical considerations of telemedicine. Sleep Med Clin. 2020;15(3):409–16. https://doi.org/10.1016/j.jsmc.2020.06.004.
85. Fujiura Y, Sugimoto C, Kohno R. BAN MAC protocol for optimization the ratio between CAP and CFP. In: Medical information and communication technology (ISMICT), 2012 6th international symposium on; 2012. p. 1–4.
86. Ganz A, Schafer JM, Yang Z, Yi J, Lord G, Ciottone G. Mobile DIORAMA-II: infrastructure-less information collection system for mass casualty incidents. In: Engineering in medicine and biology society (EMBC), 2014 36th annual international conference of the IEEE; 2014. p. 2682–5.

87. Garcia P. Telemedicine for the battlefield: present and future technologies. In: Rosen J, Hannaford B, editors. Surgical robotics. Springer US; 2010. p. 33–68. https://doi.org/10.1007/978-1-4419-1126-1_3.
88. Gerhardt RT, Berry JA, Blackbourne LH. Analysis of life-saving interventions performed by out-of-hospital combat medical personnel. J Trauma Inj Infect Crit Care. 2011;71(Suppl):109–13. https://doi.org/10.1097/TA.0b013e31822190a7.
89. Gerhardt RT, Berry JA, Mabry RL, Flournoy L, Arnold RG, Hults C, Robinson JB, Thaxton RA, Cestero R, Heiner JD, Koller AR, Cox KM, Patterson JN, Dalton WR, McKeague AL, Gilbert G, Manemeit C, Adams BD. Evaluation of contingency telemedical support to improve casualty care at a simulated military intermediate resuscitation facility: the EM-ANGEL Study. J Spec Oper Med. 2014;14(1):50–7. https://doi.org/10.55460/G0D7-OBXG.
90. Ghassemi M, Naumann T, Schulam P, Beam AL, Chen IY, Ranganath R. Practical guidance on artificial intelligence for health-care data. Lancet Digital Health. 2019;1(4):e157–9. https://doi.org/10.1016/S2589-7500(19)30084-6.
91. Gioia G, Salducci M. Medical and legal aspects of telemedicine in ophthalmology. Rom J Ophthalmol. 2019;63(3):197–205.
92. Gomez D, Berube M, Xiong W, Ahmed N, Haas B, Schuurman N, et al. Identifying targets for potential interventions to reduce rural trauma deaths: a population-based analysis. J Trauma Acute Care Surg. 2010;69(3):633–9. https://doi.org/10.1097/TA.0b013e3181b8ef81.
93. Greenhalgh T, Shaw S, Wherton J, Vijayaraghavan S, Morris J, Bhattacharya S, Hanson P, Campbell-Richards D, Ramoutar S, Collard A, Hodkinson I. Real-world implementation of video outpatient consultations at macro, meso, and micro levels: mixed-method study. J Med Internet Res. 2018;20(4):e150. https://doi.org/10.2196/jmir.9897.
94. Gríofa MÓ, Blue RS, Friedman R, Hamski P, Bhagavatula M, Jaech A, Hu SY, Savvides M. Preliminary feasibility analysis of remote subject identification during hemodynamic monitoring by radio frequency impedance. In: Proceedings of the annual international conference of the IEEE engineering in medicine and biology society (EMBC); 2011. p. 2590–3. https://doi.org/10.1109/EMBC.2011.6090715.
95. Haimi M. The tragic paradoxical effect of telemedicine on healthcare disparities—a time for redemption: A narrative review. BMC Med Inform Decis Mak. 2023;23(1):Article 95. https://doi.org/10.1186/s12911-023-02194-4.
96. Hammersley V, Donaghy E, Parker R, McNeilly H, Atherton H, Bikker A, et al. Comparing the content and quality of video, telephone, and face-to-face consultations: A non-randomised, quasi-experimental, exploratory study in UK primary care. Br J Gen Pract. 2019;69(686):e595–604. https://doi.org/10.3399/bjgp19X704573.
97. Hart LG, Larson EH, Lishner DM. Rural definitions for health policy and research. Am J Public Health. 2005;95(7):1149–55. https://doi.org/10.2105/AJPH.2004.042432.
98. Hassanalieragh M, Page A, Soyata T, Sharma G, Aktas M, Mateos G, Kantarci B. Health monitoring and management using internet-of-things (IoT) sensing with cloud-based processing: opportunities and challenges. In: 2015 IEEE international conference on services computing (SCC); 2015. p. 285–92. https://doi.org/10.1109/SCC.2015.47.
99. Hatef E, Lans D, Bandeian S, et al. Outcomes of in-person and telehealth ambulatory encounters during COVID-19 within a large commercially insured cohort. JAMA Netw Open. 2022;5(4):e228954. https://doi.org/10.1001/jamanetworkopen.2022.8954.
100. Hentschel U, Khalid F, Polze A. An approach to control transmission of medical data over cellular networks using location information. In: Object/component/service-oriented real-time distributed computing (ISORC), 2012 IEEE 15th international symposium on; 2012. p. 87–94.
101. Hernandez C, Jansa M, Vidal M, et al. The burden of chronic disorders on hospital admissions prompts the need for new modalities of care: a cross-sectional analysis in a tertiary hospital. QJM. 2009;102(3):193–202. https://doi.org/10.1093/qjmed/hcn172.
102. Hong Y, Lee SH. Effectiveness of tele-monitoring by patient severity and intervention type in chronic obstructive pulmonary disease patients: A systematic review and meta-analysis. Int J Nurs Stud. 2019;92:1–15. https://doi.org/10.1016/j.ijnurstu.2018.12.006.

103. Hong S, Kim S, Kim J, Lim D, Jung S, Kim D, et al. Portable emergency telemedicine system over wireless broadband and 3G networks. In: engineering in medicine and biology society, 2009. EMBC 2009. Annual international conference of the IEEE; 2009. p. 1250–3. https://doi.org/10.1109/IEMBS.2009.5333914.
104. Hoyt DB, Shackford SR, Fridland PH, et al. Video recording trauma resuscitations: An effective teaching technique. J Trauma. 1988;28:435–40. https://doi.org/10.1097/00005373-198804000-00003.
105. Huang K-T, Ball C, Francis J, Ratan R, Boumis J, Fordham J. Augmented versus virtual reality in education: an exploratory study examining science knowledge retention when using augmented reality/virtual reality mobile applications. Cyberpsychol Behav Soc Netw. 2019;22(2):105–10. https://doi.org/10.1089/cyber.2018.0150.
106. Hung AJ, Chen J, Shah A, Gill IS. Telementoring and telesurgery for minimally invasive procedures. J Urol. 2018;199(2):355–69.
107. Hyder MA, Razzak J. Telemedicine in the United States: an introduction for students and residents. J Med Internet Res. 2020;22:e20839. https://doi.org/10.2196/20839.
108. Inglis SC, Clark RA, McAlister FA, et al. Which components of heart failure programmes are effective? A systematic review and meta-analysis of the outcomes of structured telephone support or telemonitoring as the primary component of chronic heart failure management in 8323 patients: Abridged Cochrane review. Eur J Heart Fail. 2011;13(10):1028–40. https://doi.org/10.1093/eurjhf/hfr039.
109. Jamniczky HA, McLaughlin K, Kaminska ME, Raman M, Somayaji R, Wright B, Ma IW. Cognitive load imposed by knobology may adversely affect learners' perception of utility in using ultrasonography to learn physical examination skills, but not anatomy. Anat Sci Educ. 2015;8(3):197–204. https://doi.org/10.1002/ase.1467.
110. Janssen F, Awadallah M, Alhalabi A, Körber B, Lang R, Scibor M, Handschu R. Telemedicine in general neurology: use of audiovisual consultation for on call back-up service in an acute care hospital. J Neurol. 2018;265:880–4. https://doi.org/10.1007/s00415-018-8756-4.
111. Johansson AM, Lindberg I, Söderberg S. Patients' experiences with specialist care via video consultation in primary healthcare in rural areas. Int J Telemed Appl. 2014;2014:Article 143824. https://doi.org/10.1155/2014/143824.
112. Kalid N, Zaidan AA, Zaidan BB, Salman OH, Hashim M, Muzammil H. Based real-time remote health monitoring systems: A review on patients prioritization and related "big data" using body sensors information and communication technology. J Med Syst. 2018;42:30. https://doi.org/10.1007/s10916-017-0883-4.
113. Kamine TH, Siu M, Kramer KZ, Alouidor R, Kelly E, Deutsch A, Mader TJ, Visintainer P, Grochowski K, Jabbour N. Feasibility and acceptance of a teletrauma surgery consult service to rural and community hospitals: A pilot study. J Am Coll Surg. 2023;236(1):145–53. https://doi.org/10.1097/XCS.0000000000000460.
114. Kaplan B, Litewka S. Ethical challenges of telemedicine and telehealth. Camb Q Healthc Ethics. 2018;27(4):653–67. https://doi.org/10.1017/S0963180118000206.
115. Keelara R, Sutherland E, Almyranti M. Beyond the pandemic: leading practices for the future of telemedicine, OECD health working papers no. 173. OECD Publishing; 2025. https://doi.org/10.1787/496a8ffe-enen.pdf.
116. Keesara S, Jonas A, Schulman K. Covid-19 and healthcare's digital revolution. N Engl J Med. 2020;382(23):e82. https://doi.org/10.1056/NEJMp2005835.
117. Kepplinger J, Dzialowski I, Barlinn K, Puetz V, Wojciechowski C, Schneider H, et al. Emergency transfer of acute stroke patients within the East Saxony telemedicine stroke network: a descriptive analysis. Int J Stroke. 2014;9(2):160–5. https://doi.org/10.1111/ijs.12032.
118. Keswani SG, Woo R, Hoover SJ, Arora PK, Barber AE, Beilman G, Cooke DT, Foe LM, Hashmi ZG, Henry MCW, Huang EY, Kirby J, Liepert AE, Moriarty KP, Nikolian VC, Park C, Redan JA, Selzer DJ, Spanos WC, et al. Unlocking the potential of telehealth in surgery: a comprehensive primer for surgeons. American College of Surgeons Board of Governors Telehealth Work Group; 2024. Retrieved from https://www.facs.org/media/os0i5fyd/unlocking-the-potential-of-telehealth-in-surgery-primer.pdf

119. Khalil I, Sufi F. Real-time ECG data transmission with wavelet packet decomposition over wireless networks. In: Intelligent sensors, sensor networks and information processing, 2008. ISSNIP 2008. International conference on. IEEE; 2008. p. 267–72.
120. Khor WS, Baker B, Amin K, Chan A, Patel K, Wong J, Thamboo A. Augmented and virtual reality in surgery—the digital surgical environment: applications, limitations, and legal pitfalls. Ann Transl Med. 2019;4(23):Article 454. https://doi.org/10.21037/atm.2016.12.23.
121. Kirkpatrick AW, Tien H, Laporta AT, Lavell K, Keillor J, Wright Beatty HE, McKee JL, Brien S, Roberts DJ, Wong J, et al. The marriage of surgical simulation and telementoring for damage-control surgical training of operational first responders: a pilot study. J Trauma Acute Care Surg. 2015;79(6):741–7. https://doi.org/10.1097/TA.0000000000000829.
122. Kirkpatrick AW, McKee JL, Netzer I, McKee IA, McBeth P, et al. A randomized trial of mentored versus nonmentored military medics compared in the application of a wound clamp without prior training: when to shut up and just watch! Mil Med. 2020;185(Suppl. 1):67–72. https://doi.org/10.1093/milmed/usz251.
123. Kitamura C, Zurawel-Balaura L, Wong RKS. How effective is video consultation in clinical oncology? A systematic review. Curr Oncol. 2010;17(3):17–27. https://doi.org/10.3747/co.v17i3.513.
124. Klersy C, De Silvestri A, Gabutti G, et al. Economic impact of remote patient monitoring: An integrated economic model derived from a meta-analysis of randomized controlled trials in heart failure. Eur J Heart Fail. 2011;13(4):450–9. https://doi.org/10.1093/eurjhf/hfq232.
125. Kobayashi H, Tomozawa H, Tamura H, Shigeno H, Okada K-I. Proposal of walkable path discovery technique in triage health technology. Health Technol. 2010;9(3):679–700.
126. Koutsakis P. Scheduling for telemedicine traffic transmission over WLANs. Comput Commun. 2017;108:17–26. https://doi.org/10.1016/j.comcom.2017.04.010.
127. Kruse CS, Krowski N, Rodriguez B, Tran L, Vela J, Brooks M. Telehealth and patient satisfaction: a systematic review and narrative analysis. BMJ Open. 2017;7(8):e016242. https://doi.org/10.1136/bmjopen-2017-016242.
128. Kwak MJ, Kim JM, Shin IH, Shin SD, Song KJ, Suh GJ, et al. Real-time medical control using a wireless audio-video transmission device in a pre-hospital emergency service in Korea. J Telemed Telecare. 2009;15(8):404–8. https://doi.org/10.1258/jtt.2009.090504.
129. LaBarbera JM, Ellenby MS, Bouressa P, Burrell J, Flori HR, Marcin JP. The impact of telemedicine intensivist support and a pediatric hospitalist program on a community hospital. Telemed e-Health. 2013;19(10):760–6. https://doi.org/10.1089/tmj.2012.0303.
130. Lake R, Georgiou A, Li J, Li L, Byrne M, Robinson M, Westbrook JI. The quality, safety and governance of telephone triage and advice services: an overview of evidence from systematic reviews. BMC Health Serv Res. 2017;17(1):Article 614. https://doi.org/10.1186/s12913-017-2564-x.
131. Landercasper J, Bintz M, Cogbill TH, Bierman SL, Buan RR, et al. Spectrum of general surgery in rural America. Arch Surg. 1997;132(5):494–6. https://doi.org/10.1001/archsurg.1997.01430290040005.
132. Landolina M, Perego GB, Lunati M, Curnis A, Guenzati G, Vicentini A, Parati G, Borghi G, Zanaboni P, Valsecchi S, Marzegalli M. Remote monitoring reduces healthcare use and improves quality of care in heart failure patients with implantable defibrillators: the Evolution of Management Strategies of Heart Failure Patients With Implantable Defibrillators (EVOLVO) study. Circulation. 2012;125(24):2985–92. https://doi.org/10.1161/CIRCULATIONAHA.111.088971.
133. Langabeer JR, Gonzalez M, Alqusairi D, Champagne-Langabeer T, Jackson A, Mikhail J, Persse D. Telehealth-enabled emergency medical services program reduces ambulance transport to urban emergency departments. West J Emerg Med. 2016;17(6):713–20. https://doi.org/10.5811/westjem.2016.8.30660.
134. Lasi H, Fettke P, Kemper HG, Feld T, Hoffmann M. Industry 4.0. Business & information. Syst Eng. 2014;6(4):239–42. https://doi.org/10.1007/s12599-014-0334-4.
135. Latifi R. Telepresence and telemedicine in trauma and emergency. Stud Health Technol Inform. 2008;131:275–80. PMID: 18305337

136. Latifi R. Telemedicine for trauma and emergency care management. In: Latifi R, Doarn CR, Merrell RC, editors. Telemedicine, telehealth and telepresence. Cham: Springer; 2021. https://doi.org/10.1007/978-3-030-56917-4_18.
137. Latifi R, Ong C, Peck K, Porter J, Williams M. Telepresence and telemedicine in trauma and emergency care management. Eur Surg. 2005;37(6):293–7. https://doi.org/10.1007/s10353-005-0180-1.
138. Latifi R, Hadeed GJ, Rhee P, O'Keeffe T, Friese RS, Wynne JL, Ziemba ML, Judkins D. Initial experiences and outcomes of telepresence in the management of trauma and emergency surgical patients. Am J Surg. 2009;198(6):905–10. https://doi.org/10.1016/j.amjsurg.2009.08.011.
139. Lattimer V, George S, Thompson F, et al. Safety and effectiveness of nurse telephone consultation in out-of-hours primary care: randomized controlled trial. BMJ. 1998;317(7165):1054–9. https://doi.org/10.1136/bmj.317.7165.1054.
140. Le Tourneau FM. Sparsely populated regions as a specific geographical environment. J Rural Stud. 2020;75:70–9. https://doi.org/10.1016/j.jrurstud.2019.12.012.
141. Lee BR, Bishoff JT, Janetschek G, Bunyaratevej P, Kamolpronwijit W, et al. A novel method of surgical instruction: international telementoring. World J Urol. 1998;16(6):367–70. https://doi.org/10.1007/s003450050082.
142. Lewis ER, Thomas CA, Wilson ML, Mbarika VW. Telemedicine in acute-phase injury management: A review of practice and advancements. Telemed J E Health. 2012;18(6):434–45. https://doi.org/10.1089/tmj.2011.0199.
143. Libreros-Peña L, Quintero JA, Gelves A, Alarcón J, Morales S, Escobar MF, Valencia AM, Guzmán S, Diez-Sepulveda J. Telemedicine consultation for emergency patients' attention: A clinical experience from a high complex university hospital from Latin America. BMC Health Serv Res. 2023;23(1):559. https://doi.org/10.1186/s12913-023-09520-6.
144. Lindberg J, Bhatt R, Ferm A. Older people and rural eHealth: perceptions of caring relations and their effects on engagement in digital primary healthcare. Scand J Caring Sci. 2021;35(4):1322–31. https://doi.org/10.1111/scs.12953.
145. Lynn M. Telemedicine to manage sudden mass casualty incidents remotely. In: Lynn M, et al., editors. Disasters and mass casualty incidents. Cham: Springer; 2019. https://doi.org/10.1007/978-3-319-97361-6_17.
146. MacKenzie EJ, Rivara FP, Jurkovich GJ, Nathens AB, Frey KP, Egleston BL, Salkever DS, Scharfstein DO. A national evaluation of the effect of trauma-center care on mortality. N Engl J Med. 2006;354(4):366–78. https://doi.org/10.1056/NEJMsa052049.
147. Malasinghe LP, Ramzan N, Dahal K. Remote patient monitoring: a comprehensive study. J Ambient Intell Humaniz Comput. 2019;10(2):57–76. https://doi.org/10.1007/s12652-017-0598-x.
148. Mandel JC, Kreda DA, Mandl KD, Kohane IS, Ramoni RB. SMART on FHIR: a standards-based, interoperable apps platform for electronic health records. J Am Med Inform Assoc. 2016;23(5):899–908. https://doi.org/10.1093/jamia/ocv189.
149. Manfredi S. Congestion control for differentiated healthcare service delivery in emerging heterogeneous wireless body area networks. IEEE Wirel Commun. 2014;21(2):81–90.
150. Manski-Nankervis JA, Davidson S, Hiscock H, Hallinan C, Ride J, Lingam V, et al. Primary care consumers' experiences and opinions of a telehealth consultation delivered via video during the COVID-19 pandemic. Aust J Prim Health. 2022;28(3):224–31. https://doi.org/10.1071/PY21193.
151. Marescaux J, Rubino F. Telesurgery, telementoring, virtual surgery, and telerobotics. Curr Urol Rep. 2003;4(2):109–13. https://doi.org/10.1007/s11934-003-0036-9.
152. McCormick R, Estrada J, Whitney C, Hinrichsen M, Lee PT, Cohen AB, et al. Teleneurology comprehensive inpatient consultations expedite access to care and decreases hospital length of stay. Neurohospitalist. 2021;11(3):229–34. https://doi.org/10.1177/19418744211000951.
153. McDonald CJ, Callaghan FM, Weissman A, Goodwin RM, Mundkur M, Kuhn T. Use of internist's free time by ambulatory care electronic medical record systems. JAMA Intern Med. 2014;174(11):1860–3. https://doi.org/10.1001/jamainternmed.2014.4506.

154. McGrail KM, Ahuja MA, Leaver CA. Virtual visits and patient-centered care: results of a patient survey and observational study. J Med Internet Res. 2017;19(5):e177. https://doi.org/10.2196/jmir.7374.
155. McKinstry B, Walker J, Campbell C, Heaney D, Wyke S. Telephone consultations to manage requests for same-day appointments: a randomised controlled trial in two practices. Br J Gen Pract. 2002;52(477):306–10.
156. Medeiros de Bustos E, Vuillier F, Chavot D, Moulin T. Télémédecine: Application aux urgences neurologiques [Telemedicine: application in the neurological emergencies]. Presse Med. 2012;41(5):514–7. https://doi.org/10.1016/j.lpm.2011.11.030.
157. Meer A, Rahm P, Schwendinger M, Vock M, Grunder B, Demurtas J, Rutishauser J. A symptom-checker for adult patients visiting an interdisciplinary emergency care center and the safety of patient self-triage: real-life prospective evaluation. J Med Internet Res. 2024;26:e58157. https://doi.org/10.2196/58157.
158. Mendez I, Jong M, Keays-White D, Turner G. The use of remote presence for health-care delivery in a northern Inuit community: a feasibility study. Int J Circumpolar Health. 2013;72(1):21112. https://doi.org/10.3402/ijch.v72i0.21112.
159. Ministry of Health. Rural health services in BC: A policy framework to provide a system of quality care. 2015. Retrieved from http://www.health.gov.bc.ca/library/publications/year/2015/rural-health-policy-paper.pdf.
160. Mock C, Lormand JD, Goosen J, Joshipura M, Peden M. Guidelines for essential trauma care. Geneva: World Health Organization; 2004. Retrieved from https://iris.who.int/bitstream/handle/10665/42565/9241546409_eng.pdf
161. Mohr NM, Vakkalanka JP, Harland KK, Bell A, Skow B, Shane DM, Ward MM. Telemedicine use decreases rural emergency department length of stay for transferred North Dakota trauma patients. Telemed e-Health. 2018;24(3):194–202. https://doi.org/10.1089/tmj.2017.0083.
162. Morales-García D, Docobo-Durantez F, Capitán Vallvey JM, Suarez-Grau JM, Campo-Cimarras ME, González-Vinagre S, Hidalgo-Grau LA, Puigcercos-Fusté JM, Zaragoza-Fernández C, Valera-Sánchez Z, Vega-Ruiz V. Consensus of the Ambulatory Surgery Committee section of the Spanish Association of Surgeons on the role of ambulatory surgery in the SARS-CoV-2 pandemic. Cirugía Española (English Edition). 2022;100(3):115–24. https://doi.org/10.1016/j.cireng.2022.02.014.
163. Morozov S, Guseva E, Ledikhova N, et al. Telemedicine-based system for quality management and peer review in radiology. Insights Imaging. 2018;9(3):337–41. https://doi.org/10.1007/s13244-018-0629-y.
164. Moya M, Valdez J, Yonas H, Alverson DC. The impact of a telehealth web-based solution on neurosurgery triage and consultation. Telemed e-Health. 2010;16(9):945–9. https://doi.org/10.1089/tmj.2010.0044.
165. Mueller KJ, Potter AJ, MacKinney AC, Ward MM. Lessons from tele-emergency: improving care quality and health outcomes by expanding support for rural care systems. Health Aff. 2014;33(2):228–34. https://doi.org/10.1377/hlthaff.2013.1016.
166. Munro J, Nicholl J, O'Cathain A, Knowles E. Impact of NHS direct on demand for immediate care: observational study. BMJ. 2000;321(7254):150–3. https://doi.org/10.1136/bmj.321.7254.150.
167. Munusamy A, Sridharan D. Priority based AODV routing protocol for critical data in wireless body area network. In: Proceedings of the 2015 international conference on soft-computing and network security (ICSCN); 2015. p. 1–5. https://doi.org/10.1109/ICSCN.2015.7219885.
168. Murphy RR, Srinivasan V, Henkel Z, Suarez J, Minson M, Straus J, et al. Interacting with trapped victims using robots. In: Technologies for Homeland Security (HST), 2013 IEEE international conference on; 2013. p. 32–7.
169. Nadar M, Jouvet P, Tucci M, Toledano B, Sicotte C. Impact of synchronous telemedicine models on clinical outcomes in pediatric acute care settings: a systematic review. Pediatr Crit Care Med. 2018;19(12):e662–71. https://doi.org/10.1097/PCC.0000000000001733.

170. Napi NM, Zaidan AA, Zaidan BB, et al. Medical emergency triage and patient prioritisation in a telemedicine environment: a systematic review. Health Technol. 2019;9:679–700. https://doi.org/10.1007/s12553-019-00357-w.
171. National Center for Biotechnology Information (NCBI). Remote consultation–MeSH–NCBI. 2016. Retrieved from http://www.ncbi.nlm.nih.gov/mesh?Db=mesh&term=Remote+Consultation
172. Negrini S, Donzelli S, Negrini A, Negrini A, Romano M, Zaina F. Feasibility and acceptability of telemedicine to substitute outpatient rehabilitation services in the COVID-19 emergency in Italy: an observational everyday clinical-life study. Arch Phys Med Rehabil. 2020;101(11):2027–32. https://doi.org/10.1016/j.apmr.2020.08.001.
173. Nettesheim N, Powell D, Vasios W, Mbuthia J, Davis K, et al. Telemedical support for military medicine. Mil Med. 2018;183(11–12):e462–70. https://doi.org/10.1093/milmed/usy127.
174. Netzer I, Kirkpatrick AW, Nissan M, McKee JL, McBeth P, Dobron A, Glassberg E. Rubrum Coelis: the contribution of real-time telementoring in acute trauma scenarios—a randomized controlled trial. Telemed e-Health. 2019;25(11):1108–14. https://doi.org/10.1089/tmj.2018.0173.
175. Nijland N, Cranen K, Verlinden SF, Kelders SM, Boer H, van Gemert-Pijnen JE. eTELEMED'09. In: Proceedings of the international conference on eHealth, telemedicine, and social medicine; 2009. p. 129–35.
176. Nittari G, Pippa L, Zaffina S, Al-Khafaji H. Telemedicine practice: review of the current ethical and legal challenges. Telemed e-Health. 2020;26(12):1427–37. https://doi.org/10.1089/tmj.2019.0158.
177. Noah B, Keller MS, Mosadeghi S, Stein L, Johl S, Delshad S. Impact of remote patient monitoring on clinical outcomes: an updated meta-analysis of randomized controlled trials. NPJ Digit Med. 2014;1(1):20172. https://doi.org/10.1038/s41746-017-0002-4.
178. Obermeyer Z, Emanuel EJ. Predicting the future—Big data, machine learning, and clinical medicine. N Engl J Med. 2016;375(13):1216–9. https://doi.org/10.1056/NEJMp1606181.
179. OECD. Health at a glance 2023: OECD indicators. Paris: OECD Publishing; 2023. https://doi.org/10.1787/7a7afb35-en.
180. Orlando JF, Beard M, Kumar S. Systematic review of patient and caregivers' satisfaction with telehealth videoconferencing as a mode of service delivery in managing patients' health. PLoS One. 2019;14(8):e0221848. https://doi.org/10.1371/journal.pone.0221848.
181. Otsu Y, Choh T, Yamazaki I, Kosaka K, Iguchi M, Nakajima I. Experiments on the quick-relief medical communications via Japan's domestic communication satellite CS-2 for the case of disasters and emergencies. Acta Astronaut. 1986;13(6–7):459–66. https://doi.org/10.1016/0094-5765(86)90099-8.
182. Pamplin J, Nemeth CP, Serio-Melvin ML, Murray SJ, Rule GT, Veinott ES, Veazey SR, Hamilton AJ, Fenrich CA, Laufersweiler DE, Salinas J. Improving clinician decisions and communication in critical care using novel information technology. Mil Med. 2020;185(1–2):e254–61. https://doi.org/10.1093/milmed/usz151.
183. Pan American Health Organization (PAHO). Eight guiding principles for digital transformation of the health sector. 2021. https://iris.paho.org/handle/10665.2/54256.
184. Park K, Park J, Lee J. An IoT system for remote monitoring of patients at home. Appl Sci. 2017;7(3):260. https://doi.org/10.3390/app7030260.
185. Park JP, Montreuil J, Nooh A, Martineau PA. Telemedicine-guided forearm emergency decompressive fasciotomy for compartment syndrome. J Telemed Telecare. 2023;29(1):28–32. https://doi.org/10.1177/1357633X20964359.
186. Parthiban N, Esterman A, Mahajan R, Twomey DJ, Pathak RK, Lau DH, Roberts-Thomson KC, Young GD, Sanders P, Ganesan AN. Remote monitoring of implantable cardioverter-defibrillators: A systematic review and meta-analysis of clinical outcomes. J Am Coll Cardiol. 2015;65(24):2591–600. https://doi.org/10.1016/j.jacc.2015.04.029.
187. Patel S, Park H, Bonato P, Chan L, Rodgers M. A review of wearable sensors and systems with application in rehabilitation. J Neuroeng Rehabil. 2012;9(1):21. https://doi.org/10.1186/1743-0003-9-21.

188. Piccini JP, Mittal S, Snell J, et al. Impact of remote monitoring on clinical events and associated healthcare utilization: A nationwide assessment. Heart Rhythm. 2016;13(12):2279–86. https://doi.org/10.1016/j.hrthm.2016.08.024.
189. Polinski JM, Barker T, Gagliano N, Sussman A, Brennan TA, Shrank WH. Patients' satisfaction with and preference for telehealth visits. JAMA Netw Open. 2016;3(7):e208786. https://doi.org/10.1007/s11606-015-3489-x.
190. Polygerinos P, Correll N, Morin SA, et al. Soft robotics: review of fluid-driven intrinsically soft devices; manufacturing, sensing, control, and applications. Adv Eng Mater. 2017;19(12):1700016. https://doi.org/10.1002/adem.201700016.
191. Putra EH, Supriyanto E, Din JB, Satria H. Cross-layer design of wireless LAN based on H.264/SVC and IEEE 802.11e. In: Electrical engineering and informatics (ICEEI), 2011 international conference on. IEEE; 2011. p. 1–6.
192. Qiao L, Koutsakis P. Guaranteed bandwidth allocation and QoS support for mobile telemedicine traffic. In: Sarnoff symposium, 2008. IEEE; 2008. p. 1–5.
193. Qiao L, Koutsakis P. Fair and efficient scheduling for telemedicine traffic transmission over wireless cellular networks. In: Vehicular technology conference, 2009. VTC spring 2009. IEEE 69th. IEEE; 2009. p. 1–5.
194. Radhakrishnan S, Duvvuru A, Kamarthi SV. Investigating discrete event simulation method to assess the effectiveness of wearable health monitoring devices. Procedia Econ Finance. 2014;11:838–56.
195. Rafiq A, Moore JA, Zhao X, Doarn CR, Merrell RC. Digital video capture and synchronous consultation in open surgery. Ann Surg. 2004;239(4):567–73. https://doi.org/10.1097/01.sla.0000118749.24645.45.
196. Rajkomar A, Oren E, Chen K, Dai AM, Hajaj N, Hardt M, Liu PJ, Liu X, Marcus J, Sun M, Sundberg P, Yee H, Zhang K, Zhang Y, Flores G, Duggan GE, Irvine J, Le Q, Litsch K, et al. Scalable and accurate deep learning with electronic health records. NPJ Digit Med. 2018;1:Article 18. https://doi.org/10.1038/s41746-018-0029-1.
197. Raposo VL. Telemedicine: the legal framework (or the lack of it) in Europe. GMS Health Technol Assess. 2016;12:1–8. https://doi.org/10.3205/hta000126.
198. Reed-Fox A. Patient online: putting patients in the driving seat of their care. Br J Community Nurs. 2015;20(4):181. https://doi.org/10.12968/bjcn.2015.20.4.181.
199. Rezvani S, Ghorashi SA. Context aware and channel-based resource allocation for wireless body area networks. IET Wireless Sens Syst. 2013;3:16–25. https://doi.org/10.1049/iet-wss.2012.0100.
200. Ricci MA, Caputo M, Amour J, Rogers FB, Sartorelli K, Callas PW, Malone PT. Telemedicine reduces discrepancies in rural trauma care. Telemed J E Health. 2003;9(1):3–11. https://doi.org/10.1089/153056203763317602.
201. Richards DA, Meakins J, Tawfik J, Godfrey L, Dutton E, Richardson G, Russell D. Nurse telephone triage for same day appointments in general practice: multiple interrupted time series trial of effect on workload and costs. BMJ. 2002;325(7374):1214.
202. Richards DA, Meakins J, Tawfik J, Godfrey L, Dutton E, Heywood P. Quality monitoring of nurse telephone triage: pilot study. J Adv Nurs. 2004;47(5):551–60. https://doi.org/10.1111/j.1365-2648.2004.03132.x.
203. Richards DA, Godfrey L, Tawfik J, et al. NHS direct versus general practice-based triage for same-day appointments in primary care: cluster randomized controlled trial. BMJ. 2004;329(7469):774–8. https://doi.org/10.1136/bmj.38226.605995.55.
204. Riva G, Gamberini L. Virtual reality in telemedicine. Telemed e-Health. 2000;6(3):327–40. https://doi.org/10.1089/153056200750040183.
205. Rockwood M, Joshi V, Sullivan K, Goubran R. Using a real-time operating system for multitasking in remote patient monitoring. In: Medical measurements and applications (MeMeA), 2014 IEEE international symposium on. IEEE; 2014. p. 1–5.
206. Rodriguez D, Heuer S, Guerra A, Stork W, Weber B, Eichler M. Towards automatic sensor-based triage for individual remote monitoring during mass casualty incidents. In:

Bioinformatics and biomedicine (BIBM), 2014 IEEE international conference on; 2014. p. 544–51.
207. Rogers FB, Ricci M, Caputo M, Shackford S, Sartorelli K, Callas P. The use of telemedicine for real-time video consultation between trauma center and community hospital in a rural setting improves early trauma care: preliminary results. J Trauma Acute Care Surg. 2001;51(6):1037–41. https://doi.org/10.1097/00005373-200112000-00002.
208. Rojas-Muñoz E, Lin C, Sanchez-Tamayo N, Cabrera ME, Andersen D, Popescu V, Barragan JA, Zarzaur B, Murphy P, Anderson K, Douglas T, Griffis C, McKee J, Kirkpatrick AW, Wachs JP. Evaluation of an augmented reality platform for austere surgical telementoring: A randomized controlled crossover study in cricothyroidotomies. NPJ Digital Med. 2020;3:Article 75. https://doi.org/10.1038/s41746-020-0284-9.
209. Rosser JC, Bell RL, Harnett B, Rodas E, Murayama M, Merrell R. Use of mobile low-bandwidth telemedical techniques for extreme telemedicine applications. J Am Coll Surg. 1999;189(4):397–404. https://doi.org/10.1016/s1072-7515(99)00185-4.
210. Rothenberg SS, Yoder S, Kay S, Ponsky T. Initial experience with surgical telementoring in pediatric laparoscopic surgery using remote presence technology. J Laparoendosc Adv Surg Tech A. 2009;19(Suppl. 1):219–22. https://doi.org/10.1089/lap.2008.0133.supp.
211. Rubin MN, Wellik KE, Channer DD, Demaerschalk BM. Systematic review of teleneurology: Neurohospitalist neurology. Neurohospitalist. 2013;3(3):120–4. https://doi.org/10.1177/1941874413483754.
212. Sabo RR. Surgical practice in rural communities: challenges and opportunities. Bull Am Coll Surg. 1994 Apr;79(4):6–10.
213. Sadang KG, Centracchio JA, Turk Y, Park E, Feliciano JL, Chua IS, Blackhall L, Silveira MJ, Fischer SM, Rabow M, Zachariah F, Grey C, Campbell TC, Strand J, Temel JS, Greer JA. Clinician perceptions of barriers and facilitators for delivering early integrated palliative care via telehealth. Cancers (Basel). 2023;15(22):5340. https://doi.org/10.3390/cancers15225340.
214. Salmoiraghi A, Hussain S. A systematic review of the use of telepsychiatry in acute settings. J Psychiatr Pract. 2015;21(5):389–93. https://doi.org/10.1097/PRA.0000000000000103.
215. Santoso APA, Soares D, Fauzi F, Amallia SD. Telemedicine: international law comparison. Easta J Law Hum Rights. 2024;2(03):116–26. https://doi.org/10.58812/eslhr.v2i03.286.
216. Sarria Guerrero JA, Luaces Cubells C, Jiménez Fàbrega FX, Villamor Ordozgoiti A, Isla Pera MPMP, Guix Comellas EM. Pediatric televisits and telephone triage: impact on use of a hospital emergency department. Emergencias. 2019;31(4):257–60.
217. Satava RM, Jones SB. Virtual reality and telemedicine: exploring advanced concepts. Telemed J. 1996;2(3):195–200. https://doi.org/10.1089/tmj.1.1996.2.195.
218. Schreiber MA, Zink K, Underwood S, Sullenberger L, Kelly M, Holcomb JB. A comparison between patients treated at a combat support hospital in Iraq and a level I trauma center in the United States. J Trauma Injury Infect Crit Care. 2008;64(Suppl):118–22. https://doi.org/10.1097/TA.0b013e318160869d.
219. Schreier G, Eckmann H, Hayn D, et al. Web versus APP: compliance of patients in a telehealth diabetes management programme using two different technologies. J Telemed Telecare. 2012;18(8):476–80. https://doi.org/10.1258/jtt.2012.gth112.
220. Schulam PG, Docimo SG, Saleh W, Breitenbach C, Moore RG, Kavoussi L. Telesurgical mentoring: initial clinical experience. Surg Endosc. 1997;11(10):1001–5. https://doi.org/10.1007/s004649900511.
221. Seeber A, Mitterer M, Gunsilius E, Mazzoleni G, Giovannetti R, Farsad M, Eisterer W, Gastl G, Pall G, Wieser A, Lukas P, Wimmer M, Spizzo G. Feasibility of a multidisciplinary lung cancer videoconference between a peripheral hospital and a comprehensive cancer centre. Oncology. 2013;84(3):186–90. https://doi.org/10.1159/000345314.
222. Seto E. Cost comparison between telemonitoring and usual care of heart failure: a systematic review. Telemed e-Health. 2008;14(7):679–86. https://doi.org/10.1089/tmj.2007.0114.

223. Sharifi Kia A, Rafizadeh M, Shahmoradi L. Telemedicine in the emergency department: an overview of systematic reviews. J Public Health. 2023;31:1193–207. https://doi.org/10.1007/s10389-021-01684-x.
224. Sharma T, Bamford M, Dodman D. Person-centred care: An overview of reviews. Contemp Nurse. 2015;51(2–3):107–20. https://doi.org/10.1080/10376178.2016.1150192.
225. Sharma SK, Woungang I, Anpalagan A, Chatzinotas S. Toward tactile internet in beyond 5G era: recent advances, current issues, and future directions. IEEE Access. 2020;8:56948–91.
226. Sheltami TR, Mahmoud AS, Abu-Amara MH. An ad hoc wireless sensor network for telemedicine applications. Arab J Sci Eng. 2007;32(2):131–46.
227. Shenai MB, Tubbs RS, Guthrie BL, Cohen-Gadol AA. Virtual interactive presence for real-time, long-distance surgical collaboration during complex microsurgical procedures: technical note. J Neurosurg. 2014;121(2):277–84. https://doi.org/10.3171/2014.4.JNS131805.
228. Shin DH, Dalag L, Azhar RA, Santomauro M, Satkunasivam R, Metcalfe C, Dunn M, Berger A, Djaladat H, Nguyen M, Desai MM, Aron M, Gill IS, Hung AJ. A novel interface for the telementoring of robotic surgery. BJU Int. 2015;116(2):302–8. https://doi.org/10.1111/bju.12985Sibley.
229. Snyderman CH, Gardner PA, Lanisnik B, Ravnik J. Surgical telementoring: a new model for surgical training. Laryngoscope. 2016;126(6):1334–8. https://doi.org/10.1002/lary.25753.
230. Soltane HB, Lazrak I, Chelly S, et al. Place of telemedicine in the organization of emergency care: feasibility and benefits. BMC Emerg Med. 2024;24:160. https://doi.org/10.1186/s12873-024-01074-y.
231. Spradley P. Telemedicine: the law is the limit. Tulane J Technol Intellect Prop. 2011;14:307–18.
232. Switzer JA, Hall C, Gross H, Waller J, Nichols FT, Wang S, Adams RJ, Hess DC. A web-based telestroke system facilitates rapid treatment of acute ischemic stroke patients in rural emergency departments. J Emerg Med. 2009;36(1):12–8. https://doi.org/10.1016/j.jemermed.2007.06.041.
233. Tang YM, Chau KY, Kwok APK, Zhu T, Ma X. A systematic review of immersive technology applications for medical practice and education: trends, application areas, recipients, teaching contents, evaluation methods, and performance. Educ Res Rev. 2022;35:100429. https://doi.org/10.1016/j.edurev.2021.100429.
234. Taylor ML, Thomas EE, Snoswell CL, Smith AC, Caffery LJ. Does remote patient monitoring reduce acute care use? A systematic review. BMJ Open. 2021;11(3):e040232. https://doi.org/10.1136/bmjopen-2020-040232.
235. Tolia V, Castillo E, Guss D. EDTITRATE (emergency department telemedicine initiative to rapidly accommodate in times of emergency). J Telemed Telecare. 2017;23(4):484–8. https://doi.org/10.1177/1357633X16648535.
236. Tomozawa H, Oguchi K, Shigeno H, Okada K. Message sending method using patients' priority for medical sensor network. In: Paper presented at 2009 29th IEEE international conference on distributed computing systems workshops, ICDCS, 09, Montreal, QC, Canada; 2009. p. 194–200. https://doi.org/10.1109/ICDCSW.2009.43.
237. Topol EJ. High-performance medicine: the convergence of human and artificial intelligence. Nat Med. 2019;25(1):44–56. https://doi.org/10.1038/s41591-018-0300-7.
238. Torppa MA, Timonen O, Keinänen-Kiukaanniemi S, Larivaara P, Leiman M. Patient-nurse-doctor interaction in general practice teleconsultations: A qualitative analysis. J Telemed Telecare. 2006;12(6):306–10. https://doi.org/10.1258/135763306778558196.
239. Traub SJ, Butler R, Chang YH, Lipinski C. Emergency department physician telemedical triage. Telemed J E Health. 2013;19(11):841–5. https://doi.org/10.1089/tmj.2013.0026.
240. Trondsen MV, Bolle SR, Stensland GØ, Tjora A. Video-confidence: a qualitative exploration of videoconferencing for psychiatric emergencies. BMC Health Serv Res. 2014;14:Article 544. https://doi.org/10.1186/s12913-014-0544-y.
241. Truong M, Yeganeh L, Cook O, Crawford K, Wong P, Allen J. Using telehealth consultations for healthcare provision to patients from non-indigenous racial/ethnic minorities: a systematic review. J Am Med Inform Assoc. 2022;29:970–82. https://doi.org/10.1093/jamia/ocac015.

242. Tsou C, Robinson S, Boyd J, Jamieson A, Blakeman R, Yeung J, McDonnell J, Waters S, Bosich K, Hendrie D. Effectiveness of telehealth in rural and remote emergency departments: systematic review. J Med Internet Res. 2021;23(11):e30632. https://doi.org/10.2196/30632.
243. Tuetken M, Hamlin S, Spaulding S. Implementation of a tele-triage protocol in an emergency department setting (Doctor of Nursing Practice project, Southern Illinois University Edwardsville). Doctor of Nursing Practice Projects, 187. 2022. https://www.siue.edu/nursing/academic-programs/graduate/pdf_dnp/Program2022.pdf.
244. Tulloh B, Clifforth S, Miller I. Caseload in rural general surgical practice and implications for training. ANZ J Surg. 2001;71(4):215–7. https://doi.org/10.1046/j.1440-1622.2001.02075.x.
245. Turner J, O'Cathain A, Knowles E, Nicholl J. Impact of the urgent care telephone service NHS 111 pilot sites: a controlled before and after study. BMJ Open. 2013;3(11):e003451. https://doi.org/10.1136/bmjopen-2013-003451.
246. Uscher-Pines L, Kahn JM. Barriers and facilitators to pediatric emergency telemedicine in the United States. Telemed e-Health. 2014;20(11):990–6. https://doi.org/10.1089/tmj.2014.0015.
247. Uscher-Pines L, Fischer S, Chari R. The promise of direct-to-consumer telehealth for disaster response and recovery. Prehosp Disaster Med. 2016;31(4):454–6. https://doi.org/10.1017/s1049023x16000558.
248. Vårdanalys. Tre perspektiv på digitala vårdbesök/Three perspectives on digital care visits. 2023. Retrieved from https://www.vardanalys.se/rapporter/tre-perspektiv-pa-digitala-vardbesok/.
249. Vegesna A, Tran M, Angelaccio M, Arcona S. Remote patient monitoring via non-invasive digital technologies: a systematic review. Telemed e-Health. 2017;23(1):3–17. https://doi.org/10.1089/tmj.2016.0051.
250. Ventola CL. Medical applications for 3D printing: current and projected uses. P&T. 2014;39(10):704–11.
251. Villa L, Matz O, Olaciregui Dague K, Kluwig D, Rossaint R, Brokmann JC. The assessment of dermatological emergencies in the emergency department via telemedicine is safe: a prospective pilot study. Intern Emerg Med. 2020;15(7):1275–9. https://doi.org/10.1007/s11739-020-02323-1.
252. Wachs JP, Kölsch M, Stern H, Edan Y. Vision-based hand-gesture applications. Commun ACM. 2011;54(2):60–71. https://doi.org/10.1145/1897816.1897838.
253. Wachs JP, Kirkpatrick AW, Tisherman SA. Procedural telementoring in rural, underdeveloped, and austere settings: origins, present challenges, and future perspectives. Annu Rev Biomed Eng. 2021;23:115–39. https://doi.org/10.1146/annurev-bioeng-083120-023315.
254. Wake E, Atkins H, Willock A, Hawkes A, Dawber J, Weir KA. Telehealth in trauma: a scoping review. J Telemed Telecare. 2020;28(6):412–22. https://doi.org/10.1177/1357633X20940868.
255. Wang X-D, Wang Z-Z, Li Z-Z, Zhou Y. Performance analysis of multi-priority buffer queue and its application of data transmission system in remote monitoring system. In: Information engineering and computer science (ICIECS), 2009 international conference on. IEEE; 2009. p. 1–5.
256. Wang TT, Li JM, Zhu CR, Hong Z, An DM, Yang HY, Ren JC, Zou XM, Huang C, Chi XS, Chen JN, Hong Z, Wang WZ, Xu CG, He L, Li WM, Zhou D. Assessment of utilization and cost-effectiveness of telemedicine program in western regions of China: a 12-year study of 249 hospitals across 112 cities. Telemed J E Health. 2016;22(11):909–20. https://doi.org/10.1089/tmj.2015.0213.
257. Wani S, Rabah S, AlFadil S, Dewanjee N, Najmi Y. Efficacy of communication amongst staff members at plastic and reconstructive surgery section using smartphone and mobile whatsapp. Indian J Plast Surg. 2013;46(03):502–5. https://doi.org/10.4103/0970-0358.121990.
258. Waran V, Selladurai BM, Bahuri NF, George GJ, Lim GP, Khine M. Teleconferencing using multimedia messaging service (MMS) for long-range consultation of patients with neurosurgical problems in an acute situation. J Trauma. 2008;64(2):362–5; discussion 365. https://doi.org/10.1097/TA.0b013e318070cc88.
259. Ward MM, Jaana M, Natafgi N. Systematic review of telemedicine applications in emergency rooms. Int J Med Inform. 2015;84(9):601–16. https://doi.org/10.1016/j.ijmedinf.2015.05.009.

260. Weibel N, Gasques D, Johnson J, Sharkey T, Xu ZR, Zhang X, Zavala E, Yip M, Davis K. Artemis: mixed-reality environment for immersive surgical telementoring. In: Extended abstracts of the 2020 CHI conference on human factors in computing systems. ACM; 2020. p. 1–4. https://doi.org/10.1145/3334480.3382834.
261. Sibley LM, Weiner JP. An evaluation of access to health care services along the rural-urban continuum in Canada. BMC Health Serv Res. 2011;11:20. https://doi.org/10.1186/1472-6963-11-20.
262. Whitehouse CR, Long JA, Maloney LM, et al. Feasibility of diabetes self-management telehealth education for older adults during transitions in care. Res Gerontol Nurs. 2020;13(3):138–45. https://doi.org/10.3928/19404921-20191210-03.
263. WHO Global Observatory for eHealth. Telemedicine: opportunities and developments in member states: report on the second global survey on eHealth. World Health Organization; 2010. https://iris.who.int/handle/10665/44497
264. Wilson N, Couper I, De Vries E, Reid S, Fish T, Others. A critical review of interventions to redress the inequitable distribution of healthcare professionals to rural and remote areas. Rural Remote Health. 2009;2(9):1060. https://pubmed.ncbi.nlm.nih.gov/19530891/
265. Witkowska-Zimny M, Nieradko-Iwanicka B. Telemedicine in emergency medicine in the COVID-19 pandemic: experiences and prospects—a narrative review. Int J Environ Res Public Health. 2022;19(13):8216. https://doi.org/10.3390/ijerph19138216.
266. Wood D. No surgeon should operate alone: how telementoring could change operations. Telemed e-Health. 2011;17(3):150–2. https://doi.org/10.1089/tmj.2011.9986.
267. Wood EW, Strauss RA, Janus C, Carrico CK. Telemedicine consultations in oral and maxillofacial surgery: a follow-up study. J Oral Maxillofac Surg. 2016;74(2):262–8. https://doi.org/10.1016/j.joms.2015.09.026.
268. Wood T, Freeman S, Banner D, Martin-Khan M, Hanlon N, Flood F. Factors associated with utilization of teletrauma services in rural areas: a review of the literature. Rural Remote Health. 2021;21:Article 6354. https://doi.org/10.22605/RRH6354.
269. World Health Organization. Global strategy on digital health 2020–2025. WHO; 2021. https://apps.who.int/iris/bitstream/handle/10665/344249/9789240020924-eng.pdf
270. Xiong W, Bair A, Sandrock C, Wang S, Siddiqui J, Hupert N. Implementing telemedicine in medical emergency response: concept of operation for a regional telemedicine hub. J Med Syst. 2012;36:1651–60. https://doi.org/10.1007/s10916-010-9626-5.
271. Yellowlees P, Nakagawa K, Pakyurek M, Hanson A, Elder J, Kales HC. Rapid conversion of an outpatient psychiatric clinic to a 100% virtual telepsychiatry clinic in response to COVID-19. Psychiatr Serv. 2020;71(7):749–52. https://doi.org/10.1176/appi.ps.202000230.
272. Zhou L, Bao J, Watzlaf V, Parmanto B. Barriers to and facilitators of the use of mobile health apps from a security perspective: mixed-methods study. JMIR Mhealth Uhealth. 2019;7(4):e11223. https://doi.org/10.2196/11223.
273. Zvikhachevskaya A, Markarian G, Mihailova L. Quality of service consideration for the wireless telemedicine and e-health services. In: Wireless communications and networking conference, 2009. WCNC 2009. IEEE; 2009. p. 1–6.

Part III

Imaging Technologies, Surgical Robotics, Automation, Monitoring in Emergency General Surgery

Overview of Surgical Robotics and Automation Technologies Applications in Acute Care and Emergency Surgery (Robotic Emergency Surgery)

11

Francesco Marchegiani, Carlo Alberto Schena, and Nicola de'Angelis

11.1 Introduction

Since its introduction in 2001 and over the past 20 years, robotic surgery has rapidly grown, and its application now involves multiple surgical specialties [1]. General surgery benefitted from the adoption of robotics in several domains with some proven technical advantages that supported its progressive implementation despite the initial limited body of evidence [2]. This trend is probably changing, and several clinical trials are now available [3].

For more than 20 years, the most diffused robotic platform on the market has been the Intuitive Surgical® Da Vinci® system. The company produced five different generations of robots and registered the majority of the patents in this field [4]. Today, following the expiration of several patents, new competitors have arrived on the market, proposing alternative robotic platforms with different characteristics and architectures [4].

Acute care surgery was not kept out from the robotic revolution, and a recent analysis performed over 8 years in the United States showed a trend of an increasing adoption of robotic platforms in the field of emergency general surgery [5]. In 2021, the World Society of Emergency Surgery (WSES) published a position paper proposing recommendations for the adoption of robotic surgery in emergency settings [6]. The majority of the studies reporting on robotic emergency surgery were

F. Marchegiani
Unit of Colorectal and Digestive Surgery, Beaujon University Hospital (AP-HP) and University Paris Cité, Clichy, France

C. A. Schena · N. de'Angelis (✉)
Unit of General Surgery, Fondazione Poliambulanza Hospital, Brescia, Italy
e-mail: carloalberto.schena@ospfe.it; nicola.deangelis@unife.it

B. De Simone et al. (eds.), *New Technologies, Precision Medicine, and AI in Emergency General Surgery*, Hot Topics in Acute Care Surgery and Trauma,
https://doi.org/10.1007/978-3-032-09357-8_11

performed with the Intuitive Surgical® da Vinci® system, but more recently, and in parallel with the evolution of the market, several reports on new robotic platforms are now available [4].

This chapter aims to provide an overview of surgical robotics and automation technologies' applications that are currently adopted in acute care and emergency surgery.

11.2 Overview of Robotics and Automation Technology in Surgery

The robotic platforms are composed of a surgeon-controlled console, a patient cart, and a central tower generally accommodating the visualization system (vision cart, in this case), the insufflation system and, in some cases, the electrosurgical generator.

Nowadays, robotic platforms available for general surgery can be classified according to the patient cart or the console architecture.

11.2.1 Patient Cart

The patient cart is the interface between the machine and the patient. The available robots are classified as single-cart multi-arm when the cart is single and usually bulky, holding all three or four arms on itself. The other available architecture is the multi-cart modular one when the carts are multiples, and each one holds a specific instrument. A special mention should be made for the single-port systems, which are composed of a single cart with single or multiple arms accommodating flexible instruments. New architectures are emerging on the market, such as the Virtual Incision Mira, which is the first portable robotic device conceived as a single access, two-arms robot.

11.2.2 Surgeon Console

The surgeon's console is the control interface of all the master-slave robotic systems available on the market. The operating surgeon can manage the camera movements, the surgical instruments, and the energy. In some cases, and with model-specific procedures, the console allows to personalize all the robot settings. Each company adopted a different visualization system and command system.

The console architecture can be classified as closed or opened. The first type presents an immersive stereoscopic vision with the advantage of reducing the distraction coming from the surrounding environment and the light variations. The second type offers an increased perception of the operative theater, a less claustrophobic interface, and improved communication with the entire team.

Another crucial point in the console architecture is the ergonomics, which varies between the different models, with the possibility to adjust the arms, foot, and headrests depending on the specific product [7]. One platform, the CMR Versius®, offers the opportunity to operate in a standup position and does not have pedals because the energy commands are located on the joysticks.

The joysticks adopted to control the instruments are different according to the specific model, but they usually have multiple degrees of freedom, allowing them to articulate the instruments' tips and to grasp, as the robotic instrument could replicate the natural movement of the fingertips. The only exception is the Asensus Senhance,® which adopted a laparoscopic-like joystick with a reduced degree of freedom.

A common characteristic of robotic surgery is that systems are conceived for the telemanipulation, and the first operating surgeon (console surgeon) is not scrubbed. Some exceptions are new in this field with the advent of more recent products, such as the Distalmotion Dexter, which allows its use in a sterile field, facilitating hybrid procedures and allowing the surgeon to operate in first person on the patient and to rapidly sit in the console for the robotic time.

11.2.3 Three-Dimensional Visualization Systems

The shared characteristic of the robotic platform is the three-dimensional (3D) view. Two main options are currently proposed by the manufacturers. The closed console systems offer a stereoscopic vision projecting the correspondent's eye image on a different screen. The open console systems adopt a flat screen and polarized glasses to guarantee stereoscopic vision.

The assistant surgeon can benefit from an open 3D vision if the system is endowed with a 3D screen or a conventional bi-dimensional (2D) vision, which is still the standard in the majority of the operating theaters.

A new concept of a 3D-4K glassless vision, known as autostereoscopy, was recently mentioned by Asensus Surgical but never unveiled nor tested [8]. This technology could be a meeting point between the head-mounted devices for augmented or virtual reality and the conventional 3D screens with polarized views [9].

11.2.4 Trocars, Instruments, and Trocars' Disposition

The available robotic platforms adopt commercial or dedicated trocars. The dedicated ones are usually motivated by the need to dock the robot to the trocar in the way that the cannula acts as a fulcrum. The commercial trocars are more adopted by robots whose instruments constantly slide into the cannula with no fixed fulcrum.

The implication of a commercial trocar is related to the possibility of easily switching from a full robotic procedure to a hybrid laparoscopic and robotic procedure, which can be useful in emergency surgery. Furthermore, commercial trocars are usually less expensive than dedicated ones but have a major impact in terms of carbon footprint [10].

The instruments adopted by the robotic platforms are always specific and dedicated. The concepts proposed by the different companies are opposite: the disposable instruments on one side and the sterilizable instruments on the other.

The disposable instruments are proposed as more precise and less influenced by repetitive use and processing. The reusable instruments are less precise with the ongoing usage, but they are less impactful in terms of costs and carbon footprint. Unfortunately, the manufacturers propose different visions behind the sterilization and the carbon footprint, which are difficult to analyze in a generic context, always bearing in mind that minimally invasive surgery has a major impact in terms of pollution [4, 11].

The presence of advanced instruments such as clip appliers, staplers, and advanced energy is not a standard in robotic surgery. At the present moment, only Intuitive Surgical® can offer a complete set of instruments, while some other producers, such as MicroPort® MedBot™, offer robotic clipping and advanced stapling. In addition, rigid ultrasonic devices are currently offered by some robots such as the Wego Micro Hand S, the Asensus Senhance®, and the Meerecompany Inc. Revo-i™.

The trocar disposition is defined by the robot-specific model, but two main patterns can be defined: the linear or semi-linear disposition of the trocars and the triangulated or semi-triangulated disposition. The linear disposition conditions the surgeon in the case of hybrid laparoscopic and robotic surgery because the absence of triangulation reduces the surgeon's dexterity [12]. For this reason, the modular platforms can be considered more appropriate for hybrid procedures.

11.2.5 Platforms Adopted for Emergency General Surgery

Since 2012, the majority of the reports concerned Intuitive Surgical® platforms of third and fourth generation (namely da Vinci® Si™, da Vinci® Xi™, and da Vinci® X™) [13].

According to de'Angelis et al., in 2021 only ten studies reported outcomes of emergency general surgery in different domains: colorectal surgery [14–16], hiatal hernia surgery [17, 18], gallbladder surgery [19, 20], bariatric surgery [21, 22], and abdominal wall surgery [23].

A more recent systematic review, including case reports and small series, documented 50 papers describing the adoption of robotic surgery in an emergency setting [13]. In total, 955 urgent surgical procedures were analyzed by the authors. The majority of the patients were operated on with an Intuitive Surgical® da Vinci®. Only 3.6% of the patients were treated with a platform different from the Intuitive Surgical® one.

According to Reinisch et al., the reported areas of application for emergency robotic surgery are the following: appendectomies, cholecystectomies, hernias, and gastrointestinal procedures.

The appendectomies were realized with several generations of the Intuitive Surgical® da Vinci® [24, 25], with the CMR Versius® [26] and with the Wego Micro

Hand S [27, 28]. The cholecystectomies were realized with several generations of the Intuitive Surgical® da Vinci® [19, 20, 24, 28–50]. The hernia surgeries were performed with several generations of the Intuitive Surgical® da Vinci® [18, 23, 32, 51–55]. The gastrointestinal procedures were reported with several generations of the Intuitive Surgical® da Vinci® [14–16, 21, 22, 56–60] and with the Wego Micro Hand S [27, 28, 61]. One splenectomy was reported with the use of a first-generation Intuitive Surgical® da Vinci® [32].

With the advent of new robotic platforms, several new cases were published in the literature. In a recent analysis, 8.8% of the reported procedures were non-elective cases [4]. The retrieved information is related to the pathological condition, and few explications were granted by the authors regarding the real clinical condition of the patient or the setting of the intervention. According to the study, incarcerated hernias were operated on with the Intuitive Surgical® da Vinci® SP™ and the Asensus Senhance® [62, 63], one gastric peptic ulcer was operated on with the Wego Micro Hand S [64], seven acute appendicitis were treated with the CMR Versius® and the Wego Micro Hand S [26, 64], 99 acute cholecystitis were operated on with the Asensus Senhance®, the CMR Versius®, the Intuitive Surgical® da Vinci® SP™ and the Wego Micro Hand S [28, 63, 65–70].

The reported cases are progressively increasing worldwide. Two cases of acute-on-chronic cholecystitis, operated on with the Medtronic Hugo RAS™ robot, were reported by Belyaev et al. [71]. The authors described several technical limitations regarding the difficult grasping of the thickened gallbladder and the risk of damaging the delicate scissors.

More recently, papers reporting advanced procedures are being published, such as an emergency liver resection for a ruptured hepatocellular carcinoma [72], a subtotal colectomy for an inflammatory bowel disease [73], and a total colectomy for a refractory graft-versus-host disease colitis [74]. All three procedures were performed with an Intuitive Surgical® da Vinci®.

All the cited robots are presented below. (Fig. 11.1).

11.2.5.1 Intuitive Surgical® da Vinci® Xi™

Intuitive Surgical® has dominated the market for more than 20 years. The da Vinci® Xi™, the fourth-generation master-slave robot, was released in 2014, revolutionizing the robotic surgery field with several crucial novelties.

It's composed of the shared Intuitive Surgical® console with a closed architecture, a control tower that accommodates all the components, and a multi-arm patient single-cart with four arms.

The introduction of the rotating boom-mounted architecture eliminated the need for a perpendicular approach of the robot to the patient, allowing the entire system to rotate around a central fulcrum, according to the planned procedure. This novelty facilitated upper GI, hepatobiliary, and pelvic procedures without the need to occupy the head or the pelvis of the patient with the presence of the bulky machine. In addition, the multi-quadrant surgery became simpler thanks to the possibility of rotating the entire system during the procedure.

	Single-cart Multi-arm	Multi-cart Modular	Single-cart Single-port
	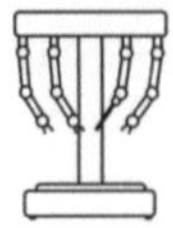	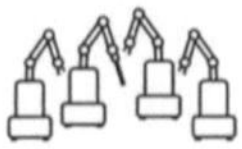	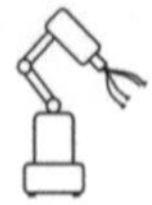
Platforms adopted in non-elective setting	Intuitive Surgical® da Vinci® Xi™ Wego Micro Hand S	Asensus Senhance® CMR Versius® Medtronic Hugo®	Intuitive Surgical® da Vinci® SP™

Fig. 11.1 Robotic platform adopted in non-elective setting, according to their architecture

The da Vinci® Xi™ introduced the linear trocar disposition and a light 8 mm camera with the same diameter as all the instruments (except for the 12 mm stapler) and the possibility to continuously switch the instruments' position from one arm to the others with no limitations.

Another useful feature was the introduction of the integrated table motion when used with the Trumpf Medical TruSystem® 7000dV operating table (TRUMPF Medizin Systeme GmbH & Co. KG, Saalfeld, Germany). The table motion allows for intraoperative patient movement, under the direct control of the operating surgeon, without the need to undock the entire platform.

The robot uses reusable instruments with a variable number of usages. Furthermore, several instruments are disposable.

11.2.5.2 Asensus Senhance®

This master-slave robotic platform was created by SOFAR S.p.A., an Italian pharmaceutical company that sold the entire division to TransEnterix Inc. in 2015. The platform gained both the CE mark in 2014 and the FDA approval in 2017. The product was first commercialized with the name ALF-X® and then rebranded to Senhance®. The company changed the name to Asensus Surgical and commercialized a robot composed of a console with an open architecture, a 3D screen, and an adjustable seat to provide better ergonomics. The controls are not flexible joysticks but rather semi-rigid laparoscopic handles. The machine was the first on the market to offer haptic feedback, an eye-tracking camera control, and the opportunity to use small 3-mm or 5-mm instruments, possibly expanding the applications of robotic surgery.

The modular carts enter from different directions to reach the patient and occupy the space around the table.

The company is struggling in the market expansion due to some limitations of the current platform, but a new model, called Luna system®, is under development to fill the gap with the competitors.

11.2.5.3 CMR Versius®

The CMR Surgical, a United Kingdom-based company, was founded in 2014, and it released in 2019 its first robotic platform called Versius®. The study behind the development of this platform took into consideration the limits of the closed console architecture and proposed an open console with a completely adjustable posture that allows the use in a standup position. No pedal is present, and the whole system is commanded through joysticks. The 3D screen is a solution shared with laparoscopy. The modular system is composed of four bedside units of limited weight and dimension, which are interfaced with the patient through commercial trocars with no need for trocar docking. The visualization system, the energy system, and the insufflation system are not dedicated, which allows to reduce the costs of the installation by adopting a preexisting laparoscopic tower. Recently, some novelties were introduced by the producer under the name Versius Plus®, such as an advanced near-infrared fluorescence system (named vLimeLite).

CMR can account for more than 20,000 procedures completed all over the world by more than 140 robotic platforms [75, 76].

11.2.5.4 Wego Micro Hand S

The platform was a joint venture project between Wego, a Chinese leader company in the healthcare sector, Tianjin University, and Central South University. The robot is sometimes referred to as "WEGO Miaoshou." In 2013, the project started with a prototype, and the evolution brought it to a national approval in 2021. The master-slave platform has an open console with 3D vision and a multi-arm cart accommodating three arms, which has, like the da Vinci® Xi™, a rotating system. Despite the literature regarding the robot and its comparison with the da Vinci® robot, little information exists on the specific model, mainly conceived for the domestic market.

11.2.5.5 Medtronic Hugo RAS™

Medtronic is a leader in the surgical field, and in 2021, it launched its first robotic device named Hugo RAS™. The development of this robot started in 2013 thanks to the licensing from the National Aeronautics and Space Research Center of the Federal Republic of Germany (DLR). The product received the CE mark and was commercialized, starting to be adopted in different domains in the last months. The Medtronic Hugo RAS™ is a master-slave system that is composed of an open surgeon console with 3D vision, four single-arm modular units approaching the patient from all directions, and a visualization cart that integrates the laparoscopic technology by Karl Storz company and the electrosurgical generator from Medtronic. The company did not develop dedicated advanced robotic instruments, but it offers a complete set of Covidien advanced laparoscopic tools, such as the Signia™ stapler, the LigaSure™ advanced bipolar system, and the Sonicision™ ultrasonic system.

11.2.5.6 Intuitive Surgical® da Vinci® SP™

As a leader in the market, Intuitive Surgical® developed its first single-port system starting its research project in 2006. The first in vivo test with a single-port system was realized in 2010 in Lille (France) but following the launch of the fourth generation of the robot (namely, the da Vinci® Xi™) the project was revisited, and the actual version of the da Vinci® SP™ was officially launched in the United States in 2018.

The robot shares the surgeon's console and the central tower with the other da Vinci® models, as well as the 3D high-definition vision. The patient cart, instead, is totally different, with a single arm accommodating the optics and three instruments. All of them are flexible and can pass through the 25-mm dedicated reusable cannula before deploying into the abdominal cavity.

For the complex procedures, the dedicated cannula is inserted in a disposable single-port commercial or dedicated system.

11.2.6 Single-Incision Surgery

A special mention, when reporting emergency robotic surgery, should be made for the single-port surgery. In 2011, Intuitive Surgical® launched the Single-Site™ system which is a five-lumen 25-mm silicon port holding two 5-mm dedicated semi-curved trocars for the instruments and one 8.5-mm straight trocar for the optics. The system is recognized by the robot software, and it offers the opportunity to perform single-port operations with a multiport robot. It was first adopted for the da Vinci® Si™ robot then it was updated for da Vinci® Xi™, in 2016.

The Single-Site™ system was adopted for more than 10 years, even in emergency procedures such as cholecystectomies [19]. This has nothing in common with the above-mentioned da Vinci® SP™ platform.

11.2.7 New Platforms

Several new robotic platforms are diffusing all around the world, and more procedures performed with these emerging platforms are progressively reported in the literature [4]. A recent review showed that the majority of the new platforms are still in the early phases of the IDEAL framework [77]. Indeed, the expanding competition among industries could be responsible for a more rapid adoption of new robots despite the lack of an extensive evaluation of their clinical performance. Several trials are ongoing, and it is known that several additional platforms will be available in different markets in the near future, including the Kangduo robot® KD-SR-01 Surgical System, the Medicaroid Corporation Hinotori™, the Meerecompany Revo-i, the MicroPort® MedBot™ Toumai™, theEdge® Medical Robotics MP1000 and SP1000, the Distalmotion® Dexter, the avateramedical Avatera® system, the SSi Mantra, the Virtual Incision MIRA Surgical System, the Shurui Robot, the Rob-Surgical Bitrack System, the Ronovo Surgical Carina™, the Titan Medical Enos™ and the Vicarious Surgical robot.

In addition, new concepts such as the robotic-assisted laparoscopy are emerging, and the Moon Surgical Maestro is a good example of a product that could rapidly integrate the laparoscopic workflow even in an emergency setting.

Each of these platforms has specific features that make it unique and requires clinical tests to evaluate their safety and efficacy.

11.2.8 Geographical Availability of the Robotic Platforms

The known robotic surgical platforms are not globally available; some of them have a limited market considering that each country has a specific regulatory policy for new medical devices.

Moreover, the access to robotic surgery may be influenced by healthcare reimbursement policies, which also differ depending on the country/state [78]. In the context of acute care surgery, the access is even more limited.

The commercialization and diffusion of new robotic platforms may contribute to increase in a significant way the access to minimally invasive surgery also in mid- or low-income countries and in the case of complex procedures [79].

Whether the new platforms produced in Asia will be available or not in Europe is not known, but several encouraging signals come from the authorities. For instance, the MicroPort® MedBot™ Toumai™ received the CE mark in May 2024, becoming the first Chinese product to be potentially adoptable in general surgery in Europe.

11.2.9 Automation Technologies

Autonomous actions in surgery can be classified on six different levels ranging from no autonomy to full automation, according to Gumbs et al. [80].

Emergency general surgery is not the ideal field for innovative scientific investigations due to the variability of the patient's clinical presentation and the organizational constraints. However, this field could benefit from the introduction of autonomous action, especially in basic gestures such as vessel and hollow organ sealing.

For this reason, two possible targets were identified by De Simone et al.: the stapling and the advanced energy [81].

These devices can be considered semi-autonomous and intelligent when performing calculations targeted to read the tissue depth and apply the optimal sealing energy or stapling time, aiming to reduce the failure rate.

These two categories of instruments are currently adopted in robotic surgery even if, as before stated, only a few robotic platforms offer a complete set of advanced tools.

Intuitive Surgical® produces an advanced stapler (named SureForm™) that is endowed with an intelligent system able to continuously read the compression during the tissues' approximation and to adapt the clamping and the stapling time to achieve an optimal result [82].

The same company produces two energy devices named Vessel Sealer Extend™ and SynchroSeal™ which are automatic advanced bipolar, rapid, and low-temperature instruments. Few scientific data are available concerning the mentioned devices, mainly presented by the producer in order to compare them with laparoscopic instruments.

Few other reports exist in the literature concerning semi-autonomous instruments in robotic surgery, such as the three systems (Asensus Senhance®; Wego Micro Hand S; Meerecompany Inc. Revo-i™) which offer advanced rigid ultrasonic energy [4] or the MicroPort® MedBotTM Toumai™ adopting an advanced stapling system [83].

Unfortunately, the majority of the available data are extracted from case reports, and the producers do not provide clear explanations concerning the technology behind the automation, mainly for intellectual property issues.

The future of automation necessarily requires the adoption of artificial intelligence in robotic surgery. Encouraging signals come from the robotic market, such as the recent FDA approval of the Intelligent Surgical Unit™ by Asensus Surgical [84], the growing collaborations between the informatics industry and healthcare [85], and the release of the latest Intuitive Surgical® da Vinci® 5 which is endowed with a huge computational power to enable AI-integration and possibly to augment the automation in several surgical steps [86].

At the present moment, no clinical results are available in robotic emergency surgery.

11.3 Feasibility of Robotic Emergency Surgery

11.3.1 Recent Evidence Behind Emergency Robotic Surgery

Despite the great interest in emergency robotic surgery, the scientific evidence is slowly growing, and it is not free from criticism.

Appendectomies are described as an unjustified intervention in the majority of the cases because the dissection time does not allow to exploit the benefits of the robotic surgery while the procedural cost remains prohibitive [87].

Difficult cholecystectomies were widely addressed in literature with discording results [5, 19, 88, 89]. A recent review highlighted the potential of fluorescence imaging in robotic surgery but suggested caution while adopting robotics in acute care surgery [90].

Diaphragmatic hernia management was recently reviewed by the WSES, which considering the reduced number of reported cases [91, 92], suggested that the potential adoption of the robot should be proportioned to the patient's condition and the surgical team's experience [93].

Abdominal wall surgery, such as ventral and inguinal hernia repair in an emergency setting, has a promising potential, but it is not as well explored as in elective surgery [23, 94, 95].

Acute diverticulitis is a field of investigation that showed positive results defining the robotic approach as safe as the laparoscopic one and highlighting some benefits when compared to laparoscopic surgery, such as a significantly reduced anastomotic leak rate and conversion rate [96–98]. Unfortunately, the robotic approach is still not the standard in emergency colorectal surgery, with a recent trial, endorsed by the WSES, reporting only six (0.49%) cases approached by robotic surgery for acute diverticulitis.

Inflammatory bowel diseases are often operated on with a robotic approach, but little evidence is available concerning the non-elective treatment. The urgent robotic subtotal colectomy for severe acute ulcerative colitis can be considered comparable to laparoscopic surgery [16]. A suggested benefit for this patient could come from the advanced energy available when using the robotic platform [99].

Other surgical areas are not sufficiently explored to draw any conclusion. The main limitation behind the retrospective review of the literature is the description of the cases, which does not allow us to understand the real clinical presentation of the reported patients.

11.3.2 Advantages and Limits of Robotic Emergency Surgery

The documented advantages of robotic surgery in an emergency scenario are not different from those reported during elective operations. The augmented dexterity in narrow spaces, the ability to intuitively suture as in open surgery, the tremor filtering, the motion scaling, and the reduced stress for the operating surgeon are of mainstay importance during difficult procedures. Furthermore, the adoption of a platform capable of standardizing the suite of wristed instruments (ranging from the suction irrigator to the robotic stapler), the imaging quality integrating the advanced near-infrared fluorescence, and the adoption of the latest technology can be of great help in an emergency scenario.

Furthermore, a great potential advantage, which is still not explored in acute care surgery, is the concept of telesurgery. Robotic surgery is a real telemanipulation gesture performed inside the operative theater. Thanks to the connection protocols, such as 5G, this limited gesture could become a distant operation. The present technology is ready for future applications such as the telestration and telementoring.

Telesurgery has shown its potential in several ways, and it could represent a future alternative to connect remote areas needing the surgical management of a medical emergency. Even during natural disasters, telesurgery could represent a potential benefit [100].

Thanks to the growing expertise in robotic surgery by several specialties, even the management of difficult intraoperative complications can be realized by a robotic approach [101].

Most of the emerging platforms are endowed with 5G connections for future developments [102–104].

Another factor to consider as beneficial is the supposed reduced surgical stress of robotic surgery when compared to laparoscopy. No data are available in the emergency setting, but a recent paper comparing the initial experience with the Asensus Senhance® robot highlighted a reduced stress for the operating surgeon in the robotic group, evoking its advantageous application for acute cholecystectomies [105]. Furthermore, the work-related musculoskeletal injuries, which are often reported during a surgical career, could be reduced by the adoption of open robotic platforms [7].

Despite all the mentioned advantages, which are constantly under investigation, the adoption of the robotic approach in emergency surgery posed several concerns for the higher costs, the organization issues, and the reduced current scientific evidence.

The robotic platform availability is not always guaranteed, and the surgical team can be composed of unprepared surgeons, nurses, or anesthesiologists, thus limiting the robotic adoption even in favorable cases [6]. The costs, which will be reduced by the competition starting on the market, remain the principal limitation even in the presence of all the favorable factors, and the robotic procedure should be motivated by real beneficial results [106, 107]. A deep analysis, concentrating not only on the feasibility of the technical gesture but rather on the long-term outcomes and the patient-reported outcomes, should be performed to sustain the emergency robotic practice [108].

In addition, security and ethics issues are not yet explored when dealing with a disruptive innovation such as emergency robotic telesurgery. The political and regulatory barriers could constitute an obstacle to its development [109].

11.3.3 Training in Robotic Emergency Surgery

More than 20 years after its adoption, robotic surgery training and credentialing are still under investigation in elective surgery [110]. Little evidence exists concerning the learning curve in emergency surgery, with a recent position paper by the WSES proposing an integration of elective and emergency surgery to support the adoption of this advanced technology in emergency settings [111].

One possible limiting factor in emergency surgery is the limited confidence with minimally invasive techniques, as assessed by a recent survey of the WSES [112]. In the literature, acute care surgery has been described as an extension of trauma surgery. It was suggested that an acute care surgeon should be exposed to a wide range of operative procedures and techniques, with a high operative load and with special attention to the research in this field, which is neglected [113].

The key to a successful robotic acute care surgery program was recently documented by Torres et al. in an exhaustive paper that established three main steps: first, the application of minimally invasive surgery to simple cases; then the inclusion of more complex patients but at the right time of the day; and finally, the "around the clock" robotic surgery adoption, according to the clinical condition, irrespective of the time or the day [114].

The integration of the elective curriculum in the emergency one is difficult, but it is the only practical way to be exposed to a sufficient range of technical gestures [115].

11.4 Conclusion

The increasing use of robotics in acute care surgery may contribute to increase the rate of interventions performed with a minimally invasive approach [116]. Several obstacles are still present, but with the spread of this technology and the growing familiarization of the surgical teams, the majority of the laparoscopic emergency procedures could potentially become robotic surgeries [117]. Robotic technology will play a pivotal role in the future evolution of emergency surgery [118].

Clinical trials are ongoing to clarify the role of robotics in emergency surgery.

References

1. Lu H, Han T, Li F, Yang J, Hou Z. Global trends and hotspots in research of robotic surgery in oncology: A bibliometric and visual analysis from 2002 to 2021. Front Oncol. 2022;12:1055118. https://doi.org/10.3389/fonc.2022.1055118.
2. Sheetz KH, Claflin J, Dimick JB. Trends in the adoption of robotic surgery for common Surgical procedures. JAMA Netw Open. 2020;3(1):e1918911. https://doi.org/10.1001/jamanetworkopen.2019.18911.
3. Tan WS, Ta A, Kelly JD. Robotic surgery: getting the evidence right. Med J Aust. 2022;217(8):391–3. https://doi.org/10.5694/mja2.51726.
4. Marchegiani F, Siragusa L, Zadoroznyj A, Laterza V, Mangana O, Schena CA, et al. New robotic platforms in general surgery: what's the current clinical scenario? Medicina (Kaunas). 2023;59(7) https://doi.org/10.3390/medicina59071264.
5. Lunardi N, Abou-Zamzam A, Florecki KL, Chidambaram S, Shih IF, Kent AJ, et al. Robotic technology in emergency general surgery cases in the era of minimally invasive surgery. JAMA Surg. 2024;159(5):493–9. https://doi.org/10.1001/jamasurg.2024.0016.
6. de'Angelis N, Khan J, Marchegiani F, Bianchi G, Aisoni F, Alberti D, et al. Robotic surgery in emergency setting: 2021 WSES position paper. World J Emerg Surg. 2022;17(1):4. https://doi.org/10.1186/s13017-022-00410-6.
7. Dixon F, Vitish-Sharma P, Khanna A, Keeler BD, Group VT. Robotic assisted surgery reduces ergonomic risk during minimally invasive colorectal resection: the VOLCANO randomised controlled trial. Langenbecks Arch Surg. 2024;409(1):142. https://doi.org/10.1007/s00423-024-03322-y.
8. Surgical A: ASXC 2022 annual report. 2023. https://ir.asensus.com/static-files/058b67f6-6036-4064-a8ec-44267cc2d453. Accessed 20 May 2024.
9. Zhang X, Otoo EM, Fan Y, Tao C, Wang T, Rhode K. Autostereoscopic 3D augmented reality navigation for laparoscopic surgery: a preliminary assessment. IEEE Trans Biomed Eng. 2023;70(4):1413–21. https://doi.org/10.1109/TBME.2022.3217481.
10. Rizan C. Environmental impact of hybrid (reusable/single-use) ports versus single-use equivalents in robotic surgery. J Robot Surg. 2024;18(1):155. https://doi.org/10.1007/s11701-024-01899-6.
11. de'Angelis N, Conso C, Bianchi G, Rodriguez AGB, Marchegiani F, Carra MC, et al. Systematic review of carbon footprint of surgical procedures. J Visc Surg. 2024;161(2S):7–14. https://doi.org/10.1016/j.jviscsurg.2023.03.002.
12. Pisani Ceretti A, Mariani NM, Perego M, Giovenzana M, Salaj A, Formisano G, et al. Proposal of set-up standardization for general surgery procedures with the CMR Versius system, a new robotic platform: our initial experience. Langenbecks Arch Surg. 2024;409(1):107. https://doi.org/10.1007/s00423-024-03291-2.
13. Reinisch A, Liese J, Padberg W, Ulrich F. Robotic operations in urgent general surgery: a systematic review. J Robot Surg. 2023;17(2):275–90. https://doi.org/10.1007/s11701-022-01425-6.

14. Felli E, Brunetti F, Disabato M, Salloum C, Azoulay D, De'angelis N. Robotic right colectomy for hemorrhagic right colon cancer: a case report and review of the literature of minimally invasive urgent colectomy. World J Emerg Surg. 2014;9:32. https://doi.org/10.1186/1749-7922-9-32.
15. Pedraza R, Ragupathi M, Martinez T, Haas EM. Robotic-assisted laparoscopic primary repair of acute iatrogenic colonic perforation: case report. Int J Med Robot. 2012;8(3):375–8. https://doi.org/10.1002/rcs.1447.
16. Anderson M, Lynn P, Aydinli HH, Schwartzberg D, Bernstein M, Grucela A. Early experience with urgent robotic subtotal colectomy for severe acute ulcerative colitis has comparable perioperative outcomes to laparoscopic surgery. J Robot Surg. 2020;14(2):249–53. https://doi.org/10.1007/s11701-019-00968-5.
17. Hosein S, Carlson T, Flores L, Armijo PR, Oleynikov D. Minimally invasive approach to hiatal hernia repair is superior to open, even in the emergent setting: a large national database analysis. Surg Endosc. 2021;35(1):423–8. https://doi.org/10.1007/s00464-020-07404-y.
18. Ceccarelli G, Pasculli A, Bugiantella W, De Rosa M, Catena F, Rondelli F, et al. Minimally invasive laparoscopic and robot-assisted emergency treatment of strangulated giant hiatal hernias: report of five cases and literature review. World J Emerg Surg. 2020;15(1):37. https://doi.org/10.1186/s13017-020-00316-1.
19. Kubat E, Hansen N, Nguyen H, Wren SM, Eisenberg D. Urgent and elective robotic single-site cholecystectomy: analysis and learning curve of 150 consecutive cases. J Laparoendosc Adv Surg Tech A. 2016;26(3):185–91. https://doi.org/10.1089/lap.2015.0528.
20. Milone M, Vertaldi S, Bracale U, D'Ambra M, Cassese G, Manigrasso M, et al. Robotic cholecystectomy for acute cholecystitis: three case reports. Medicine (Baltimore). 2019;98(30):e16010. https://doi.org/10.1097/MD.0000000000016010.
21. Robinson TD, Sheehan JC, Patel PB, Marthy AG, Zaman JA, Singh TP. Emergent robotic versus laparoscopic surgery for perforated gastrojejunal ulcers: a retrospective cohort study of 44 patients. Surg Endosc. 2022;36(2):1573–7. https://doi.org/10.1007/s00464-021-08447-5.
22. Sudan R, Desai SS. Emergency and weekend robotic surgery are feasible. J Robot Surg. 2012;6(3):263–6. https://doi.org/10.1007/s11701-011-0289-0.
23. Kudsi OY, Bou-Ayash N, Chang K, Gokcal F. Perioperative and midterm outcomes of emergent robotic repair of incarcerated ventral and incisional hernia. J Robot Surg. 2021;15(3):473–81. https://doi.org/10.1007/s11701-020-01130-2.
24. Cadiere GB, Himpens J, Germay O, Izizaw R, Degueldre M, Vandromme J, et al. Feasibility of robotic laparoscopic surgery: 146 cases. World J Surg. 2001;25(11):1467–77. https://doi.org/10.1007/s00268-001-0132-2.
25. Kibar Y, Yalcin S, Kopru B, Kaya E, Topuz B, Ebiloglu T. Robot-assisted laparoscopic repair of spontaneous Appendicovesical fistula. J Endourol Case Rep. 2016;2(1):111–3. https://doi.org/10.1089/cren.2016.0063.
26. Kelkar D, Borse MA, Godbole GP, Kurlekar U, Slack M. Interim safety analysis of the first-in-human clinical trial of the Versius surgical system, a new robot-assisted device for use in minimal access surgery. Surg Endosc. 2021;35(9):5193–202. https://doi.org/10.1007/s00464-020-08014-4.
27. Yi B, Wang G, Li J, Jiang J, Son Z, Su H, et al. The first clinical use of domestically produced Chinese minimally invasive surgical robot system "Micro Hand S". Surg Endosc. 2016;30(6):2649–55. https://doi.org/10.1007/s00464-015-4506-1.
28. Yi B, Wang G, Li J, Jiang J, Son Z, Su H, et al. Domestically produced Chinese minimally invasive surgical robot system "Micro Hand S" is applied to clinical surgery preliminarily in China. Surg Endosc. 2017;31(1):487–93. https://doi.org/10.1007/s00464-016-4945-3.
29. Buzad FA, Corne LM, Brown TC, Fagin RS, Hebert AE, Kaczmarek CA, et al. Single-site robotic cholecystectomy: efficiency and cost analysis. Int J Med Robot. 2013;9(3):365–70. https://doi.org/10.1002/rcs.1507.
30. Chung PJ, Huang R, Policastro L, Lee R, Schwartzman A, Alfonso A, et al. Single-site robotic cholecystectomy at an inner-city academic center. JSLS. 2015;19(3) https://doi.org/10.4293/JSLS.2015.00033.

31. Daskalaki D, Fernandes E, Wang X, Bianco FM, Elli EF, Ayloo S, et al. Indocyanine green (ICG) fluorescent cholangiography during robotic cholecystectomy: results of 184 consecutive cases in a single institution. Surg Innov. 2014;21(6):615–21. https://doi.org/10.1177/1553350614524839.
32. Giulianotti PC, Coratti A, Angelini M, Sbrana F, Cecconi S, Balestracci T, et al. Robotics in general surgery: personal experience in a large community hospital. Arch Surg. 2003;138(7):777–84. https://doi.org/10.1001/archsurg.138.7.777.
33. Gonzalez AM, Rabaza JR, Donkor C, Romero RJ, Kosanovic R, Verdeja JC. Single-incision cholecystectomy: a comparative study of standard laparoscopic, robotic, and SPIDER platforms. Surg Endosc. 2013;27(12):4524–31. https://doi.org/10.1007/s00464-013-3105-2.
34. Honaker MD, Paton BL, Stefanidis D, Schiffern LM. Can robotic surgery be done efficiently while training residents? J Surg Educ. 2015;72(3):377–80. https://doi.org/10.1016/j.jsurg.2014.11.008.
35. Jeong Jang E, Kang SH, Kim KW. Early outcomes of robotic single site cholecystectomy using the DaVinci Xi(R) system. JSLS. 2021;25(1) https://doi.org/10.4293/JSLS.2020.00082.
36. Konstantinidis KM, Hirides P, Hirides S, Chrysocheris P, Georgiou M. Cholecystectomy using a novel Single-Site((R)) robotic platform: early experience from 45 consecutive cases. Surg Endosc. 2012;26(9):2687–94. https://doi.org/10.1007/s00464-012-2227-2.
37. Kulaylat AN, Richards H, Yada K, Coyle D, Shelby R, Onwuka AJ, et al. Comparative analysis of robotic-assisted versus laparoscopic cholecystectomy in pediatric patients. J Pediatr Surg. 2021;56(10):1876–80. https://doi.org/10.1016/j.jpedsurg.2020.11.013.
38. Li YP, Wang SN, Lee KT. Robotic versus conventional laparoscopic cholecystectomy: a comparative study of medical resource utilization and clinical outcomes. Kaohsiung J Med Sci. 2017;33(4):201–6. https://doi.org/10.1016/j.kjms.2017.01.010.
39. Mattei P. Single-site robotic-assisted laparoscopic cholecystectomy in children and adolescents: a report of 20 cases. Surg Endosc. 2018;32(5):2402–8. https://doi.org/10.1007/s00464-017-5939-5.
40. Rosales-Velderrain A, Alkhoury F. Single-port robotic cholecystectomy in pediatric patients: single institution experience. J Laparoendosc Adv Surg Tech A. 2017;27(4):434–7. https://doi.org/10.1089/lap.2016.0484.
41. Schertz P, Misra S, Livert D, Mulligan J, Rohatgi C. Comparison of intraoperative outcomes between single-incision robotic cholecystectomy and multi-incision robotic cholecystectomy. Cureus. 2019;11(8):e5386. https://doi.org/10.7759/cureus.5386.
42. Su WL, Huang JW, Wang SN, Lee KT. Comparison study of clinical outcomes between single-site robotic cholecystectomy and single incision laparoscopic cholecystectomy. Asian J Surg. 2017;40(6):424–8. https://doi.org/10.1016/j.asjsur.2016.03.005.
43. Svoboda S, Qaqish TR, Wilson A, Park H, Youssef Y. Robotic single-site cholecystectomy in the obese: outcomes from a single institution. Surg Obes Relat Dis. 2015;11(4):882–5. https://doi.org/10.1016/j.soard.2014.11.016.
44. Tao Z, Emuakhagbon VS, Pham T, Augustine MM, Guzzetta A, Huerta S. Outcomes of robotic and laparoscopic cholecystectomy for benign gallbladder disease in veteran patients. J Robot Surg. 2021;15(6):849–57. https://doi.org/10.1007/s11701-020-01183-3.
45. Vidovszky TJ, Carr AD, Farinholt GN, Ho HS, Smith WH, Ali MR. Single-site robotic cholecystectomy in a broadly inclusive patient population: a prospective study. Ann Surg. 2014;260(1):134–41. https://doi.org/10.1097/SLA.0000000000000295.
46. Hanisch E, Markus B, Gutt C, Schmandra TC, Encke A. Robot-assisted laparoscopic cholecystectomy and fundoplication–initial experiences with the Da Vinci system. Chirurg. 2001;72(3):286–8. https://doi.org/10.1007/s001040051307.
47. Bustos R, Mashbari H, Gangemi A. First report of gallbladder volvulus managed with a robotic approach. Case Rep Surg. 2019;2019:2189890. https://doi.org/10.1155/2019/2189890.
48. Ayloo S, Roh Y, Choudhury N. Laparoscopic versus robot-assisted cholecystectomy: a retrospective cohort study. Int J Surg. 2014;12(10):1077–81. https://doi.org/10.1016/j.ijsu.2014.08.405.

49. Balachandran B, Hufford TA, Mustafa T, Kochar K, Sulo S, Khorsand J. A comparative study of outcomes between single-site robotic and multi-port laparoscopic cholecystectomy: An experience from a tertiary care center. World J Surg. 2017;41(5):1246–53. https://doi.org/10.1007/s00268-016-3799-0.
50. Bibi S, Rahnemai-Azar AA, Coralic J, Bayoumi M, Khorsand J, Farkas DT, et al. Single-site robotic cholecystectomy: the timeline of Progress. World J Surg. 2015;39(10):2386–91. https://doi.org/10.1007/s00268-015-3135-0.
51. Bou-Ayash N, Gokcal F, Kudsi OY. Robotic inguinal hernia repair for incarcerated hernias. J Laparoendosc Adv Surg Tech A. 2021;31(8):926–30. https://doi.org/10.1089/lap.2020.0607.
52. Cubas R, Garcia M, Mukherjee K. Robotic repair of incarcerated morgagni hernia in an adult on the acute care surgery service. Rev Fac Cien Med Univ Nac Cordoba. 2021;78(1):91–4. https://doi.org/10.31053/1853.0605.v78.n1.28299.
53. John M, Michael H, Matthew S, Anthony U, David D, Pablo G, et al. Identification and repair of left-sided Paraduodenal hernia using both laparoscopic and robotic techniques. Case Rep Surg. 2020;2020:7569530. https://doi.org/10.1155/2020/7569530.
54. Muysoms F, Vierstraete M, Nachtergaele F, Van Garsse S, Pletinckx P, Ramaswamy A. Economic assessment of starting robot-assisted laparoscopic inguinal hernia repair in a single-Centre retrospective comparative study: the EASTER study. BJS Open. 2021;5(1) https://doi.org/10.1093/bjsopen/zraa046.
55. Smith MT, Wong NC, Coleman JA. Inguinal hernia of the distal ureter causing hydronephrosis: A rare case. Urol Case Rep. 2021;35:101549. https://doi.org/10.1016/j.eucr.2020.101549.
56. Beltzer C, Knoerzer L, Bachmann R, Axt S, Dippel H, Schmidt R. Robotic versus laparoscopic sigmoid resection for diverticular disease: a single-center experience of 106 cases. J Laparoendosc Adv Surg Tech A. 2019;29(11):1451–5. https://doi.org/10.1089/lap.2019.0451.
57. Guerra F, Petrelli F, Stortoni P, Patriti A. Acute large bowel malignant obstruction of the splenic flexure: fully robotic resection with central ligation and intracorporeal anastomosis – a video vignette. Colorectal Dis. 2021;23(1):325. https://doi.org/10.1111/codi.15384.
58. Kudsi OY, Gokcal F. Urgent robotic mesocolic excision for obstructing proximal transverse colon cancer – a video vignette. Color Dis. 2019;21(9):1093–4. https://doi.org/10.1111/codi.14714.
59. Kudsi OY, Bou-Ayash N. Bleeding sigmoid diverticulosis – urgent stapleless totally robotic sigmoidectomy-a video vignette. Color Dis. 2020;22(9):1205. https://doi.org/10.1111/codi.15051.
60. Kudsi OY, Bou-Ayash N. Caecal volvulus – urgent totally robotic right colectomy – a video vignette. Color Dis. 2020;22(10):1448–9. https://doi.org/10.1111/codi.15068.
61. Sun L, Tang S. Perioperative nursing for gastric perforation repair operation performed by the first domestic surgical robot. Zhong Nan Da Xue Xue Bao Yi Xue Ban. 2015;40(4):453–6. https://doi.org/10.11817/j.issn.1672-7347.2015.04.019.
62. Kim D, Lee CS. Single-port robotic totally extraperitoneal(TEP) inguinal hernia repair using the da Vinci SP platform: A video vignette. Asian J Surg. 2022;45(10):2062–3. https://doi.org/10.1016/j.asjsur.2022.04.101.
63. de Beche-Adams T, Eubanks WS, de la Fuente SG. Early experience with the Senhance(R)-laparoscopic/robotic platform in the US. J Robot Surg. 2019;13(2):357–9. https://doi.org/10.1007/s11701-018-0893-3.
64. Yao Y, Liu Y, Li Z, Yi B, Wang G, Zhu S. Chinese surgical robot micro hand S: A consecutive case series in general surgery. Int J Surg. 2020;75:55–9. https://doi.org/10.1016/j.ijsu.2020.01.013.
65. Aggarwal R, Winter Beatty J, Kinross J, von Roon A, Darzi A, Purkayastha S. Initial experience with a new robotic Surgical system for cholecystectomy. Surg Innov. 2020;27(2):136–42. https://doi.org/10.1177/1553350619890736.
66. Kelkar DS, Kurlekar U, Stevens L, Wagholikar GD, Slack M. An early prospective clinical study to evaluate the safety and performance of the Versius Surgical system in robot-assisted cholecystectomy. Ann Surg. 2023;277(1):9–17. https://doi.org/10.1097/SLA.0000000000005410.

67. Khanna S, Barua A. Robotic assisted cholecystectomy – a retrospective cohort study of experience of 106 first robotic cholecystectomies in versius robotic platform. Int J Surg Open. 2022;47:100554. https://doi.org/10.1016/j.ijso.2022.100554.
68. Melling N, Barr J, Schmitz R, Polonski A, Miro J, Ghadban T, et al. Robotic cholecystectomy: first experience with the new Senhance robotic system. J Robot Surg. 2019;13(3):495–500. https://doi.org/10.1007/s11701-018-0877-3.
69. Bianco FM, Dreifuss NH, Chang B, Schlottmann F, Cubisino A, Mangano A, et al. Robotic single-port surgery: preliminary experience in general surgery. Int J Med Robot. 2022;18(6):e2453. https://doi.org/10.1002/rcs.2453.
70. Kang YH, Kang JS, Cho YS, Kim HS, Lee M, Han Y, et al. A retrospective multicentre study on the evaluation of perioperative outcomes of single-port robotic cholecystectomy comparing the Xi and SP versions of the da Vinci robotic surgical system. Int J Med Robot. 2022;18(1):e2345. https://doi.org/10.1002/rcs.2345.
71. Belyaev O, Fahlbusch T, Slobodkin I, Uhl W. Safety and feasibility of cholecystectomy with the Hugo(TM) RAS: proof of setup guides and first-in-human German experience. Visc Med. 2023;39(3–4):76–86. https://doi.org/10.1159/000531595.
72. Conticchio M, Delvecchio A, Ferraro V, Stasi M, Casella A, Chetta N, et al. Robotic emergency liver resection of ruptured hepatocellular carcinoma. Int J Med Robot. 2023;19(5):e2537. https://doi.org/10.1002/rcs.2537.
73. Ferrari L, Nicolaou S, Adams K. Implementation of a robotic surgical practice in inflammatory bowel disease. J Robot Surg. 2024;18(1):57. https://doi.org/10.1007/s11701-023-01750-4.
74. Ziegler O, Jikaria NR, Cioccio J, Scow JS. A case report of refractory graft-versus-host disease colitis managed with robotic Total abdominal colectomy. Cureus. 2024;16(4):e57829. https://doi.org/10.7759/cureus.57829.
75. Surgical C: Press information. https://cmrsurgical.com/news. 2024. Accessed 20 May 2024.
76. Huscher C, Marchegiani F, Cobellis F, Tejedor P, Pastor C, Lazzarin G, et al. Robotic oncologic colorectal surgery with a new robotic platform (CMR Versius): hope or hype? A preliminary experience from a full-robotic case-series. Tech Coloproctol. 2022;26(9):745–53. https://doi.org/10.1007/s10151-022-02626-9.
77. Boal M, Di Girasole CG, Tesfai F, Morrison TEM, Higgs S, Ahmad J, et al. Evaluation status of current and emerging minimally invasive robotic surgical platforms. Surg Endosc. 2024;38(2):554–85. https://doi.org/10.1007/s00464-023-10554-4.
78. Childers CP, Uppal A, Tillman M, Chang GJ, Tran Cao HS. Insurance disparities in access to robotic surgery for colorectal cancer. Ann Surg Oncol. 2023;30(6):3560–8. https://doi.org/10.1245/s10434-023-13354-1.
79. Mehta A, Cheng Ng J, Andrew Awuah W, Huang H, Kalmanovich J, Agrawal A, et al. Embracing robotic surgery in low- and middle-income countries: potential benefits, challenges, and scope in the future. Ann Med Surg (Lond). 2022;84:104803. https://doi.org/10.1016/j.amsu.2022.104803.
80. Gumbs AA, Alexander F, Karcz K, Chouillard E, Croner R, Coles-Black J, et al. Erratum: White paper: definitions of artificial intelligence and autonomous actions in clinical surgery. Artif Intell Surg. 2022;2(3):120–1. https://doi.org/10.20517/ais.2022.17.
81. De Simone B, Chouillard E, Gumbs AA, Loftus TJ, Kaafarani H, Catena F. Artificial intelligence in surgery: the emergency surgeon's perspective (the ARIES project). Discov Health Syst. 2022;1(1):9. https://doi.org/10.1007/s44250-022-00014-6.
82. Johnson CS, Kassir A, Marx DS, Soliman MK. Performance of da Vinci Stapler during robotic-assisted right colectomy with intracorporeal anastomosis. J Robot Surg. 2019;13(1):115–9. https://doi.org/10.1007/s11701-018-0828-z.
83. Huang J, Zhu H, Lu P, Li J, Tian Y, Takase Y, et al. Comparison of lobectomy performed through Toumai((R)) surgical robot and da Vinci surgical robot in early-stage non-small cell lung cancer: a retrospective study of early perioperative results. Transl Lung Cancer Res. 2023;12(11):2219–28. https://doi.org/10.21037/tlcr-23-603.
84. Inc. AS: Asensus Surgical Receives FDA 510(k) Clearance for Expansion of Machine Vision Capabilities. https://ir.asensus.com/news-releases/news-release-details/

asensus-surgical-receives-fda-510k-clearance-expansion-machine. 2021. Accessed 20 May 2024.
85. Nvidia: NVIDIA Medical Edge AI computing platform selected by top robotic and digital surgery startups. https://blogs.nvidia.com/blog/igx-clara-holoscan-edge-ai-robotic-surgery/. 2022. Accessed 20 May 2024.
86. Surgical I: Da Vinci 5. https://www.intuitive.com/en-us/products-and-services/da-vinci/5. 2024. Accessed 20 May 2024.
87. Arang H, El Boghdady M. Robotic appendicectomy: a review of feasibility. Sultan Qaboos Univ Med J. 2023;23(4):440–6. https://doi.org/10.18295/squmj.7.2023.043.
88. Kalata S, Thumma JR, Norton EC, Dimick JB, Sheetz KH. Comparative safety of robotic-assisted vs laparoscopic cholecystectomy. JAMA Surg. 2023;158(12):1303–10. https://doi.org/10.1001/jamasurg.2023.4389.
89. Campbell S, Lee SH, Liu Y, Wren SM. A retrospective study of laparoscopic, robotic-assisted, and open emergent/urgent cholecystectomy based on the PINC AI Healthcare Database 2017-2020. World J Emerg Surg. 2023;18(1):55. https://doi.org/10.1186/s13017-023-00521-8.
90. Seshadri A, Peitzman AB. The difficult cholecystectomy: what you need to know. J Trauma Acute Care Surg. 2024; https://doi.org/10.1097/TA.0000000000004337.
91. Jambhekar A, Robinson S, Housman B, Nguyen J, Gu K, Nakhamiyayev V. Robotic repair of a right-sided Bochdalek hernia: a case report and literature review. J Robot Surg. 2018;12(2):351–5. https://doi.org/10.1007/s11701-017-0705-1.
92. Hunter LM, Mozer AB, Anciano CJ, Oliver AL, Iannettoni MD, Speicher JE. Robotic-assisted thoracoscopic repair of right-sided Bochdalek hernia in adults: a two-case series. Innovations (Phila). 2019;14(1):69–74. https://doi.org/10.1177/1556984518823642.
93. Giuffrida M, Perrone G, Abu-Zidan F, Agnoletti V, Ansaloni L, Baiocchi GL, et al. Management of complicated diaphragmatic hernia in the acute setting: a WSES position paper. World J Emerg Surg. 2023;18(1):43. https://doi.org/10.1186/s13017-023-00510-x.
94. Murgante Testa N, Mongelli F, Sabbatini F, Iaquinandi F, Prouse G, Pini R, et al. Safety and feasibility of emergency robot-assisted transabdominal preperitoneal repair for the treatment of incarcerated inguinal hernia: A retrospective study. World J Surg. 2024;48(3):622–8. https://doi.org/10.1002/wjs.12063.
95. de'Angelis N, Schena CA, Moszkowicz D, Kuperas C, Fara R, Gaujoux S, et al. Robotic surgery for inguinal and ventral hernia repair: a systematic review and meta-analysis. Surg Endosc. 2024;38(1):24–46. https://doi.org/10.1007/s00464-023-10545-5.
96. Curfman KR, Jones IF, Conner JR, Neighorn CC, Wilson RK, Rashidi L. Robotic colorectal surgery in the emergent diverticulitis setting: is it safe? A review of large national database. Int J Color Dis. 2023;38(1):142. https://doi.org/10.1007/s00384-023-04436-3.
97. Arnott SM, Arnautovic A, Haviland S, Ng M, Obias V. Safety of robotic surgical management of non-elective colectomies for diverticulitis compared to laparoscopic surgery. J Robot Surg. 2023;17(2):587–95. https://doi.org/10.1007/s11701-022-01452-3.
98. Maertens V, Stefan S, Rawlinson E, Ball C, Gibbs P, Mercer S, et al. Emergency robotic colorectal surgery during COVID-19 pandemic: A retrospective case series study. Laparosc Endosc Robot Surg. 2022;5(2):57–60. https://doi.org/10.1016/j.lers.2022.03.001.
99. Aydinli HH, Anderson M, Hambrecht A, Bernstein MA, Grucela AL. Robotic ileocolic resection with intracorporeal anastomosis for Crohn's disease. J Robot Surg. 2021;15(3):465–72. https://doi.org/10.1007/s11701-020-01125-z.
100. Lokmic-Tomkins Z, Bhandari D, Bain C, Borda A, Kariotis TC, Reser D. Lessons learned from natural disasters around digital health technologies and delivering quality healthcare. Int J Environ Res Public Health. 2023;20(5) https://doi.org/10.3390/ijerph20054542.
101. de'Angelis N, Schena CA, Marchegiani F, Reitano E, De Simone B, Wong GYM, et al. WSES guidelines for the prevention, detection, and management of iatrogenic urinary tract injuries (IUTIs) during emergency digestive surgery. World J Emerg Surg. 2023;18(1):45. https://doi.org/10.1186/s13017-023-00513-8.

102. Wang Y, Ai Q, Zhao W, Gao Y, Liu Q, Shi T, et al. Safety and reliability of a robot-assisted laparoscopic Telesurgery system: expanding indications in urological surgery. Eur Urol. 2024;85(5):506–7. https://doi.org/10.1016/j.eururo.2023.11.002.
103. Li J, Yang X, Chu G, Feng W, Ding X, Yin X, et al. Application of improved robot-assisted laparoscopic Telesurgery with 5G Technology in Urology. Eur Urol. 2023;83(1):41–4. https://doi.org/10.1016/j.eururo.2022.06.018.
104. Fan S, Xu W, Diao Y, Yang K, Dong J, Qin M, et al. Feasibility and safety of dual-console Telesurgery with the KangDuo Surgical Robot-01 system using fifth-generation and wired networks: An animal experiment and clinical study. Eur Urol Open Sci. 2023;49:6–9. https://doi.org/10.1016/j.euros.2022.12.010.
105. Menke V, Hansen O, Schmidt J, Dechantsreiter G, Staib L, Davliatov M, et al. The stress for surgeons: exploring stress entities with the robotic senhance surgical system. J Robot Surg. 2024;18(1):94. https://doi.org/10.1007/s11701-024-01853-6.
106. Liatsikos E, Tsaturyan A, Kyriazis I, Kallidonis P, Manolopoulos D, Magoutas A. Market potentials of robotic systems in medical science: analysis of the Avatera robotic system. World J Urol. 2022;40(1):283–9. https://doi.org/10.1007/s00345-021-03809-z.
107. Grimsley EA, Janjua HM, Herron T, Read MD, Lorch S, Cha JY, et al. Patient outcomes and cost in robotic emergency general surgery. J Robot Surg. 2023;17(6):2937–44. https://doi.org/10.1007/s11701-023-01739-z.
108. Sheetz KH, Telem DA, Feldman LS. Robotics for emergency general surgery-selecting the right tool. JAMA Surg. 2024;159(5):500. https://doi.org/10.1001/jamasurg.2024.0023.
109. Patel V, Saikali S, Moschovas MC, Patel E, Satava R, Dasgupta P, et al. Technical and ethical considerations in telesurgery. J Robot Surg. 2024;18(1):40. https://doi.org/10.1007/s11701-023-01797-3.
110. Stefanidis D, Huffman EM, Collins JW, Martino MA, Satava RM, Levy JS. Expert consensus recommendations for robotic surgery credentialing. Ann Surg. 2022;276(1):88–93. https://doi.org/10.1097/SLA.0000000000004531.
111. de'Angelis N, Marchegiani F, Schena CA, Khan J, Agnoletti V, Ansaloni L, et al. Training curriculum in minimally invasive emergency digestive surgery: 2022 WSES position paper. World J Emerg Surg. 2023;18(1):11. https://doi.org/10.1186/s13017-023-00476-w.
112. Ceresoli M, Pisano M, Abu-Zidan F, Allievi N, Gurusamy K, Biffl WL, et al. Minimally invasive surgery in emergency surgery: a WSES survey. World J Emerg Surg. 2022;17(1):18. https://doi.org/10.1186/s13017-022-00419-x.
113. Tian BW. The rise of ACS and its importance. World J Emerg Surg. 2024;19(1):9. https://doi.org/10.1186/s13017-024-00538-7.
114. Torres CM, Florecki K, Haghshenas J, Manukyan M, Kent A, Lawrence C, et al. The evolution and development of a robotic acute care surgery program. J Trauma Acute Care Surg. 2023;95(4):e26–30. https://doi.org/10.1097/TA.0000000000004020.
115. Tian BWCA. Can acute care surgery sustain as a specialty in Singapore? Discov Health Sys. 2023;2(1):7. https://doi.org/10.1007/s44250-023-00023-z.
116. Kirkpatrick J, Wang Y, Greene M, Armstrong D, Srinivasa S, Koea J. The increasing use of minimally invasive surgery in acute general surgical conditions: A decade of results from a national data set. Surgery. 2024;175(4):1205–11. https://doi.org/10.1016/j.surg.2023.11.023.
117. Friedman G. Robotics for acute Care in Colorectal Surgery. Clin Colon Rectal Surg. 2021;34(5):328–33. https://doi.org/10.1055/s-0041-1726448.
118. Sermonesi G, Tian B, Vallicelli C, Abu-Zidan FM, Damaskos D, Kelly MD, et al. Cesena guidelines: WSES consensus statement on laparoscopic-first approach to general surgery emergencies and abdominal trauma. World J Emerg Surg. 2023;18(1):57. https://doi.org/10.1186/s13017-023-00520-9.

12 Autonomous Robotics and AI in Trauma and Emergency Care for Space Medicine

Lidia Al-Zogbi, Axel Krieger, Thorsten Fleiter, Mathias Unberath, Jacopo Martellucci, Carlo Bergamini, Belinda De Simone, and Desiree Pantalone

12.1 Trauma and Emergency Care in Space Medicine

The National Aeronautics and Space Administration (NASA) has long envisioned the expansion of human space travel beyond Low Earth Orbit (LEO). With the Artemis missions under active development, NASA is planning to establish a sustainable human presence on the Moon, which will usher in the discovery of new scientific knowledge, open possible commercial activity, and help prepare for exploration missions to Mars [1]. Private aerospace companies are also on the rise, with six major companies emerging just in the US since 2000 [2]. SpaceX, for

L. Al-Zogbi · A. Krieger
Department of Mechanical Engineering, Johns Hopkins University, Baltimore, MD, USA

T. Fleiter
Department of Diagnostic Radiology, R Adams Cowley Shock Trauma Center, School of Medicine, University of Maryland, Baltimore, MD, USA

M. Unberath
Department of Computer Science, Johns Hopkins University, Baltimore, MD, USA

J. Martellucci · C. Bergamini
Emergency Surgery Unit-Trauma Team, level 1 Trauma Center, Emergency and Admission Department, University Hospital Careggi, Florence, Italy

B. De Simone
Department of Emergency and General Minimally Invasive Surgery, Level I Trauma Center, Bufalini Hospital, AUSL Romagna, Cesena, Italy

Department of Theoretical and Applied Sciences, eCampus University, Novedrate, Como, Italy

D. Pantalone (✉)
Emergency Surgery Unit-Trauma Team, level 1 Trauma Center, Emergency and Admission Department, University Hospital Careggi, Florence, Italy

Department of Experimental and Clinical Medicine, University of Florence, Florence, Italy
e-mail: desire.pantalone@unifi.it

B. De Simone et al. (eds.), *New Technologies, Precision Medicine, and AI in Emergency General Surgery*, Hot Topics in Acute Care Surgery and Trauma,
https://doi.org/10.1007/978-3-032-09357-8_12

example, is currently partnering with NASA on some of the Artemis missions [3], while also leading efforts on deep space travel for future Mars colonization missions [4].

With deep space human exploration becoming a reality, preparing to manage health emergencies aboard a spacecraft is paramount. In fact, Schneider et al. published a summary of the "Spaceflight for Everybody" symposium focusing on identifying health risks and corresponding countermeasures for long-duration space travel [5]. A "traffic light" rating scale was proposed to classify the severity of adverse event risks based on mission length, distance from Earth, and space radiation exposure. While missions in LEO typically see risks classified as green or yellow, with only about 15% categorized as red, Mars missions—whether in orbit or on the surface—see nearly half of the risks fall into the yellow or red categories, foreboding more severe consequences [6]. This approach to risk assessment in space missions mirrors the challenges in similarly isolated environments, like on US submarines, where crew injuries were found to be the primary cause of morbidity and downtime [7]. Similarly, in remote areas like Antarctica, comprehensive mass casualty incident response and aeromedical evacuation plans are in place due to the region's extreme remoteness and heightened risk [8].

Medical interventions are deemed necessary within space programs to address emergency conditions [9]. Although numerous studies have indicated that illnesses and injuries requiring major surgery during spaceflight are expected to be rare [10], the occurrence of such events can have a detrimental impact on the mission, resulting in compromised returns to Earth and mission aborts. As we venture further into space and for longer periods of time, understanding what injuries and illnesses astronauts might sustain becomes crucial for effective preparation and response.

12.1.1 Injury and Emergency Profiles in Prolonged Space Exploration

Astronauts undergo extensive screening for chronic and heritable diseases. Traumatic injuries, however, can be sustained unexpectedly even by the healthiest individuals. The primary concern with injuries in microgravity is hemorrhage, which becomes life-threatening if it progresses to major traumatic hemorrhage. Hemorrhages are classified as compressible or non-compressible based on their location and responsiveness to simple compression methods [11, 12]. Non-compressible torso hemorrhages, which may arise from major vascular trauma, pulmonary parenchyma, solid abdominal organs, or pelvic disruptions, are particularly perilous as they are often occult [12]. Managing such injuries presents profound challenges despite diagnostic advancements using ultrasound (US), and immediate surgical intervention is frequently necessary before precise localization of the bleeding source is even possible [9]. During the construction phase of the International Space Station (ISS), there was a heightened risk of trauma, including crush injuries, lacerations, and thermal and electrical burns [13, 14]. Through careful planning of crew safety, astronauts have only experienced minor injuries, such as lacerations and finger pinching [14]. While there have been several catastrophic fatalities, to date, no evacuations due to serious trauma have been required in space [9]. The most common medical incidents reported in the Shuttle-*Mir* orbital program involved only minor traumatic injuries to the skin and mucous membranes [15].

Deep space exploration, however, exacerbates existing conditions. Research has shown that the medical event rate is directly proportional to the mission duration [16]. A correlation was also identified between extravehicular activity (EVA) and the onset of illnesses and injuries, particularly relating to fractures, trauma, and radiation exposure from solar particle events [17]. Future long-duration missions to the Moon or Mars will require up to 24 h of EVA per week, compared to the typical 3–4 h during a 6-month stay on the ISS [18]. Additionally, in environments with reduced gravity—such as those with a third or sixth of Earth's gravity—objects may seem deceptively light due to weightlessness. Yet, they still retain their mass, potentially enabling serious crush injuries. Hardened protective gear can help shield astronauts from serious thoracoabdominal injuries [11], but their use may impose excessive musculoskeletal strain, thereby elevating the risk of emergency skeletal injuries [9]. Renal stone formation among astronauts is another well-documented condition, with evidence pointing to a higher risk during longer missions [19]. Lastly, emergency medical conditions such as appendicitis and cholecystitis remain concerns in space, as highlighted by reports of sudden abdominal pain among astronauts [9]. The risks and benefits of prophylactic procedures are a topic of debate, meaning that these conditions must still be carefully considered in planning for long-duration space travel.

12.1.2 Challenges of Trauma and Emergency Care in Space

Although astronauts may experience injuries and illnesses during space missions that are similar to those on Earth, the complexity of patient care in long-duration space missions is compounded by multiple factors. We categorize these factors into three distinct areas, namely environmental conditions, human factors, and technological limitations.

12.1.2.1 Environmental Conditions

Physiological Changes Space travel has profound physiological effects on astronauts, which can complicate any injury or surgical scenario. Certain physiological changes, particularly those affecting the body's ability to withstand and recover from major systemic trauma, are especially critical in emergency medical care. One significant concern is the loss of bone mineral density (BMD) during periods of weightlessness due to reduced loading stimuli. BMD in astronauts decreases at an average rate of 1–1.5% per month, which is ten times the rate observed in osteoporosis [20]. Furthermore, bone resorption and possible decrease in bone formation are only partially responsive to non-pharmacological countermeasures such as exercise and adjusted diet [20]. With bone weakening, the risk of fractures is heightened. The thoracic cage, for instance, protects vital thoracic and abdominal organs like the heart, liver, and spleen. Its weakening means even minor blunt trauma can lead to organ injury and uncontrolled internal hemorrhage, requiring immediate surgical intervention. Moreover, the calcium released from bone resorption is excreted in the urine, which can lead to the formation of renal stones [21].

Cardiovascular changes have also been observed in microgravity. In a recent publication, Gallo et al. developed and validated a 1D-0D multiscale model to study the cardiovascular response to long-term zero gravity (0G) spaceflight in comparison to the 1G supine reference condition [22]. The authors found that the cardiac work, oxygen consumption, contractility indexes, and central mean and pulse pressures were reduced in microgravity. Additionally, the exercise tolerance of a spaceflight traveler was shown to be comparable to that of an untrained person with a sedentary lifestyle [22]. Other studies have also reported evidence of cardiac remodeling due to conditions of weightlessness [23]. In particular, cardiac atrophy was linked to reductions in metabolic demand and oxygen uptake [24]. Another study documented a 9.1% decrease in left ventricular mass among astronauts [25]. Hemostasis is also adversely affected by gravity reduction, making bleeding a general concern and potentially necessitating novel approaches for effective blood loss control. Fluid redistribution and diuresis in space result in a 10–23% blood volume reduction before any injury even occurs, which is equivalent to a Class I Advanced Trauma Life Support (ATLS) hemorrhage on Earth [26]. Such a reduction decreases cardiac reserve, and the autonomic nervous system's reset increases beta receptor sensitivity, potentially inhibiting effective vasoconstriction [13]. Additionally, the combined effects of microgravity and radiation on human cardiovascular functions are not yet well understood.

Microgravity also dysregulates the human immune system. The number and function of white blood cells are altered, with studies showing a redistribution of peripheral leukocytes, diminished function of specific leukocyte subpopulations, and skewed cytokine profiles in many astronauts [27]. While the adaptive immunity is dysregulated during space flight, some aspects of the general immunity are heightened, with an altered interaction observed between the two [27]. Wound healing was shown to be impaired in space as well, with studies on rat abdominal incisions demonstrating greater inflammatory responses [28]. With a potentially weakened immune system, the greater bacterial growth observed in weightless environments becomes a further complication [29]. Bacteria were shown to develop thicker cell walls and increased resistance to antibiotics, as evidenced by post-flight samples collected from the crew of the Apollo-Soyuz Project [30]. The effect of increased radiation exposure, which also affects the astronaut's immunity and proliferation of rapidly dividing cells, has not been adequately studied either.

Procedural Changes Microgravity complicates surgical interventions from a procedural standpoint, too, affecting both the human body's physical response to the surgery and the execution of the surgery itself. For instance, arterial bleeding can form droplet streams, and venous bleeding can form domes, which swell like balloons before leaving the vessel [26]. Blood drops can also adhere to surgical instruments and wound areas due to surface tension. Precise surgical maneuvers are more difficult to execute, as organs that normally rest in place now float in space. Laparotomy, which entails creating a wide incision in the abdomen to access the peritoneal cavity, is often performed on emergency trauma patients but may not be practical in 0G conditions. Similar challenges are observed in laparoscopy. A laparoscopic porcine study showed that in weightlessness, the bowel in the supine position does not remain posteriorly retracted and exerts pressure on the anterior abdominal wall [31]. The anterior bowel flotation, compounded by floating blood, bodily fluids, and debris, can obscure the surgical field and increase the risk of contamination. Maintaining sterility in the surgical workspace is another concern. The spacecraft environment increases the risk of infection due to the possible presence of floating bodily fluids and surgical debris. The limited space onboard means that the surgical area might be uncomfortably close to the non-sterile galley or exercise facilities [32]. Furthermore, patients, surgical personnel, and hardware must all be securely restrained to prevent unintended movement, introducing additional discomfort and risks.

12.1.2.2 Human Factors

Personnel Availability Presently on the ISS, a Crew Medical Officer (CMO) is responsible for the healthcare of astronauts. A CMO is not necessarily a physician but is an astronaut who has received 40–60 h of medical training [33]. CMOs must be proficient in key medical procedures, such as those outlined by the ATLS protocols [34], including intravenous insertions for infusions, endotracheal intubation, and chest tube placement [8]. While trained in a wide range of medical and non-medical subjects, CMOs lack the specialized surgical skills that would be needed, particularly for more complex clinical cases. The general consensus is that surgical trauma procedures in space would be best handled by two surgeons [35]. However, the presence of even one space surgeon in future long-duration missions may not be guaranteed [35]. Non-physician CMOs are currently favored over surgeons because they can undertake a variety of activities other than medical treatment, making their versatility a key asset in the constrained and resource-limited environment of a spacecraft. At the same time, this compromises the CMO's capacity to devote time and attention to medical emergencies. Additionally, trauma and emergency surgery on Earth require the support of an entire medical team. Space missions do not have the luxury of nurses, anesthetists, and other support personnel who play critical roles in providing medical care on Earth.

Personnel Training To better prepare astronauts, space missions are emulated on Earth through various analog environments, simulations, and training programs. Analog missions such as NASA Extreme Environment Missions Operations (NEEMO) underwater off the coast of Florida [36], *Hawaii* Space Exploration Analog and Simulation (HI-SEAS) on the slopes of Mauna Loa in Hawaii [37] and missions on the Concordia Station in Antarctica [38] provide valuable opportunities for astronauts to experience the isolation, confinement, and operational challenges of long-duration space travel. However, training for surgical procedures in microgravity remains particularly challenging. While various setups exist to test equipment for space missions, realistic surgical training in reduced gravity can only be achieved through parabolic testing [39]. Parabolic testing takes place on an aircraft executing a series of parabolic maneuvers, ascending and descending at 45° angles to create 20–30 s of microgravity during each transition, repeated 30–40 times [40]. Multiple studies have demonstrated the feasibility of laparoscopic surgeries on porcine models during these flights [31, 39]. Thoracoscopic surgeries, however, proved to be more difficult and were less successful [39]. Although parabolic flights are useful for simulating microgravity, the duration of weightlessness provided is insufficient to realistically replicate the complexity of performing a full surgical procedure in space. To date, only minor medical procedures, such as treatment of superficial lacerations, have been performed on the ISS. Future trips to the ISS for surgical training are unlikely, as they are prohibitively expensive and time-consuming. Virtual Reality (VR) could augment surgical training capabilities, though the ecological validity of this approach is currently only partially understood. Additionally, the unpredictability of space travel makes comprehensive preparation and training extremely challenging.

12.1.2.3 Technological Limitations

Distance and Communication Space missions to date have primarily taken place on the ISS. On these missions, astronauts are a select group of healthy individuals who attend a weekly private medical teleconference with a flight surgeon on Earth who monitors their health status [35]. The astronauts can also evacuate to a Soyuz capsule from LEO and return to Earth within a few hours if a critical condition arises [35]. However, for future missions involving greater distances, immediate communication and evacuation to Earth will not be feasible. For instance, a return trip from the Moon to Earth can take 6–7 days, while a journey from Mars will last anywhere between 18 and 24 months [35]. Communication between the Earth and Moon, with an average distance between the two of about 384,400 km, experiences a delay of approximately 1.28 s each way [41]. This delay increases dramatically for Mars missions, where the distance to Earth ranges from 54.6 million to 44 million kilometers, resulting in a communication latency of about 6–24 min [35]. The "golden hour" rule, for example, stipulates that critically injured patients must receive definitive care within one hour of sustaining an injury to reduce the risk of death or disability [42]. Communication delays that span tens of minutes can easily surpass this critical timeframe, making timely patient stabilization even more challenging. Furthermore, the limited bandwidth for data transmission restricts the amount and quality of data that can be sent to Earth. Such limitations render Earth-based telemedicine support to astronauts in space impractical in critical situations.

Mass, Volume, and Power In space travel, mass limitations are dictated by the rocket's payload capacity. Every additional kilogram requires more fuel not only to leave LEO but also to enter, maintain orbit around, and leave the surface of the Moon or Mars. Current estimates for NASA's space shuttle launch are US$54,000 per kg. With a payload of 27,500 kg, this amounts to a total of US$1.5 billion per launch [43]. For context, the da Vinci Xi surgical system, including the surgeon console, patient cart, and vision cart, weighs a total of 1344 kg [44], adding approximately US$72.5 million in costs if transported aboard a spacecraft. Although commercial launch systems such as SpaceX's Falcon 9 have reduced launch costs by about four times, the need for specialized equipment increases the costs and reduces the payload capacity [43]. In tandem with mass restrictions, the volume of items to be transported is also limited, given the confined space of the shuttle. Power limitations result from the finite amount of energy available, typically supplied by solar panels and batteries. Efficient energy management is critical to ensure that essential systems, including life support, communication, and scientific instruments, operate continuously. As spacecraft travel farther away from the Sun, they require larger solar panels to capture sufficient energy, which adds weight and further limits the amount of equipment that can be carried on board.

Equipment and Auxiliary Support As a direct outcome of mass, volume, and power limitations, only specific medical equipment and systems can be transported aboard a spacecraft. Devices such as Computed Tomography (CT) scanners are currently excluded from long-duration space missions. Magnetic Resonance Imaging (MRI) scanners present even greater challenges, weighing approximately 11 tons and requiring constant helium cooling of their superconducting magnets. The emitted stray magnetic fields from MRI scanners can also interfere with spacecraft operations [45]. Initiatives have been undertaken to miniaturize robotic systems and streamline their designs to include only essential components [46], but these systems remain in the experimental phase.

The variety and quantity of medical and surgical tools that can be carried are also restricted. Medications, blood, and fluids are limited and subject to expiration. On the ISS, the only available resuscitation fluids are 4 L of normal saline [47]. Methods to generate crystalloids in flight are still under investigation [48]. Blood transfusion, whether for surgical support or standalone treatment, is currently not possible. Only lyophilized blood components, such as plasma, which may be stored for up to a year, are suitable [47]. An alternative involves hemoglobin-based oxygen carriers, which are artificial substitutes for red blood cells that can deliver oxygen and provide volume expansion [47]. These substitutes are convenient as they require minimal preparation, but they have similar mass and volume to packed red cells and will thus consume a lot of space. They also utilize significant refrigeration power and have a short shelf life of 35 days at 1–6 °C [47].

These limitations undermine the synergistic ecosystem of healthcare present in hospitals on Earth. Effective patient care on Earth relies on the seamless coordination of multiple departments, equipped with diverse facilities, tools, and expertise. In space, the absence of readily available auxiliary support, such as on-demand clinical laboratories and pharmacies, may jeopardize clinical decision support and the quality of long-term patient care.

Data and Testing Much of what we know about the specific challenges posed by space exploration is based on research conducted on the ISS. The actual needs and hazards of performing surgical procedures in deep space remain largely speculative and untested. The collection and interpretation of physiological data from astronauts is far from perfect, as monitoring health conditions in space is, at best, limited and often outright impossible. Furthermore, all existing physiological data is obtained from astronauts who had spent no more than 6–7 months in LEO. Few astronauts have remained in microgravity for longer durations, and those who have participated in extended missions have not been studied extensively to assess potential changes or adverse effects on their anatomy and physiology [5]. Long-duration space exploration missions to Mars, for example, can last at least 34 months, which is more than twice the record for the number of consecutive days spent in space by any astronaut [49]. Lastly, developing effective strategies for testing new space technologies on Earth is crucial for verifying their suitability for future missions, especially in terms of their performance in microgravity. The six main experimental systems for ground verification of a microgravity environment are air-bearing, neutral buoyancy, free-fall, parabolic flight, suspension, and hardware-in-the-loop systems [50]. Each of these systems has limitations, and some are not even suitable for medical and surgical applications. For instance, neutral buoyancy requires submerging the system in water, making it impractical for surgical testing or training.

12.1.3 Procedures for Trauma and Emergency Care in Space

Despite studies on the viability of emergency procedures in microgravity [9, 51], the complex pathophysiology of hemorrhagic shock in space remains poorly understood. In the next section, we will examine procedures for patient stabilization, reconstructive surgery, and acute care that hold promise for adaptation from terrestrial to space missions.

12.1.3.1 Patient Stabilization

Damage control resuscitation (DCR) is a strategy for early initiation of blood product transfusions, crystalloid fluid administration, permissive hypotension, and damage control surgery (DCS). It can be delivered to a critically ill patient in any location (emergency department, interventional radiology suite, operating theater, and/or intensive care unit) [52]. The equivalent protocol designed specifically for austere environments is the Remote Damage Control Resuscitation (RDCR) [12, 53]. In this scenario, permissive hypotension is a valuable support, allowing the control of exsanguination by lowering blood pressure while ensuring vital organ perfusion [54]. This approach requires careful monitoring of the patient's radial pulse and mental status while maintaining a systolic blood pressure (SBP) between 80 and 100 mmHg. Traumatic brain injury needs a higher SBP (>100 mm Hg for ages 50–69 and >110 mm Hg for ages 15–49) to preserve cerebral perfusion and avoid a secondary ischemic injury to the brain [12, 53]. The early use of blood products, fresh warm whole blood, and other blood components [47] also reflects DCR and RDCR practices. For limb and extremity trauma, tourniquets or hemostatic dressings may be adequate to stabilize the patient [55]. Non-compressible torso hemorrhage is better managed using medical devices such as abdominal aortic and junctional tourniquets, injectable hemostatic sponge, resuscitative endovascular balloon occlusion of the aorta (REBOA), intra-abdominal self-expanding foam, and expandable hemostatic sponges [56, 57].

Topical hemostatics can also play a crucial role in managing medical emergencies in space. A systematic review in 2018 identified four primary categories of topical hemostatics: (1) adhesives (liquid fibrin adhesives and fibrin patches), (2) mechanical hemostats, (3) sealants, and (4) hemostatic dressings (mineral and polysaccharides) [58]. The choice of hemostatic agent largely depends on the patient's endogenous coagulation state. For instance, mechanical agents are preferred after surgical hemostasis or packing if coagulation is normal. For ongoing arterial or high-flow bleeding, adhesive agents with a patch are recommended because they can be directly applied at the bleeding site. Sealant agents are particularly useful for controlling bleeding in organs, such as the liver, pancreas, and kidney, or for sealing lung wounds. Hemostatic dressings are indicated for junctional and non-compressible hemorrhages, such as those in the neck, groin, or axilla. Recent advances have also seen the clinical application of novel hemostats, like self-assembling peptide nanofibers and chitosan nanofibers [58–60].

DCS helps manage severe intra-abdominal hemorrhage, organ damage, and other serious injuries that cannot be treated through non-operative means. DCS also aims to minimize the number of surgical interventions while safeguarding a patient's physiological reserves. This approach not only restricts surgical operations to those that are absolutely necessary but also reduces the need for extensive surgical equipment. Once the patient is prepared for surgery, rapid evaluation and control of bleeding sources are paramount. This may involve techniques such as packing, ligation, or resection of damaged tissues. Temporary abdominal closure techniques, such as the use of negative pressure wound therapy or Bogota bags, help prevent abdominal compartment syndrome and facilitate re-exploration. For managing solid organ injuries, techniques such as splenectomy, hepatorrhaphy, and nephrectomy may be necessary. These procedures require precise surgical skills to control bleeding while preserving as much organ function as possible. If the patient is hemodynamically stable, angiography with selective embolization of bleeding vessels might be performed. Advances in minimally invasive techniques, such as laparoscopic surgery, are increasingly being incorporated into trauma care to reduce recovery time and postoperative complications.

12.1.3.2 Postoperative and Definitive Surgical Care

Postoperative complications following DCS are detected through a combination of laboratory tests, clinical assessment, and imaging studies [61–63]. The patient is monitored for signs of instability, such as changes in vital signs, increased abdominal pain, or decreased urine output, indicating issues like bleeding or infection. Laboratory tests, including complete blood count, coagulation profiles, and blood cultures, provide information on the patient's physiological status and help identify infections or ongoing hemorrhage. Imaging studies using US or CT can detect complications like intra-abdominal abscesses or anastomotic leaks [61, 62]. Postoperative bleeding frequently requires surgical re-exploration. Surgeons may perform methods such as repacking of the abdominal cavity, selective vascular ligation, or bleeding site suture. Angioembolization may be used for specific arterial bleeding identified on angiography, especially if re-exploration poses a significant risk [61]. In cases of intra-abdominal sepsis or abscess formation, surgical intervention involves drainage of pus collections, which can be performed percutaneously via imaging or through open surgical drainage. When an anastomotic leak is detected, surgeons may need to resect the leaking section of the bowel and create a new anastomosis. In some cases, especially if the patient is unstable or the tissue is not healthy enough for a new anastomosis, a diverting stoma, such as an ileostomy or colostomy, is created to facilitate fecal diversion and tissue healing [63]. Contaminated wounds may require surgical debridement to remove infected tissue, followed by wound care procedures such as negative pressure wound therapy [64]. Abdominal compartment syndrome is another potential complication. It is characterized by increased intra-abdominal pressure that can impair organ function. Surgical decompression through laparotomy is often necessary to restore blood supply to vital organs and prevent further organ damage [65]. It is not uncommon for patients to require future definitive surgeries following DCS.

12.1.3.3 Acute Care

Appendectomies are critical interventions that will be required if an astronaut develops appendicitis during a mission [66]. There are two primary surgical techniques for performing an appendectomy: open surgery and laparoscopic surgery. Traditionally, open surgery was the standard approach, requiring an incision to access and remove the appendix. However, over the past few decades, laparoscopic surgery has become the preferred method for treating both nonperforated and perforated appendicitis due to its minimally invasive nature and associated benefits, such as reduced postoperative pain, shorter recovery times, and lower infection rates [66]. Similarly, cholecystitis, an inflammation of the gallbladder often caused by gallstones, requires surgical intervention to remove the gallbladder. This surgery can also be performed using either the open or laparoscopic approach [67]. The management of renal stones in space is also crucial. While small stones can often be passed naturally with the aid of muscle relaxant medications containing alpha-blockers, larger stones require more advanced interventions [68]. One non-invasive approach is extracorporeal shock wave lithotripsy, where high-energy sound waves are used to break down the stones into smaller fragments that can be excreted naturally in the urine. Ureteroscopy is routinely used to treat stones located in the bladder or lower ureters. This treatment involves introducing a small, flexible ureteroscope through the urethra and bladder to allow direct visualization and removal or fragmentation of the stone using specialized instruments. Percutaneous nephrolithotomy is a minimally invasive surgical alternative for larger stones found within the kidney.

12.2 Autonomous Robotics for Trauma and Emergency Care in Space

Autonomous robotic systems are poised to play a pivotal role in support of trauma and emergency care in long-duration space missions. At its core, a robotic system is a programmable machine engineered to automate tasks traditionally performed by humans. Over time, these systems have been augmented with various sensors, including vision devices like 2D and 3D cameras, accelerometers, inertial measurement units, proximity sensors, and force sensors. The most transformative development in robotics, however, has resulted from the integration of AI, which enabled three key components: perception, decision-making, and learning. Robots can now perceive their environment much like humans do, make informed decisions, and learn from past experiences to continuously improve their performance, thus growing into increasingly intelligent and autonomous systems. In the medical field, these systems transform into dynamic agents capable of working alongside healthcare providers. They can assist in clinical procedures, expand the operational capacity of medical professionals, and autonomously manage specific tasks within a surgical workflow [69].

In space, autonomous medical robotics can emerge as a particularly powerful tool. These systems have shown promise to enhance the accuracy, precision, and repeatability of healthcare delivery [70, 71]. These attributes are critical in environments where errors can have dire consequences, and managing health complications poses significant challenges. Autonomous robots can also improve clinical support by assessing injuries, providing diagnostics, and autonomously executing surgical interventions, either partially or in full. This capability is invaluable for optimizing the use of limited medical resources on a spacecraft and addressing extreme scenarios where healthcare providers may become unavailable. Furthermore, AI-powered robotics excel at adapting to new environments, continuously learning from each operation to improve their performance in future, unforeseen scenarios. This behavior is beneficial as we venture into the unknown realms of space, where the exact medical challenges are largely unknown.

Although commercial systems have achieved some level of autonomy, they still heavily rely on human input [69]. Deep space missions, with their extreme conditions and operational constraints, will demand more autonomous systems to ensure that medical care is delivered effectively and in a timely manner. Thus, the remainder of this chapter will look at the latest advancements in autonomous medical robotics research, with a particular emphasis on innovations that can be useful during space travel. Given the widespread use of AI in healthcare, our discussion will only include AI algorithms that support robotic system autonomy.

12.2.1 History of Medical Robotics in Space

Much of modern robotic surgery can be traced back to early NASA initiatives to promote space exploration [72]. In the 1970s, researchers at NASA's Ames Research

Center proposed providing medical support to astronauts in space via a robotic system operated by clinicians on Earth, a concept known as teleoperation [72]. Although the project remained unfunded for over a decade, it eventually gained the support of the US military, which recognized its potential for use on battlefields, environments similarly characterized by remoteness and austerity. When NASA researchers created the first prototype of a teleoperated robotic system, they rapidly recognized the limitations posed by time delays in space teleoperation [72]. This realization redirected research efforts toward shorter distance teleoperation, ultimately catalyzing the development of the first commercial surgical robotic systems, including AESOP, da Vinci, and Zeus [73]. Among these, the da Vinci Surgical System has been particularly transformative, utilized in over 11 million procedures worldwide since 2000, including 1.5 million surgeries in 2021 alone [74]. Following these pioneering systems, other robotic platforms have been effectively employed across a variety of surgical procedures, including minimally invasive biopsies, orthopedic surgery, radiosurgery, urological surgeries, cardiology interventions, and neurosurgery.

Despite years of scientific progress, robotic surgery in space has remained largely experimental and untested in actual missions. The first and only surgical robotic system to reach LEO is the Miniaturized In Vivo Robotic Assistant, known as spaceMIRA, developed by Virtual Incision and the University of Nebraska [75]. SpaceMIRA, a 2-pound device, builds on its Earth-bound predecessor, MIRA, which was created for colectomy procedures [76]. Unlike traditional teleoperated robotic systems, MIRA features two miniaturized robotic arms, one for grasping and one for cutting, that operate directly inside the patient's body through a single incision. In February 2024, MIRA received the de novo classification from the Food and Drug Administration as a table-mounted miniature electromechanical surgical system. SpaceMIRA was further miniaturized for space surgeries, reducing its overall length by about 3 inches compared to MIRA's. On February 22, 2024, spaceMIRA successfully carried out the first-ever simulated robotic surgery aboard the ISS. The study involved two types of experiments simulating surgery on rubber bands: one was a pre-programmed run for a semi-autonomous operation, and the other was a teleoperated session where a surgeon on Earth controlled the robot. While the outcomes of the semi-autonomous operation remain unpublished, reports indicate that during teleoperation, despite communication delays ranging from 0.6 to 0.8 s, the surgeon successfully cut through the rubber bands, thereby compensating for the delays using their expertise [75].

Despite the scarcity of space-based robotic surgery trials, significant progress is being made on Earth toward autonomous medical procedures and surgeries. These developments lay the groundwork for future space medicine and will be the focus of our next discussion.

12.2.2 State-of-the-Art Robotics for Trauma and Emergency Care

When an emergency patient is treated, the process starts with an assessment of vital signs such as heart rate (HR), blood pressure (BP), respiratory rate (RR), oxygen saturation (SpO_2), and body temperature (BT). This initial triage determines the severity of the patient's condition and identifies immediate threats. Following that, a diagnostic evaluation, including imaging and blood testing, is conducted to identify underlying issues. Based on these findings, interventional procedures, ranging from medication administration to surgery, are performed. We will thus divide our overview of autonomous medical robotics into three areas, each corresponding to these key steps in emergency medical treatment: initial assessment and triage, robotic diagnostic evaluation, and robotic interventional procedures, as illustrated in Fig. 12.1.

12.2.2.1 Initial Assessment and Triage

Vital signs are often measured using separate instruments like sphygmomanometers, thermometers, and pulse oximeters. Over the years, compact wearable devices have emerged for longitudinal and ambulatory vital sign monitoring, capable of measuring several physiological parameters with a single device [77]. US miniaturization led to the development of adhesive US patches the size of a postage stamp that can measure BP and even collect US images of organs like the lungs and heart [78]. While these wearables are useful for continuous health monitoring, they have drawbacks such as limited battery life, potential discomfort for the wearer, and susceptibility to damage from impact or wear and tear. As a result, remote photoplethysmography (rPPG) technology, which enables contactless measurement of patient vital signs, is becoming increasingly popular [79]. Clinically used for measuring SpO_2 and pulse rate, photoplethysmography (PPG) works by measuring the amount of light absorbed or reflected by human tissues using contact devices such as electronic pulse oximeters. Signal processing advances have enabled visual contactless physiological monitoring by consumer RGB cameras that extract PPG signals from facial or abdominal skin [80]. Once the PPG signal is obtained, deep learning can be used to estimate vital signs such as HR [81, 82], BP [81, 83], RR [81, 84], and SpO_2 [82] with an accuracy comparable to that of standard contact devices [84–86]. Although most of these algorithms are designed to extract a single vital sign from the PPG signal at a time, the development of large-scale, multi-task AI models capable of estimating multiple vital signals simultaneously has been deemed feasible [80]. In addition to rPPG-based vitals monitoring, thermal imaging using infrared (IR) signals can detect body temperature and help localize wounds from active bleeding, which is particularly useful in trauma cases [87]. Dual RGB/thermal cameras, such as the Teledyne FLIR Hadron 320, can facilitate comprehensive care in space, where minimizing the number of devices is critical.

Most rPPG algorithms were evaluated on high-quality video data collected in controlled environments [80, 84] In real-world emergencies, it is impossible to maintain consistent and continuous visual access to the patient's skin from a single location. Mounting cameras and sensors on mobile robots offers a dynamic

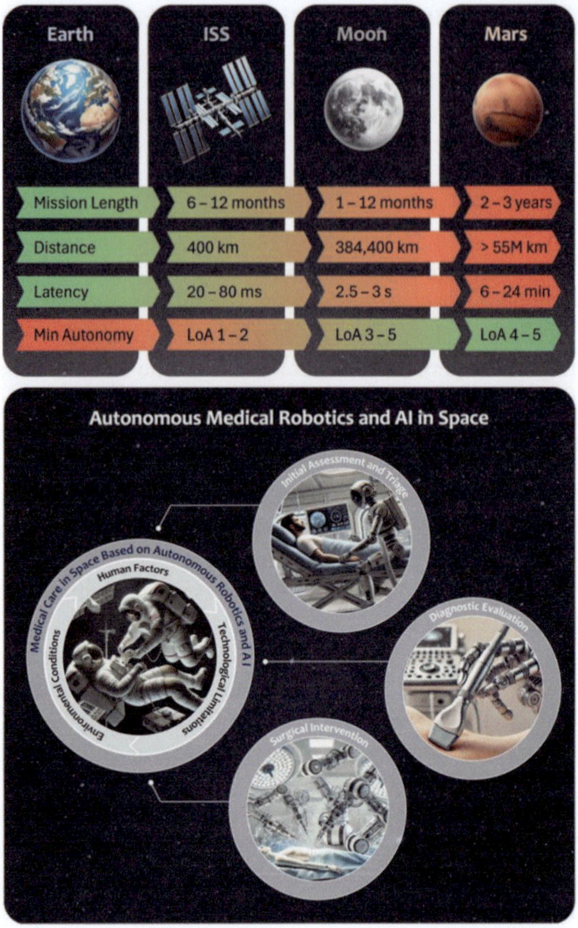

Fig. 12.1 The figure illustrates the relationship between increasing distance from Earth to the ISS, the Moon, and Mars. As missions venture farther from Earth, the length of the mission extends, communication delays increase, and the need for highly autonomous robotic systems becomes critical. These systems are pivotal in addressing the three major challenges in space medicine by: (1) performing initial assessment and triage, (2) conducting diagnostic evaluations, and (3) executing surgical interventions, thereby ensuring the health and safety of crew members in deep space exploration missions. (AI generated image created with OpenAI Inc., DALL-E 3, 2024)

platform for improved patient access. During the COVID-19 pandemic, Huang et al. developed a quadruped robotic system for contactless vital signs monitoring in hospitals [88]. The system uses IR and multimonochrome cameras to automatically track individuals and measure skin temperature, HR, and RR, while also screening for fever, tachypnea, and tachycardia. Mobile quadruped robots have been a popular platform for collecting patient data in hospitals and public spaces [89, 90], as well as in more challenging settings like rescue missions [91]. Similarly, drones have been experimentally deployed to accident sites to autonomously assess a subject's vital signs and identify life-threatening wounds [92]. Advanced algorithms for skin segmentation [93], object tracking [94], and robot motion planning [95] facilitate capturing high-quality patient video data using visual servoing. This technique ensures that the best skin area remains in the robot's field of view long enough to reliably extract vital signs. In space, mounting cameras on mobile robotic platforms or manipulators can help autonomously collect critical data for patient triage.

Machine-learning algorithms, including logistic regression, random forests, and deep learning, have been developed to streamline patient triage by predicting the likelihood of acute outcomes in emergency scenarios [96]. Input for these models often includes vital signs, medical history, and primary complaints [97]. Studies have shown that such "electronic" triage accurately classifies emergency severity index level 3 patients and highlights opportunities for using predictive analytics to support early triage decisions [98]. Building on mobile robots' ability to collect contact-free vital signs in space, predictive triage can augment the attending provider's capacity by assisting with critical decision-making and giving them more time to prepare for urgent surgical procedures.

12.2.2.2 Robotic Diagnostic Evaluation

If the patient's vital signs are stable, medical imaging is employed next to assess the severity of the injury and diagnose the patient's condition. US is the primary medical imaging modality used on the ISS due to its lightweight, compact design, and low power requirements. It is also used in the primary assessment of trauma patients in search of abdominal hemorrhaging via the extended Focused Assessment with Sonography for Trauma (eFAST) exam. Currently, all US scanning procedures on the ISS are manually performed by the crew members themselves, guided remotely by a physician on Earth [99]. Attaching a US probe to a robotic arm is the most intuitive approach for enabling autonomous robotic US scanning.

First, the robotic system must identify the patient's body via 2D and 3D cameras. Before attempting to collect US images of the abdomen, the robot must locate scannable skin, which entails differentiating healthy skin from wounds, bandages, and clothing. Solutions specific to abdominal skin segmentation were proposed using a UNet network [100], alongside more advanced algorithms for generic skin segmentation [93]. Wound delineation has also been investigated [101, 102], as has clothing segmentation from colored images [103]. While most of these algorithms have not yet been integrated or tested specifically on trauma patients, deep learning's current capabilities should be sufficient for these applications, given access to adequate training data. Another method of interest involves using body surface information to infer key internal organ markers, such as the femoral artery bifurcation point or the center of the femoral head. Siemens Healthineers developed a convolutional neural network that can generate a patient-specific avatar model (DARWIN) from a depth camera snapshot [104]. This patient model was used to map a relationship between the body's surface geometry and select 3D internal anatomical markers with high accuracy [105, 106]. A total of 60 predicted markers on the rib cage, for example, had a mean Euclidean error of 14.8 mm [107]. These internal landmarks can be used to avoid imaging certain areas under US or to help the robot locate specific organs, including the liver, spleen, and femoral artery. Researchers have also developed methods to estimate a patient's pose in real time [108] and predict eFAST locations on a patient's body [108, 109].

Several robotic systems have been developed for teleoperated abdominal US scanning [109–111], with more recent work focusing on autonomous operation to decrease the dependency on operator skills and availability. A team at Johns Hopkins

University demonstrated preliminary feasibility of autonomous point-of-care US scanning for lung diagnosis and staging, with and without pre-operative patient CT data. Their system comprises a 3D RGB camera, a force sensor, and a wireless US probe, mounted on a six-degrees-of-freedom robotic manipulator [106]. To avoid obstruction of US images by ribs, the internal markers prediction algorithm [105] was used to estimate landmarks on the ribcage using only surface body scans. A study on a full torso US phantom [112] showed that using only the predicted landmarks and force feedback, 87.5% of autonomously acquired US images without preliminary CT data were interpretable. Other studies have reported successful autonomous robotic US scanning of solid abdominal organs such as the liver [113] and vascular structures like the jugular artery [114]. Raina et al. proposed a solution that uses demonstrations from expert sonographers to train robots to acquire high-quality US scans [115]. The team used Bayesian optimization with domain expertise to predict and scan regions where US images are of the best quality. Experiments on urinary bladder phantoms showed an accuracy of 98.7% in probe positioning and 97.8% in force application [115]. Others have also explored advanced learning frameworks for autonomous robotic US manipulation, such as imitation learning and reinforcement learning [116, 117]. These various learning frameworks have both advantages and disadvantages, which will be discussed in the following sections.

Although eFAST is an effective tool for detecting pneumothorax and free fluid in abdominal cavities, patients with positive scans typically undergo CT imaging to assess hemorrhage volume and classify trauma severity. Given that the miniaturization of CT scanners for space applications is still in the experimental phase [118], robotic US scanning combined with US image analysis can be a valuable diagnostic alternative. Most current algorithms concentrate on the binary identification of abdominal free fluid [119] or pneumothorax [120] in US images. Some US segmentation models exist for delineating organs such as the liver [121], heart compartments [122], and blood vessels [123], but they are limited in number primarily due to the scarcity of labeled US datasets. To address this, US data simulation from 3D imaging modalities was proposed [124]. State-of-the-art deep learning models, capable of identifying over 100 different organs from CT [125] and MRI data [126], can help generate extensive datasets of high-quality annotated US images. These datasets can be leveraged to develop more sophisticated US segmentation algorithms [127, 128], enable volumetric interpretation of US data [127, 128], and train robots to dynamically adjust probe placement based on US image analysis [129]. Moreover, novel multi-modal registration techniques [130] can integrate astronauts' pre-existing medical imaging data with intraoperative images, further enhancing the accuracy and precision of autonomous robotic diagnostic procedures in space.

12.2.2.3 Robotic Interventional Procedures

Levels of Robotic Autonomy Innovations driven by research in AI have gradually increased robotic autonomy in various surgical tasks. Autonomous features in surgical robotics have shown superior performance compared to expert surgeons in both synthetic and living tissues [131]. Some of these features are already integrated into clinically approved surgical systems. However, robotic autonomy encompasses a broad spectrum, ranging from entirely teleoperated systems to autonomous "robotic surgeons" that require no human supervision [132]. Over the years, the definition of the different levels of autonomy has been refined to include a formal framework based on four cognition-related functions of a system: generating an option, executing an option, monitoring an option, and selecting an option from many [133]. The number and type of these functions performed by the robot help classify the system into a specific level of autonomy [134].

To this end, the standard classification for surgical robotics currently comprises five levels of autonomy [132, 134]. At Level 0, robots operate as tools controlled entirely by humans, such as teleoperated robots and prosthetic devices that respond directly to user commands. The Intuitive da Vinci system exhibits Level 0 autonomy, utilizing "transparent" teleoperation, where the surgeon's movements on the control interface are exactly replicated by the surgical instruments on the patient side [135]. At Level 1, robots provide cognitive and physical assistance, offering mechanical guidance or support while the human operator maintains continuous control. Examples include surgical robots with virtual fixtures and haptic feedback, such as MAKO by Stryker and ROSA ONE by Zimmer Biomet for knee arthroplasty. Level 2 robots achieve task autonomy, performing specific tasks initiated by a human with discrete control, such as robotic surgical suturing. Examples of such systems include the Senhance robot by Asensus Surgical for laparoscopic procedures and the CorPath GRX by Corindus for percutaneous coronary interventions and vascular procedures. Level 3, or conditional autonomy, allows robots to generate and adjust task strategies during execution, requiring human approval for strategy selection but performing tasks with minimal oversight. As of 2024, the only robotic systems to achieve Level 3 autonomy and receive the FDA's 510(k) clearance are the iSR'obot Mona Lisa 2.0 (Biobot), TSolution One (Think Surgical), and ARTAS iX System (Venus Concept). At Level 4, robots exhibit high autonomy, making medical decisions and executing complex procedures under the supervision of a qualified healthcare professional. Finally, Level 5 represents full autonomy, where robots can perform entire surgeries independently, making all necessary medical decisions without any human intervention. To date, no commercially available surgical systems have reached Levels 4 or 5 autonomy. However, these advanced levels are actively being researched at various institutions, which we will discuss next.

Autonomous Surgical Robotics The Veebot system (Veebot LLC) is a Level 4 autonomous robot designed for vascular access [136]. The procedure begins by positioning the patient's arm through an archway over a padded surface, followed by constricting the arm using an inflatable cuff to enhance vein visibility. The system then employs infrared (IR) light to illuminate the inner elbow, and software algorithms compare the camera's view against a vascular anatomy model to select the optimal vein for puncture. US imaging then confirms the selected vein's location and suitability. A robotic arm aligns the needle with the vein and performs the insertion, completing the procedure within approximately one minute. Human intervention is limited to attaching appropriate collection tubes or intravenous bags to the syringe. While this system is not yet commercially available, it has demonstrated successful cannulation in 83% of veins [137]. Chen et al. developed a comparable robotic phlebotomy device [138]. Their system combines near-IR and US imaging to create a 3D model of the patient's vasculature and uses miniaturized robotics for precise needle placement. The platform was later augmented by adding a sample handling station and a centrifuge-based blood analyzer, enabling fully automated, point-of-care diagnostic blood testing on-site [139]. The current iteration of this system supports a 3-part white blood cell differential and hemoglobin measurement. While initially conceived for blood sample collection, these autonomous systems have potential applications beyond phlebotomy, including critical care interventions such as the placement of REBOA for patient stabilization [140].

Recent research focuses on advancing autonomous robots with Level 3 autonomy and higher for surgical tasks such as suturing and tumor removal. The Smart Tissue Autonomous Robot (STAR) is one research platform that uses machine learning for tissue tracking to autonomously complete small bowel anastomosis [131, 141]. STAR consists of a suturing tool, an imaging system that combines near-IR and 3D plenoptic imaging, and supervised-autonomy control. A comparative study evaluating the efficiency and efficacy of STAR against state-of-the-art master-follower robotic (da Vinci) and manual laparoscopic techniques demonstrated remarkable improvements. STAR achieved a five-fold and nine-fold reduction in operation time compared to robotic and manual techniques, respectively, while exhibiting four times greater consistency in suturing planar phantoms with one knot and nine running sutures [141]. Moreover, STAR pioneered pre-clinical supervised autonomous robotic anastomosis of porcine small intestines in both open and laparoscopic surgeries, outperforming expert surgeons' manual and robotically assisted surgery in terms of consistency and accuracy [131]. Concurrently, the Autonomous System for Tumor Resection (ASTR) has been developed for supervised autonomous tumor excision [142]. ASTR consists of two robotic manipulators, one equipped with an electrosurgical instrument and the other with a vacuum grasping tool. ASTR also employs a dual-camera vision system to detect color inks and near-IR fluorescent markers used to delineate tumor margins. The robot autonomously plans and executes trajectories to excise a tumor. Using glossectomy as a case study, ASTR successfully performed six consecutive supervised autonomous pseudotumor resections on ex vivo porcine tongues without positive tumor margins, with an accuracy comparable to manual pseudotumor glossectomy performed by an experienced otolaryngologist. Current research is exploring the system's generalizability to partial nephrectomy procedures [143].

While the STAR and ASTR systems represent significant advancements in autonomous surgical robotics, they rely on physical tissue markers to guide their operations [131, 142]. Although effective for certain tasks, these methods cannot be used for all actions in surgical procedures, such as tissue manipulation and knot tying, which are challenging to reduce to a set of motion primitives and require dynamic adaptability to the environment. The broader field of robotics has greatly benefited from learning frameworks that enable robots to "learn" through two primary approaches: reinforcement learning (RL) and imitation learning (IL). RL is a framework where the robot teaches itself certain actions by directly interacting with an environment, while IL enables the robot to mimic expert behavior without the trial-and-error exploration that is characteristic of RL. These approaches have gained popularity in tasks such as walking, grasping, and tabletop object manipulation by industrial robots [144, 145]. Surgical tasks, however, present unique challenges that demand more precise and delicate manipulation of deformable soft tissues, coupled with the need to overcome perceptual difficulties caused by occlusions and inconsistent lighting. Despite the relatively recent application of RL and IL in surgical robotics, progress has been promising. Recent research has demonstrated the successful application of combined RL and IL for automatic laparoscope motion control, trained on a 3D-rendered surgical scene derived from real-world collected surgical videos [146]. The learned robot policy for laparoscope control was shown to outperform baseline IL approaches and generalize well to unseen environments. Scheikl et al. adopted IL to perform gentle manipulation of deformable objects while requiring fewer demonstrations, addressing a common challenge with these algorithms [147]. Their approach was successfully tested in a real-world task on a porcine liver with an attached latex gallbladder, where one laparoscopic robotic instrument learned to manipulate the gallbladder to expose a target point, which was then autonomously touched by a second laparoscopic robotic instrument [147]. In another study, Kim et al. demonstrated IL's capabilities in training a da Vinci system using 3D colored videos and the robot's kinematics data to autonomously perform surgical tasks that include lifting soft tissue, picking up and transferring a needle between two surgical tools, and tying knots [148]. The system's generalizability was successfully validated on both phantoms and ex vivo animal tissues that were not used in training.

12.2.3 Future Technological Directions

Despite promising results, certain technological advancements are necessary to make these robotic systems viable for providing autonomous care in space, particularly addressing the unique challenges outlined at the beginning of this chapter. A major issue in autonomous surgical robotics is the ability to extrapolate to environments that were not seen in training. This concern is amplified in space applications, where both patient physiology and tissue behavior differ substantially from terrestrial norms, and relevant data is scarce. While developing algorithms with enhanced extrapolation capabilities is essential, it remains insufficient without comprehensive validation. A promising solution lies in a dual approach: generating high-fidelity simulated data that closely approximates real-world scenarios while simultaneously advancing learning algorithms to enhance the generalizability from simulated environments to real conditions. This approach necessitates advanced augmentation techniques beyond simple rotation, scaling, and flipping to maximize the utility of limited real-world surgical data. Deep networks, such as generative adversarial networks, should be further improved to synthesize realistic surgical scenes, while style transfer techniques can be adapted to represent more diverse surgical conditions and patient anatomies. Researchers would thus be able to leverage a limited number of surgical videos recorded in microgravity to generate novel, stylistically consistent simulations based on terrestrial surgical procedures. These artificial demonstrations can in turn be utilized to train robotic systems using IL, with the development of advanced methods to ensure effective generalization from simulated to real-world data. Such methodology does present some caveats, however. In IL, a policy—defined as a strategy that maps observations to actions—guides the robot's behavior. Robots are penalized during training if their execution diverges from the expert's demonstrations. A critical consideration is that artificial data may not consistently provide optimal expert demonstrations. This limitation is further compounded by the fact that robotic systems, with their unique mechanical designs and dynamics, may achieve task optimality differently from human experts. For instance, a robotic arm, with its increased degrees of freedom, can manipulate surgical tools in ways that exceed human anatomical capabilities. Additionally, altered gravitational conditions might necessitate modified kinematic strategies to execute a surgical task. Delving into the mathematical foundations of IL-based frameworks becomes essential to estimate better policies that can effectively balance the importance of task outcomes with the accuracy of behavior imitation. A key advantage in advancing IL is the potential to learn from not only manual expert demonstrations but also teleoperated robotic interventions, rendering the learning process more intuitive and organic for a robot.

An alternative approach for artificial data generation is to utilize realistic simulation platforms that employ physics laws and AI to create virtual representations of the real world, rather than relying on prior surgical videos. Current simulators, constrained by simplifying assumptions, struggle to model the complex, non-linear behaviors of biological tissues. Future research should focus on enhancing the fidelity of soft tissue deformation, cutting, and suturing simulations, incorporating factors such as anisotropy, viscoelasticity, and patient-specific variations. For space surgery simulations, microgravity-induced physical dynamics must also be accounted for. Additionally, improving photorealism is crucial, as visually unconvincing training data will hinder a robot's ability to generalize to real-world scenarios. In surgical robotics, enhanced simulations can be leveraged to train RL-based algorithms, addressing the persistent "sim-to-real" gap where performance in simulated environments often fails to translate effectively to real-world clinical scenarios. To further bridge this gap, domain adaptation methods that align feature distributions between simulated and real data, combined with progressive neural networks for sequential task learning, offer promising solutions. Meta-learning algorithms for quick task adaptation can enhance the generalizability of surgical robotic solutions. Developing hybrid sim-to-real training pipelines, where robots are initially trained in simulation and fine-tuned on limited real-world data, can also be adopted. Even though utilizing simulation to reliably train robots for real-world surgeries will be quite difficult, improvements in simulations can still be leveraged to aid the robot in decision-making tasks, for instance, by predicting future tissue state and interaction with surgical tools. Online learning algorithms capable of updating tissue models in real time during surgical procedures are valuable for immediate adaptation to patient-specific variations and unexpected scenarios. Realistic simulations also show tremendous potential to improve the medical preparedness of CMOs. Advanced VR environments that emulate space conditions can become particularly powerful platforms for medical training on Earth itself. Enhancing VR immersiveness with realistic tactile feedback will enable CMOs to practice for medical procedures as if they were operating under microgravity and physical constraints, while also preparing them psychologically for the distinct challenges of providing care in the demanding environment of space.

The constraints of spacecraft transportation necessitate innovative design solutions for medical equipment and robotic systems. Miniaturization emerges as a paramount consideration, not only reducing the invasiveness of surgical procedures but also enabling novel interventions while potentially lowering power requirements. Concurrently, the exploration of lightweight yet robust materials for robotic components and surgical tools is crucial. Developing modular robotic designs capable of accommodating various medical instruments can maximize system versatility in the resource-limited confines of a spacecraft. Advancements in additive manufacturing, particularly in rapid production capabilities and multi-material printing, present transformative possibilities for on-demand fabrication of surgical tools, robot replacement parts, and patient-specific devices. This approach, guided by optimized design algorithms, could significantly enhance the autonomy of space-based medical care. Equally critical is the integration of novel sensing technologies to provide rich, multi-modal information about the surgical field, addressing the unique challenges posed by microgravity environments. Miniaturized force sensors, multi-modal cameras, and spectroscopic sensors can offer unprecedented insight into tissue properties and composition. The integration of flexible and stretchable electronic sensors into surgical instruments or artificial tissues represents a frontier in sensory feedback. The true value lies not only in the development of these advanced technologies but also in the integration of sophisticated algorithms capable of efficiently fusing and interpreting multi-modal data streams in real time, thereby enabling more informed and precise surgical interventions.

12.3 Conclusions

The integration of autonomous robotics and AI into space-based trauma and emergency care represents a paradigm shift in medical capabilities for future space missions. The unique challenges of space environments—microgravity, isolation, and limited resources—necessitate innovative solutions that enhance robotic autonomy and decision-making capabilities. Communication delays and limited availability of trained personnel necessitate real-time analysis and adaptive responses to medical emergencies. As we advance toward longer and more complex space missions, ensuring astronaut health and safety through autonomous medical interventions will be paramount. Current technological progress offers potential solutions, but the isolation of space missions demands extensive redundancy and fail-safe features to ensure reliable operation. This raises important questions about liability and decision-making authority in critical situations, highlighting the need for developing clear regulatory guidelines and protocols. Collaboration between space agencies, medical institutions, and technology developers will be crucial in addressing remaining technical, ethical, and legal challenges.

Autonomous medical robotics and AI not only promise to revolutionize space exploration but also offer transformative insights for medical care on Earth, potentially improving healthcare delivery in remote or resource-limited settings. The development of autonomous medical robotics for space applications represents a frontier of innovation with far-reaching implications. As we continue to push the boundaries of human space exploration, balancing technological innovation with ethical considerations will be essential to ensure these increasingly autonomous systems remain aligned with human values and medical best practices. The journey toward fully autonomous medical care in space is complex and challenging, but its potential benefits for both space exploration and terrestrial healthcare make it a pursuit of utmost importance and promise.

Acknowledgments This review was written within the activities of the ESA-Topical Team's research on "Tissue Healing in Space: Techniques for Promoting and Monitoring Tissue Repair and Regeneration"; the ESA-MAP Project "WHISPER-Wound Healing In Space: Problems and Perspectives for Tissue Regeneration and Engineering" Sci Space Microgravity Application Promotion Program, ESA Contract Number 4000130928/20/NL/PG/pt.; the SUTURE in SPACE experiment, selected by ESA (ESAAO-ILSRA-2014) and supported by ASI (ASI Contract N. 2018-14-U.O). This work was also supported by the National Institutes of Health under award number R56EB033807 and the National Science Foundation under CAREER identification number 2144348. The content is solely the responsibility of the authors and does not necessarily represent the official views of the National Institutes of Health or the National Science Foundation.

References

1. Creech S, Guidi J, Elburn D. Artemis: an overview of NASA's activities to return humans to the moon. In: In 2022 IEEE Aerospace Conference (aero). IEEE; 2022. p. 1–7.
2. Seedhouse E. The commercial spaceflight market. In: Commercial astronauts: the next generation of spacefarers. Springer; 2024. p. 15–25.
3. Smth M, Craig D, Herrman N, Mahoney E, Krezel J, McIntyre N, Goodliff N. The Artemis program: an overview of NASA's activities to return humans to the moon. IEEE Aerospace Conference, Big Sky, MT, USA, 2020; 2020. p. 1–10. https://doi.org/10.1109/AERO47225.2020.9172323.
4. Harris WL, Wonglimpiyarat J. Complexity model and Mars colonization. Foresight. 2023;25(6):753–68.
5. Schneider V, Siegel B, Allen JR. Human health on the moon and beyond and the results of the spaceflight for "everybody symposium". Aerosp Med Hum Perform. 2023;94(8):634–43.
6. Antonsen EL, Connell E, Anton W, Reynolds RJ, Buckland DM, Van Baalen M. Updates to the NASA human system risk management process for space exploration. npj Microgravity. 2023;9:72. https://doi.org/10.1038/s41526-023-00305-z.
7. Thomas TL, Garland FC, Molé D, Cohen BA, Gudewicz TM, Spiro RT, Zahm SH. Health of US navy submarine crew during periods of isolation. Aviat Space Environ Med. 2003;74(3):260–5.

8. Mills CN, Mills GH. Mass casualty incident response and aeromedical evacuation in Antarctica. West J Emerg Med. 2011;12(1):37.
9. Kirkpatrick AW, Ball CG, Campbell M, Williams DR, Parazynski SE, Mattox KL, Broderick TJ. Severe traumatic injury during long duration spaceflight: light years beyond ATLS. J Trauma Manag Outcomes. 2009;3:1–11.
10. Tansey W, Wilson JM, Schaefer K. Analysis of health data from 10 years of polaris submarine patrols. Undersea Biomed Res. 1979;6:S217–46.
11. Kirkpatrick AW, Campbell MR, Jones JA, Broderick TJ, Ball CG, McBeth PB, Mc-Swain NE, Hamilton DR, Holcomb JB. Extraterrestrial hemorrhage control: terrestrial developments in technique, technology, and philosophy with applicability to traumatic hemorrhage control in long-duration spaceflight. J Am Coll Surg. 2005;200(1):64–76.
12. Kirkpatrick AW, McKee JL, Tien H, LaPorta AJ, Lavell K, Leslie T, King DR, McBeth PB, Brien S, Roberts DJ, et al. Damage control surgery in weightlessness: a comparative study of simulated torso hemorrhage control comparing terrestrial and weightless conditions. J Trauma Acute Care Surg. 2017;82(2):392–9.
13. Kirkpatrick AW, Campbell MR, Novinkov OL, Goncharov IB, Kovachevich IV. Blunt trauma and operative care in microgravity: a review of microgravity physiology and surgical investigations with implications for critical care and operative treatment in space. J Am Coll Surg. 1997;184(5):441–53.
14. Alexander DJ. Trauma and surgical capabilities for space exploration. In: Trauma Team Dynamics: A Trauma Crisis Resource Management Manual; 2016. p. 253–66.
15. Gontcharov IB, Kovachevich IV, Pool SL, Navinkov OL, Barratt MR, Bogomolov VV, House N. In-flight medical incidents in the NASA-Mir program. Aviat Space Environ Med. 2005;76(7):692–6.
16. Assad A, de Weck OL. Model of medical supply and astronaut health for long-duration human space flight. Acta Astronaut. 2015;106:47–62.
17. A. E. Nicogossian, C. L. Huntoon, S. L. Pool, and P. Johnson, "Space physiology and medicine," 1988.
18. Belobrajdic B, Melone K, Diaz-Artiles A. Planetary extravehicular activity (EVA) risk mitigation strategies for long-duration space missions. npj Microgravity. 2021;7(1):16.
19. Pietrzyk RA, Jones JA, Sams CF, Whitson PA. Renal stone formation among astronauts. Aviat Space Environ Med. 2007;78(4):A9–A13.
20. Vico L, van Rietbergen B, Vilayphiou N, Linossier M-T, Locrelle H, Normand M, Zouch M, Gerbaix M, Bonnet N, Novikov V, et al. Cortical and trabecular bone microstructure did not recover at weight-bearing skeletal sites and progressively deteriorated at non-weight-bearing sites during the year following international space station missions. J Bone Miner Res. 2017;32(10):2010–21.
21. Thamer S, Stevanovic M, Buckey JC. Pre-flight body weight effects on urinary calcium excretion in space. npj Microgravity. 2023;9(1):45.
22. Gallo C, Ridolfi L, Scarsoglio S. Cardiovascular deconditioning during long-term spaceflight through multiscale modeling. npj Microgravity. 2020;6(1):27.
23. Patel S. The effects of microgravity and space radiation on cardiovascular health: from low-earth orbit and beyond. IJC Heart Vasc. 2020;30:100595.
24. Perhonen MA, Franco F, Lane LD, Buckey JC, Blomqvist CG, Zerwekh JE, Peshock RM, Weatherall PT, Levine BD. Cardiac atrophy after bed rest and spaceflight. J Appl Physiol. 2001;91(2):645–53.
25. Summers RL, Martin DS, Meck JV, Coleman TG. Mechanism of spaceflight-induced changes in left ventricular mass. Am J Cardiol. 2005;95(9):1128–30.
26. McCuaig KE, Houtchens BA. Management of trauma and emergency surgery in space. J Trauma Acute Care Surg. 1992;33(4):610–26.
27. Crucian BE, Chouker A, Simpson RJ, Mehta S, Marshall G, Smith SM, Zwart SR, Heer M, Ponomarev S, Whitmire A, et al. Immune system dysregulation during spaceflight: potential countermeasures for deep space exploration missions. Front Immunol. 2018;9:1437.

28. Daun S, Rubin J, Vodovotz Y, Roy A, Parker R, Clermont G. An ensemble of models of the acute inflammatory response to bacterial lipopolysaccharide in rats: results from parameter space reduction. J Theor Biol. 2008;253(4):843–53.
29. Kacena M, Merrell G, Manfredi B, Smith E, Klaus D, Todd P. Bacterial growth in space flight: logistic growth curve parameters for escherichia coli and bacillus subtilis. Appl Microbiol Biotechnol. 1999;51:229–34.
30. Taylor PW. Impact of space flight on bacterial virulence and antibiotic susceptibility. Infect Drug Resist. 2015;8:249–62.
31. Campbell MR, Billica RD, Johnston S 3rd. Animal surgery in microgravity. Aviat Space Environ Med. 1993;64(1):58–62.
32. Gernhardt M, Chappell S, Beaton K, Litaker H, Bekdash O, Newton C, Stoffel J. Deep space habitability design guidelines based on the NASA next step phase 2 ground test program. Tech Rep. 2019;
33. Bacal K, Beck G, McSwain NE Jr. A concept of operations for contingency medical care on the international space station. Mil Med. 2004;169(8):631–41.
34. Parrino CR, Fransman RB, Varone AJ, Galvagno SM Jr. Advanced trauma life support. In: Recent strategies in high risk surgery. Springer; 2024. p. 171–94.
35. Roslee MF. Review of medical capabilities requirements for manned missions on lunar and martian surfaces base activities. REACH. 2021;23:100042.
36. Reagan M. The NEEMO project: a report on how NASA utilizes the"aquarius"undersea habitat as an analog for long-duration space flight.
37. Engler S, Binsted K, Leung H. Hi-seas habitat energy requirements and forecasting. Acta Astronaut. 2019;162:50–5.
38. Pagel JI, Chouker A. Effects of isolation and confinement on humans-implications for manned space explorations. J Appl Physiol. 2016;120:1449.
39. Campbell M, Kirkpatrick A, Billica R, Johnston S, Jennings R, Short D, Hamilton D, Dulchavsky S. Endoscopic surgery in weightlessness. Surg Endosc. 2001;15(12):1413.
40. Shelhamer M. Parabolic flight as a spaceflight analog. J Appl Physiol. 2016;120(12):1442–8.
41. de Curtò J, de Zarzà I, Calafate CT. Uwb and mb-ofdm for lunar rover navigation and communication. Mathematics. 2023;11(18):3835.
42. Murdock DB. Trauma: when there's no time to count. AORN J. 2008;87(2):322–8.
43. Jones H, The recent large reduction in space launch cost, 48th International Conference on Environmental Systems, 2018.
44. da Vinci Xi Surgical System, da Vinci Xi Surgical System readiness guide, tech. rep., 2024.
45. Sarty GE, Obenaus A. Magnetic resonance imaging of astronauts on the international Space Station and into the solar system. Canad Aeronaut Space J. 2012;58(1):60–8.
46. Rentschler ME, Platt SR, Berg K, Dumpert J, Oleynikov D, Farritor SM. Miniature in vivo robots for remote and harsh environments. IEEE Trans Inf Technol Biomed. 2008;12(1):66–75.
47. Nowak ES, Reyes DP, Bryant BJ, Cap AP, Kerstman EL, Antonsen EL. Blood transfusion or deep space exploration. Transfusion. 2019;59(10):3077–83.
48. McQuillen JB, McKay TL, Griffin DW, Brown DF, Zoldak JT. Final report for intravenous fluid generation (ivgen) spaceflight experiment. tech. rep; 2011.
49. Charles JB, Pietrzyk RA. A year on the international space station: implementing a long-duration biomedical research mission. Aerosp Med Hum Perform. 2019;90(1):4–11.
50. Ma B, Jiang Z, Liu Y, Xie Z. Advances in space robots for on-orbit servicing: a comprehensive review. Adv Intell Syst. 2023;5(8):2200397.
51. Campbell MR. A review of surgical care in space erase 1 at the end of the title. J Am Coll Surg. 2002;194(6):802–12.
52. Ball CG. Damage control resuscitation: history, theory and technique. Can J Surg. 2014;57(1):55.
53. Chang R, Eastridge BJ, Holcomb JB. Remote damage control resuscitation in austere environments. Wilderness Environ Med. 2017;28(2 suppl):S124–34.
54. Lamb C, MacGoey P, Navarro A, Brooks A. Damage control surgery in the era of damage control resuscitation. Br J Anaesth. 2014;113(2):242–9.

55. Rappold JF, Bochicchio GV. Surgical adjuncts to noncompressible torso hemorrhage as tools for patient blood management. Transfusion. 2016;56:S203–7.
56. Gordy SD, Rhee P, Schreiber MA. Military applications of novel hemostatic devices. Expert Rev Med Devices. 2011;8(1):41–7.
57. Jenkins DH, Rappold JF, Badloe JF, Berséus O, Blackbourne CL, Brohi KH, Butler FK, Cap LAP, Cohen MJ, Davenport R, et al. Trauma hemostasis and oxygenation research position paper on remote damage control resuscitation: definitions, current practice, and knowledge gaps. Shock. 2014;41:3–12.
58. Chiara O, Cimbanassi S, Bellanova G, Chiarugi M, Mingoli A, Olivero G, Ribaldi S, Tugnoli G, Basilico S, Bindi F, et al. A systematic review on the use of topical hemostats in trauma and emergency surgery. BMC Surg. 2018;18:1–20.
59. Chaturvedi A, Dowling MB, Gustin JP, Scalea TM, Raghavan SR, Pasley JD, Narayan M. Hydrophobically modified chitosan gauze: a novel topical hemostat. J Surg Res. 2017;207:45–52.
60. Tompeck AJ, Dowling M, Johnson SB, Barie PS, Winchell RJ, King D, Scalea TM, Britt L, Narayan M, et al. A comprehensive review of topical hemostatic agents: the good, the bad, and the novel. J Trauma Acute Care Surg. 2020;88(1):e1–e21.
61. Jacobs D, Christmas A. Surgical techniques for managing hepatic injury. 2022, Uptodate: literature review: Mar 2025, Topic last updated: February 28; 2024.
62. Maung AA, Kaplan LJ. Surgical management of splenic injury in the adult trauma patient, UpToDate, Post, TW (Ed). UpToDate, Waltham, MA. Accessed on 15 Jan 2017; 2023.
63. McMahon KR, Balasubramanya R. Intestinal trauma. In: StatPearls [Internet]. StatPearls Publishing; 2023.
64. Attinger CE, Bulan E, Blume PA. Surgical debridement: the key to successful wound healing and reconstruction. Clin Pediatric Med Surg. 2000;17(4):599–630.
65. Newman RK, Dayal N, Dominique E. Abdominal compartment syndrome. In: StatPearls [Internet]. StatPearls Publishing; 2023.
66. Nguyen NT, Zainabadi K, Mavandadi S, Paya M, Stevens CM, Root J, Wilson SE. Trends in utilization and outcomes of laparoscopic versus open appendectomy. Am J Surg. 2004;188(6):813–20.
67. Eldar S, Sabo E, Nash E, Abrahamson J, Matter I. Laparoscopic versus open cholecystectomy in acute cholecystitis. Surg Laparosc Endosc Percutan Tech. 1997;7(5):407–14.
68. Tzelves L, Geraghty RM, Hughes T, Juliebø-Jones P, Somani BK. Innovations in kidney stone removal. Research and Reports in Urology. 2023:131–9.
69. Lee A, Baker TS, Bederson JB, Rapoport BI. Levels of autonomy in FDA-cleared surgical robots: a systematic review. NPJ Digit Med Nature Group. 2024;7(1):103.
70. Thai MT, Phan PT, Hoang TT, Wong S, Lovell NH, Do TN. Advanced intelligent systems for surgical robotics. Adv Intell Syst. 2020;2(8):1900138.
71. Morris B. Robotic surgery: applications, limitations, and impact on surgical education. Medscape Gen Med. 2005;7(3):72.
72. Takács Á, Nagy DA, Rudas I, Haidegger T. Origins of surgical robotics: from space to the operating room. Acta Polytechnica Hungarica. 2016;13(1):13–30.
73. Takács Á, Jordán S, Nagy DÁ, Tar JK, Rudas IJ, Haidegger T. Surgical robotics—born in space. In: in 2015 IEEE 10th Jubilee International symposium on applied computational intelligence and informatics. IEEE; 2015. p. 547–51.
74. Intuitive Surgical, "Da vinci robotic surgery," 2023. Accessed: 10 July 2024.
75. Nicioli T, Fisher K. MIRA robot performs first surgery in space. Accessed: 10 July 2024; 2024. https://edition.cnn.com/2024/02/13/world/mira-robot-first-surgery-in-space-scn.
76. Marks JH, Keller DS, Lagares-Garcia JA, Schoonyoung HP, Farritor SM, Oleynikov D, Jobst MA. Safety and efficacy of a novel miniaturized robotic assisted surgery system in colectomy: a prospective, investigational device exemption clinical study using the ideal framework. Dis Colon Rectum. 2024:10–1097.
77. Konijnenburg M, Stanzione S, Yan L, Jee D-W, Pettine J, Van Wegberg R, Kim H, Van Liempd C, Fish R, Schuessler J, et al. A multi (BIO) sensor acquisition system with integrated

processor, power management, 8x8 LED drivers, and simultaneously synchronized ECG, BIO-Z, GSR, and two PPG readouts. IEEE J Solid-State Circuits. 2016;51(11):2584–95.
78. Wang C, Li X, Hu H, Zhang L, Huang Z, Lin M, Zhang Z, Yin Z, Huang B, Gong H, et al. Monitoring of the central blood pressure waveform via a conformal ultrasonic device. Nat Biomed Eng. 2018;2(9):687–95.
79. Kim S, Kim J-A, Lee JY. International trend of non-contact healthcare and related changes due to covid-19 pandemic. Yonsei Med J. 2022;63(Suppl):S22.
80. Huang B, Hu S, Liu Z, Lin C-L, Su J, Zhao C, Wang L, Wang W. Challenges and prospects of visual contactless physiological monitoring in clinical study. NPJ Digit Med. 2023;6(1):231.
81. El Boussaki H, Latif R, Saddik A. A review on video-based heart rate, respiratory rate and blood pressure estimation. In: International Conference of Machine Learning and Computer Science Applications. Springer; 2022. p. 129–40.
82. Zheng Y. Heart rate and oxygen level estimation from facial videos using a hybrid deep learning model. In: Multimodal Image Exploitation and Learning 2024, vol. 13033. SPIE; 2024. p. 48–59.
83. Panwar M, Gautam A, Biswas D, Acharyya A. PP-net: a deep learning framework for PPG-based blood pressure and heart rate estimation. IEEE Sensors J. 2020;20(17):10000–11.
84. Bian D, Mehta P, Selvaraj N. Respiratory rate estimation using PPG: a deep learning approach. In: in 2020 42nd Annual International Conference of the IEEE engineering in Medicine & Biology Society (EMBC). IEEE; 2020. p. 5948–52.
85. Allado E, Poussel M, Renno J, Moussu A, Hily O, Temperelli M, Albuisson E, Chenuel B. Remote photoplethysmography is an accurate method to remotely measure respiratory rate: a hospital-based trial. J Clin Med. 2022;11(13):3647.
86. Tohma A, Nishikawa M, Hashimoto T, Yamazaki Y, Sun G. Evaluation of remote photoplethysmography measurement conditions toward telemedicine applications. Sensors. 2021;21(24):8357.
87. West C, Kaus B, Sullivan SO, Schneider H, Seifert O. Using infrared cameras in drones to detect bleeding events. BMC Emerg Med. 2023;23(1):142.
88. Huang H-W, Chen J, Chai PR, Ehmke C, Rupp P, Dadabhoy FZ, Feng A, Li C, Thomas AJ, da Silva M, et al. Mobile robotic platform for contactless vital sign monitoring. Cyborg and Bionic Systems. 2022;2022
89. Khalid WB, Anwar A, Waheed OT. Contactless vitals measurement robot. In: in 2022 8th International Conference on Automation, Robotics and Applications (ICARA). IEEE; 2022. p. 91–6.
90. Hussain MN, Idrissi M. Contactless vital signs monitoring in hospital wards: a quadruped robot approach. In: in 2024 10th International Conference on Automation, Robotics and Applications (ICARA). IEEE; 2024. p. 75–80.
91. Huang R, Su W, Jian R, Li S, Xie P, Zhang S, Qin W. Non-contact vital signals measurement on a mobile rescue robot. In: in 2019 3rd International Conference on Data Science and Business Analytics (ICDSBA). IEEE; 2019. p. 443–7.
92. Wong KH, Lo S-CB, Lin C-F, Lasser B, Mun SK. Imaging components for a robotic casualty evaluation system. In: in 2009 Annual International Conference of the IEEE Engineering in Medicine and Biology Society. IEEE; 2009. p. 467–70.
93. Nanni L, Loreggia A, Lumini A, Dorizza A. A standardized approach for skin detection: analysis of the literature and case studies. J Imag. 2023;9(2):35.
94. Li P, Wang D, Wang L, Lu H. Deep visual tracking: review and experimental comparison. Pattern Recogn. 2018;76:323–38.
95. Allotta B, Fioravanti D. 3d motion planning for image-based visual servoing tasks. Proceedings of the 2005 IEEE International Conference on Robotics and Automation, pp. 2173–2178, IEEE; 2005.
96. Sanchez-Salmeron R, Gomez-Urquiza JL, L. Albend´ın-Garc´ıa, M. Correa-Rodr´ıguez, M. B. Martos-Cabrera, A. Velando-Soriano, and N. Suleiman-Martos. Machine learning methods applied to triage in emergency services: a systematic review. Int Emerg Nurs. 2022;60:101109.

97. Xie F, Ong MEH, Liew JNMH, Tan KBK, Ho AFW, Nadarajan GD, Low LL, Kwan YH, Goldstein BA, Matchar DB, et al. Development and assessment of an interpretable machine learning triage tool for estimating mortality after emergency admissions. JAMA Netw Open. 2021;4(8):e2118477–67.
98. Levin S, Toerper M, Hamrock E, Hinson JS, Barnes S, Gardner H, Dugas A, Linton B, Kirsch T, Kelen G. Machine-learning-based electronic triage more accurately differentiates patients with respect to clinical outcomes compared with the emergency severity index. Ann Emerg Med. 2018;71(5):565–74.
99. Sargsyan AE, Hamilton DR, Melton SL, Young J. The international space station ultrasound imaging capability overview for prospective users. NASA/TP. 2006:2006–213731.
100. Topiwala A, Al-Zogbi L, Fleiter T, Krieger A. Adaptation and evaluation of deep learning techniques for skin segmentation on novel abdominal dataset. In: in 2019 IEEE 19th International Conference on Bioinformatics and Bioengineering (BIBE). IEEE; 2019. p. 752–9.
101. Carrión H, Jafari M, Bagood MD, Yang H-y, Isseroff RR, Gomez M. Automatic wound detection and size estimation using deep learning algorithms. PLoS Comput Biol. 2022;18(3):e1009852.
102. Wang C, Anisuzzaman D, Williamson V, Dhar MK, Rostami B, Niezgoda J, Gopalakrishnan S, Yu Z. Fully automatic wound segmentation with deep convolutional neural networks. Sci Rep. 2020;10(1):21897.
103. Zhang H, Sun Y, Liu L, Wang X, Li L, Liu W. Clothingout: a category-supervised Gan model for clothing segmentation and retrieval. Neural Comput & Applic. 2020;32:4519–30.
104. Singh V, Ma K, Tamersoy B, Chang Y-J, Wimmer A, O'Donnell T, Chen T. Darwin: Deformable patient avatar representation with deep image network. in Medical Image Computing and Computer-Assisted Intervention-MICCAI 2017: 20th International Conference, Quebec City, QC, Canada, September 11–13, 2017, Proceedings, Part II 20, pp. 497–504, Springer; 2017.
105. Teixeira B, Singh VK, Tamersoy B, Chen T, Ma K, Krauss A, Wimmer A. Internal body marker prediction from surface data in medical imaging. Dec. 31 2019. US Patent 10,521,927; 2019.
106. Teixeira B, Singh V, Chen T, Ma K, Tamersoy B, Wu Y, Balashova E, Comaniciu D. Generating synthetic x-ray images of a person from the surface geometry. Proceedings of the IEEE conference on computer vision and pattern recognition, pp. 9059–9067; 2018.
107. Al-Zogbi L, Singh V, Teixeira B, Ahuja A, Bagherzadeh PS, Kapoor A, Saeidi H, Fleiter T, Krieger A. Autonomous robotic point-of-care ultrasound imaging for monitoring of covid-19–induced pulmonary diseases. Front Robot AI. 2021;8:645756.
108. Lee J, Quist E, German S, Kim M, Fisher N. Neural network model of eFAST target prediction for robotic ultrasound diagnostics in austere environments. In: 2022 19th International Conference on Ubiquitous Robots (UR). IEEE; 2022. p. 153–8.
109. Mathur B, Topiwala A, Schaffer S, Kam M, Saeidi H, Fleiter T, Krieger A. A semi-autonomous robotic system for remote trauma assessment. In: 2019 IEEE 19th International conference on bioinformatics and bioengineering (BIBE). IEEE; 2019. p. 649–56.
110. Raina D, Singh H, Saha SK, Arora C, Agarwal A, Chandrashekhara S, Rangarajan K, Nandi S. Comprehensive telerobotic ultrasound system for abdominal imaging: development and in-vivo feasibility study. In: 2021 International Symposium on Medical Robotics (ISMR). IEEE; 2021. p. 1–7.
111. Duan B, Xiong L, Guan X, Fu Y, Zhang Y. Tele-operated robotic ultrasound system for medical diagnosis. Biomed Signal Proc Control. 2021;70:102900.
112. Al-Zogbi L, Bock B, Schaffer S, Fleiter T, Krieger A. A 3-d-printed patient-specific ultrasound phantom for fast scan. Ultrasound Med Biol. 2021;47(3):820–32.
113. Mustafa ASB, Ishii T, Matsunaga Y, Nakadate R, Ishii H, Ogawa K, Saito A, Sugawara M, Niki K, Takanishi A. Development of robotic system for autonomous liver screening using ultrasound scanning device. In: 2013 IEEE International Conference on Robotics And Biomimetics (ROBIO). IEEE; 2013. p. 804–9.
114. Suligoj F, Heunis CM, Sikorski J, Misra S. RobUSt–an autonomous robotic ultrasound system for medical imaging. IEEE access. 2021;9:67456–65.

115. Raina D, Chandrashekhara S, Voyles R, Wachs J, Saha SK. Robotic sonographer: autonomous robotic ultrasound using domain expertise in bayesian optimization. In: 2023 IEEE International Conference on Robotics and Automation (ICRA). IEEE; 2023. p. 6909–15.
116. Jiang Z, Salcudean SE, Navab N. Robotic ultrasound imaging: state-of-the-art and future perspectives. Med Image Anal. 2023;89:102878.
117. Ning G, Zhang X, Liao H. Autonomic robotic ultrasound imaging system based on reinforcement learning. IEEE Trans Biomed Eng. 2021;68(9):2787–97.
118. Cramer A, Hecla J, Wu D, Lai X, Boers T, Yang K, Moulton T, Kenyon S, Arzoumanian Z, Krull W, et al. Stationary computed tomography for space and other resource-constrained environments. Sci Rep. 2018;8(1):14195.
119. Sjogren AR, Leo MM, Feldman J, Gwin JT. Image segmentation and machine learning for detection of abdominal free fluid in focused assessment with sonography for trauma examinations: a pilot study. J Ultrasound Med. 2016;35(11):2501–9.
120. Mehanian C, Kulhare S, Millin R, Zheng X, Gregory C, Zhu M, Xie H, Jones J, Lazar J, Halse A, et al. Deep learning-based pneumothorax detection in ultrasound videos. Smart Ultrasound Imaging and Perinatal, Preterm and Paediatric Image Analysis: First International Workshop, SUSI 2019, and 4th International Workshop, PIPPI 2019, Held in Conjunction with MICCAI 2019, Shenzhen, China, October 13 and 17, 2019, Proceedings 4, pp. 74–82, Springer; 2019.
121. Hiransakolwong N, Hua KA, Vu K, Windyga PS. Segmentation of ultrasound liver images: an automatic approach. In: 2003 International Conference on Multimedia and Expo. ICME'03. Proceedings (Cat. No. 03TH8698), vol. 1. IEEE; 2003. p. 1–573.
122. Carneiro G, Nascimento JC, Freitas A. The segmentation of the left ventricle of the heart from ultrasound data using deep learning architectures and derivative-based search methods. IEEE Trans Image Process. 2011;21(3):968–82.
123. Mishra D, Chaudhury S, Sarkar M, Manohar S, Soin AS. Segmentation of vascular regions in ultrasound images: a deep learning approach. In: 2018 IEEE International Symposium on Circuits and Systems (ISCAS). IEEE; 2018. p. 1–5.
124. Kutter O, Shams R, Navab N. Visualization and gpu-accelerated simulation of medical ultrasound from CT images. Comput Methods Prog Biomed. 2009;94(3):250–66.
125. Wasserthal J, Breit H-C, Meyer MT, Pradella M, Hinck D, Sauter AW, Heye T, Boll DT, Cyriac J, Yang S, et al. Totalsegmentator: robust segmentation of 104 anatomic structures in CT images. Radiol Artif Intell. 2023;5(5)
126. Geißler K, Mensing D, Wenzel M, Hirsch JG, Heldmann S. Towards total segmentator for MRI data leveraging gin data augmentation. In: Medical Imaging 2024: Image Processing, vol. 12926. SPIE; 2024. p. 13–22.
127. Gooding MJ, Kennedy S, Noble JA. Volume segmentation and reconstruction from freehand three- dimensional ultrasound data with application to ovarian follicle measurement. Ultrasound Med Biol. 2008;34(2):183–95.
128. Treece G, Prager R, Gee A, Berman L. 3d ultrasound measurement of large organ volume. Med Image Anal. 2001;5(1):41–54.
129. Li K, Xu Y, Meng MQ-H. An overview of systems and techniques for autonomous robotic ultrasound acquisitions. IEEE Trans Med Robotic Bionics. 2021;3(2):510–24.
130. Wei W, Haishan X, Alpers J, Rak M, Hansen C. A deep learning approach for 2d ultrasound and 3d CT/MR image registration in liver tumor ablation. Comput Methods Prog Biomed. 2021;206:106117.
131. Saeidi H, Opfermann JD, Kam M, Wei S, Léonard S, Hsieh MH, Kang JU, Krieger A. Autonomous robotic laparoscopic surgery for intestinal anastomosis. Sci Robotics. 2022;7(62):eabj2908.
132. Yang G-Z, Cambias J, Cleary K, Daimler E, Drake J, Dupont PE, Hata N, Kazanzides P, Martel S, Patel RV, et al. Medical robotics—regulatory, ethical, and legal considerations for increasing levels of autonomy. Sci Robot. 2017;2

133. Kaber DB, Endsley MR. The effects of level of automation and adaptive automation on human performance, situation awareness and workload in a dynamic control task. Theor Issues Ergon Sci. 2004;5(2):113–53.
134. Haidegger T. Autonomy for surgical robots: concepts and paradigms. IEEE Trans Med Robotics Bionics. 2019;1(2):65–76.
135. DiMaio S, Hanuschik M, Kreaden U. The da vinci surgical system. In: Surgical robotics: systems applications and visions; 2011. p. 199–217.
136. Harris RJ, Mygatt JB, Harris SI. Systems and methods for autonomous intravenous needle insertion. June 14 2016. US Patent 9,364,171; 2016.
137. Perry TS. Profile: veebot [resources start-ups]. IEEE Spectr. 2013;50(8):23–33.
138. Chen AI, Balter ML, Maguire TJ, Yarmush ML. Real-time needle steering in response to rolling vein deformation by a 9-dof image-guided autonomous venipuncture robot. In: 2015 IEEE/RSJ International Conference on Intelligent Robots and Systems (IROS). IEEE; 2015. p. 2633–8.
139. Balter ML, Leipheimer JM, Chen AI, Shrirao A, Maguire TJ, Yarmush ML. Automated end-to-end blood testing at the point-of-care: integration of robotic phlebotomy with downstream sample processing. Technology. 2018;6(02):59–66.
140. Zevallos N, Harber E, Patel K, Gu Y, Sladick K, Guyette F, Weiss L, Pinsky MR, Gomez H, Galeotti J, et al. Toward robotically automated femoral vascular access. In: 2021 International Symposium on Medical Robotics (ISMR). IEEE; 2021. p. 1–7.
141. Shademan A, Decker RS, Opfermann JD, Leonard S, Krieger A, Kim PC. Supervised autonomous robotic soft tissue surgery. Sci Transl Med. 2016;8(337):337ra64.
142. Ge J, Kam M, Opfermann JD, Saeidi H, Leonard S, Mady LJ, Schnermann MJ, Krieger A. Autonomous system for tumor resection (ASTR)-dual-arm robotic midline partial glossectomy. IEEE Robotics and Automation Letters. 2023;
143. Hendrich P, Liu J, Ge J, Schmidgall S, Shepard L, Ghazi A, Mathis-Ullrich F, Krieger A. Tracking tumors under deformation from partial point clouds using occupancy networks. In: 2024 IEEE/RSJ Interna-tional Conference on Intelligent Robots and Systems (IROS). IEEE; 2024.
144. Han D, Mulyana B, Stankovic V, Cheng S. A survey on deep reinforcement learning algorithms for robotic manipulation. Sensors. 2023;23(7):3762.
145. Zare M, Kebria PM, Khosravi A, Nahavandi S. A survey of imitation learning: Algorithms, recent developments, and challenges. IEEE Transactions on Cybernetics. 2024;
146. Li B, Wei R, Xu J, Lu B, Yee CH, Ng CF, Heng P-A, Dou Q, Liu Y-H. 3d perception based imitation learning under limited demonstration for laparoscope control in robotic surgery. In: 2022 International Conference on Robotics and Automation (ICRA). IEEE; 2022. p. 7664–70.
147. Scheikl PM, Schreiber N, Haas C, Freymuth N, Neumann G, Lioutikov R, Mathis-Ullrich F. Movement primitive diffusion: learning gentle robotic manipulation of deformable objects. IEEE Robot Autom Lett. 2024;9:5338.
148. Kim JW, Zhao TZ, Schmidgall S, Deguet A, Kobilarov M, Finn C, Krieger A. Surgical robot transformer (SRT): Imitation learning for surgical tasks. arXiv preprint arXiv:2407.12998; 2024.

Principles of Advancements in Imaging Modalities for Acute Care Surgery

13

Abid Qureshi, Kinjal Kasbawala, Timothy Gichuru, and Luca Milone

13.1 Introduction

In the United States, acute care surgery involves approximately 20% of the hospital inpatient adult population and 25% of total inpatient costs [1]. Acute care surgery, by definition, according to the American Association for the Surgery of Trauma (AAST), consists of three divisions, including trauma surgery, emergency surgery, and surgical critical care. These heavily involved subsets of surgical specialties require fast-paced assessment and patient management. As such, with budding technologies, advancements in imaging modalities are sought continuously for expedited patient care and diagnostic accuracy. In recent years, imaging has progressively improved in a logarithmic fashion in conjunction with the introduction of artificial intelligence and hybrid techniques, ranging from X-rays to sonograms to laparoscopies.

Beginning in 1895, the era of medical imaging underwent a revolution with the foundation of X-rays developed by Wilhelm Conrad Roentgen. This led to pictures of bones, less visualization of soft tissue, and even less fatty tissue. As this technology grew to find itself harboring groundbreaking utilization in the medical field, Roentgen was granted the Nobel Prize in Physics in 1901. Soon after, the field of acute care surgery began to use X-ray devices in hospital settings for traumatic injuries and in the military as well for diagnosing combat injuries. Innovations in techniques and tools started to develop further using this technology [2]. Currently, the vast utility of X-rays makes them among the most commonly acquired tests in acute care settings, providing imaging for clinicians to make many diagnoses.

Although medical ultrasonics began during World War II, it was first used in 1947 by Dr. Karl Theodore Dussik, an Austrian neurologist, to investigate brain

A. Qureshi · K. Kasbawala · T. Gichuru · L. Milone (✉)
Department of Surgery, The Brooklyn Hospital Center, Brooklyn, NY, USA
e-mail: aqureshi@tbh.org; k.kasbawala@saba.edu; tgichuru@tbh.org; lmilone@tbh.org

B. De Simone et al. (eds.), *New Technologies, Precision Medicine, and AI in Emergency General Surgery*, Hot Topics in Acute Care Surgery and Trauma,
https://doi.org/10.1007/978-3-032-09357-8_13

ventricular changes due to tumor growth. However, only over the last three decades have acute care surgeons used ultrasound technology. Ultrasound is operator-dependent, fast, portable, and highly versatile in the examination of acute care pathology. Using a piezoelectric transducer to effectively convert electricity to sound waves, which are then converted back to electricity via lead zirconate titanate crystals, ultrasound produces vibrations through the electrically stimulated crystals, producing ultrasound waves [3]. Most commonly in trauma settings, surgeons use ultrasound for the Focused Assessment of Sonogram Examination of the Trauma Patient (FAST) exam as a rapid diagnostic assessment of torso injuries. In both trauma and non-trauma acute care settings, sonography provides technology as an adjunct for procedures, visualizing complications, and supplementing quick imaging for a suspected diagnosis based on physical examination.

The computed tomography (CT) scanner was invented in 1972 by Godfrey Hounsfield, an electrical engineer from Great Britain, alongside Dr. Allan Cormack, a South African-American physicist. Both were jointly awarded the Nobel Prize in Physiology and Medicine for their CT technology in 1979. Initially known as the EMI scanner, it was created in the EMI Laboratories in 1972, but various names have been known for it over the years. The CT scanner has paved its way in acute care settings as arguably the most critical imaging that physicians can obtain. Using 360-degree X-ray beams, computer production of three-dimensional imaging allows for a detailed cross-sectional view of organs and body structures with an accuracy as high as 95% in the acute abdomen [4]. Expertise in having CT technology in acute care surgery becomes apparent when non-specific symptoms need searching for a localized contributor, which surgeons rely on to configure an exact etiology.

Magnetic resonance imaging (MRI) first came to fruition in the medical field in 1980, when John Mallard, an English physicist and professor, used it clinically to examine primary and secondary cancers. Following this, the performance of MRI technology has evolved with image reconstruction, data processing, and computing. Diffusion MRI (dMRI), nuclear magnetic resonance (NMR), and MR elastography (MRE) are all variations of MRI technology used for different reasons. An added benefit of MRI is exemplified in acute care surgery for the reliable diagnosis of brain and spinal cord injuries. However, its use is limited by greater scan times, hospital costs, and the need for trained professionals [5].

Laparoscopy, a technique first used experimentally on dogs in 1901, was first introduced in a trauma setting for intra-abdominal examination for hemoperitoneum and visceral rupture in the 1920s [6]. Although in the past, it had been a relative contraindication for trauma and acute abdominal pathology, it has since grown in popularity with modern concepts, considering it safe with decreases in hospitalization, financial burdens, and unnecessary laparotomies. The benefit of laparoscopy is not only due to the above; it is also more safely used now in many acute care pathologies, such as appendicitis, cholecystitis, and bowel obstruction, among others.

Within busy healthcare systems, artificial intelligence has provided different avenues by which hospital care has met the demands of enlarging patient populations. This chapter discusses acute care surgery, with the roles of artificial intelligence in image interpretation, image guidance, precision targeting during interventions, and hybrid imaging techniques assisting in improved diagnoses and therapies.

13.2 The Role of Artificial Intelligence in Image Interpretation and Analysis

Artificial intelligence (AI) in its application for medical imaging has grown expeditiously, percolating the field over the last two decades. The development of machine learning, inspired by the human brain, is a collaborative effort of various fields, including mathematics, physics, and engineering. This interdisciplinary nature has paved the way for more accurate diagnostic and therapeutic technologies in radiology. With the addition of new algorithms and software, the innovation of AI has had profound effects on the development of the interpretation of medical data, including imaging, as well as continuous learning and adaptation to novel pathologies. AI in radiology is involved via radiomics, which utilizes machine learning along with its subset, deep learning (DL).

Radiomics is an emerging field of research surrounding medical imaging involving AI that focuses on capturing and defining tissue features and separating the normal from abnormal by characterizing specific shapes and heterogeneity of lesions. In general, radiomics aims to produce reliable information and imaging analysis, including configuring highly complex quantitative data patterns that may only sometimes be identifiable to radiologists. The utility of radionics is visibly noticeable when applied to large amounts of mineable data by convertible imaging, which can provide a deeper understanding of disease processes involving tougher variables. The fundamentals of radiomics comprise a stepwise progression when undertaking any proposed study design: clinical data collection, image acquisition and transfer, image preparation, image annotation, performance evaluation, model validation, feature selection, and feature extraction [7].

To simplify this, the radiomics workflow starts by evaluating a clinical hypothesis with a background literature review. The next step is data collection of preprocessed raw images via a given imaging modality, such as X-ray or CT. These raw images are then transferred via data exporting programs, which also involve removing any identifiable patient data. All data undergoes analysis for incompletion and inconsistencies requiring correction. The images then go through preprocessing, further designed to enhance quality by image filtration, optimization, and standardization. Imaging undergoes segmentation for feature selection, entailing defining regions of interest manually by a medical expert or automatically via programs. Feature selection is followed by feature extraction by programs utilizing algorithms, such as Python scripts, generating various geometric radiomic features. Reproducible radiomic features are then grouped to produce statistical models for model validation, which can be internally tested for external validation for final results [7–9].

Now, how is AI directly involved? In radiomics, it is through the branch of machine learning (ML), which is composed of statistical models using previously observed world data, that inferences are further provided based on explicit instructions provided by human beings. ML is further broken down into different divisions: supervised learning, unsupervised learning, semi-supervised learning, and reinforcement learning. Supervised learning analyzes and uses labeled datasets to design algorithms to predict outcomes. On the other hand, unsupervised learning uses unlabeled datasets to explore patterns without human intervention. Semi-supervised learning combines supervised and unsupervised learning, which offers the benefit of using a smaller group of labeled data with a more significant amount of unlabeled data for analysis and providing conclusions. Reinforcement learning utilizes trial and error to make decisions for maximized results [10].

Deep learning (DL), a specialized branch of ML, can revolutionize radiology. Unlike traditional machine learning, DL can process raw data and identify complex patterns without human intervention. As the field of radiology continues to evolve, DL is poised to become a powerful prognostic technology, capable of diagnosing conditions as quickly and accurately as human experts, while also reducing healthcare costs and improving accessibility [11].

The most commonly used networks branching from DL are the deep convolutional neural networks (DCNN), which allow for swift pattern recognition in imaging. Using any number of data, the automated DCNN produces the necessary information based on the training given. The benefit of these networks stems from the sheer volume of data analysis they can generate, with which humans cannot compete [12]. The networks over the last decade have also vastly improved to be more precise than humans, with some studies showing that DL's abilities surpass those of humans in minimizing errors in performing tasks, and these networks will only continue to improve in the future [13].

Now, how does AI integrate with radiology to benefit emergency surgery? The cornerstone of the field of emergency radiology relies on diagnostic accuracy and efficient timing, with improved performance necessary for patient management. Prosperous advances in AI have led emergency radiology healthcare professionals to increasingly rely on models to improve workflow efficiency and prioritization via chatbots, patient triaging and study selection, image acquisition and reconstruction, structured categorization via classification systems, and patient positioning. Radiologists can use these applications to detect diseases and diagnose them more quickly than before. Later in the chapter, we discuss hybrid imaging in conjunction with AI.

13.2.1 Chatbots and Automation of Triaging

Since the creation of Chat Generative Pre-Trained Transformer (ChatGPT), an integrative AI chat interface developed by the AI research development company OpenAI, it has been a unique tool with its ability to take large measures of intricate data to aid physicians in making the correct diagnoses. The benefit of such technology comes with constantly adapting and learning new datasets for updated performances in medical case analysis and preoperative diagnosis, even guiding and improving the speed of providing medical or surgical treatments. Previously, the

ChatGPT (ChatGPT-3) version proved diagnostic accuracy for ten differential diagnoses greater than 90% [14]. However, the study showed accuracy as inferior to physicians, and despite the limitation of the study testing limited pathologies, the system is continuously growing with transparency of building on itself. The ability to assist in making surgical plans, identifying preoperative and postoperative complications, and guiding complex cases makes chatbots very useful.

There are various challenges involving the use of this technology. First, medical professionals must consistently oversee its use to avoid misdiagnosis. They should not replace them regardless of timely efficiency due to the lack of testability of bots and lower diagnostic accuracy compared to physicians. There is also a question of patient privacy, which raises ethical issues. The protection of patient data should be respected, and consent should be obtained to use this technology as an aid, as well as to ensure its reliability.

With chest radiographs and CT imaging being among the most frequently ordered examinations in the emergency department in high-volume settings, it is essential to have fast triaging to improve workflow efficiency and timely diagnoses, avoiding significant delays. Previously, studies have shown that DL-based electronic triaging differentiates patients based on clinical outcomes in emergency severity with greater accuracy than older systems [15]. These predictive AI-based analyses play an increased role in allowing patients to receive quicker emergent imaging and possible surgical treatment.

13.2.2 Imaging Selection and Protocoling

Image selection and protocols ensure the correct study is selected for the clinical indication based on various parameters such as the type of modality required, the anatomic region of interest, and acquisition parameters that determine how the sequences of the study are performed, such as image dimensionality, perspective, and granularity. The process can be time consuming, with many co-existing options to target clinical issues, and the workflow can become less effective. Natural language processing (NLP) is a subfield of AI that enables data processing, interrogation, and interpretation of human language. NLP technology, a type of DCNN, has been shown to automate image protocoling effectively. Not to mention, this technology is vital in allowing for decreased healthcare costs and waste due to the selection of correct imaging protocols.

Previously, NLP models were tested for clinical decision-making with MRI technology to assess the brain with an accuracy of 82.9% for examination protocoling and 88.2% for prioritization tasks [16]. A study comparing DCNN protocoling with musculoskeletal radiologists for MRI examinations for routine versus tumor protocol demonstrated an accuracy of 94.2% [17]. Recent studies have also consistently shown that AI models have superiority in image selection and protocoling over previous traditional machine learning models. Although this technology is of use, it does come with limitations, such as keeping the patient data safe with continuous, systematic input and access required for utmost performance.

13.2.3 Image Acquisition and Reconstruction

Neural networking algorithms surrounding the emergency radiology field help by acquiring enhanced imaging quality, as well as reduced performance times and radiation dosages. With the harmful effects of radiation on cells for both adults and even more so on children, it is an area of concern to reduce radiation dosages when obtaining scans. Radiologic practices are now more than ever centered around the principle of ALARA, or "As Low As Reasonably Achievable," specifically focusing on decreasing the ionizing radiation in image production [18]. With the introduction of diagnostic reference levels initiatives for radiology practices introduced by the International Commission on Radiological Protection, studies involving AI networking models have shown radiation dose optimization while maintaining and even producing improved imaging quality with DL reconstruction [19, 20].

Improved imaging reconstruction relies on reductions in noise and artifacts while keeping spatial resolution intact. In medical imaging, "noise" refers to random variations or interference in the image data that do not represent the actual structure or composition of the subject being imaged. Imaging involving CT or MR technologies has previously relied upon the simpler filtered back projection (FBP) analytical models, with the benefit of utilizing low computational power, but with the adverse effects of increased noise and artifacts when trying to reduce radiation doses, leading to poorer imaging quality [21]. Model-based iterative reconstruction (MBIR) and hybrid iterative reconstruction (HIR) techniques were further introduced with principles of reducing these noises and artifacts and producing higher-quality images even when doses of radiation were lowered [21]. The DL reconstruction techniques ideally are hybridizations of direct models, those that reconstruct sinograms directly into an image without using FBP or HIR, in combination with the following indirect models, which use either FBP or HIR [21]. Studies have shown that using CT technology, these DL reconstruction algorithms display more vital computational abilities, with significant noise reduction of 30–71%, artifact reduction, preserved spatial resolution, radiation dose reduction of 36–70%, and improved image quality [21, 22].

MRI is particularly valuable in emergencies due to its excellent soft-tissue contrast and comprehensive structural and functional imaging capabilities. However, its lengthy examination times can increase patient discomfort and motion artifacts, which are problematic in urgent situations. Traditional methods like compressed sensing and dictionary learning have been employed to reduce MRI acquisition time to reconstruct high-quality images from undersampled data. However, these methods are computationally intensive [23].

Recent advancements in DL offer promising alternatives. Recurrent neural networks and DCNNs have successfully accelerated dynamic MRI reconstruction, making it feasible for emergency settings. Variational networks enable real-time image reconstruction, outperforming traditional methods and providing near-instantaneous diagnostic images. Generative adversarial networks, a form of DL, have created augmented compressed sensing frameworks that produce high-quality reconstructions from sparsely sampled data [24].

Applying these technologies in emergency surgery can significantly reduce the time needed for accurate imaging, allowing for faster decision-making and treatment initiation. However, thorough evaluation is required to ensure these techniques meet the rigorous demands of clinical settings, including quantitative accuracy across different tracers, pathologies, and scanner configurations.

13.2.4 Radiomics in Emergency Surgery

The field of radiomics is emerging in emergency surgery, both in acute care and trauma settings. It can identify complex and assessable features in imaging indiscernible to the unaided eye, with great clinical benefits.

Let's take acute appendicitis, for example, which can appear on imaging as simple with inflammatory changes or complicated with perforation or gangrenous changes. Previously, studies utilizing developed radiomic models have been conducted in diagnosing acute appendicitis by analyzing either regions of interest covering the end of the cecum and appendix or identifying the appendix by coronal slicing of CT imaging [25, 26]. Both studies showed radiomics with successful prediction for diagnosing acute appendicitis and further differentiating between simple and complicated appendicitis. Another multicenter study using a combined DL and radiomics DCNN model to differentiate uncomplicated appendicitis from complicated appendicitis demonstrated superiority compared to even the radiologists' visual diagnosis [26].

In the pediatric population less than 36 months of age, intussusception is an abdominal emergency, constituting the most common cause of bowel obstruction [27]. Pathology involves a portion of the intestine telescoping into itself. DL algorithms, or DCNN statistical models, were developed in a retrospective multicenter study to detect intussusception with plain abdominal radiographs as a screening tool [28, 29]. DCNN models in the study were trained by identifying regions of interest (ranging from the diaphragm to upper and lateral margins of the acetabulum) to configure a probability of being an intussusception, with an external validity of 0.65 [29]. The study extrapolated and identified the use of superfluous ultrasonography, preventing increased healthcare costs and resources. Another study developed DL models based on image standardization, enhancement, and analysis, assisting junior sonographers in diagnosing intussusception. Results of the study showed that the least experienced junior sonographers, with the aid of DL models, were superior in diagnosing pathology to intermediate sonographers and on par with senior sonographers [30].

A significant cause of an acute abdomen is intestinal obstruction, which can involve a segment of the large intestine but most commonly involves the small bowel. Postoperative adhesive bowel obstruction is the leading cause of intestinal obstruction, followed by cancers and hernias [31]. Prolonged obstruction can lead to incarceration and, subsequently, strangulation, causing severe intestinal ischemia and bowel necrosis. Due to strangulation being a surgical emergency, it is imperative to identify it, and it can be a life-saving measure. Radiomic clinical models, with evaluation of CT scans, have assessed for strangulation using clinical and imaging features and significantly demonstrated substantial predictive numbers for ischemic intestinal necrosis [32]. The study highlighted the ability of radiomic models to validate bowel strangulation risks, with the most important feature being the presence of mesenteric fluid on imaging, further elucidating that surgical intervention would be required.

AI-integrated ML models in the field of radiomics have previously been studied in trauma settings, particularly the liver and spleen. Automated assessment of traumatic injuries can provide patients with swift and enhanced outcomes and can be applicable in emergencies. The AAST classifies both liver and spleen injuries by grading scales. For both organ injuries, contrast-enhanced CT is the gold standard for diagnosis.

Liver injuries most commonly occur in trauma settings. DL radiomic models in association with blunt liver trauma, focusing on percentage segmentation of hepatic parenchymal damage on CT imaging, have previously evaluated major hepatic arterial injuries to identify populations that required angiographic intervention, excluding unstable patients that required emergent intervention [33]. These models were able to elicit a predictive accuracy rate of 84% [33]. Another study showed the ability of trained algorithms in the segmentation of injured liver parenchymal regions due to trauma, accurately yielding percentages with a linear regression of 0.95 [34]. The models were designed as an alternative to the current grading scales, quantifying further methods to assess liver injury.

When discussing abdominal trauma, the spleen has been found to account for the most common solid organ injury. Splenic trauma, like the liver, can include insults that are parenchymal, subcapsular, vascular, or a combination of such. The detection of splenic lacerations has previously been shown by automated ML software designed to analyze CT imaging via localization and segmentation, allowing for feature extraction and assessing splenic injuries with great accuracy [35]. In the same study, DL models were compared but were subpar to the automated software. However, a limitation of the study was its small sample size [35]. Further studies need to be conducted on DL models and radiomics to explore the various categories of splenic trauma.

Future directions of radiomics in emergency surgery need to expand on the models developed to assess for the above-mentioned causes. Other directions should explore models in association with pancreatic and renal trauma, in addition to other common abdominal surgical emergencies.

13.3 Image-Guidance and Precision Targeting During Interventions

In its simplest terms, image-guided surgery (IGS) refers to any invasive intervention performed with the assistance of images of the targeted organ. Imaging modalities include endoscopy, fluoroscopy, intraoperative CT or MRI, ultrasound, and stereotaxis [36]. Image-guidance routinely identifies blood vessels, lymph nodes, bony structures, and macroscopic tumor lesions [37]. CT and MRI are the most utilized imaging modalities for obtaining preoperative images due to their high spatial resolution and versatility. Ultrasound imaging, however, allows for real-time intraoperative imaging acquisition [38].

In IGS, the surgeon plays a pivotal role in digitally integrating preoperative high-quality imaging into a computerized workstation. This integration allows the surgeon to generate a 3D visual localization of surgical instrumentation and its position within the operating field. It's a testament to the surgeon's skill and adaptability that they can use these advanced tools to enhance their surgical precision [39].

IGS or image-guided systems commonly consist of the following essential components: image acquisition, planning, registration, instrument tracking, and visualization [36, 40]. Briefly, image acquisition refers to obtaining preoperative imaging studies from various modalities. Planning is merging these preoperative images to allow for a surgical roadmap through computer software. Registration integrates coordinate systems in real and digital space or intraoperatively and volumetric reconstruction of preoperative imaging, respectively. Essentially, registration aligns different images taken at various points in time of the same underlying tissue into a standard reference frame [37,42]. Instrument tracking provides a surgical tool's current location and projected trajectory within the working field. There are three methods of monitoring: electromagnetic, optical, and image-based [42]. Lastly, visualization pertains to displaying the anatomic location of the target of interest. This can be done through traditional views such as axial, coronal, or sagittal, and more advanced views such as 3D reconstruction, among others, depending on the type of image-guidance system.

13.3.1 Ultrasound-Based Guidance

Ultrasound is a noninvasive, relatively inexpensive, real-time imaging modality widely applied to many surgical procedures. It best characterizes soft tissue and blood flow; as such, it is routinely seen in tumor ablation, central line placement, and soft-tissue biopsies that include breast, thyroid, and lymph nodes [36]. Ultrasound is highly user-dependent, as imaging is obtained at arbitrary orientations in 2D, using free-hand scanning, forcing a mental reconstruction of the underlying anatomical structures. This subjective interpretation brought on the idea of a navigation system such that each user could precisely identify the underlying anatomy, known as tracked ultrasound guidance systems [43]. These tracking systems have significantly progressed, with 3D imaging recreation gaining popularity. There are two approaches to obtaining 3D ultrasound data. First, using a standard probe and a one-dimensional detector transducer, 2D images are paired with their positional information [41]. Second, a 2D detector transducer was used to obtain 3D volumetric images directly.

Intraoperative contrast-enhanced ultrasound (CEUS) guidance is also an attractive type of ultrasound guidance system. Ultrasound contrast agents are gas-filled microspheres that reflect sound waves and enhance the ultrasound image. They are typically stabilized within a lipoprotein shell and remain within the vascular system [44]. Ultrasound contrast agents can be given intravenously to identify enhancement patterns of focal lesions in the urinary bladder to detect and grade vesicoureteral reflux and endocavitary for drainage or detect abnormal communication between two cavities [42, 44]. CEUS also has applications in the assessment of hepatic tumors at the time of resection; studies have shown a strong correlation between CEUS parameters and histological features of the tumor lesions [44]. Malignant focal liver lesions have variable arterial enhancement patterns based on their etiology; metastatic lesions may have rim enhancement in the arterial phase and show washout, appearing hypoechoic in the venous or late phases [45]. Similarly, neurosurgery has assisted in defining margins between variable intracranial tumors and adjacent healthy parenchyma. Another unique feature of CEUS is its ability to provide real-time visualization of the vascular pattern in higher-grade tumors, allowing for more aggressive margins during resection [44].

Another type of ultrasound guidance navigation is ultra-high-frequency ultrasound (UHFUS), which is attributed to the development of novel matrix transducers that can produce ultra-high-frequency emission. This allows for higher spatial resolution and improved imaging quality for superficial layers. UHFUS has applications in dermatology, vascular analysis, lymphatic channel identification, and musculoskeletal evaluation of hand anatomy for presurgical planning [42, 44].

13.3.2 Fluorescence-Guided Surgery

In its simplest form, the fluorescence-guided surgery (FSG) system consists of a light source that excites a fluorescence contrast agent; the emitted fluorescence signal from the probe is then passed through appropriate emission filters to remove unwanted excitation light and autofluorescence. Next, using collection optics, the filtered fluorescence signal is focused on a detector, which transfers the signal to a computer for visualization [43, 46].

Fluorescent probes provide contrast in FGS between the targeted tissue and its surroundings. Fluorescent probes can be intrinsic or extrinsic. Intrinsic probes are endogenous fluorophores that fluoresce in their native form. At the same time, irrelevant probes are specifically designed molecules that fluoresce under certain conditions to provide a fluorescent signal where one usually does not exist [44]. One of the most well-known FDA-approved extrinsic fluorescent probes is indocyanine green (ICG). It is a water-soluble, rapidly excreted contrast agent used in various surgical procedures. It was initially approved for determining cardiac output, hepatic blood flow, and ophthalmic angiography [46]. ICG also has promising off-label applications in vascular anatomy, lymphatic vessels, hepatobiliary visualization, and defining surgical margins during tumor resections, among others. When administered intravenously, ICG is confined to the vascular compartment by binding to plasma proteins with an intravascular half-life of 3 min. It is hepatically cleared, leading to its application in fluorescence cholangiography as an adjunct for laparoscopic cholecystectomy [43, 46].

A recent systematic review conducted by Fransvea et al. discusses the application of ICG in FGS for abdominal emergencies, specifically highlighting its use in acute cholecystitis, mesenteric ischemia, and trauma surgery. In the emergency setting, one of the most common surgeries is a cholecystectomy for acute cholecystitis. However, bile duct injuries remain among the most feared complications. Fransvea et al. found that ICG fluorescence clearly identified biliary structures in 48% of cases analyzed in distorted anatomy, leading to a safer surgical procedure. Similarly, in acute bowel ischemia, the researchers found that ICG fluorescence angiography led to modifications in surgical decision-making for resection margins in 36.6% of cases analyzed. In some instances, a more conservative approach was utilized with no resection or less extended resection; in other cases, a more aggressive approach was required with an extended resection. ICG is administered intraoperatively to identify areas of viable bowel by green fluorescence, whereas ischemic bowel segments do not fluoresce [46]. It appears that ICG is a useful tool in assessing bowel viability by detecting blood supply in mesenteric ischemia. Lastly, the use of ICG in trauma surgery was analyzed. In this setting, ICG has been applied to assess bowel or parenchymatous organ viability, evaluate perfusion-related tissue impairment in craniofacial or extremity trauma, and reassess vascularization in certain surgical procedures. ICG injection led to modifications in surgical decisions in 23.9% of the cases analyzed [46].

Another application of ICG angiography has been described as a tool to assess indeterminate burn wounds, which are second-degree burn wounds where the distinction of dermal involvement, either superficial or deep, cannot be made by observation alone [47, 48]. In a study conducted by Wongkietkachorn et al., the accuracy of ICG angiography compared to clinical assessment was evaluated to determine if indeterminate burn wounds are superficial or deep second-degree burns. The identification of superficial or deep would dictate the subsequent intervention. They found that among the 30 assessed burn sites, ICG angiography was 100% accurate, whereas clinical assessment was only 50%. ICG is used with laser fluorescence videography to capture dye uptake and clearance as an indicator of tissue perfusion. As such, ICG video angiography can determine dermal viability since impaired circulation and tissue perfusion are directly associated with tissue necrosis. In a subsequent study, Wongkietkachorn et al. used ICG angiography to characterize indeterminate burn wounds as either superficial or deep second-degree burns, and the latter was marked for surgical excision using ICG angiography. They found that marking with ICG angiography with subsequent excision and skin grafting led to favorable outcomes in complete wound closures defined as 100% reepithelialization or graft uptake. Short-term complete wound closure at 21 days was found to be as high as 96.7%, and long-term complete wound closure at two months was 100% [47, 48].

13.3.3 Augmented Reality

Immersive technology, such as augmented/virtual/mixed reality (AR/VR/MR), provides medical image visualization realistically and interactively to aid in preoperative planning, intraoperative navigation, and surgical training [40]. The immersive technologies differ in the views displayed for the user. AR provides a view of the natural world with an overlay of digital elements. VR provides an entirely immersive digital environment. MR combines aspects of AR and VR where, in real-time, the user, the real world, and virtual reality may interact [40, 41]. In the surgical context, AR refers to enhancing the physical world with virtual data by superimposing computer-generated visual information onto a real-world surface and displaying the combination of these on a screen, allowing for stereoscopic visualization [44, 49]. Surgical AR comprises three leading technologies: image registration, tracking, and visual rendering. The visual information from the superimposed image largely depends on the target organ's color or shape. CT is often used to construct a volume-rendering image overlaid over the abdominal wall [42]. In this fashion, the overlay of intraperitoneal organs helps determine port insertion in laparoscopic surgery. On the other hand, surface-rendering imaging is optically vivid and more understandable, making it better suited for overlay display [49, 50].

Image registration refers to the alignment of preoperative images with the currently treated patient by combining feature points from imaging data with features within the actual patient anatomy into the exact spatial coordinates. This alignment accuracy is achieved by using a set of trackers, which determine the precise position of the camera and the patient's body. The trackers, typically an infrared optical sensor, trace fiducial markers that remain stationary during the surgery, such as the iliac crest and clavicles [39, 44].

AR can be effectively applied in preoperative planning and the completion of the surgical procedure. It is seen in tailoring individually preferred incisions, cutting planes, and optimal trocar placement to improve safety by displaying the underlying major organ components. AR also allows surgeons to maneuver challenging operating fields, specifically after neoadjuvant chemotherapy or radiation, where anatomical landmarks are incredibly skewed. While AR has applications in neurosurgery, orthopedics, and spine surgery, its application in laparoscopic surgery is growing. Minimally invasive surgery is often favored over an open surgical approach, in which laparoscopy is frequently employed due to vastly lower morbidity and shortened recovery time. It has drawbacks, such as restricted flexibility in manipulation and inadequate depth perception in a 2D display, with small incisions for laparoscopic instrument placement [42, 50]. AR can provide supplemental video images to model the targeted organ, such that the internal organ features are depicted, typically hidden with laparoscopic visualization or an extended surface view of the organ [44].

13.4 Hybrid Imaging Techniques for Improved Diagnostics and Navigation

Since the discovery of X-ray technology, noninvasive medical imaging has revolutionized disease diagnosis and therapy. CT and MRI are widely utilized to visualize anatomical changes, while ultrasound provides real-time imaging capabilities. Integrating hybrid imaging techniques has revolutionized medical imaging by seamlessly combining varying datasets and providing comprehensive information, leveraging the strengths of each modality to offer new insights into disease processes [51–54]. Early efforts involved software advancements for reconstructing structural and dynamic data [54]. The late 1990s saw the advent of hardware fusion systems, combining different imaging modalities within one gantry [53]. Hybrid imaging has become vital in accurately providing pathological diagnoses and improving patient outcomes [53]. With continued technological improvements, various advantages of these imaging techniques have emerged. This section explores how AI significantly enhances hybrid imaging in improving diagnostics and navigation in emergency general surgery through data handling, image reconstruction, and surgical guidance. Understanding the basic principles of hybrid imaging, functionality, information processing, and utilization is crucial to appreciate the implementation of AI in this field and the promising future it holds for medical imaging.

13.4.1 Basic Principles of Hybrid Imaging Techniques

Hybrid imaging techniques combine anatomical and functional imaging to provide comprehensive diagnostic information, such as the fusion of MRI with US (MRI/US) or CT with angiography (CTA). MRI/US integrates the high soft-tissue contrast of MRI with the imaging capabilities of ultrasound, making it especially beneficial in procedures requiring precision, such as tumor ablations and biopsies [55]. MRI/US enhances the visualization of lesions that might be challenging to detect with a single modality, thereby improving diagnostic accuracy and patient outcomes [56] and significantly reducing the need for multiple imaging sessions. This reduction minimizes patient exposure to radiation, a crucial safety benefit, and streamlines the workflow in emergency settings [57].

CTA, on the other hand, uniquely combines the high-resolution imaging capabilities of CT with the detailed vascular imaging provided by angiography, offering visualization of blood vessels. This feature makes it a powerful tool in acute care surgery, particularly for emergency procedures requiring vascular mapping [58]. It offers in-phase visualization of blood vessels, enhancing diagnostic accuracy and improving patient outcomes in treating conditions like aneurysms or arterial blockages [59].

13.4.2 Functionality, Information Processing, and Utilization of Hybrid Imaging Techniques

The most commonly used hybrid imaging techniques in emergency settings are MRI/US and CTA, which offer clear benefits. Examining their development, functionality, and clinical applications underscores their effectiveness, instilling confidence in their use among healthcare professionals.

MRI/US combination enhances the ability to accurately localize target tissues during procedures, reducing the likelihood of complications and improving patient outcomes [55]. AI algorithms significantly enhance the precision of MRI/US with the automated detection and matching of anatomical landmarks. New directions are instilling optimism about the future of emergency care by reducing human error and variability [60].

CTA, by integrating high-resolution anatomical detail with real-time vascular imaging, provides a comprehensive view of the patient's condition. The role of AI applications in improving the accuracy and efficiency of aligning images from different modalities is crucial, as it significantly enhances diagnostic performance and aids in complex surgical planning.

13.4.3 Artificial Intelligence in Hybrid Imaging Techniques

Hybrid imaging techniques generate a substantial amount of anatomical and functional data. Innovative extraction methods are required to attain meaningful clinical insights from these extensive, multi-dimensional datasets. AI has become particularly beneficial in medical diagnostics [24]. AI algorithms that are branches of ML, such as DL models, are adept at handling and integrating complex data streams [24]. They can combine multiparametric information to identify critical features within the data through learning more complicated and subtle patterns within imaging datasets [61]. This capability significantly improves image processing tasks such as classification and predicting future changes [24].

AI encompasses intelligent systems, like the human brain, that can solve problems creatively. DL involves systems learning to solve problems autonomously using human-annotated training data. This data contains examples of correct decisions, which guide the AI in making future inferences and decisions with new data. DL often requires the creation of "hand-engineered" features, defined by humans, for optimization and model development [24]. Extracting these features from medical imaging data is part of the emerging field of radiomics. As discussed in the earlier chapter, radiomics is the field focused on medical imaging involving AI that captures imaging details. It seeks to derive quantitative, consistent data from diagnostic images, capturing complex patterns challenging for the human eye to detect or measure [62]. Radiomics is still created via "hand-engineered" features defined by humans.

Also previously discussed in the chapter, DL eliminates the need for manual feature engineering by autonomously identifying key features from input data without human intervention. DL algorithms, the most widely utilized form being DCNNs, mimic the information processing patterns of the human brain and have already been applied to numerous challenges in medical imaging due to their strong performance [24]. They are capable of rapid pattern recognition in imaging. Based on their training, these automated networks can generate essential information from any data. The advantage of DCNNs lies in their ability to analyze immense quantities of data, far exceeding human capabilities [12].

The role of AI in MRI/US imaging cannot be overstated. AI algorithms, especially DL, have revolutionized the accuracy and efficiency of aligning images from different modalities by automatically detecting and matching anatomical landmarks, thereby reducing human error [60]. AI also provides immediate feedback during surgical procedures by dynamically adjusting imaging parameters, detecting areas of interest, and predicting intervention outcomes based on live data [63]. This capability is crucial in acute care, where timely decision-making is essential, and AI's ability to track tissue changes ensures accurate surgical guidance and reduces complications [64].

Integrating AI-enhanced MRI/US imaging in acute care surgery offers numerous benefits and challenges. Benefits include combining MRI's superior soft-tissue contrast with ultrasound imaging for accurate diagnoses and improved surgical guidance, reducing the need for multiple imaging sessions, and enhancing workflow efficiency [65]. However, challenges include the need for large, high-quality datasets to train AI models, which can be challenging to obtain in emergencies [66]. Additionally, integrating AI systems with existing hospital infrastructure requires investment in technology and training for healthcare professionals [67]. Concerns about the reliability and interpretability of AI decisions, particularly in high-stakes environments, must also be addressed to ensure the safe practice of using AI-enhanced MRI/US guidance in acute care surgery.

AI has also significantly enhanced image registration and immediate CTA analysis. DL algorithms have improved the accuracy and efficiency of aligning images from different modalities by automatically detecting and matching anatomical and vascular landmarks [60]. AI has also provided direct feedback during procedures, dynamically adjusting imaging parameters, detecting areas of interest, and predicting intervention outcomes based on real-time data [63]. Being efficient is crucial and life-saving in acute care surgery, where swift and precise decision-making is vital. Additionally, AI technology can track vascular changes during procedures, ensuring accurate guidance and reducing complications [64].

Integrating AI-enhanced CTA in acute care offers numerous benefits. Still, we are met with the same challenges as MRI/US, where a large and high-quality dataset is required to train AI models that can be scarce in emergencies, and integrating AI systems with existing hospital infrastructure may not be fiscally possible [66, 67]. There are also concerns about AI's reliability and interpretability in high-stakes environments. These concerns must be addressed to ensure the safe and effective use of AI-enhanced CTA, reassuring healthcare professionals about its potential.

13.4.4 Artificial Intelligence-Enhanced Hybrid Angiography

AI-enhanced hybrid angiography combines traditional angiography with advanced imaging technologies like fluoroscopy or CT, significantly improving the management of emergency vascular cases. This fusion technique provides comprehensive anatomical and functional insights, crucial for accurate diagnosis and treatment planning in emergencies such as aneurysms, arterial blockages, and trauma-induced vascular injuries. Hybrid angiography allows for detailed live visualization of vasculature while offering high-resolution cross-sectional images, enhancing the precision of interventions and improving patient outcomes [58, 68].

AI applications have further revolutionized hybrid angiography by significantly improving image registration and real-time analysis. AI-driven tools provide instantaneous feedback during procedures, dynamically adjusting imaging parameters, highlighting areas of interest, and predicting intervention outcomes based on live data. Moreover, AI enhances the ability to track vascular changes during procedures, ensuring accurate guidance and reducing the likelihood of complications. For instance, AI can detect even minor changes in blood flow or vessel morphology that might be missed by human operators, providing critical insights that inform surgical actions and improve patient safety [64]. The integration of AI in hybrid angiography thus optimizes workflow efficiency and contributes to better clinical outcomes.

The potential of AI-enhanced hybrid angiography to revolutionize emergency vascular cases can inspire and motivate us to continue seeking the integration of AI. However, we are presented with several challenges to this goal. Similar to AI-enhanced MRI/US and CTA, integrating AI systems with existing hospital infrastructure requires substantial technological investment and proper training for healthcare professionals [67]. The reliability and interpretability of AI decisions are significant concerns, particularly in high-stakes environments where errors could lead to severe consequences. It is essential to address all these challenges to unlock the full potential of AI-enhanced hybrid angiography in emergency vascular cases.

13.4.5 Hybrid Operating Rooms

It is essential to consider the role of Hybrid Operating Rooms (HORs), which are broader in scope and designed to accommodate both traditional surgeries and image-guided interventions across various medical disciplines. AI applications may benefit HORs by enhancing imaging accuracy and procedural outcomes in endovascular cases.

HORs present a surgical environment that blends advanced imaging technologies with surgical and interventional capabilities. A critical component of HORs is integrating AI. AI algorithms analyze data from various imaging modalities, such as MRI and CT scans, and assist surgeons during complex procedures. This integration improves targeting and navigation, reducing complications and improving patient outcomes. Importantly, AI-driven image fusion techniques combine preoperative and intraoperative images, providing a comprehensive and detailed view of the surgical site and instilling confidence in the thoroughness of the procedures. This technology is already particularly beneficial in exact procedures, such as neurosurgery and cardiovascular surgery. Still, it has also significantly impacted emergency general and vascular surgery in trauma settings [64].

Regarding precise procedures, endovascular techniques have greatly benefited from the advancements in AI within HORs. These minimally invasive procedures, which involve navigating catheters through blood vessels to treat conditions such as aneurysms, have seen significant improvement with the introduction of AI. AI enhances these procedures by providing analysis and decision support, helping interventional radiologists and surgeons make more informed decisions. For example, AI can assist in detecting blood flow anomalies and predict potential complications, leading to more effective interventions. Studies have shown that AI can significantly improve the accuracy of procedures like thrombectomies, where timely and precise actions are critical for patient outcomes [68]. The combination of AI and endovascular procedures in HORs optimizes surgical performance and expands the possibilities for treating complex vascular conditions with excellent safety and efficiency.

13.5 Challenges and Limitations

13.5.1 Real-Time Processing

AI algorithms used in imaging, including hybrid techniques, must operate in real time to provide timely guidance to surgeons, which is critical during emergency surgeries. Achieving this level of immediacy necessitates developing and implementing highly efficient computational methods capable of rapidly processing vast amounts of data. These algorithms must be designed to handle complex imaging inputs from the combined functional and structural data and convert them into clinically useful information without delay. The challenges lie in data processing speed and maintaining that speed over a short period with various data sets. High-performance resources such as optimized software and hardware are essential to meet these demands.

13.5.2 Integration with Existing Systems

The integration of AI algorithms into existing surgical workflows may be a challenge. The integration aims to harness the strengths of the chosen imaging technique to create a comprehensive, multi-faceted view of the patient's condition that can significantly enhance diagnostic and surgical precision. However, ensuring seamless integration is crucial to avoid disrupting the surgical process. Integration requires a harmonious blend of hardware and software systems to effectively provide real-time feedback to the surgical team without causing delays or distractions. It also involves developing user-friendly interfaces that allow surgical team members to interact intuitively with these complex imaging systems, minimizing the learning curve and preventing workflow interruptions. The successful integration of imaging technologies into surgical practices demands technical excellence and a deep understanding of AI-enhanced imaging to ensure that the new tools assist the surgeons' capabilities and improve patient outcomes without adding unnecessary complexity or disruption to the surgical workflow.

13.5.3 Accuracy and Reliability

AI algorithms must be accurate and reliable in interpreting complex imaging data, as emergency settings have high stakes. Rapid and precise data analysis is imperative for informed decisions that can significantly impact outcomes in these critical situations. Any errors or inaccuracies can lead to incorrect diagnoses or misguided surgical actions, potentially resulting in severe consequences such as complications, extended recovery times, or mortality. Therefore, developing and deploying AI algorithms in this context demands rigorous validation and continuous performance monitoring to warrant that they meet emergency medical care requirements. The reliability of these systems must be upheld through robust testing against diverse datasets and real-world scenarios to minimize the risk of failure. Consequently, integrating AI into emergency surgery hinges on ensuring the enhancement of the capabilities of healthcare professionals and the improvement of patient safety and outcomes.

13.5.4 Cost and Infrastructure

Deploying AI in imaging entails a significant investment in infrastructure, including high-performance computing systems and substantial data storage capacities. These technologies are essential for managing the vast amounts of data generated and the abilities of sophisticated AI algorithms to analyze them. Maintaining these systems requires ongoing investments, continuous updates, and technical support to warrant reliable performance. The cost-effectiveness and feasibility of implementing such advanced technologies in emergency surgical settings need careful consideration. Budget constraints, resource allocation, and the potential impact on overall healthcare costs must be weighed against the anticipated benefits of improved diagnostic accuracy, enhanced surgical outcomes, and increased efficiency. Decision-makers must evaluate whether the long-term gains in patient care and operational effectiveness justify the initial and recurring expenditures. Thus, while the promise of AI-enhanced imaging is substantial, its successful deployment demands a strategic approach that balances financial, technical, and clinical factors to ensure sustainable and effective integration into emergency medical care.

13.5.5 Regulatory and Ethical Considerations

Implementing AI in emergency surgery is a complex process that involves navigating a landscape of regulatory approvals and ethical considerations. Regulatory bodies play a crucial and reassuring role in ensuring that AI systems meet safety and efficacy standards before being deployed in clinical settings. This requires rigorous testing and validation to demonstrate that the AI can reliably assist in surgical decision-making without compromising patient care. However, the most challenging aspect is the ethical considerations, particularly concerning patient consent and data privacy. In emergency situations, where time is of the essence, informing patients about the use of AI in their treatment and obtaining their consent could be a challenge.

Furthermore, storing patient data safely is critical, as AI systems may require access to personal health information. Ensuring this data is stored and processed in compliance with privacy regulations is essential to keeping with HIPAA guidelines. Some liabilities arise for determining responsibility when a medical error occurs due to an AI system's involvement. Regularly updated guidelines and legal frameworks are necessary to address these issues, balancing the innovative potential of AI with the need to protect patients' rights and safety.

13.6 Conclusion

In conclusion, integrating AI in imaging techniques represents a positive direction in emergency surgery. AI-enhanced imaging can revolutionize diagnostics and surgical navigation by improving image reconstruction, reducing imaging time, and addressing issues. However, successfully implementing these technologies requires overcoming challenges related to real-time processing, seamless integration with existing surgical workflows, and substantial investment in infrastructure. Additionally, ensuring AI system accuracy, reliability, and ethical deployment is crucial to their practical use in emergencies. Navigating the regulatory landscape and maintaining patient consent and data privacy are essential considerations. Balancing these challenges with the promising benefits of AI-enhanced imaging can significantly improve patient outcomes and the overall efficiency of emergency surgical care.

References

1. Knowlton LM, Minei J, Tennakoon L, Davis KA, Doucet J, Bernard A, Haider A, Scherer LRT 3rd, Spain DA, Staudenmayer KL. The economic footprint of acute care surgery in the United States: implications for systems development. J Trauma Acute Care Surg. 2019;86(4):609–16. https://doi.org/10.1097/TA.0000000000002181. PMID: 30589750; PMCID: PMC6433481
2. Bercovich E, Javitt MC. Medical imaging: from roentgen to the digital revolution, and beyond. Rambam Maimonides Med J. 2018;9(4):e0034. https://doi.org/10.5041/RMMJ.10355. PMID: 30309440; PMCID: PMC6186003
3. Mantsevich SN, Yushkov KB. Optimization of piezotransducer dimensions for quasicollinear paratellurite AOTF. Ultrasonics. 2021;112:106335. https://doi.org/10.1016/j.ultras.2020.106335. Epub 2020 Dec 30. PMID: 33395592
4. Elmi A, Hedgire S, Harisinghani M. Computed tomography: basics. In: Butler KL, Harisinghani M, editors. Acute care surgery: imaging essentials for rapid diagnosis [Internet]. New York: McGraw-Hill Education; 2015. [cited 2024 Feb 25]. Available from: accesssurgery.mhmedical.com/content.aspx?aid=1108258923.
5. Kawakyu-O'Connor D, Bordia R, Nicola R. Magnetic resonance imaging of spinal emergencies. Magn Reson Imaging Clin N Am. 2016;24(2):325–44. https://doi.org/10.1016/j.mric.2015.11.004. Epub 2016 Feb 23. PMID: 27150322

6. Short AR. The uses of coelioscopy. Br Med J 1925;2(3371):254–255. doi: https://doi.org/10.1136/bmj.2.3371.254. PMID: 20772142; PMCID: PMC2226817.
7. Elmahdy M, Sebro R. Radiomics analysis in medical imaging research. J Med Radiat Sci. 2023;70(1):3–7. https://doi.org/10.1002/jmrs.662. Epub 2023 Feb 10. PMID: 36762402; PMCID: PMC9977659
8. Scapicchio C, Gabelloni M, Barucci A, Cioni D, Saba L, Neri E. A deep look into radiomics. Radiol Med. 2021;126(10):1296–1311. doi: https://doi.org/10.1007/s11547-021-01389-x. Epub 2021 Jul 2. PMID: 34213702; PMCID: PMC8520512.
9. Shur JD, Doran SJ, Kumar S, Ap Dafydd D, Downey K, O'Connor JPB, Papanikolaou N, Messiou C, Koh DM, Orton MR. Radiomics in oncology: a practical guide. Radiographics. 2021;41(6):1717–32. https://doi.org/10.1148/rg.2021210037. PMID: 34597235; PMCID: PMC8501897
10. Sarker IH. Machine learning: algorithms, real-world applications and research directions. SN Comput Sci. 2021;2(3):160. https://doi.org/10.1007/s42979-021-00592-x. Epub 2021 Mar 22. PMID: 33778771; PMCID: PMC7983091
11. Aggarwal R, Sounderajah V, Martin G, Ting DSW, Karthikesalingam A, King D, Ashrafian H, Darzi A. Diagnostic accuracy of deep learning in medical imaging: a systematic review and meta-analysis. NPJ Digit Med. 2021;4(1):65. https://doi.org/10.1038/s41746-021-00438-z. PMID: 33828217; PMCID: PMC8027892
12. Chan HP, Samala RK, Hadjiiski LM, Zhou C. Deep learning in medical image analysis. Adv Exp Med Biol. 2020;1213:3–21. https://doi.org/10.1007/978-3-030-33128-3_1. PMID: 32030660; PMCID: PMC7442218
13. He K, Zhang X, Ren S, Sun J. Delving deep into rectifiers: Surpassing human-level performance on imagenet classification. In Proc IEEE Int Conf Comput Vis. 2015:1026–34.
14. Hirosawa T, Harada Y, Yokose M, Sakamoto T, Kawamura R, Shimizu T. Diagnostic accuracy of differential-diagnosis lists generated by generative pretrained transformer 3 Chatbot for clinical vignettes with common chief complaints: a pilot study. Int J Environ Res Public Health. 2023;20(4):3378. https://doi.org/10.3390/ijerph20043378. PMID: 36834073; PMCID: PMC9967747
15. Levin S, Toerper M, Hamrock E, Hinson JS, Barnes S, Gardner H, Dugas A, Linton B, Kirsch T, Kelen G. Machine-learning-based electronic triage more accurately differentiates patients with respect to clinical outcomes compared with the emergency severity index. Ann Emerg Med. 2018;71(5):565–574.e2. https://doi.org/10.1016/j.annemergmed.2017.08.005. Epub 2017 Sep 6. PMID: 28888332
16. Brown AD, Marotta TR. A natural language processing-based model to automate MRI brain protocol selection and prioritization. Acad Radiol. 2017;24(2):160–6. https://doi.org/10.1016/j.acra.2016.09.013. Epub 2016 Nov 23. PMID: 27889399
17. Lee YH. Efficiency improvement in a busy radiology practice: determination of musculoskeletal magnetic resonance imaging protocol using deep-learning convolutional neural networks. J Digit Imaging. 2018;31(5):604–10. https://doi.org/10.1007/s10278-018-0066-y. PMID: 29619578; PMCID: PMC6148815
18. Frane N, Bitterman A. Radiation safety and protection. 2023 May 22. In: StatPearls [Internet]. Treasure Island (FL): StatPearls Publishing; 2024 Jan. PMID: 32491431.
19. Ng CKC, Sun Z, Parry H, Burrage J. Local diagnostic reference levels for X-ray examinations in an Australian tertiary hospital. J Med Imag Health Inform. 2014;4(2):297–302.
20. Brady SL, Trout AT, Somasundaram E, Anton CG, Li Y, Dillman JR. Improving image quality and reducing radiation dose for pediatric CT by using deep learning reconstruction. Radiology. 2021;298(1):180–8. https://doi.org/10.1148/radiol.2020202317. Epub 2020 Nov 17. PMID: 33201790
21. Koetzier LR, Mastrodicasa D, Szczykutowicz TP, van der Werf NR, Wang AS, Sandfort V, van der Molen AJ, Fleischmann D, Willemink MJ. Deep learning image reconstruction for CT: technical principles and clinical prospects. Radiology. 2023;306(3):e221257. doi: https://doi.org/10.1148/radiol.221257. Epub 2023 Jan 31. PMID: 36719287; PMCID: PMC9968777.

22. Ng CKC. Artificial intelligence for radiation dose optimization in pediatric radiology: a systematic review. Children (Basel). 2022;9(7):1044. https://doi.org/10.3390/children9071044. PMID: 35884028; PMCID: PMC9320231
23. Arun A, Thomas TJ, Rani JS, Gorthi RKSS. Efficient directionality-driven dictionary learning for compressive sensing magnetic resonance imaging reconstruction. J Med Imaging (Bellingham). 2020;7(1):014002. https://doi.org/10.1117/1.JMI.7.1.014002. Epub 2020 Jan 24. PMID: 32042856; PMCID: PMC6989772
24. Shiyam Sundar LK, Muzik O, Buvat I, Bidaut L, Beyer T. Potentials and caveats of AI in hybrid imaging. Methods. 2021;188:4–19. https://doi.org/10.1016/j.ymeth.2020.10.004. Epub 2020 Oct 15. PMID: 33068741
25. Zhao Y, Wang X, Zhang Y, Liu T, Zuo S, Sun L, Zhang J, Wang K, Liu J. Combination of clinical information and radiomics models for the differentiation of acute simple appendicitis and non simple appendicitis on CT images. Sci Rep. 2024;14(1):1854. https://doi.org/10.1038/s41598-024-52390-z. PMID: 38253872; PMCID: PMC10803326
26. Liang D, Fan Y, Zeng Y, Zhou H, Zhou H, Li G, Liang Y, Zhong Z, Chen D, Chen A, Li G, Deng J, Huang B, Wei X. Development and validation of a deep learning and radiomics combined model for differentiating complicated from uncomplicated acute appendicitis. Acad Radiol. 2024;31(4):1344–54. https://doi.org/10.1016/j.acra.2023.08.018. Epub 2023 Sep 27. PMID: 37775450
27. Stringer MD, Pablot SM, Brereton RJ. Paediatric intussusception. Br J Surg. 1992;79(9):867–76. https://doi.org/10.1002/bjs.1800790906. PMID: 1422744
28. Kim S, Yoon H, Lee MJ, Kim MJ, Han K, Yoon JK, Kim HC, Shin J, Shin HJ. Performance of deep learning-based algorithm for detection of ileocolic intussusception on abdominal radiographs of young children. Sci Rep. 2019;9(1):19420. https://doi.org/10.1038/s41598-019-55536-6. PMID: 31857641; PMCID: PMC6923478
29. Kwon G, Ryu J, Oh J, Lim J, Kang BK, Ahn C, Bae J, Lee DK. Deep learning algorithms for detecting and visualising intussusception on plain abdominal radiography in children: a retrospective multicenter study. Sci Rep. 2020;10(1):17582. https://doi.org/10.1038/s41598-020-74653-1. PMID: 33067505; PMCID: PMC7567788
30. Pei Y, Wang G, Cao H, Jiang S, Wang D, Wang H, Wang H, Yu H. A deep-learning pipeline to diagnose pediatric intussusception and assess severity during ultrasound scanning: a multicenter retrospective-prospective study. NPJ Digit Med. 2023;6(1):182. https://doi.org/10.1038/s41746-023-00930-8. PMID: 37775624; PMCID: PMC10541898
31. Ghimire P, Maharjan S. Adhesive small bowel obstruction: a review. JNMA J Nepal Med Assoc. 2023;61(260):390–6. https://doi.org/10.31729/jnma.8134. PMID: 37208871; PMCID: PMC10089019
32. Wang Z, Liu R, Liu S, Sun B, Xie W, Wang D, Lu Y. A computed tomography-based radiomic model for the prediction of strangulation risk in patients with acute intestinal obstruction. Intell Med. 2024;4(1):33–42.
33. Dreizin D, Chen T, Liang Y, Zhou Y, Paes F, Wang Y, Yuille AL, Roth P, Champ K, Li G, McLenithan A, Morrison JJ. Added value of deep learning-based liver parenchymal CT volumetry for predicting major arterial injury after blunt hepatic trauma: a decision tree analysis. Abdom Radiol (NY). 2021;46(6):2556–66. https://doi.org/10.1007/s00261-020-02892-x. Epub 2021 Jan 19. PMID: 33469691; PMCID: PMC8205942
34. Farzaneh N, Stein EB, Soroushmehr R, Gryak J, Najarian K. A deep learning framework for automated detection and quantitative assessment of liver trauma. BMC Med Imaging. 2022;22(1):39. https://doi.org/10.1186/s12880-022-00759-9. PMID: 35260105; PMCID: PMC8905785
35. Wang J, Wood A, Gao C, Najarian K, Gryak J. Automated spleen injury detection using 3D active contours and machine learning. Entropy (Basel). 2021;23(4):382. https://doi.org/10.3390/e23040382. PMID: 33804831; PMCID: PMC8063804
36. Azagury DE, Dua MM, Barrese JC, Henderson JM, Buchs NC, Ris F, Cloyd JM, Martinie JB, Razzaque S, Nicolau S, Soler L, Marescaux J, Visser BC. Image-guided surgery. Curr Probl

Surg. 2015;52(12):476–520. https://doi.org/10.1067/j.cpsurg.2015.10.001. Epub 2015 Oct 22. PMID: 26683419

37. Boekestijn I, van Oosterom MN, Dell'Oglio P, van Velden FHP, Pool M, Maurer T, Rietbergen DDD, Buckle T, van Leeuwen FWB. The current status and future prospects for molecular imaging-guided precision surgery. Cancer Imaging. 2022;22(1):48. https://doi.org/10.1186/s40644-022-00482-2. PMID: 36068619; PMCID: PMC9446692
38. Unger M, Berger J, Melzer A. Robot-assisted image-guided interventions. Front Robot AI. 2021;8:664622. https://doi.org/10.3389/frobt.2021.664622. PMID: 34322519; PMCID: PMC8312560
39. Zaffino P, Moccia S, De Momi E, Spadea MF. A review on advances in intra-operative imaging for surgery and therapy: imagining the operating room of the future. Ann Biomed Eng. 2020;48(8):2171–91. https://doi.org/10.1007/s10439-020-02553-6. Epub 2020 Jun 29. PMID: 32601951
40. Lin Z, Lei C, Yang L. Modern image-guided surgery: a narrative review of medical image processing and visualization. Sensors (Basel). 2023;23(24):9872. https://doi.org/10.3390/s23249872. PMID: 38139718; PMCID: PMC10748263
41. Maybody M, Stevenson C, Solomon SB. Overview of navigation systems in image-guided interventions. Tech Vasc Interv Radiol. 2013;16(3):136–43. https://doi.org/10.1053/j.tvir.2013.02.008. PMID: 23993075
42. Yaniv Z, Cleary K. Image-guided procedures: a review. Computer Aided Interventions and Medical Robotics. 2006;3(1–63):7.
43. Sutton PA, van Dam MA, Cahill RA, Mieog S, Polom K, Vahrmeijer AL, van der Vorst J. Fluorescence-guided surgery: comprehensive review. BJS Open. 2023;7(3):zrad049. https://doi.org/10.1093/bjsopen/zrad049.
44. Privitera L, Paraboschi I, Dixit D, Arthurs OJ, Giuliani S. Image-guided surgery and novel intraoperative devices for enhanced visualisation in general and paediatric surgery: a review. Innovative Surgical Sciences. 2022;6(4):161–72. https://doi.org/10.1515/iss-2021-0028. PMID: 35937852; PMCID: PMC9294338
45. Dietrich CF, Averkiou M, Nielsen MB, Barr RG, Burns PN, Calliada F, Cantisani V, Choi B, Chammas MC, Clevert DA, Claudon M, Correas JM, Cui XW, Cosgrove D, D'Onofrio M, Dong Y, Eisenbrey J, Fontanilla T, Gilja OH, Ignee A, Jenssen C, Kono Y, Kudo M, Lassau N, Lyshchik A, Franca Meloni M, Moriyasu F, Nolsøe C, Piscaglia F, Radzina M, Saftoiu A, Sidhu PS, Sporea I, Schreiber-Dietrich D, Sirlin CB, Stanczak M, Weskott HP, Wilson SR, Willmann JK, Kim TK, Jang HJ, Vezeridis A, Westerway S. How to perform contrast-enhanced ultrasound (CEUS). Ultrasound Int Open. 2018;4(1):E2–E15. https://doi.org/10.1055/s-0043-123931. Epub 2018 Feb 7. PMID: 29423461; PMCID: PMC5802984
46. Fransvea P, Fico V, Puccioni C, D'Agostino L, Costa G, Biondi A, Brisinda G, Sganga G. Application of fluorescence-guided surgery in the acute care setting: a systematic literature review. Langenbeck's Arch Surg. 2023;408(1):375. https://doi.org/10.1007/s00423-023-03109-7. PMID: 37743419
47. Wongkietkachorn A, Surakunprapha P, Winaikosol K, Waraasawapati S, Chaiwiriyakul S, Eua-Angkanakul K, Wongkietkachorn N, Punyavong P, Jenwitheesuk K, Chowchuen B. Indocyanine green dye angiography as an adjunct to assess indeterminate burn wounds: a prospective, multicentered, triple-blinded study. J Trauma Acute Care Surg. 2019;86(5):823–8. https://doi.org/10.1097/TA.0000000000002179. PMID: 30589753; PMCID: PMC6493689
48. Wongkietkachorn A, Surakunprapha P, Jenwitheesuk K, Eua-Angkanakul K, Winaikosol K, Punyavong P, Wongkietkachorn N, Wongkietkachorn S, Salyapongse AN. Indocyanine green angiography precise marking for indeterminate burn excision: a prospective, multicentered, double-blinded study. Plast Reconstr Surg Glob Open. 2021;9(4):e3538. https://doi.org/10.1097/GOX.0000000000003538. PMID: 33868880; PMCID: PMC8049159
49. Okamoto T, Onda S, Yanaga K, et al. Clinical application of navigation surgery using augmented reality in the abdominal field. Surg Today. 2015;45:397–406. https://doi.org/10.1007/s00595-014-0946-9.

50. Bernhardt S, et al. The status of augmented reality in laparoscopic surgery as of 2016. Med Image Anal. 2017;37:66–90. https://doi.org/10.1016/j.media.2017.01.007.
51. Cal-Gonzalez J, Rausch I, Shiyam Sundar LK, Lassen ML, Muzik O, Moser E, Papp L, Beyer T. Hybrid imaging: instrumentation and data processing. Front Phys. 2018., Sec. Medical Physics and Imaging;18 https://doi.org/10.3389/fphy.2018.00047.
52. Patton JA, Townsend DW, Hutton BF. Hybrid imaging technology: from dreams and vision to clinical devices. Semin Nucl Med. 2009;39(4):247–63. https://doi.org/10.1053/j.semnuclmed.2009.03.005. PMID: 19497402
53. Beyer T, Townsend DW, Brun T, Kinahan PE, Charron M, Roddy R, Jerin J, Young J, Byars L, Nutt R. A combined PET/CT scanner for clinical oncology. J Nucl Med. 2000;41(8):1369–79. PMID: 10945530
54. Wahl RL, Quint LE, Cieslak RD, Aisen AM, Koeppe RA, Meyer CR. "Anatometabolic" tumor imaging: fusion of FDG PET with CT or MRI to localize foci of increased activity. J Nucl Med. 1993;34(7):1190–7. PMID: 8315501
55. Xu S, et al. Targeting accuracy of MR/US fusion imaging for prostate biopsy: an analysis of large-scale clinical data. J Magn Reson Imaging. 2021;29(5):1085–90.
56. Krücker J, Xu S, Glossop N, Viswanathan A, Borgert J, Schulz H, Wood BJ. Electromagnetic tracking for thermal ablation and biopsy guidance: clinical evaluation of spatial accuracy. J Vasc Interv Radiol. 2007;18(9):1141–50. https://doi.org/10.1016/j.jvir.2007.06.014. PMID: 17804777; PMCID: PMC2555977
57. Koh WS, et al. Clinical value of MRI/ultrasound fusion-guided prostate biopsy in patients with previous negative biopsy results. Korean J Urol. 2020;61(7):432–9.
58. Mokin M, et al. Impact of interventional thrombectomy on acute ischemic stroke outcomes: a review of recent literature. J NeuroIntervent Surg. 2016;8(2):211–6.
59. Nandalur KR, et al. Diagnostic performance of computed tomographic angiography in peripheral arterial disease: a systematic review and meta-analysis. J Vasc Interv Radiol. 2014;18(7):849–57.
60. Haskins G, et al. Deep learning in medical image registration: a survey. Mach Vis Appl. 2020;31(1):8.
61. De Simone B, Chouillard E, Gumbs AA, Loftus TJ, Kaafarani H, Catena F. Artificial intelligence in surgery: the emergency surgeon's perspective (the ARIES project). Discov Health Syst. 2022;1(1):9. https://doi.org/10.1007/s44250-022-00014-6. Published online 2022 Dec 6. PMCID: PMC9734362, PMID: 37521114
62. Mayerhoefer ME, Materka A, Langs G, Häggström I, Szczypiński P, Gibbs P, Cook G. Introduction to radiomics. J Nucl Med. 2020;61(4):488–95. https://doi.org/10.2967/jnumed.118.222893.
63. Litjens G, et al. A survey on deep learning in medical image analysis. Med Image Anal. 2017;42:60–88.
64. Esteva A, et al. Deep learning-enabled medical computer vision. NPJ Digital Med. 2021;4(1):5.
65. Thakor AS, et al. Artificial intelligence in emergency medicine. J Emerg Med. 2020;58(3):538–44.
66. Topol EJ. High-performance medicine: the convergence of human and artificial intelligence. Nat Med. 2019;25(1):44–56.
67. Shortliffe EH, Sepúlveda MJ. Clinical decision support in the era of artificial intelligence. JAMA. 2018;320(21):2199–200.
68. Goyal M, et al. Endovascular thrombectomy after large-vessel ischaemic stroke: a meta-analysis of individual patient data from five randomised trials. Lancet. 2016;387(10029):1723–31.

14 Indocyanine Green Fluorescence-Guided Emergency Surgery: Principles for an Evidence-Based Practice

Belinda De Simone and Fausto Catena

Abbreviations

AC	acute cholecystitis
AMI	acute mesenteric ischemia
CVS	critical view of safety
DM	decision-making
FA	fluorescence angiography
FC	fluorescence cholangiography
ICG	indocyanine green
NIR	near-infrared

14.1 Introduction

Modern surgery has been revolutionized by advancements in technologies and digital models, aimed at supporting surgeons in complex decision-making (DM) and high-risk procedures. In emergency situations, where time is critical, the DM

B. De Simone (✉)
Department of Emergency and General Minimally Invasive Surgery, Level I Trauma Center, Bufalini Hospital, AUSL Romagna, Cesena, Italy

Department of Theoretical and Applied Sciences, eCampus University, Novedrate, Como, Italy

F. Catena
Dipartimento di Scienze Mediche e Chirurgiche Alma Mater Studiorum Università di Bologna, Bologna, Italy

Department of General Surgery, Level I Trauma Center, Bufalini Hospital, AUSL Romagna, Cesena, Italy

B. De Simone et al. (eds.), *New Technologies, Precision Medicine, and AI in Emergency General Surgery*, Hot Topics in Acute Care Surgery and Trauma,
https://doi.org/10.1007/978-3-032-09357-8_14

process becomes particularly challenging. Surgeons must rapidly assess a variety of clinical, diagnostic, and environmental variables, alongside the patient's overall risk of negative outcomes. This involves synthesizing information from diagnoses, available management strategies, and resources to ensure the best course of action for the patient [1–3].

Intraoperatively, a surgeon's decision to proceed with or modify a surgical plan relies heavily on their experience and visual judgment. Emergency surgeons must evaluate inflamed tissues, assess blood flow to intestinal segments, and manage conditions such as peritonitis—all while dealing with fluctuating patient hemodynamics. However, many of these visual assessments are subjective and lack reproducibility, making it difficult to standardize emergency procedures across cases [1–3].

In recent years, fluorescence imaging—and more specifically, indocyanine green (ICG) fluorescence—has emerged as a powerful tool to enhance surgical visualization [4–6].

In elective procedures, ICG fluorescence has demonstrated its value in identifying anatomical structures, ensuring adequate perfusion, and mapping lymphatic spread in oncology [4–6]. Its application in emergency surgery, where decisions must be made swiftly, has grown with the increasing use of minimally invasive techniques such as laparoscopy and robotic-assisted surgery [7, 8]. ICG fluorescence is particularly beneficial in assessing bowel viability and reducing postoperative complications in surgical diseases such as acute cholecystitis, intestinal ischemia, strangulated hernia, and volvulus [9–19].

Despite promising outcomes, the routine use of ICG fluorescence-guided surgery in emergency settings remains limited. Many emergency surgeons agree that ICG fluorescence imaging can assist in performing complex procedures in the presence of severe inflammation, such as acute cholecystitis, and assessing bowel viability. Nevertheless, concerns persist regarding the lack of training, as well as the limited accessibility and availability of the technology in emergency settings [1–3].

Recently, the World Society of Emergency Surgery released a consensus document aimed at standardizing the use of ICG fluorescence imaging in emergent and urgent surgical procedures [20]. Accordingly, this chapter summarizes practical recommendations to help surgeons safely and effectively integrate ICG fluorescence into emergency operations, ultimately improving outcomes for high-risk, critically ill patients.

14.2 Mechanism of ICG Fluorescence

ICG is a water-soluble, tricarbocyanine dye that emits fluorescence when exposed to near-infrared (NIR) light. Once injected intravenously, ICG binds quickly to plasma proteins, circulating in the bloodstream without significant diffusion into surrounding tissues. It is metabolized and excreted via the liver, which provides a short half-life (approximately 3–5 minutes), making it safe for repeated doses in a single procedure [21, 22].

The mechanism of ICG fluorescence relies on its optical properties. When exposed to NIR light, specifically in the 800 nm wavelength range, ICG absorbs the light and then re-emits it at a longer wavelength (approximately 820–840 nm), which can be detected by an NIR camera system. This fluorescence is invisible to the naked eye but can be visualized in real time on a monitor, allowing for intraoperative assessment of tissue perfusion, vascularization, and anatomical landmarks [4].

The advantage of ICG lies in its strong affinity for vascular tissues and its ability to highlight blood flow in real time, enabling surgeons to assess perfusion in tissues such as the bowel, liver, and bile ducts. This makes it a powerful tool in both elective and emergency surgeries for evaluating tissue viability, identifying bile ducts during cholecystectomy, and ensuring adequate blood supply to anastomoses [21, 22].

In clinical use, ICG's fluorescence can be triggered multiple times during the same surgery due to its short half-life and minimal risk of toxicity. This mechanism helps guide surgical decisions with greater precision, improving outcomes by reducing complications like ischemia or bile duct injury [21, 22].

14.3 Clinical Applications of ICG Fluorescence Imaging in the Emergency Setting

14.3.1 The Role of ICG Fluorescence Cholangiography in Performing Laparoscopic Cholecystectomies for Acute Cholecystitis

- **Fluorescence Cholangiography (FC) should be considered for real-time visualization of the extrahepatic biliary tree during laparoscopic cholecystectomies for acute cholecystitis.**
- **FC cholangiography improves the visualization of biliary structures during cholecystectomies for acute cholecystitis, reducing operative time, conversion to open surgery, and negative outcomes.**
- **Further research and larger trials are needed to standardize its use and confirm its benefits across broader patient populations in the emergency setting.**

Laparoscopic cholecystectomy (LC) is the gold standard for managing acute cholecystitis, yet the risk of iatrogenic bile duct injury remains significant, especially in emergency settings, with rates as high as 4% [23, 24]. Conventional intraoperative cholangiography (CC) has been a long-standing method to improve identification of the biliary anatomy. However, CC poses several challenges: it requires radiological equipment, introduces additional operative time, and carries risks of ionizing radiation exposure. These disadvantages have made the need for an alternative intraoperative technique apparent [25–30].

ICG fluorescence cholangiography (FC) provides a promising solution by allowing real time, radiation-free visualization of the biliary structures. Once injected, ICG binds to plasma proteins and highlights the biliary anatomy when exposed to near-infrared light. Recent studies have demonstrated that ICG cholangiography facilitates quicker identification of critical anatomical structures in Calot's triangle, reducing the risk of bile duct injury.

Although there is limited high-quality data on ICG use specifically in emergency cholecystectomies, single-center experiences have shown favorable outcomes.

Di Maggio et al. reported reduced conversion rates to open surgery and shorter operative times with the use of ICG during emergency cholecystectomies. Surgeons felt more confident operating beyond the traditional 72-hour safety window for acute cholecystitis when ICG imaging was available [15]. Similarly, a randomized controlled trial by She et al. found no significant difference in complication rates between conventional LC and LC with ICG cholangiography, though a trend toward fewer complications in the ICG group was noted. The small sample size of this study limited its power to detect statistically significant differences [31].

ICG cholangiography shows promise as a useful tool for improving outcomes in emergency cholecystectomies, particularly in challenging cases of severe acute cholecystitis. It provides enhanced visualization of biliary structures without the need for radiation, potentially reducing intraoperative complications. However, further research and larger trials are needed to standardize the use of near-infrared ICG imaging and confirm its benefits across broader patient populations [32–39].

14.3.2 The Role of ICG Fluorescence Angiography in Managing Intestinal Ischemia and Strangulated Bowel

- **Fluorescence Angiography (FA) provides real-time perfusion data, helping to identify viable bowel segments, reducing the risk of inadequate resection, and preserving as much healthy tissue as possible.**
- **FA can be performed safely in the emergency setting, and it is a useful tool in the setting of acute intestinal ischemia and strangulated bowel.**
- **Emergency surgeons should consider its use to guide intraoperative DM in patients presenting with intestinal ischemia and strangulated bowels in order to define resection margins and anastomosis, when it is available.**
- **Despite its advantages, further research is needed to standardize interpretation methods and optimize its use.**

The intraoperative application of ICG fluorescence angiography (FA) has proven to be an effective tool in guiding the identification of the optimal resection site and assessing the blood supply of visceral anastomosis in both upper gastrointestinal and colorectal surgeries. The rationale behind ICG fluorescence angiography is that, upon systemic injection, the dye highlights only vascularized tissues, making it a valuable method for evaluating tissue perfusion and viability in real time [39].

Intestinal ischemia is a surgical emergency, and its incidence varies based on the population and the underlying risk factors. Acute mesenteric ischemia (AMI) is rare but has high mortality, estimated to affect around 0.1% of hospital admissions, especially in older populations. Chronic forms of ischemia, such as chronic mesenteric ischemia (CMI), often manifest in patients with atherosclerosis and are typically underdiagnosed. It occurs when blood flow to the intestines is reduced, leading to insufficient oxygen supply to intestinal tissues. This condition can cause significant morbidity and mortality if not diagnosed and managed promptly. Intestinal ischemia is generally classified into two major categories: occlusive and non-occlusive [40, 41].

Occlusive intestinal ischemia (OMI) occurs when a blood clot or embolus blocks a major artery or vein supplying the intestines. Common causes include embolism or thrombosis in the mesenteric arteries or veins. It can also result from mechanical obstruction of the bowel, such as in strangulated hernias or volvulus. OMI tends to have an acute presentation with severe abdominal pain, vomiting, and signs of shock, especially when large areas of bowel are affected [40, 41].

Non-occlusive mesenteric ischemia (NOMI) occurs without a clear blockage in the blood vessels. Instead, it arises due to a reduction in blood flow caused by systemic conditions like heart failure, hypovolemia, or vasoconstriction associated with shock, sepsis, or certain medications. NOMI often occurs in critically ill patients and may present more insidiously, leading to delayed diagnosis and worse outcomes [42].

The mortality rates for untreated intestinal ischemia are particularly high, with occlusive ischemia carrying a 60–80% mortality rate depending on how quickly it is diagnosed and treated. NOMI is also associated with high mortality, often due to its occurrence in critically ill patients and the difficulty of diagnosing the condition early [40–42].

Understanding the types and risks of intestinal ischemia is essential in managing and reducing complications. Early diagnosis, which may include imaging techniques like CT scans or ICG angiography, along with surgical or medical intervention, can improve outcomes significantly [14, 43–47].

Surgical exploration and bowel resection are often required, with intraoperative evaluation of intestinal perfusion remaining subjective and challenging. ICG angiography can be particularly useful in these cases by providing objective perfusion assessment, helping to define resection margins more accurately, and improving decision-making. Studies have shown that ICG angiography may reveal discrepancies between traditional visual assessment and actual perfusion, leading to better management of bowel resection and improved surgical outcomes. For instance, *Sheridan* et al. reported that the accuracy of prediction of intestinal viability using clinical criteria, such as intestinal color, arterial perfusion, and peristalsis, was only 57.7%. They measured tissue oxygen tension using miniaturized polarographic oxygen electrodes in 134 segments of rats' small intestines of varying degrees of ischemia. Histological examination revealed that most of the specimens ($n = 111$) were potentially viable, as evidenced by no or minimal damage. The use of clinical criteria alone correctly identified all 23 histologically compromised segments. Of the 111 histologically non-compromised segments, however, only 40 (36%) were felt to be viable using clinical parameters [43]. Karampinis et al. analyzed the use of ICG fluorescence angiography in 52 patients with acute mesenteric ischemia and found that it provided supplemental information to traditional macroscopic evaluation in 34.6% of cases, leading to significant changes in operative strategy [44]. Additionally, Ryu et al. compared ICG angiography with surgeon palpation during bowel resections for strangulated bowel obstruction. They enrolled 38 patients who underwent emergency surgery for strangulated bowel obstruction. Two groups were compared: (I) the ICG + group, in which ICG was used during laparoscopic surgery, and (II) the ICG − group, in which palpation without ICG was used during open surgery. Although there were fewer intestinal resections in the ICG + group, the rate of pathological necrosis of the removed specimens tended to be high, and there were no complications due to ineligibility in the intestinal preservation group. In the ICG − group, the demarcation line was not distinct under normal light observation, and bowel resection was performed slightly more carefully for safety. In conclusion, ICG provided more accurate identification of ischemic bowel segments [16].

During surgery for a strangulated bowel or OMI, the viability of the bowel must be carefully evaluated after treating the underlying obstruction or occlusion. In cases of necrosis or perforation, bowel resection is mandatory, but determining the exact resection margins can be difficult. The surgeon typically relies on visual and tactile cues, such as bowel color, peristalsis, temperature, and mesenteric pulsations, all of which have limited sensitivity and reproducibility [47]. ICG angiography offers an objective method to assess intestinal blood flow, even during laparoscopic procedures, where traditional methods may fall short. This real-time technique can highlight well-perfused areas and help surgeons determine safe resection lines and assess anastomotic viability. *Guerra* et al. [48] analyzed 71 patients with acute small bowel obstruction who received surgery via a laparoscopic approach. They concluded that the selective use of ICG angiography provides a direct, objective tool for assessing bowel viability and supports the surgeon in the intraoperative decision-making. Compared with other methods for assessing bowel viability, ICG angiography requires only a dedicated camera and can be done in no more than 2–3 minutes [48].

ICG fluorescence angiography is particularly beneficial in laparoscopic surgery for assessing bowel perfusion in strangulated bowel or occlusive mesenteric ischemia cases. It allows surgeons to identify the extent of tissue necrosis or ischemia and determine appropriate resection margins with high precision. Compared to other methods, ICG angiography is quick, non-invasive, and can be performed using a dedicated camera within minutes [14, 43–48].

14.3.3 The Role of ICG Fluorescence Angiography in Preventing Anastomotic Leakage After Emergency Surgical Procedures

- **Emergency surgeons may consider the use of fluorescence angiography to assess anastomotic perfusion following emergency intestinal resection, when appropriate equipment and expertise are available, as an adjunct to support intraoperative decision-making and potentially reduce the risk of anastomotic leakage.**

Anastomotic leakage (AL) is one of the most serious complications in gastrointestinal surgery, particularly following bowel resection, and it is associated with significant morbidity and mortality. The etiology of AL is multifactorial, with inadequate vascular perfusion (hypoperfusion) being a key factor in its pathogenesis [49–53]. In emergency surgical settings, patients frequently present with hemodynamic instability due to conditions like peritonitis, sepsis, or septic shock, all of which further impair tissue perfusion and elevate the risk of AL.

Indocyanine green (ICG) fluorescence angiography has gained recognition as a useful tool for intraoperative assessment of tissue perfusion. It provides real time, objective feedback on vascular integrity at the anastomotic site, aiding surgeons in determining whether the perfusion is adequate for creating a safe anastomosis. Studies in elective colorectal surgery have shown that using ICG angiography to assess blood flow at anastomotic sites significantly reduces the risk of anastomotic leakage. While most of these studies are from elective settings, the same principles apply in the emergency setting, where tissue perfusion is often compromised due to shock, hypoxia, or other complications [54–62].

Intraoperative clinical assessment, such as the surgeon's evaluation of bowel color, bleeding at the edges, and mesenteric pulsations, has been the traditional method to gauge perfusion. However, this approach is highly subjective and depends on the surgeon's experience and judgment. By contrast, NIR-ICG offers an objective method to visualize perfusion, reducing the risk of misjudging the vascular supply in edematous or ischemic tissues, which are frequently encountered in emergency bowel resections or after strangulated hernia repair [63–89].

While the use of ICG angiography has been well-documented in elective surgeries, its application in emergency settings remains less extensively studied. However, early case reports and retrospective analyses suggest that it may reduce postoperative complications and improve outcomes by providing more accurate perfusion assessments. For example, studies have demonstrated that ICG fluorescence can help prevent AL by highlighting areas of poor perfusion that may not be apparent through clinical assessment alone [63–89].

In conclusion, ICG fluorescence angiography provides a valuable, real-time assessment of tissue perfusion, especially in high-risk emergency situations. Its use in preventing anastomotic leakage in emergency surgery is promising, though further randomized studies are needed to confirm its efficacy in this context.

14.3.4 The Role of ICG Fluorescence Angiography in Managing Abdominal Blunt and Penetrating Trauma

- **The use of fluorescence angiography (FA) in patients with abdominal trauma undergoing surgical exploration, either open or laparoscopic, may assist surgeons in assessing bowel viability in the presence of mesenteric lacerations or hematomas.**
- **In selected haemodynamically stable patients, the use of fluorescence angiography (FA) may support emergency and trauma surgeons in evaluating blood perfusion of high-risk intestinal segments affected by mesenteric injuries, thereby assisting intraoperative decision-making.**

For hemodynamically stable patients undergoing surgical exploration for abdominal trauma, ICG fluorescence imaging can significantly enhance intraoperative decision-making [90–93]. Afifi and colleagues have demonstrated that ICG fluorescence is a valuable real-time tool for assessing bowel perfusion in trauma cases [94]. It enables visualization of blood flow in high-risk bowel segments with mesenteric lacerations, assisting surgeons in determining the optimal approach for repair. Additionally, it helps assess the viability of anastomotic edges and identifies ischemic intestinal segments that may otherwise appear perfused, thereby reducing the risk of postoperative complications and the need for planned reoperations [95, 96].

The use of intraoperative fluorescent angiography has also been reported in the context of war-related trauma, where it assists in evaluating tissue perfusion and optimizing the management of patients with bowel injuries [95]. While the application of ICG fluorescence in abdominal trauma shows promise and appears beneficial, the current quality of evidence is insufficient to support definitive clinical guidelines.

14.4 ICG Fluorescence Cholangiography and Angiography: Protocols of Administration

14.4.1 General Technical Tips for Practice

The intensity of the ICG fluorescence signal depends on several factors, including:

- **The device used;**
- **The distance from the tip of the laparoscope to its target;**
- **The amount of covering tissue.**

Kono et al. demonstrated that the fluorescence signal intensity decreases by 50% when the distance between the laparoscope and the target increases from 5 cm to 15 cm. Additionally, the tip of the laparoscope should be held perpendicular (at a 90-degree angle) to the target, particularly when visualizing Calot's triangle, to maximize the direct exposure of light to the bile ducts and optimize fluorescence signals. When using a 30-degree laparoscope, it should be positioned at a 120-degree angle to achieve the highest fluorescence intensity [97].

In emergency settings, where equipment availability may vary, these factors can affect the quality of imaging. The surgeon's knowledge and familiarity with fluorescence imaging technology are critical for obtaining optimal results. It is essential for surgeons to understand that achieving the best fluorescence signal may require temporary adjustments to both the distance and angle of the laparoscope.

Key factors to consider for effective ICG fluorescence imaging include:

- *Timing of ICG administration*: Administering ICG either too early or too late relative to the surgical procedure can result in suboptimal visualization. In emergency situations, careful coordination is required to ensure that the fluorescence peaks precisely at the time of image acquisition [98, 99].
- *Dose and dilution of ICG*: Using an insufficient dose may produce weak fluorescence signals, while excessive dosing can cause excessive background fluorescence, making it challenging to distinguish target structures. The dilution should be optimized according to the specific clinical scenario and patient characteristics [100, 101].
- *Angle and Distance of Laparoscope*: For optimal fluorescence signal, the laparoscope tip should be positioned perpendicular (90 degrees) to the target, particularly when visualizing Calot's triangle. If using a 30-degree laparoscope, it should be angled at 120 degrees to enhance fluorescence intensity [97].

14.5 Recommendations for an Effective ICG Fluorescence Cholangiography in the Emergency Setting

Timing of Administration

- For optimal results, ICG should be administered intravenously at the induction of general anesthesia, 45–60 minutes before surgery. This approach ensures sufficient dye uptake by the biliary structures before dissection begins.
- In cases where IV administration is not feasible or additional visualization is needed, ICG can be injected directly into the gallbladder during surgery. This should be done before starting gallbladder dissection to enhance visualization.

Dose of Administration

- A single IV dose of 5 mg of ICG is recommended for fluorescent cholangiography during urgent laparoscopic cholecystectomy. In patients who are obese or have severe cholecystitis, additional doses may improve visibility. However, the cumulative dose should not exceed 2 mg/kg to prevent adverse effects.
- When opting for intra-gallbladder administration, it is suggested to use an ICG concentration of 2.5 mg/mL. This involves diluting 9 mL of bile with 1 mL of ICG solution (prepared with sterile water at a concentration of 0.25 mg/mL) and injecting it into the gallbladder before dissection. This achieves an ICG concentration of 0.025 mg/mL within the gallbladder.

Dilution of ICG

For IV administration, ICG should be diluted with sterile water. While some authors report using albumin or saline solution, sterile water is generally preferred to maintain fluorescence intensity.

Administration Route
The choice of ICG administration route should be tailored to the specific clinical scenario. Intravenous injection is more commonly used and provides systemic visualization, while intra-gallbladder injection offers enhanced localized fluorescence in challenging cases, such as acute inflammation or anatomical variations.

Timing of Image Acquisition
Fluorescence images should be captured at key points:

- Before initiating gallbladder dissection.
- During dissection of Calot's Triangle.
- Prior to clipping or dividing any structures.

Additional images can be taken as needed, based on the surgeon's assessment, to confirm the anatomy or clarify uncertain structures.

Quantitative and Qualitative Interpretation of ICG Fluorescence
Current evidence highlights the potential benefits of both quantitative and qualitative methods for assessing ICG fluorescence cholangiography. However, there is a need for further research to develop standardized protocols for the objective interpretation of ICG images. Future studies should focus on refining these protocols to enhance accuracy and utility, especially in emergency settings.

14.5.1 The ICG Fluorescence Cholangiography in the Emergency Setting: How to Perform It

ICG fluorescent cholangiography is widely recognized as a safe technique, primarily because it does not involve radiation exposure and carries an exceptionally low risk of adverse reactions to ICG injection (approximately 0.003% at doses above 0.5 mg/kg). This method can be safely employed in patients with mild iodine allergies, a population for whom radiographic intraoperative cholangiography (IOC) may be contraindicated. This safety is due to the minimal iodine content in ICG (less than 0.1 mg/mL) compared to the much higher concentrations found in standard radio-contrast agents (50–300 mg/mL) [102, 103].

In a retrospective cohort study by Losurdo et al. [104], comparing emergency laparoscopic cholecystectomy (LC) performed with and without ICG cholangiography, the use of ICG was shown to significantly reduce operative time ($P = 0.002$). Furthermore, the intra- and postoperative complication rates were 4.17% in the ICG group versus 15.8% in the non-ICG group. After adjusting for confounding factors such as cholangitis and cholecystitis, the ICG group demonstrated a reduced trend in postoperative bile duct injury and other complications. Notably, ICG use was found to be protective against intra- and postoperative complications, as well as bile duct injuries (HR 0.037, $P = 0.337$ and HR 0.039, $P = 0.647$; HR 0.288, $P = 0.05$ and HR 0.635, $P = 0.687$, respectively) [104].

14.5.2 Key Factors Influencing Fluorescence Cholangiography Outcomes

The effectiveness of ICG cholangiography during LC is influenced by the dosage, timing, and route of administration [105–142]. A practical and essential step-by-step guide is provided in Table 14.1.

Table 14.1 The step-by-step guide to performing an ICG fluorescent cholangiography in the emergency setting

Step	Details
1. Dilution of ICG	*Preparation*: Reconstitute a 25 mg vial of ICG with 10 mL of sterile water or normal saline to create a solution with a concentration of 2.5 mg/mL.
	Mixing: Thoroughly mix the solution to achieve a consistent concentration. Protect it from light to prevent degradation.
2. Dose of Administration	*Recommended Dose*: Administer ICG at 0.2 to 0.5 mg/kg body weight.
	Standard Protocol: Typically, 5 mg of ICG is administered for an average adult, depending on the patient's weight and surgical scenario.
3. Timing of Administration	*Timing Before Surgery*: Inject ICG intravenously at least 45–60 minutes before imaging or surgery to allow absorption by the liver and excretion into the bile ducts.
	Emergency Adjustments: In emergencies, the time can be shortened to 30 minutes, potentially affecting fluorescence intensity.
4. Injection Point	*Intravenous Injection*: Inject ICG intravenously, preferably through a central line or large peripheral vein, to ensure rapid distribution.
5. Time Acquisition of Images	*Imaging Window*: Start near-infrared (NIR) fluorescence imaging 45 minutes after ICG administration for optimal biliary tree visualization.
	Real-Time Imaging: Perform intraoperative imaging in real time to dynamically assess biliary anatomy during dissection.
6. Interpretation	*Qualitative Interpretation*:
	Visualization of Anatomy: Bright fluorescence should outline biliary structures (cystic duct, common bile duct, hepatic ducts).
	Anomalies: Absence or poor fluorescence may indicate biliary obstruction, inadequate timing, or imaging equipment issues.
	Quantitative Interpretation:
	Fluorescence Intensity: Measure the intensity of fluorescence in bile ducts; lower intensity may indicate reduced liver function or incomplete excretion.
	Flow Assessment: Dynamic imaging allows for bile flow assessment, with quantitative measures potentially correlating with obstruction severity.

14.5.3 Timing of ICG Administration

The "bile duct-to-liver ratio" (BLR) is a crucial metric in ICG cholangiography, comparing the fluorescence intensity of the bile duct against the liver. This ratio enhances visualization of the biliary anatomy by differentiating the bile duct from the liver background. Achieving a BLR greater than 1 is essential for optimal imaging, but the best timing for this remains debated. The timing of ICG administration varies, with reports ranging from 25 hours to as little as 5 minutes before surgery when administered intravenously, or during surgery via local gallbladder injection [104–142].

Verbeek et al. [135] demonstrated that administering ICG 24 hours before surgery significantly improved the signal-to-background ratio by reducing liver fluorescence. Conversely, a recent study from the European Fluorescence Image-Guided Surgery (FIGS) registry highlighted inconsistencies in dosing practices, emphasizing that timing is often more critical than dosage [136]. Boogerd et al. reported that the optimal BLR was achieved 3 to 7 hours after administering 5 mg of ICG or 5 to 25 hours after a 10 mg dose [132]. Zarrinpar et al. [133] conducted a prospective study demonstrating that higher doses (0.25 mg/kg) and longer intervals (at least 45 minutes before imaging) improved biliary visualization.

14.5.4 Dose of ICG Administration

The standard ICG dose ranges from 0.1 to 0.5 mg/kg, with a commonly used dose of 0.2 to 0.25 mg/kg, allowing for effective imaging while minimizing side effects. In their study, Zarrinpar et al. [132] found that increasing the dose from 0.02 to 0.25 mg/kg improved the visualization score from 1.9 to 3.4 out of 5 ($P < 0.05$). The EURO-FIGS registry data suggested that administering a lower dose of 5 mg is adequate for most cases, with administration 30–45 minutes prior to surgery being both practical and effective [136].

In certain scenarios, such as when surgery must be performed urgently, administering ICG 30–60 minutes before the procedure is often sufficient. However, when feasible, administering the dose 2–6 hours prior yields the best visualization results [33, 132–137].

14.5.5 Dilution and Administration Techniques

ICG is typically diluted with sterile water for injection. The standard preparation involves diluting 25 mg of ICG in 10 mL of sterile water to achieve a concentration of 2.5 mg/mL. For intravenous administration, the recommended dose is adjusted based on patient weight, ranging from 5 to 10 mg [106, 107]. Some studies have also experimented with diluting ICG using albumin, though sterile water remains the most common solvent due to its consistency in clinical outcomes [34, 136].

Local administration of ICG directly into the gallbladder has been explored as an alternative technique. Škrabec et al. [137] demonstrated that local injection provides superior visualization of the cystic duct and gallbladder neck without the interference of liver background fluorescence. This technique can be especially beneficial in emergency settings, as it allows for immediate and clear visualization of critical anatomical landmarks, even if administered at the time of surgery.

14.5.6 Timing of Image Acquisition

The acquisition of ICG cholangiography images should occur at key points during laparoscopic cholecystectomy: while exposing the critical view of safety (CVS), during dissection of Calot's triangle, and before clipping the cystic duct [138–140]. Some authors also advocate for imaging after clipping to check for bile leakage [141, 142].

14.5.7 Quantitative and Qualitative Images Interpretation

ICG fluorescence cholangiography is primarily used qualitatively to enhance the visualization of the biliary tree during LC. Surgeons rely on visual cues to guide dissection and avoid bile duct injuries, which have been associated with reduced conversion rates and fewer complications. The subjective interpretation of fluorescence patterns is dependent on the surgeon's experience and proficiency with this technique.

While qualitative interpretation is currently the standard, the development of quantitative metrics is gaining traction. Emerging technologies, such as the SPY fluorescence imaging platform, aim to provide objective measurements of fluorescence intensity, potentially improving the accuracy and reproducibility of ICG cholangiography [143]. Further research is needed to establish standardized quantitative methods that could enhance surgical decision-making and patient safety.

14.6 Recommendations for an Effective ICG Fluorescence Angiography in the Emergency Setting

Timing of ICG Administration

In the emergency setting, ICG should be administered intravenously approximately 1–2 minutes before the intended imaging, ideally just prior to surgical resection. The optimal timing will depend on factors such as the patient's hemodynamic status, the tissue being assessed, and the specific clinical scenario. Adjustments may be required to account for conditions like shock or reduced perfusion, where circulation time may be prolonged.

Dose of ICG Administration

A single intravenous dose of 5 mg is generally recommended for fluorescence angiography. Care should be taken not to exceed a maximum dose of 2 mg/kg. Alternatively, a weight-adjusted dose between 0.1 mg/kg and 0.5 mg/kg can be used, with adjustments based on patient weight, clinical condition, and specific imaging requirements. Emergency surgeons should be mindful of dose limitations, especially in patients with liver dysfunction.

ICG Dilution

ICG should be diluted using sterile water for injection to ensure optimal fluorescence. While some studies have reported using albumin or saline solutions for dilution, sterile water remains the most reliable choice to prevent precipitation and ensure clear imaging.

Route of Administration

For ICG fluorescent angiography, intravenous administration is the standard route, which can be performed through either a peripheral or central venous catheter. This approach allows for rapid distribution and clear visualization of tissue perfusion.

Timing of Image Acquisition

Surgeons should acquire fluorescence images within 30 seconds to 3 minutes after ICG injection, as fluorescence typically becomes visible within seconds and peaks between 1 and 2 minutes. This window provides the best opportunity to assess tissue perfusion before making critical decisions, such as proceeding with bowel resection.

Interpretation of ICG Fluorescence Angiography in Different Clinical Scenarios in the Emergency Setting

In emergency situations like acute mesenteric ischemia, bowel obstruction, incarcerated hernia, or bowel anastomosis, the interpretation of ICG fluorescence is primarily qualitative, relying on the surgeon's visual assessment. While this qualitative approach aids in real-time intraoperative decision-making, it remains subjective and may vary based on the surgeon's experience. To enhance accuracy and reproducibility, further research is needed to develop standardized protocols and softwares for quantitative analysis of ICG fluorescence, particularly in the emergency setting.

14.6.1 ICG Fluorescent Angiography in the Emergency Setting: How to Perform It

ICG fluorescent angiography has become an indispensable tool in the emergency surgical setting for assessing bowel viability, especially in cases where rapid and accurate evaluation is critical. Traditionally, clinicians relied on clinical judgment, Doppler ultrasound, or direct visual inspection to assess bowel viability—methods that are often subjective and can lack accuracy. In contrast, ICG fluorescent angiography provides a more objective and dynamic approach by enabling real-time visualization of tissue perfusion. This technology enhances the ability to assess blood flow adequacy, thereby helping predict areas of ischemia or necrosis [16, 129, 144–157].

In emergencies such as acute mesenteric ischemia (AMI), strangulated hernias, or damage control surgeries, the timely use of ICG fluorescent angiography can significantly impact surgical decision-making. It guides resections and reduces the risk of postoperative complications by providing clear, real-time insights into tissue viability. For example, a retrospective study of 52 patients with acute mesenteric non-occlusive ischemia revealed that fluorescence angiography provided additional information beyond macroscopic evaluation, resulting in a major change in surgical decisions in 18 (34.6%) patients, ultimately leading to significant clinical benefit [44]. In a prospective study of 56 patients, the use of fluorescence angiography for bowel viability assessment in cases of intestinal ischemia and mechanical obstruction resulted in changes to the surgical plan in 32% of cases (18/56), with 67% (12/18) of these patients avoiding unnecessary resections [153].

The benefits of ICG fluorescence angiography extend to reducing the incidence of anastomotic leakage after colorectal surgery. The FLAG single-center randomized trial, involving 377 patients undergoing colorectal anastomosis, compared outcomes between those assessed with ICG fluorescence and those without. The study found that impaired blood perfusion was identified in 19% of patients using ICG, resulting in a lower rate of anastomotic leaks (9.1% in the ICG group vs. 16.3% in the control group, $P = 0.04$). Additionally, for low colorectal anastomoses (4–8 cm), the leak rate was reduced to 14.4% with ICG versus 25.7% without ICG ($P = 0.04$) [11].

Similarly, an Italian multicenter randomized study involving 240 patients (118 in the ICG group vs. 122 controls) assessed the role of ICG fluorescence angiography in laparoscopic left-sided colon and rectal resections. This study detected impaired perfusion in 11% of cases, with a lower but not statistically significant rate of anastomotic leaks in the ICG group (5%) compared to the control group (9%) [12]. Two systematic reviews and meta-analyses further support these findings. The first review, which included 27 studies with 8786 patients, showed significantly lower odds of anastomotic leaks and other complications when ICG fluorescence was used [73]. The second meta-analysis, incorporating 3 randomized controlled trials (RCTs) with 964 patients, confirmed that ICG angiography significantly reduced the risk of anastomotic leaks (RR 0.67, 95% CI 0.46–0.99, $P = 0.04$) [157].

In emergency surgeries for intestinal ischemia, ICG fluorescence angiography demonstrated its value in a multicenter retrospective analysis of 93 patients, influencing surgical management in 29% of cases [10]. However, it is essential to note that while ICG angiography is effective for identifying arterial ischemia, it does not reliably assess venous ischemia. The efficacy of this technology depends on several factors, including proper timing of ICG administration, patient hemodynamics, and accurate interpretation of fluorescence patterns [16, 129, 144–159].

A practical and essential step-by-step guide is provided in Table 14.2.

14.6.2 Timing of ICG Administration

ICG is typically administered intravenously a few minutes prior to imaging. The exact timing varies based on factors such as patient hemodynamic status and the clinical scenario. In most cases, an injection 1–2 minutes before imaging allows

Table 14.2 A step-by-step guide to performing ICG fluorescence angiography in the Emergency Setting

Step	Description
1. Dilution of ICG	*Preparation*: Reconstitute the ICG vial with sterile water or normal saline according to the manufacturer's instructions to achieve the desired concentration.
	Mixing: Ensure the solution is thoroughly mixed for consistent concentration. Protect the solution from light to prevent degradation.
2. Dose of Administration	*Recommended Dose*: Administer ICG at a dose of 0.2 to 0.5 mg/kg adjusted based on body weight and the clinical scenario. In practice, a 5 mg bolus dose is administered.
3. Timing of Administration	*Timing Before Imaging*: Inject ICG intravenously 30 seconds to 2 minutes before imaging, as fluorescence appears rapidly post-injection.
	Emergency Adjustments: Administer ICG as early as possible in critical situations, adjusting timing based on the urgency of the clinical situation.
4. Injection Point	*Intravenous Injection*: Administer ICG through an intravenous line, preferably via a central line or large peripheral vein for rapid distribution.
5. Time Acquisition of Images	*Imaging Window*: Begin acquiring images immediately after ICG administration, as fluorescence peaks within 1 to 2 minutes, providing optimal visualization.
	Real-Time Imaging: Perform real-time intraoperative imaging to assess tissue perfusion dynamically during the procedure.
6. Interpretation	*Qualitative Interpretation*:
	Visualization of Perfusion: Successful ICG angiography shows bright fluorescence in well-perfused tissues, helping to identify viable areas.
	Anomalies: Areas with reduced or absent fluorescence suggest compromised blood flow, requiring further evaluation or immediate intervention.
	Quantitative Interpretation:
	Fluorescence Intensity Measurement: Quantify fluorescence intensity to objectively assess tissue perfusion. Lower intensity may indicate ischemia.
	Time-to-Peak Fluorescence: Measure the time taken for fluorescence to peak post-injection. Prolonged times suggest compromised perfusion.

sufficient time for the dye to circulate, achieving peak fluorescence in perfused tissues. In hyperdynamic states, this window may be narrower, requiring earlier or repeated doses. Conversely, in patients with compromised perfusion, such as those in shock, the dye may take longer to reach the tissues, necessitating a longer wait time before imaging. The goal is to capture images at peak fluorescence, typically observed within 30–60 seconds after injection, for optimal differentiation between viable and ischemic tissues [16, 44, 143–149].

14.6.3 Dose and Dilution of ICG

The standard dose of ICG for fluorescent angiography ranges from 0.1 to 0.5 mg/kg, with 0.2 to 0.25 mg/kg being the most commonly used in clinical practice. Adjustments may be needed based on the patient's condition. For example, lower doses are advisable for patients with liver dysfunction, as ICG is metabolized by the liver. The dye is typically diluted in sterile water for injection to ensure optimal fluorescence without precipitation [129, 150–155].

14.6.4 Route and Timing of Image Acquisition

ICG is administered as an intravenous bolus, typically followed by a saline flush to ensure rapid distribution. The fluorescence usually appears within seconds and peaks within 1 to 2 minutes. The recommended imaging window is generally between 30 seconds and 3 minutes post-injection, depending on the specific vascular application [152–154].

14.6.5 Quantitative and Qualitative Images Interpretation

In conditions such as AMI, bowel obstruction, incarcerated hernias, and bowel anastomosis, both quantitative and qualitative interpretations of ICG fluorescence play a crucial role.

In AMI, the decreased or absent fluorescence indicates severe ischemia, guiding the resection of non-viable bowel segments. Delayed or patchy fluorescence suggests compromised blood flow, requiring further assessment [129, 149–155].

In bowel obstruction, reduced fluorescence indicates partial strangulation and bowel vascular souffrance, while the absence of fluorescence suggests complete ischemia. The pattern of fluorescence helps distinguish reversible from irreversible changes [16, 144–148].

In assessing incarcerated hernias, low fluorescence intensity indicates impaired perfusion, guiding resection decisions. Delayed patterns can reveal compromised flow despite a seemingly viable bowel on visual inspection [16, 144–148].

In evaluating bowel anastomosis, strong, uniform fluorescence indicates good perfusion, reducing the risk of anastomotic leaks. Conversely, reduced fluorescence may necessitate revision of the anastomosis [9–11, 67, 72, 73, 86, 158].

In a study assessing bowel perfusion in patients with strangulated bowel obstruction, fluorescence patterns were categorized by intensity, with non-fluorescent patterns indicating necrosis. Resection was necessary in cases showing a perivascular pattern, as confirmed by histopathology [13].

Emerging technologies, such as the SPY fluorescence imaging platform and quantitative algorithms like fluorescence-based enhanced reality (FLER) and Q-ICG, aim to enhance the accuracy of ICG fluorescence interpretation, although further validation in clinical practice is required [143].

Understanding these protocols and interpretations is crucial for optimizing the use of ICG fluorescence angiography, particularly in the emergency setting, where timely and accurate decisions can significantly impact patient outcomes.

14.7 Optimizing the Quality of ICG Fluorescence Imaging in Urgent Surgical Conditions: Addressing Limitations in the Emergency Setting

ICG angiography and cholangiography are valuable tools that can significantly enhance surgical decision-making in urgent cases. However, certain challenges in the emergency setting can impact the quality and utility of ICG imaging. Understanding these limitations is crucial for maximizing its effectiveness.

14.7.1 Factors Impacting the Quality of ICG Imaging in Emergency Surgery

- ***Patient-specific variables potentially affecting ICG fluorescence imaging:***
  A. *Liver Function*: Since ICG is metabolized by the liver, impaired hepatic function can reduce fluorescence intensity.
  B. *Cardiac Output*: Low cardiac output can limit ICG distribution, leading to suboptimal fluorescence.
  C. *Microangiopathy and Tissue Edema*: Conditions like severe inflammation (e.g., acute cholecystitis) or microvascular disease can reduce the penetration of fluorescence, particularly in thickened tissues.
  D. *Body Mass Index (BMI)*: In obese patients, fluorescence may not penetrate deep tissues effectively, reducing the clarity of images.
- ***Hemodynamic instability***
  - Low blood pressure, compromised respiratory function, or the use of vasopressors can decrease tissue perfusion, affecting the visibility of fluorescence.

– The patient's hemodynamic status is critical in deciding whether to perform intestinal resection and anastomosis in cases of acute intestinal ischemia and strangulated hernias, although ICG imaging can support decision-making.

14.7.2 Contraindications and Precautions for ICG Use

Absolute Contraindication ICG should not be administered to patients with known allergies to iodides or iodinated contrast agents due to the risk of anaphylaxis.

Relative Contraindication Following ICG use, radioactive iodine uptake studies should be deferred for at least 1 week, as ICG may interfere with results.

Practical Recommendations for Enhancing ICG Imaging Quality in the Emergency Setting

- *Training and Preparation*: Ensure that the surgical team and OR staff are well-trained in the use of ICG technology to optimize its effectiveness in urgent scenarios.
- *Preoperative Assessment*: Consider patient-specific factors (e.g., liver function, cardiac status, BMI) to anticipate and mitigate potential challenges with ICG imaging.
- *Intraoperative Monitoring*: Regularly assess the patient's hemodynamic status throughout the procedure to enhance the accuracy of ICG imaging.
- *Allergy Checks*: Always screen for iodide allergies before ICG administration to prevent adverse reactions.

14.8 Safety Issues of ICG Administration in the Emergency Setting

The intravenous administration of ICG is generally considered safe, with a rapid onset of action that provides real-time visualization to support surgical DM. ICG is a water-soluble anionic dye that, after intravenous injection, binds to albumin without altering its structure. It is primarily cleared by the liver, with nearly complete excretion into bile within approximately 8 minutes in patients with normal liver function. The reported toxicity of ICG is minimal, with adverse reactions occurring in only 1 in 40,000 cases [99, 100]. The standard clinical dose (0.1–0.5 mg/mL/kg) is well below the established toxicity threshold.

However, due to the presence of iodine in the ICG molecule, its use is contraindicated in patients with thyrotoxicosis or known iodine allergies, which may trigger non-immunological histamine release and cause severe allergic reactions [99, 100, 160].

14.8.1 Renal Function and Its Impact on ICG Imaging

While ICG is primarily excreted by the liver, conditions such as edema and fluid overload, often seen in patients with renal impairment, can affect tissue perfusion and the quality of fluorescence imaging. Despite these challenges, current evidence supports the safe use of ICG in elderly patients, those with impaired liver function, patients on inotropes, and individuals with renal dysfunction in emergency settings [160–162].

14.8.2 Pediatric and Obstetric Considerations

Most available studies on ICG focus on elective surgeries rather than emergency procedures. A systematic review indicated that ICG is generally safe for infants under 3 months, with no reports of serious adverse events [163–165]. Minor side effects, such as temporary dye retention or skin discoloration, resolved spontaneously [166, 167].

In pregnant patients, there is no evidence to suggest that ICG poses significant risks to the mother or fetus. ICG does not significantly cross the placenta, likely due to its minimal transplacental transfer, similar to how rifampin behaves [168]. Wang et al. concluded that the placenta acts as an effective barrier, protecting the fetus from ICG exposure [139].

14.8.3 Risk of Allergic Reactions

The incidence of serious allergic reactions to ICG, including anaphylaxis, is less than 0.05%, demonstrating a high level of safety [102, 103]. However, because ICG contains traces of iodine, it may be contraindicated in patients with known allergies to iodinated contrast agents, such as those used in CT imaging. A prospective study involving 1414 endometrial cancer patients who received ICG for sentinel lymph node mapping found that, despite 65 patients having iodine or contrast allergies, only three experienced mild allergic reactions, none of which were anaphylactic [169].

14.9 Patients' Factors Influencing Fluorescence Imaging Quality in the Emergency Setting

14.9.1 Hepatic Function

Liver function plays a crucial role in the metabolism and clearance of ICG. In patients with liver dysfunction (e.g., cirrhosis or acute liver failure), altered pharmacokinetics can lead to prolonged fluorescence or reduced signal intensity, complicating image interpretation during surgery [170, 171]. The ICG plasma disappearance rate (ICGPDR) and retention rate at 15 minutes (ICGR15) are valuable indicators of liver function, although their correlation with fluorescence quality in emergency surgeries remains underexplored [172, 173].

14.9.2 Body Mass Index

Obesity poses a significant challenge to fluorescence imaging due to increased tissue thickness, which limits light penetration and reduces image clarity. Studies have shown that higher BMI decreases the visualization of biliary structures during ICG cholangiography, particularly for deeper ducts like the common hepatic duct [97, 139, 174–178]. In patients with severe cholecystitis or obesity, ICG fluorescence may be insufficient for delineating biliary anatomy before dissecting Calot's Triangle [97].

14.9.3 Age and Comorbidities

Elderly patients and those with multiple comorbidities may experience reduced fluorescence due to age-related changes in tissue composition, such as increased collagen density and decreased elasticity. Additionally, comorbid conditions like diabetes and peripheral vascular disease can impair tissue perfusion, further reducing imaging quality [179–181].

14.9.4 Hemodynamic Status

The patient's hemodynamic stability is a critical factor influencing ICG imaging quality:

- Hypotension or shock can delay ICG delivery to tissues, resulting in poor fluorescence signals.
- Conversely, in hyperdynamic states, rapid circulation may reduce the imaging window due to quicker dye clearance.

Emerging technologies like fluorescence-based enhanced reality (FLER) and laser speckle contrast imaging (LSCI) offer potential solutions by providing quantitative assessments of tissue perfusion. Studies by D'Urso et al. [182] and Al-Taher et al. [183] suggest that these advanced techniques can enhance the precision of perfusion measurements, even in patients receiving vasopressors.

14.10 The Use of ICG Fluorescence Imaging in Emergency and Trauma Surgery: Benefits, Limitations, and Practical Considerations

ICG fluorescence imaging has gained significant popularity in emergency and trauma surgery due to its ability to provide real time, dynamic visualization of tissue perfusion and anatomical structures. However, like any advanced technology, its application comes with advantages, disadvantages, contraindications, limitations, and considerations regarding cost-effectiveness.

14.10.1 ICG Angiography in Trauma Surgery: Bowel Perfusion Assessment

In cases of blunt or penetrating abdominal trauma, assessing bowel viability, determining resection margins, and evaluating the feasibility of bowel anastomosis are critical. The use of ICG fluorescence imaging in this context is expanding, particularly for evaluating bowel perfusion [134, 158, 184, 185]. Despite the lack of large prospective studies, recent case series have highlighted its utility in trauma settings. Osterkamp et al. [186] conducted a study on 20 patients undergoing emergency laparotomy for penetrating abdominal trauma. Using the System Usability Scale (SUS), they evaluated the practicality of ICG angiography, noting that it influenced surgical decisions in 14 out of 20 cases. The technique helped correct underestimations of perfusion, allowing surgeons to avoid unnecessary colonic diversion, and identified areas needing further resection due to inadequate perfusion. In eight cases, it led to modifications in resection margins. Additionally, ICG angiography facilitated the identification of previously undetected small and large bowel injuries. Undiagnosed hollow viscus injuries are a significant cause of relaparotomies, associated with high morbidity and mortality [187, 188]. Similarly, Afifi et al. [94] reported on the effectiveness of ICG in cases of blunt abdominal trauma, showing that its use extended resection margins and optimized the creation of well-perfused bowel anastomoses. ICG also helped prevent unnecessary extensive bowel resections by accurately assessing tissue viability, thereby potentially reducing the need for second-look laparotomies.

14.10.2 ICG Angiography in Evaluating Mesenteric Ischemia and Strangulated Bowel

ICG fluorescence imaging is particularly beneficial in mesenteric ischemia, where accurate assessment of bowel perfusion is crucial for patient outcomes [40, 44, 189]. Traditional methods of assessing bowel viability often rely heavily on the surgeon's experience, which can be subjective and prone to error [43, 47, 49].

Karampinis et al. reported in a case series of 52 patients that ICG fluorescence led to changes in surgical management in 11% of cases. In some instances, it avoided extensive resections by identifying adequate perfusion, while in others, it guided additional resection based on real-time perfusion data [44].

For incarcerated and strangulated hernias, assessing bowel viability is critical. Case studies, such as those by Ahmed et al., demonstrated that ICG angiography could prevent unnecessary resections in patients with edematous but viable bowel that would traditionally appear non-viable due to discoloration and lack of peristalsis [190].

14.10.3 ICG Cholangiography for Biliary Surgery

ICG cholangiography is particularly advantageous in laparoscopic cholecystectomy, where clear delineation of the biliary anatomy is essential to avoid bile duct injuries [190–192]. The technique enables visualization of the gallbladder, cystic duct, and biliary tract, minimizing the risk of injury to these structures. However, the effectiveness of ICG cholangiography can be compromised in cases of severe acute cholecystitis, obesity, or impaired liver function, where proper excretion of the dye into the biliary tree may be delayed [193]. Additionally, while ICG can help outline biliary anatomy, it is not effective for diagnosing biliary obstructions, such as choledocholithiasis.

14.10.4 Limitations and Challenges in Emergency Settings

One current limitation of ICG angiography is its reliance on qualitative assessment, which can lead to variability in evaluating perfusion adequacy. This subjectivity may impact decision-making, especially in less experienced hands [153].

The timing of ICG administration is critical, especially in patients with impaired liver function, as delayed excretion can affect imaging results. Additionally, ICG has limited tissue penetration (5–10 mm), making it less effective in patients with significant inflammation, scarring, or obesity [97, 139, 177].

14.10.5 Cost-Effectiveness Considerations

The cost of implementing ICG fluorescence imaging, including the purchase and maintenance of specialized equipment, must be balanced against its potential benefits in reducing postoperative complications and hospital stays. To date, there are no comprehensive studies evaluating the cost-effectiveness of ICG in the urgent or emergency setting.

In Table 14.3, a summary of the advantages, disadvantages, and limitations of the ICG fluorescent imaging in emergency settings is provided.

Table 14.3 Summary of the advantages, disadvantages, contraindications, limitations, and cost-effectiveness of Indocyanine Green (ICG) implementation in emergency and trauma surgery

Category	Details
Advantages	*Real-Time Assessment*: Provides immediate visualization of tissue perfusion, enabling quicker and more accurate decision-making.
	Enhanced Visualization: Improves clarity of critical structures (e.g., blood vessels, bile ducts) in complex anatomical situations, reducing the risk of surgical errors.
	Minimally Invasive: Compatible with laparoscopic and robotic surgery, leading to faster recovery times and fewer complications compared to open surgery.
	Low Risk of Allergic Reactions: Generally safe with a low incidence of allergic reactions, making it suitable for a wide range of patients.
	No Ionizing Radiation: Safer for patients and surgical staff, as it avoids the risks associated with ionizing radiation, especially in cases requiring multiple imaging sessions.
Disadvantages	*Limited Tissue Penetration*: Effective only for shallow tissues, limiting its use in assessing deeper structures or organs.
	Short Imaging Window: Requires precise timing for imaging, which can be challenging in emergency settings.
	Need for Specialized Equipment: Requires access to near-infrared cameras and other specialized tools, which may not be available in all surgical settings.
	Operator Dependence: The effectiveness of ICG is highly dependent on the operator's experience and skill, which can lead to variability in results.
Absolute Contraindications	*Allergy to Iodine or ICG*: Patients with known allergies to iodine or ICG should not be administered this dye due to the risk of severe allergic reactions.
Relative Contraindications	*Liver Dysfunction*: Patients with significant liver impairment may have altered clearance of ICG, affecting fluorescence results.
	Renal Impairment: Although ICG is not primarily excreted by the kidneys, caution is advised in patients with severe renal dysfunction.
	Pregnancy and Breastfeeding: While not strictly contraindicated, there is limited data on the safety of ICG in pregnant or breastfeeding women, warranting caution.
Limitations	*Limited Penetration Depth*: ICG fluorescence is less effective for evaluating perfusion in large or deep structures, which may be critical in some surgical cases.
	Cost and Accessibility: High cost of ICG dye and necessary imaging equipment may limit its use, especially in resource-limited settings or low-volume centers.
	Risk of Misinterpretation: Variability in tissue perfusion, timing, and equipment settings can lead to potential misinterpretation, affecting surgical decisions.
Cost-Effectiveness	*Initial Cost*: The expense of ICG and specialized equipment can be high, but this may be offset by improved outcomes and reduced complication rates in high-volume centers.
	Long-Term Savings: Potential for reduced surgical complications, shorter operative times, and quicker recovery could translate to overall cost savings in the long term.
	Resource-Limited Settings: In settings with limited resources, the high cost of implementation may not be justified if the technology is underutilized or alternatives are available.

14.11 Conclusions

ICG-guided surgery includes the concept of precision surgery by tailoring surgical treatment plans to the unique characteristics of each patient, thereby improving overall surgical outcomes. Fluorescence-guided emergency surgery, whether performed through minimally invasive techniques or open procedures, supports surgeons in a range of critical scenarios. It allows for real-time assessment of bowel perfusion and enhances the intraoperative visualization of critical structures during laparoscopic cholecystectomies.

The combination of minimally invasive techniques—such as laparoscopy and robotic-assisted surgery—with advanced imaging technologies for intraoperative navigation in emergency settings enables surgeons to quickly identify and perform the most appropriate surgical procedure tailored to each patient and clinical situation. This integrated approach not only reduces postoperative complications but also decreases the length of hospital stays.

Acknowledgements Not applicable

Declarations

Ethics approval Not applicable.

Consent to participate Not applicable.

Consent for publication Not applicable.

Availability of data and materials Supplemental materials are available.

Competing interests The authors have no competing interests in this study.

Funding Not applicable.

References

1. De Simone B, Abu-Zidan FM, Saeidi S, et al. Knowledge, attitudes and practices of using Indocyanine Green (ICG) fluorescence in emergency surgery: an international web-based survey in the ARtificial Intelligence in Emergency and trauma Surgery (ARIES)—WSES project. Updat Surg. 2024; https://doi.org/10.1007/s13304-024-01853-z.
2. De Simone B, Abu-Zidan FM, Gumbs AA, et al. Knowledge, attitude, and practice of artificial intelligence in emergency and trauma surgery, the ARIES project: an international web-based survey. World J Emerg Surg. 2022;17:10. https://doi.org/10.1186/s13017-022-00413-3.
3. De Simone B, Chouillard E, Gumbs AA, et al. Artificial intelligence in surgery: the emergency surgeon's perspective (the ARIES project). Discov Health Syst. 2022;1:9. https://doi.org/10.1007/s44250-022-00014-6.
4. Diana M. Enabling precision digestive surgery with fluorescence imaging. Transl Gastroenterol Hepatol. 2017;2:97. https://doi.org/10.21037/tgh.2017.11.06.

5. Cassinotti E, Boni L, Baldari L. Application of indocyanine green (ICG)-guided surgery in clinical practice: lesson to learn from other organs-an overview on clinical applications and future perspectives. Updat Surg. 2023;75(2):357–65. https://doi.org/10.1007/s13304-022-01361-y. Epub 2022 Oct 6.
6. Diana M, Agnus V, Halvax P, Liu YY, Dallemagne B, Schlagowski AI, Geny B, Diemunsch P, Lindner V, Marescaux J. Intra- operative fluorescence-based enhanced reality laparoscopic real- time imaging to assess bowel perfusion at the anastomotic site in an experimental model. Br J Surg. 2015;102:e169–76.
7. de'Angelis N, Khan J, Marchegiani F, et al. Robotic surgery in emergency setting: 2021 WSES position paper. World J Emerg Surg. 2022;17:4.
8. Sermonesi G, Tian BWCA, Vallicelli C, et al. Cesena guidelines: WSES consensus statement on laparoscopic-first approach to general surgery emergencies and abdominal trauma. World J Emerg Surg. 2023;18:57. https://doi.org/10.1186/s13017-023-00520-9.
9. Ris F, Hompes R, Cunningham C, Lindsey I, Guy R, Jones O, George B, Cahill RA, Mortensen NJ. Near-infrared (NIR) perfusion angiography in minimally invasive colorectal surgery. Surg Endosc. 2014;28:2221–6. https://doi.org/10.1007/s00464-014-3432-y.
10. Jafari MD, Wexner SD, Martz JE, McLemore EC, Margolin DA, Sherwinter DA, Lee SW, Senagore AJ, Phelan MJ, Stamos MJ. Perfusion assessment in laparoscopic left-sided/anterior resection (PILLAR II): a multi-institutional study. J Am Coll Surg. 2015;220:82–92.e81. https://doi.org/10.1016/j.jamcollsurg.2014.09.015.
11. Alekseev M, Rybakov E, Shelygin Y, Chernyshov S, Zarodnyuk I. A study investigating the perfusion of colorectal anastomoses using fluorescence angiography: results of the FLAG randomized trial. Color Dis. 2020;22(9):1147–53. https://doi.org/10.1111/codi.15037. Epub 2020 Apr 6. PMID: 32189424.
12. De Nardi P, Elmore U, Maggi G, Maggiore R, Boni L, Cassinotti E, Fumagalli U, Gardani M, De Pascale S, Parise P, Vignali A, Rosati R. Intraoperative angiography with indocyanine green to assess anastomosis perfusion in patients undergoing laparoscopic colorectal resection: results of a multicenter randomized controlled trial. Surg Endosc. 2020;34(1):53–60. https://doi.org/10.1007/s00464-019-06730-0. Epub 2019 Mar 21. PMID: 30903276.
13. Joosten JJ, Longchamp G, Khan MF, Lameris W, van Berge Henegouwen MI, Bemelman WA, Cahill RA, Hompes R, Ris F. The use of fluorescence angiography to assess bowel viability in the acute setting: an international, multi-centre case series. Surg Endosc. 2022;36(10):7369–75. https://doi.org/10.1007/s00464-022-09136-7. Epub 2022 Feb 23. PMID: 35199204; PMCID: PMC9485089.
14. Nakashima K, Ryu S, Okamoto A, Hara K, Ishida K, Ito R, Nakabayashi Y. Usefulness of blood flow evaluation with indocyanine green fluorescence imaging during laparoscopic surgery for strangulated bowel obstruction: a cohort study. Asian J Surg. 2022;45(3):867–73. https://doi.org/10.1016/j.asjsur.2021.08.020. Epub 2021 Sep 10. PMID: 34518078.
15. Di Maggio F, Hossain N, De Zanna A, Husain D, Bonomo L. Near-infrared fluorescence cholangiography can be a useful adjunct during emergency cholecystectomies. Surg Innov. 2022;29(4):526–31. https://doi.org/10.1177/1553350620958562. Epub 2020 Sep 16.
16. Ryu S, Hara K, Goto K, Okamoto A, Kitagawa T, Marukuchi R, Ito R, Nakabayashi Y. Fluorescence angiography vs. direct palpation for bowel viability evaluation with strangulated bowel obstruction. Langenbeck's Arch Surg. 2022;407(2):797–803. https://doi.org/10.1007/s00423-021-02358-8. Epub 2021 Oct 19.
17. Stolz MP, Foxhall EN, Gibson BH, Gill S, McNamee MM. Improving the safety of laparoscopic cholecystectomy with indocyanine green dye using critical view of safety plus. Am Surg. 2023;89(7):3136–9. https://doi.org/10.1177/00031348231161659. Epub 2023 Mar 1.
18. D'Acapito F, Cucchetti A, Solaini L, Serenari M, Framarini M, Ercolani G. Fluorescence cholangiography using indocyanine green improves the identification of biliary structures during laparoscopic cholecystectomy. World J Surg. 2023;47(3):666–73. https://doi.org/10.1007/s00268-022-06854-w. Epub 2022 Dec 2.
19. van den Bos J, Schols RM, Boni L, Cassinotti E, Carus T, Luyer MD, Vahrmeijer AL, Mieog JSD, Warnaar N, Berrevoet F, van de Graaf F, Lange JF, Van Kuijk SMJ, Bouvy ND, Stassen

LPS. Near-infrared fluorescence cholangiography assisted laparoscopic cholecystectomy (FALCON): an international multicentre randomized controlled trial. Surg Endosc. 2023; https://doi.org/10.1007/s00464-023-09935-6. Epub ahead of print. PMID: 36849564.

20. Speich R, Saesseli B, Hoffmann U, Neftel KA, Reichen J. Anaphylactoid reactions after indocyanine-green administration. Ann Intern Med. 1988;109(4):345–6. https://doi.org/10.7326/0003-4819-109-4-345_2.
21. Yoneya S, Saito T, Komatsu Y, Koyama I, Takahashi K, Duvoll-Young J. Binding properties of indocyanine green in human blood. Invest Ophthalmol Vis Sci. 1998;39(7):1286–90.
22. De Simone B, Abu-Zidan FM, Boni L, et al. Indocyanine green fluorescence-guided surgery in the emergency setting: the WSES international consensus position paper. World J Emerg Surg. 2025;20:13. https://doi.org/10.1186/s13017-025-00575-w.
23. Flum DR, Dellinger EP, Cheadle A, Chan L, Koepsell T. Intraoperative cholangiography and risk of common bile duct injury during cholecystectomy. JAMA. 2003;289(13):1639–44.
24. Z'Graggen K, Wehrli H, Metzger A, Buehler M, Frei E, Klaiber C. Complications of laparoscopic cholecystectomy in Switzerland. A prospective 3-year study of 10,174 patients. Swiss association of laparoscopic and thoracoscopic surgery. Surg Endosc. 1998;12(11):1303–10. Crossref. PubMed.
25. Fletcher DR, Hobbs MST, Tan P, et al. Complications of cholecystectomy: risks of the laparoscopic approach and protective effects of operative cholangiography: a population-based study. Ann Surg. 1999;229(4):449–57. Crossref PubMed ISI.
26. Nuzzo G, Giuliante F, Giovannini I, et al. Bile duct injury during laparoscopic cholecystectomy: results of an Italian national survey on 56 591 cholecystectomies. Arch Surg. 2005;140(10):986–92. Crossref PubMed.
27. Waage A, Nilsson M. Iatrogenic bile duct injury: a population-based study of 152 776 cholecystectomies in the Swedish inpatient registry. Arch Surg. 2006;141(12):1207–13. Crossref PubMed.
28. Bandoh T, Shiraishi N, Yamashita Y, et al. Endoscopic surgery in Japan: the 12th national survey(2012-2013) by the Japan society for endoscopic surgery. Asian J Endosc Surg. 2017;10(4):345–53. Crossref PubMed.
29. Ausania F, Holmes LR, Ausania F, Iype S, Ricci P, White SA. Intraoperative cholangiography in the laparoscopic cholecystectomy era: why are we still debating? Surg Endosc. 2012;26(5):1193–200. Crossref PubMed.
30. Ford JA, Soop M, Du J, Loveday BPT, Rodgers M. Systematic review of intraoperative cholangiography in cholecystectomy. Br J Surg. 2012;99(2):160–7. Crossref. PubMed. ISI.
31. She WH, Cheung TT, Chan MY, Chu KW, Ma KW, Tsang SHY, Dai WC, Chan ACY, Lo CM. Routine use of ICG to enhance operative safety in emergency laparoscopic cholecystectomy: a randomized controlled trial. Surg Endosc. 2022;36(6):4442–51. https://doi.org/10.1007/s00464-021-08795-2. Epub 2022 Feb 22.
32. Lim SH, Tan HTA, Shelat VG. Comparison of indocyanine green dye fluorescent cholangiography with intra-operative cholangiography in laparoscopic cholecystectomy: a meta-analysis. Surg Endosc. 2021;35:1511–20. https://doi.org/10.1007/s00464-020-08164-5.
33. Pesce A, Piccolo G, Lecchi F, Fabbri N, Diana M, Feo CV. Fluorescent cholangiography: an up-to-date overview twelve years after the first clinical application. World J Gastroenterol. 2021;27(36):5989–6003. https://doi.org/10.3748/wjg.v27.i36.5989. PMID: 34629815; PMCID: PMC8476339.
34. Boni L, David G, Mangano A, Dionigi G, Rausei S, Spampatti S, Cassinotti E, Fingerhut A. Clinical applications of indocyanine green (ICG) enhanced fluorescence in laparoscopic surgery. Surg Endosc. 2015;29(7):2046–55. https://doi.org/10.1007/s00464-014-3895-x. Epub 2014 Oct 11. PMID: 25303914; PMCID: PMC4471386.
35. Vu VQ, Le VT, Nguyen HNA, Dang KK, Luong MVA. Preliminary results of laparoscopic cholecystectomy using real-time indocyanine green fluorescence: a cross-sectional study. Ann Med Surg (Lond). 2023;85(3):402. https://doi.org/10.1097/MS9.0000000000000261. PMID: 36923758; PMCID: PMC10010799.

36. Ankersmit M, van Dam DA, van Rijswijk AS, van den Heuvel B, Tuynman JB, Meijerink WJHJ. Fluorescent imaging with indocyanine green during laparoscopic cholecystectomy in patients at increased risk of bile duct injury. Surg Innov. 2017;24(3):245–52. https://doi.org/10.1177/1553350617690309. Epub 2017 Feb 8. PMID: 28178882; PMCID: PMC5431362.
37. Stolz MP, Foxhall EN, Gibson BH, Gill S, McNamee MM. Improving the safety of laparoscopic cholecystectomy with indocyanine green dye using critical view of safety plus. Am Surg. 2023:31348231161659. https://doi.org/10.1177/00031348231161659. Epub ahead of print.
38. Vlek SL, van Dam DA, Rubinstein SM, de Lange-de Klerk ESM, Schoonmade LJ, Tuynman JB, Meijerink WJHJ, Ankersmit M. Biliary tract visualization using near- infrared imaging with indocyanine green during laparoscopic cholecystectomy: results of a systematic review. Surg Endosc. 2017;31(7):2731–42. https://doi.org/10.1007/s00464-016-5318-7. Epub 2016 Nov 14. PMID: 27844236; PMCID: PMC5487840.
39. Baiocchi GL, Diana M, Boni L. Indocyanine green-based fluorescence imaging in visceral and hepatobiliary and pancreatic surgery: state of the art and future directions. World J Gastroenterol. 2018;24(27):2921–30. https://doi.org/10.3748/wjg.v24.i27.2921. PMID: 30038461; PMCID: PMC6054946.
40. Adaba F, et al. Mortality after acute primary mesenteric infarction: a systematic review and meta-analysis of observational studies. Color Dis. 2015;17(7):566–77.
41. Groesdonk HV, Klingele M, Schlempp S, et al. Risk factors for nonocclusive mesenteric ischemia after elective cardiac surgery. J Thorac Cardiovasc Surg. 2013;145:1603–10.
42. Mazzei MA, Volterrani L. Nonocclusive mesenteric ischaemia: think about it. Radiol Med. 2015;120:85–95.
43. Sheridan WG, Lowndes RH, Williams GT, Young HL. Determination of a critical level of tissue oxygenation in acute intestinal ischaemia. Gut. 1992;33(6):762–6. https://doi.org/10.1136/gut.33.6.762. PMID: 1624156; PMCID: PMC1379332.
44. Karampinis I, Keese M, Jakob J, Stasiunaitis V, Gerken A, Attenberger U, Post S, Kienle P, Nowak K. Indocyanine green tissue angiography can reduce extended bowel resections in acute mesenteric ischemia. J Gastrointest Surg. 2018;22(12):2117–24. https://doi.org/10.1007/s11605-018-3855-1. Epub 2018 Jul 10.
45. Kassahun WT, et al. Unchanged high mortality rates from acute occlusive intestinal ischemia: six year review. Langenbeck's Arch Surg. 2008;393(2):163–71.
46. Mamode N, Pickford I, Leiberman P. Failure to improve outcome in acute mesenteric ischaemia: seven-year review. Eur J Surg. 1999;165(3):203–8.
47. Nerup N, Svendsen MBS, Rønn JH, Konge L, Svendsen LB, Achiam MP. Quantitative fuorescence angiography aids novice and experienced surgeons in performing intestinal resection in well-perfused tissue. Surg Endosc. 2021; https://doi.org/10.1007/s00464-021-08518-7.
48. Guerra F, Coletta D, Greco PA, Eugeni E, Patriti A. The use of indocyanine green fluorescence to define bowel microcirculation during laparoscopic surgery for acute small bowel obstruction. Color Dis. 2021;23(8):2189–94. https://doi.org/10.1111/codi.15680. Epub 2021 May 5.
49. Karliczek A, Harlaar NJ, Zeebregts CJ, Wiggers T, Baas PC, van Dam GM. Surgeons lack predictive accuracy for anastomotic leakage in gastrointestinal surgery. Int J Color Dis. 2009;24:569–76. https://doi.org/10.1007/s00384-009-0658-6.
50. Hyman N, Manchester TL, Osler T, Burns B, Cataldo PA. Anastomotic leaks after intestinal anastomosis: it's later than you think. Ann Surg. 2007;245:254–8.
51. Jannasch O, Klinge T, Otto R, Chiapponi C, Udelnow A, Lippert H, et al. Risk factors, short and long term outcome of anastomotic leaks in rectal cancer. Oncotarget. 2015;6:36884–93.
52. Kang J, Choi GS, Oh JH, et al. Multicenter analysis of long-term oncologic impact of anastomotic leakage after laparoscopic total mesorectal excision: the Korean Laparoscopic Colorectal Surgery Study Group. Medicine (Baltimore). 2015;94:e1202.
53. Vignali A, Gianotti L, Braga M, Radaelli G, Malvezzi L, Di Carlo V. Altered micro perfusion of the rectal stump is predictive for rectal anastomotic leak. Dis Colon Rectum. 2000;30:867–71.

54. Jafari MD, Lee KH, Halabi WJ, Mills SD, Carmichael JC, Stamos MJ, Pigazzi A. The use of indocyanine green fuorescence to assess anastomotic perfusion during robotic assisted laparoscopic rectal surgery. Surg Endosc. 2013;27:3003–8. https://doi.org/10.1007/s00464-013-2832-8.
55. Sherwinter DA. Transanal near-infrared imaging of colorectal anastomotic perfusion. Surg Laparosc Endosc Percutan Tech. 2012;22:433–6. https://doi.org/10.1097/SLE.0b013e3182601eb8.
56. Kudszus S, Roesel C, Schachtrupp A, Höer JJ. Intraoperative laser fuorescence angiography in colorectal surgery: a noninvasive analysis to reduce the rate of anastomotic leakage. Langenbecks Arch Surg. 2010;395:1025–30. https://doi.org/10.1007/s00423-010-0699-x.
57. Wada T, Kawada K, Takahashi R, Yoshitomi M, Hida K, Hasegawa S, Sakai Y. ICG fuorescence imaging for quantitative evaluation of colonic perfusion in laparoscopic colorectal surgery. Surg Endosc. 2017;31:4184–93. https://doi.org/10.1007/s00464-017-5475-3.
58. Ryu S, Suwa K, Kitagawa T, Aizawa M, Ushigome T, Okamoto T, Eto K, Yanaga K. Evaluation of anastomosis with ICG fuorescence method using VISERA ELITE2 during laparoscopic colorectal cancer surgery. Anticancer Res. 2020;40:373–7. https://doi.org/10.21873/anticanres.13962.
59. Son GM, Kwon MS, Kim Y, Kim J, Kim SH, Lee JW. Quantitative analysis of colon perfusion pattern using indocyanine green (ICG) angiography in laparoscopic colorectal surgery. Surg Endosc. 2019;33:1640–9. https://doi.org/10.1007/s00464-018-6439-y.
60. Boni L, David G, Dionigi G, Rausei S, Cassinotti E, Fingerhut A. Indocyanine green-enhanced fuorescence to assess bowel perfusion during laparoscopic colorectal resection. Surg Endosc. 2016;30:2736–42. https://doi.org/10.1007/s00464-015-4540-z.
61. Wada T, Kawada K, Hoshino N, Inamoto S, Yoshitomi M, Hida K, Sakai Y. The efects of intraoperative ICG fuorescence angiography in laparoscopic low anterior resection: a propensity score-matched study. Int J Clin Oncol. 2019;24:394–402. https://doi.org/10.1007/s10147-018-1365-5.
62. Watanabe J, Ishibe A, Suwa Y, Suwa H, Ota M, Kunisaki C, Endo I. Indocyanine green fuorescence imaging to reduce the risk of anastomotic leakage in laparoscopic low anterior resection for rectal cancer: a propensity score-matched cohort study. Surg Endosc. 2020;34:202–8. https://doi.org/10.1007/s00464-019-06751-9.
63. Hagiwara C, Wakabayashi T, Tsutsui A, Sakamoto J, Fujita S, Fujiyama Y, Okamoto N, Omura K, Naitoh T, Wakabayashi G. Time required for indocyanine green fluorescence emission for evaluating bowel perfusion in left-sided colon and rectal cancer surgery. Surg Endosc. 2023;37(10):7876–83. https://doi.org/10.1007/s00464-023-10356-8.
64. Marquardt C, Kalev G, Schiedeck T. Intraoperative fuorescence angiography with indocyanine green: retrospective evaluation and detailed analysis of our single-center 5-year experience focused on colorectal surgery. Innov Surg Sci. 2020;5:35–42.
65. Ris F, et al. Multicentre phase II trial of near-infrared imaging in elective colorectal surgery. Br J Surg. 2018;105:1359–67.
66. Blanco-Colino R, Espin-Basany E. Intraoperative use of ICG fluorescence imaging to reduce the risk of anastomotic leakage in colorectal surgery: a systematic review and meta-analysis. Tech Coloproctol. 2018;22(1):15–23. https://doi.org/10.1007/s10151-017-1731-8. Epub 2017 Dec 11.
67. Meijer RPJ, Faber RA, Bijlstra OD, Braak JPBM, Meershoek-Klein Kranenbarg E, Putter H, Mieog JSD, Burggraaf K, Vahrmeijer AL, Hilling DE, AVOID study group. AVOID; a phase III, randomised controlled trial using indocyanine green for the prevention of anastomotic leakage in colorectal surgery. BMJ Open. 2022;12(4):e051144. https://doi.org/10.1136/bmjopen-2021-051144. PMID: 35365509; PMCID: PMC8977759.
68. Liu D, Liang L, Liu L, Zhu Z. Does intraoperative indocyanine green fluorescence angiography decrease the incidence of anastomotic leakage in colorectal surgery? A systematic review and meta-analysis. Int J Color Dis. 2021;36(1):57–66. https://doi.org/10.1007/s00384-020-03741-5. Epub 2020 Sep 18.

69. Song M, Liu J, Xia D, Yao H, Tian G, Chen X, Liu Y, Jiang Y, Li Z. Assessment of intraoperative use of indocyanine green fluorescence imaging on the incidence of anastomotic leakage after rectal cancer surgery: a PRISMA-compliant systematic review and meta-analysis. Tech Coloproctol. 2021;25(1):49–58. https://doi.org/10.1007/s10151-020-02335-1. Epub 2020 Sep 3.
70. Tang G, Du D, Tao J, Wei Z. Effect of indocyanine green fluorescence angiography on anastomotic leakage in patients undergoing colorectal surgery: a meta-analysis of randomized controlled trials and propensity-score-matched studies. Front Surg. 2022;9:815753. https://doi.org/10.3389/fsurg.2022.815753. PMID: 35372484; PMCID: PMC8964518.
71. Zhang W, Che X. Effect of indocyanine green fluorescence angiography on preventing anastomotic leakage after colorectal surgery: a meta-analysis. Surg Today. 2021;51(9):1415–28. https://doi.org/10.1007/s00595-020-02195-0. Epub 2021 Jan 11.
72. Mok HT, Ong ZH, Yaow CYL, Ng CH, Buan BJL, Wong NW, Chong CS. Indocyanine green fluorescent imaging on anastomotic leakage in colectomies: a network meta-analysis and systematic review. Int J Color Dis. 2020;35(12):2365–9. https://doi.org/10.1007/s00384-020-03723-7. Epub 2020 Aug 26.
73. Emile SH, Khan SM, Wexner SD. Impact of change in the surgical plan based on indocyanine green fluorescence angiography on the rates of colorectal anastomotic leak: a systematic review and meta-analysis. Surg Endosc. 2022;36(4):2245–57. https://doi.org/10.1007/s00464-021-08973-2. Epub 2022 Jan 13.
74. Lin J, Zheng B, Lin S, Chen Z, Chen S. The efficacy of intraoperative ICG fluorescence angiography on anastomotic leak after resection for colorectal cancer: a meta-analysis. Int J Color Dis. 2021;36(1):27–39. https://doi.org/10.1007/s00384-020-03729-1. Epub 2020 Sep 4.
75. Jafari MD, Pigazzi A, McLemore EC, Mutch MG, Haas E, Rasheid SH, Wait AD, Paquette IM, Bardakcioglu O, Safar B, Landmann RG, Varma MG, Maron DJ, Martz J, Bauer JJ, George VV, Fleshman JW Jr, Steele SR, Stamos MJ. Perfusion assessment in left-sided/low anterior resection (PILLAR III): a randomized, controlled, parallel, multicenter study assessing perfusion outcomes with PINPOINT near-infrared fluorescence imaging in low anterior resection. Dis Colon Rectum. 2021;64(8):995–1002. https://doi.org/10.1097/DCR.0000000000002007.
76. Pang HY, Chen XL, Song XH, Galiullin D, Zhao LY, Liu K, Zhang WH, Yang K, Chen XZ, Hu JK. Indocyanine green fluorescence angiography prevents anastomotic leakage in rectal cancer surgery: a systematic review and meta-analysis. Langenbeck's Arch Surg. 2021;406(2):261–71. https://doi.org/10.1007/s00423-020-02077-6. Epub 2021 Jan 7.
77. Lauricella S, Peyser D, Carrano FM, Sylla P. Intraluminal anastomotic assessment using indocyanine green near-infrared imaging for left-sided colonic and rectal resections: a systematic review. J Gastrointest Surg. 2023;27(3):615–25. https://doi.org/10.1007/s11605-022-05564-x. Epub 2023 Jan 5.
78. Li Z, Zhou Y, Tian G, Liu Y, Jiang Y, Li X, Song M. Meta-analysis on the efficacy of indocyanine green fluorescence angiography for reduction of anastomotic leakage after rectal cancer surgery. Am Surg. 2021;87(12):1910–9. https://doi.org/10.1177/0003134820982848. Epub 2020 Dec 30.
79. Safiejko K, Tarkowski R, Kozlowski TP, Koselak M, Jachimiuk M, Tarasik A, Pruc M, Smereka J, Szarpak L. Safety and efficacy of indocyanine green in colorectal cancer surgery: a systematic review and meta-analysis of 11,047 patients. Cancers (Basel). 2022;14(4):1036. https://doi.org/10.3390/cancers14041036. PMID: 35205784; PMCID: PMC8869881.
80. Degett TH, Andersen HS, Gögenur I. Indocyanine green fluorescence angiography for intraoperative assessment of gastrointestinal anastomotic perfusion: a systematic review of clinical trials. Langenbeck's Arch Surg. 2016;401(6):767–75. https://doi.org/10.1007/s00423-016-1400-9. Epub 2016 Mar 11.
81. Shen Y, Yang T, Yang J, Meng W, Wang Z. Intraoperative indocyanine green fluorescence angiography to prevent anastomotic leak after low anterior resection for rectal cancer: a meta-analysis. ANZ J Surg. 2020;90(11):2193–200. https://doi.org/10.1111/ans.15809. Epub 2020 Mar 11.

82. Rausa E, Zappa MA, Kelly ME, Turati L, Russo A, Aiolfi A, Bonitta G, Sgroi LG. A standardized use of intraoperative anastomotic testing in colorectal surgery in the new millennium: is technology taking over? A systematic review and network meta-analysis. Tech Coloproctol. 2019;23(7):625–31. https://doi.org/10.1007/s10151-019-02034-6. Epub 2019 Jul 13.
83. Mizrahi I, Wexner SD. Clinical role of fluorescence imaging in colorectal surgery - a review. Expert Rev Med Devices. 2017;14(1):75–82. https://doi.org/10.1080/17434440.2017.1265444. Epub 2016 Dec 5.
84. Gosvig K, Jensen SS, Qvist N, Agnus V, Jensen TS, Lindner V, Marescaux J, Diana M, Ellebæk MB. Remote computer-assisted analysis of ICG fluorescence signal for evaluation of small intestinal anastomotic perfusion: a blinded, randomized, experimental trial. Surg Endosc. 2020;34(5):2095–102. https://doi.org/10.1007/s00464-019-06990-w. Epub 2019 Jul 22.
85. Deng J, Hu W, Li Y, Xiong K, Yue T, Lai X, Xiao T. Meta analysis of indocyanine green fluorescence in patients undergoing laparoscopic colorectal cancer surgery. Front Oncol. 2022;12:1010122. https://doi.org/10.3389/fonc.2022.1010122. PMID: 36387166; PMCID: PMC9645423.
86. Han SR, Lee CS, Bae JH, Lee HJ, Yoon MR, Al-Sawat A, Lee DS, Lee IK, Lee YS. Quantitative evaluation of colon perfusion after high versus low ligation in rectal surgery by indocyanine green: a pilot study. Surg Endosc. 2022;36(5):3511–9. https://doi.org/10.1007/s00464-021-08673-x. Epub 2021 Aug 9.
87. Trastulli S, Munzi G, Desiderio J, Cirocchi R, Rossi M, Parisi A. Indocyanine green fluorescence angiography versus standard intraoperative methods for prevention of anastomotic leak in colorectal surgery: meta-analysis. Br J Surg. 2021;108(4):359–72. https://doi.org/10.1093/bjs/znaa139.
88. Arezzo A, Bonino MA, Ris F, Boni L, Cassinotti E, Foo DCC, Shum NF, Brolese A, Ciarleglio F, Keller DS, Rosati R, De Nardi P, Elmore U, Fumagalli Romario U, Jafari MD, Pigazzi A, Rybakov E, Alekseev M, Watanabe J, Vettoretto N, Cirocchi R, Passera R, Forcignanò E, Morino M. Intraoperative use of fluorescence with indocyanine green reduces anastomotic leak rates in rectal cancer surgery: an individual participant data analysis. Surg Endosc. 2020;34(10):4281–90. https://doi.org/10.1007/s00464-020-07735-w. Epub 2020 Jun 18.
89. Baiocchi GL, Guercioni G, Vettoretto N, Scabini S, Millo P, Muratore A, Clementi M, Sica G, Delrio P, Longo G, Anania G, Barbieri V, Amodio P, Di Marco C, Baldazzi G, Garulli G, Patriti A, Pirozzi F, De Luca R, Mancini S, Pedrazzani C, Scaramuzzi M, Scatizzi M, Taglietti L, Motter M, Ceccarelli G, Totis M, Gennai A, Frazzini D, Di Mauro G, Capolupo GT, Crafa F, Marini P, Ruffo G, Persiani R, Borghi F, de Manzini N, Catarci M. ICG fluorescence imaging in colorectal surgery: a snapshot from the ICRAL study group. BMC Surg. 2021;21(1):190. https://doi.org/10.1186/s12893-021-01191-6. PMID: 33838677; PMCID: PMC8035779.
90. Pekkari P, Bylund PO, Lindgren H, Öman M. Abdominal injuries in a low trauma volume hospital: a descriptive study from northern Sweden. Scand J Trauma Resusc Emerg Med. 2014;22:48.
91. Arikanoglu Z, et al. Factors afecting morbidity and mortality in hollow visceral injuries following blunt abdominal trauma. Clin Ter. 2014;165:23–6. when compared to elective resection. All these factors also impair bowel perfusion and are recognised as risk factors for AL.
92. Swaid F, et al. Concomitant hollow viscus injuries in patients with blunt hepatic and splenic injuries: an analysis of a National Trauma Registry database. Injury. 2014;45:1409–12.
93. Abbasi HR, et al. Pattern of traumatic injuries and injury severity score in a major trauma center in Shiraz, Southern Iran. Bull Emerg Trauma. 2013;1:81–5.
94. Afifi I, Abdelrahman H, El-Faramawy A, Mahmood I, Khoschnau S, Al-Naimi N, El-Menyar A, Al-Thani H, Rizoli S. The use of Indocyanine green fluorescent in patients with abdominal trauma for better intraoperative decision-making and less bowel anastomosis leak: case series. J Surg Case Rep. 2021;2021(6):rjab235. https://doi.org/10.1093/jscr/rjab235. PMID: 34150193; PMCID: PMC8208799.

95. Green JM 3rd, Sabino J, Fleming M, Valerio I. Intraoperative fluorescence angiography: a review of applications and outcomes in war-related trauma. Mil Med. 2015;180:37–43.
96. Yamaguchi K, Abe T, Nakajima K, Watanabe C, Kawamura Y, Suwa H, Minami Y, Nojiri K, Ono H, Yoshida K, Masui H, Doi T, Takeuchi I. Use of near-infrared imaging using indocyanine green associates with the lower incidence of postoperative complications for intestinal and mesenteric injury. Sci Rep. 2021;11(1):23880. https://doi.org/10.1038/s41598-021-03361-1. PMID: 34903816; PMCID: PMC8669015.
97. Kono Y, Ishizawa T, Tani K, Harada N, Kaneko J, Saiura A, Bandai Y, Kokudo N. Techniques of fluorescence cholangiography during laparoscopic cholecystectomy for better delineation of the bile duct anatomy. Medicine (Baltimore). 2015;94:e1005.
98. Soares AS, Bano S, Clancy NT, Stoyanov D, Lovat LB, Chand M. Multisensor perfusion assessment cohort study: preliminary evidence toward a standardized assessment of indocyanine green fluorescence in colorectal surgery. Surgery. 2022;172(1):69–73. https://doi.org/10.1016/j.surg.2021.12.021. Epub 2022 Feb 12.
99. Moskovitz AH, Bush WH Jr, Horvath KD. Anaphylactoid reaction to intraoperative cholangiogram. Report of a case review of the literature, and guidelines for prevention. Surg Endosc. 2001;15:1227. https://doi.org/10.1007/s004640042036.
100. Heeman W, Steenbergen W, van Dam G, Boerma EC. Clinical applications of laser speckle contrast imaging: a review. J Biomed Opt. 2019;24(8):1–11. https://doi.org/10.1117/1.JBO.24.8.080901. PMID: 31385481; PMCID: PMC6983474.
101. Nwaiwu CA, Buharin VE, Mach A, et al. Feasibility and comparison of laparoscopic laser speckle contrast imaging to near-infrared display of indocyanine green in intraoperative tissue blood flow/tissue perfusion in preclinical porcine models. Surg Endosc. 2023;37:1086–95. https://doi.org/10.1007/s00464-022-09583-2.
102. Meira J, Marques ML, Falcão-Reis F, Rebelo Gomes E, Carneiro Â. Immediate reactions to fluorescein and indocyanine green in retinal angiography: review of literature and proposal for patient's evaluation. Clin Ophthalmol. 2020;14:171–8. https://doi.org/10.2147/OPTH.S234858. PMID: 32021082; PMCID: PMC6980835.
103. Kwiterovich KA, Maguire MG, Murphy RP, et al. Frequency of adverse systemic reactions after fluorescein angiography. Results of a prospective study. Ophthalmology. 1991;98(7):1139–42. https://doi.org/10.1016/S0161-6420(91)32165-1.
104. Losurdo P, Giunta C, Modica A, de Manzini N, Bortul M. Near-infrared indocyanine green fluorescent cholangiography in urgent and emergency laparoscopic cholecystectomy: a preliminary study after propensity score-matched study. Eur J Trauma Emerg Surg. 2024;50(1):275–81. https://doi.org/10.1007/s00068-023-02340-7. Epub 2023 Aug 4. PMID: 37540247; PMCID: PMC10924024.
105. von Kroge PH, Russ D, Rieß HC, Debus ES, Pinnschmidt HO, Izbicki JR, Mann O, Wipper SH, Duprée A. The impact of nitroglycerine and volume on gastric tube microperfusion assessed by indocyanine green fluorescence imaging. Sci Rep. 2022;12(1):22394. https://doi.org/10.1038/s41598-022-26545-9. PMID: 36575280; PMCID: PMC9794817.
106. Chen Q, Zhou R, Weng J, et al. Extrahepatic biliary tract visualization using near-infrared fluorescence imaging with indocyanine green: optimization of dose and dosing time. Surg Endosc. 2021;35(10):5573–82. https://doi.org/10.1007/s00464-020-08058-6.
107. Aranda FP, Škrabec CG, López-Sánchez J, Pinedo AZ, Álvarez FE, Pérez MC, López JN, Vicente CH, Piñeiro LV, Andorrà EC. Indocyanine green (ICG) fluorescent cholangiography in laparoscopic cholecystectomy: simplifying time and dose. Dig Liver Dis. 2023;55(2):249–53. ISSN 1590-8658. https://doi.org/10.1016/j.dld.2022.10.023.
108. Liu H, Kuang J, Xu Y, et al. Investigation of the optimal indocyanine green dose in real-time fluorescent cholangiography during laparoscopic cholecystectomy with an ultra-high-definition 4K fluorescent system: a randomized controlled trial. Updat Surg. 2023;75:1903–10. https://doi.org/10.1007/s13304-023-01557-w.
109. Tagaya N, Shimoda M, Kato M, Nakagawa A, Abe A, Iwasaki Y, et al. Intraoperative exploration of biliary anatomy using fluorescence imaging of indocyanine green in experimental and clinical cholecystectomies. J Hepatobiliary Pancreat Sci. 2010;17(5):595–600.

110. Zroback C, Chow G, Meneghetti A, Warnock G, Meloche M, Chiu CJ, et al. Fluorescent cholangiography in laparoscopic cholecystectomy: the initial Canadian experience. Am J Surg. 2016;211(5):933–7.
111. Igami T, Nojiri M, Shinohara K, Ebata T, Yokoyama Y, Sugawara G, et al. Clinical value and pitfalls of fluorescent cholangiography during single-incision laparoscopic cholecystectomy. Surg Today. 2016;46(12):1443–50.
112. Schols RM, Bouvy ND, Masclee AA, van Dam RM, Dejong CH, Stassen LP. Fluorescence cholangiography during laparoscopic cholecystectomy: a feasibility study on early biliary tract delineation. Surg Endosc. 2013;27(5):1530–6.
113. Ishizawa T, Bandai Y, Ijichi M, Kaneko J, Hasegawa K, Kokudo N. Fluorescent cholangiography illuminating the biliary tree during laparoscopic cholecystectomy. Br J Surg. 2010;97(9):1369–77.
114. Aoki T, Murakami M, Yasuda D, Shimizu Y, Kusano T, Matsuda K, et al. Intraoperative fluorescent imaging using indocyanine green for liver mapping and cholangiography. J Hepatobiliary Pancreat Sci. 2010;17(5):590–4.
115. Mitsuhashi N, Kimura F, Shimizu H, Imamaki M, Yoshidome H, Ohtsuka M, et al. Usefulness of intraoperative fluorescence imaging to evaluate local anatomy in hepatobiliary surgery. J Hepato-Biliary-Pancreat Surg. 2008;15(5):508–14.
116. Haritoglou C, Gandorfer A, Schaumberger M, Tadayoni R, Gandorfer A, Kampik A. Light-absorbing properties and osmolarity of indocyanine-green depending on concentration and solvent medium. Invest Ophthalmol Vis Sci. 2003;44(6):2722–9.
117. Broderick RC, Lee AM, Cheverie JN, et al. Fluorescent cholangiography significantly improves patient outcomes for laparoscopic cholecystectomy. Surg Endosc. 2021;35(10):5729–39. https://doi.org/10.1007/s00464-020-08045-x.
118. Gadiyaram S, Thota RK. Near-infrared fluorescence guided laparoscopic cholecystectomy in the spectrum of complicated gallstone disease. Medicine (United States). 2022;101(42):E31170. https://doi.org/10.1097/MD.0000000000031170.
119. Larsen SS, Schulze S, Bisgaard T. Non-radiographic intraoperative fluorescent cholangiography is feasible. Dan Med J. 2014;61(8):1–5.
120. Dip F, Roy M, Menzo EL, Simpfendorfer C, Szomstein S, Rosenthal RJ. Routine use of fluorescent incisionless cholangiography as a new imaging modality during laparoscopic cholecystectomy. Surg Endosc. 2015;29(6):1621–6. https://doi.org/10.1007/s00464-014-3853-7.
121. Dip FD, Nahmod M, Alle L, Sarotto L, Anzorena FS, Ferraina P. Fluorescence cholangiography in laparoscopic cholecystectomy experience in Argentina. In: Fluorescent imaging: treatment of hepatobiliary and pancreatic diseases, vol. 31. S. Karger AG; 2013. p. 80–5. https://doi.org/10.1159/000348621.
122. Quaresima S, Balla A, Palmieri L, et al. Routine near infra-red indocyanine green fluorescent cholangiography versus intraoperative cholangiography during laparoscopic cholecystectomy: a case-matched comparison. Surg Endosc. 2020;34(5):1959–67. https://doi.org/10.1007/s00464-019-06970-0.
123. Hiwatashi K, Okumura H, Setoyama T, et al. Evaluation of laparoscopic cholecystectomy using indocyanine green cholangiography including cholecystitis: a retrospective study. Medicine (United States). 2018;97(30) https://doi.org/10.1097/MD.0000000000011654.
124. Martinez-Onate A d J, Martinez-Salas A d J, Cazares-Garcia V. Fluorescence guided cholecystectomy by a single group: initial 47 procedures experience in Mexico. J Soc Laparoendosc Surg. 2022;26(3) https://doi.org/10.4293/JSLS.2022.00043.
125. Daskalaki D, Fernandes E, Wang X, et al. Indocyanine green (ICG) fluorescent cholangiography during robotic cholecystectomy: results of 184 consecutive cases in a single institution. Surg Innov. 2014;21(6):615–21. https://doi.org/10.1177/1553350614524839.
126. Tsutsui N, Yoshida M, Ito E, Ohdaira H, Kitajima M, Suzuki Y. Laparoscopic cholecystectomy using the PINPOINT® Endoscopic Fluorescence Imaging System with intraoperative fluorescent imaging for acute cholecystitis: a case report. Ann Med Surg. 2018;35:146–8. https://doi.org/10.1016/j.amsu.2018.09.019.

127. Dip F, LoMenzo E, Sarotto L, et al. Randomized trial of near-infrared incisionless fluorescent cholangiography. Ann Surg. 2019;270(6):992–9. https://doi.org/10.1097/SLA.0000000000003178.
128. Schols RM, Bouvy ND, Van Dam RM, Masclee AAM, Dejong CHC, Stassen LPS. Combined vascular and biliary fluorescence imaging in laparoscopic cholecystectomy. Surg Endosc. 2013;27(12):4511–7. https://doi.org/10.1007/s00464-013-3100-7.
129. Ishizuka M, Nagata H, Takagi K, et al. Usefulness of intraoperative observation using a fluorescence imaging instrument for patients with nonocclusive mesenteric ischemia. Int Surg. 2015;100(4):593–9. https://doi.org/10.9738/INTSURG-D-14-00038.1.
130. Nitta T, Kataoka J, Ohta M, et al. Laparoscopic cholecystectomy for cholecystitis using direct gallbladder indocyanine green injection fluorescence cholangiography: a case report. Ann Med Surg. 2020;57:218–22. https://doi.org/10.1016/j.amsu.2020.07.057.
131. Liu YY, Kong SH, Diana M, et al. Near-infrared cholecysto-cholangiography with indocyanine green may secure cholecystectomy in difficult clinical situations: proof of the concept in a porcine model. Surg Endosc. 2016;30(9):4115–23. https://doi.org/10.1007/s00464-015-4608-9.
132. Boogerd LSF, Handgraaf HJM, Huurman VAL, Lam HD, Mieog JSD, Van Der Made WJ, Van De Velde CJH, Vahrmeijer AL. The best approach for laparoscopic fluorescence cholangiography: overview of the literature and optimization of dose and dosing time. Surg Innov. 2017;24:386–96.
133. Zarrinpar A, Dutson EP, Mobley C, Busuttil RW, Lewis CE, Tillou A, Cheaito A, Hines OJ, Agopian VG, Hiyama DT. Intraoperative laparoscopic near-infrared fluorescence cholangiography to facilitate anatomical identification: when to give indocyanine green and how much. Surg Innov. 2016;23:360–5. https://doi.org/10.1177/1553350616637671.
134. Tsutsui N, Yoshida M, Nakagawa H, Ito E, Iwase R, Suzuki N, Imakita T, Ohdaira H, Kitajima M, Yanaga K, Suzuki Y. Optimal timing of preoperative indocyanine green administration for fluorescent cholangiography during laparoscopic cholecystectomy using the PINPOINT® endoscopic fluorescence imaging system. Asian J Endosc Surg. 2018;11:199–205. https://doi.org/10.1111/ases.12440.
135. Verbeek FP, Schaafsma BE, Tummers QR, van der Vorst JR, van der Made WJ, Baeten CI, et al. Optimization of near-infrared fluorescence cholangiography for open and laparoscopic surgery. Surg Endosc. 2014;28(4):1076–82.
136. Agnus V, Pesce A, Boni L, et al. Fluorescence-based cholangiography: preliminary results from the IHU-IRCAD-EAES EURO-FIGS registry. Surg Endosc. 2020;34(9):3888–96. https://doi.org/10.1007/s00464-019-07157-3.
137. Gené Škrabec C, Pardo Aranda F, Espín F, et al. Fluorescent cholangiography with direct injection of indocyanine green (ICG) into the gallbladder: a safety method to outline biliary anatomy. Langenbeck's Arch Surg. 2020;405(6):827–32. https://doi.org/10.1007/s00423-020-01967-z.
138. Osayi SN, Wendling MR, Drosdeck JM, Chaudhry UI, Perry KA, Noria SF, et al. Near-infrared fluorescent cholangiography facilitates identification of biliary anatomy during laparoscopic cholecystectomy. Surg Endosc. 2015;29(2):368–75.
139. Wang C, Peng W, Yang J, Li Y, Yang J, Hu X, Xia L, Zhang L, Zhong Y, Qiao L, Pan W. Application of near-infrared fluorescent cholangiography using indocyanine green in laparoscopic cholecystectomy. J Int Med Res. 2020;48:300060520979224.
140. Morales-Conde S, Licardie E, Alarcón I, Balla A. Indocyanine green (ICG) fluorescence guide for the use and indications in general surgery: recommendations based on the descriptive review of the literature and the analysis of experience. Cir Esp. 2022;100(9):534–54. https://doi.org/10.1016/j.ciresp.2021.11.018.
141. Castagneto-Gissey L, Russo MF, Iodice A, Casella-Mariolo J, Serao A, Picchetto A, D'Ambrosio G, Urciuoli I, De Luca A, Salvati B, et al. Intracholecystic versus Intravenous Indocyanine Green (ICG) injection for biliary anatomy evaluation by fluorescent cholangiography during laparoscopic cholecystectomy: a case–control study. J Clin Med. 2022;11:3508. https://doi.org/10.3390/jcm11123508.

142. Ishizawa T, Kaneko J, Inoue Y, Takemura N, Seyama Y, Aoki T, et al. Application of fluorescent cholangiography to single-incision laparoscopic cholecystectomy. Surg Endosc. 2011;25(8):2631–6.
143. Madsen MH, Svendsen LB, Achiam MP. Quantification of fluorescence angiography in a porcine model. Langenbeck's Arch Surg. 2017;402:655–62.
144. Gianchandani Moorjani R, Díaz García A, Rosat Rodrigo A, Barrera Gómez M. Use of ICG to evaluate the viability of intestine during laparoscopic transabdominal hernioplasty in emergency surgery of incarcerated hernia. Cir Esp. 2021;99:313–4. https://doi.org/10.1016/j.ciresp.2020.05.014.
145. Daskalopoulou D, Kankam J, Plambeck J, Ambe PC, Zarras K. Intraoperative real-time fluorescence angiography with indocyanine green for evaluation of intestinal viability during surgery for an incarcerated obturator hernia: a case report. Patient Saf Surg. 2018;12:24. https://doi.org/10.1186/s13037-018-0173-1.
146. Ryu S, Yoshida M, Ohdaira H, Tsutsui N, Suzuki N, Ito E, et al. A case of incarcerated femoral hernia with intestinal blood flow assessment by brightfield full-color near-infrared fluorescence camera: report of a case. Int J Surg Case Rep. 2016;29:234–6. https://doi.org/10.1016/j.ijscr.2016.11.041.
147. Ryu S, Yoshida M, Ohdaira H, Tsutsui N, Suzuki N, Ito E, et al. Blood flow evaluation using PINPOINT® in a case of incarcerated inguinal hernia: a case report. Asian J Endosc Surg. 2017;10:75–8.
148. Ryu S, Yoshida M, Ohdaira H, Tsutsui N, Suzuki N, Ito E, et al. Intestinal blood flow assessment by indocyanine green fluorescence imaging in a patient with the incarcerated umbilical hernia: report of a case. Ann Med Surg (Lond). 2016;8:40–2.
149. Alexander K, Ismail M, Alexander M, Ivan T, Olga V, Dmitry S, et al. Use of ICG imaging to confirm bowel viability after upper mesenteric stenting in patient with acute mesenteric ischemia: case report. Int J Surg Case Rep. 2019;61:322–6.
150. Nakagawa Y, Kobayashi K, Kuwabara S, Shibuya H, Nishimaki T. Use of indocyanine green fluorescence imaging to determine the area of bowel resection in non-occlusive mesenteric ischemia: a case report. Int J Surg Case Rep. 2018;51:352–7. https://doi.org/10.1016/j.ijscr.2018.09.024.
151. Miyashita R, Kitazawa M, Tokumaru S, et al. Importance of intraoperative indocyanine green imaging in the management of non-occlusive mesenteric ischemia: a case report. Surg Case Rep. 2023;9(1) https://doi.org/10.1186/s40792-023-01614-x.
152. Furusawa K, Yoshimitsu M, Matsukawa H, Oi K, Yunoki K, Tamura A. Precise diagnosis of acute mesenteric ischemia using indocyanine green imaging prevents small bowel resection: a case report. Int J Surg Case Rep. 2022;97 https://doi.org/10.1016/j.ijscr.2022.107463.
153. Liot E, Assalino M, Buchs NC, et al. Does near-infrared (NIR) fluorescence angiography modify operative strategy during emergency procedures? Surg Endosc. 2018;32(10):4351–6. https://doi.org/10.1007/s00464-018-6226-9.
154. Iinuma Y, Hirayama Y, Yokoyama N, et al. Intraoperative near-infrared indocyanine green fluorescence angiography (NIR-ICG AG) can predict delayed small bowel stricture after ischemic intestinal injury: report of a case. J Pediatr Surg. 2013;48(5):1123–8. https://doi.org/10.1016/j.jpedsurg.2013.03.067.
155. Irie T, Matsutani T, Hagiwara N, et al. Successful treatment of non-occlusive mesenteric ischemia with indocyanine green fluorescence and open-abdomen management. Clin J Gastroenterol. 2017;10(6):514–8. https://doi.org/10.1007/s12328-017-0779-3.
156. Nowak K, Sandra-Petrescu F, Post S, Horisberger K. Ischemic and injured bowel evaluation by fluorescence imaging. Color Dis. 2015;17:12–5. https://doi.org/10.1111/codi.13032.
157. Meyer J, Joshi H, Buchs NC, Ris F, Davies J. Fluorescence angiography likely protects against anastomotic leak in colorectal surgery: a systematic review and meta-analysis of randomised controlled trials. Surg Endosc. 2022;36(10):7775–80. https://doi.org/10.1007/s00464-022-09255-1.
158. Reinhart MB, Huntington CR, Blair LJ, Heniford BT, Augenstein VA. Indocyanine Green. Surg Innov. 2016;23(2):166–75. https://doi.org/10.1177/1553350615604053.

159. Alander JT, Kaartinen I, Laakso A, Pätilä T, Spillmann T, Tuchin VV, Venermo M, Välisuo P. A review of indocyanine green fluorescent imaging in surgery. Int J Biomed Imaging. 2012;2012:940585. https://doi.org/10.1155/2012/940585.
160. Vos JJ, Wietasch JK, Absalom AR, Hendriks HG, Scheeren TW. Green light for liver function monitoring using indocyanine green? An overview of current clinical applications. Anaesthesia. 2014;69:1364–76.
161. Haertel F, Nuding S, Reisberg D, Peters M, Werdan K, Schulze PC, Ebelt H. The prognostic value of a liver function test using Indocyanine Green (ICG) clearance in patients with Multiple Organ Dysfunction Syndrome (MODS). J Clin Med. 2024;13(4):1039. https://doi.org/10.3390/jcm13041039. PMID: 38398351; PMCID: PMC10888702.
162. Sakka SG, Reinhart K, Meier-Hellmann A. Prognostic value of the indocyanine green plasma disappearance rate in critically ill patients. Chest. 2002;122:1715–20. https://doi.org/10.1378/chest.122.5.1715.
163. Esposito C, Settimi A, Del Conte F, Cerulo M, Coppola V, Farina A, Crocetto F, Ricciardi E, Esposito G, Escolino M. Image-guided pediatric surgery using Indocyanine Green (ICG) fluorescence in laparoscopic and robotic surgery. Front Pediatr. 2020;8:314. https://doi.org/10.3389/fped.2020.00314. PMID: 32626676; PMCID: PMC7311575.
164. Wang X, Zhang Y, Yang H, Xu Y. Maternal-fetal transfer of indocyanine green: a systematic review. J Matern Fetal Neonatal Med. 2022;35(25):8181–5. https://doi.org/10.1080/14767058.2021.1966410. Epub 2021 Sep 26. PMID: 34565270.
165. Breuking EA, van Varsseveld OC, Harms M, Tytgat SHAJ, Hulscher JBF, Ruiterkamp J. Safety and feasibility of indocyanine green fluorescence angiography in pediatric gastrointestinal surgery: a systematic review. J Pediatr Surg. 2023;58(8):1534–42. https://doi.org/10.1016/j.jpedsurg.2022.10.045. Epub 2022 Oct 24.
166. Shibasaki J, Hara H, Mihara M, Adachi S, Uchida Y, Itani Y. Evaluation of lymphatic dysplasia in patients with congenital pleural effusion and ascites using indocyanine green lymphography. J Pediatr. 2014;164(5):1116–1120.e1. https://doi.org/10.1016/j.jpeds.2013.12.052. Epub 2014 Feb 8.
167. Shirotsuki R, Uchida H, Tanaka Y, et al. Novel thoracoscopic navigation surgery for neonatal chylothorax using indocyanine-green fluorescent lymphography. J Pediatr Surg. 2018;53(6):1246–9. https://doi.org/10.1016/j.jpedsurg.2018.01.019. PMID: 29486888.
168. Probst P, Paumgartner G, Caucig H, Fröhlich H, Grabner G. Studies on clearance and placental transfer of indocyanine green during labor. Clin Chim Acta. 1970;29(1):157–60. ISSN 0009-8981. https://doi.org/10.1016/0009-8981(70)90237-8.
169. Zammarrelli WA 3rd, Afonso AM, Broach V, Sonoda Y, Zivanovic O, Mueller JJ, Leitao MM Jr, Chan A, Abu-Rustum NR. Sentinel lymph node biopsy in patients with endometrial cancer and an indocyanine green or iodinated contrast reaction - A proposed management algorithm. Gynecol Oncol. 2021;162(2):262–7. https://doi.org/10.1016/j.ygyno.2021.05.009. Epub 2021 May 13. PMID: 33992449; PMCID: PMC8319058.
170. Schwarz C, Plass I, Fitschek F, et al. The value of indocyanine green clearance assessment to predict postoperative liver dysfunction in patients undergoing liver resection. Sci Rep. 2019;9:8421. https://doi.org/10.1038/s41598-019-44815-x.
171. De Gasperi A, Mazza E, Prosperi M. Indocyanine green kinetics to assess liver function: ready for a clinical dynamic assessment in major liver surgery? World J Hepatol. 2016;8(7):355–67. https://doi.org/10.4254/wjh.v8.i7.355. PMID: 26981173; PMCID: PMC4779164.
172. Halle BM, Poulsen TD, Pedersen HP. Indocyanine green plasma disappearance rate as dynamic liver function test in critically ill patients. Acta Anaesthesiol Scand. 2014;58(10):1214–9. https://doi.org/10.1111/aas.12406.
173. Mathes A, Plata C, Rensing H, Kreuer S, Fink T, Raddatz A. Plasma disappearance rate of indocyanine green for determination of liver function in three different models of shock. Diagnostics (Basel). 2019;9(3):108. https://doi.org/10.3390/diagnostics9030108. PMID: 31480421; PMCID: PMC6787744.
174. Grischke EM, Röhm C, Hahn M, Helms G, Brucker S, Wallwiener D. ICG fluorescence technique for the detection of sentinel lymph nodes in breast cancer: results of a

prospective open-label clinical trial. Geburtshilfe Frauenheilkd. 2015;75(9):935–40. https://doi.org/10.1055/s-0035-1557905. PMID: 26500370.
175. Eriksson AG, Montovano M, Beavis A, Soslow RA, Zhou Q, Abu-Rustum NR, Gardner GJ, Zivanovic O, Barakat RR, Brown CL, Levine DA, Sonoda Y, Leitao MM Jr, Jewell EL. Impact of obesity on sentinel lymph node mapping in patients with newly diagnosed uterine cancer undergoing robotic surgery. Ann Surg Oncol. 2016;23(8):2522–8. https://doi.org/10.1245/s10434-016-5134-2. Epub 2016 Feb 23. PMID: 26905542.
176. Insalaco G, Incognito GG, Genovese F, et al. Impact of obesity in the identification of the sentinel lymph node in endometrial cancer: a retrospective, monocentric study and literature review. Arch Gynecol Obstet. 2024; https://doi.org/10.1007/s00404-024-07386-5.
177. Koong JK, Ng GH, Ramayah K, Koh PS, Yoong BK. Early identification of the critical view of safety in laparoscopic cholecystectomy using indocyanine green fluorescence cholangiography: a randomised controlled study. Asian J Surg. 2021;44:537–43.
178. Dip F, Nguyen D, Montorfano L, et al. Accuracy of near infrared-guided surgery in morbidly obese subjects undergoing laparoscopic cholecystectomy. Obes Surg. 2016;26:525–30. https://doi.org/10.1007/s11695-015-1781-9.
179. Liu YY, Liao CH, Diana M, Wang SY, Kong SH, Yeh CN, et al. Near-infrared cholecystocholangiography with direct intragallbladder indocyanine green injection: preliminary clinical results. Surg Endosc. 2017;32(3):15061514.
180. Vinegoni C, Botnaru I, Aikawa E, Calfon MA, Iwamoto Y, Folco EJ, Ntziachristos V, Weissleder R, Libby P, Jaffer FA. Indocyanine green enables near-infrared fluorescence imaging of lipid-rich, inflamed atherosclerotic plaques. Sci Transl Med. 2011;3(84):84ra45. https://doi.org/10.1126/scitranslmed.3001577. PMID: 21613624; PMCID: PMC3112179.
181. Rother U, Amann K, Adler W, et al. Quantitative assessment of microperfusion by indocyanine green angiography in kidney transplantation resembles chronic morphological changes in kidney specimens. Microcirculation. 2019;26:e12529.
182. D'Urso A, Agnus V, Barberio M, et al. Computer-assisted quantification and visualization of bowel perfusion using fluorescence-based enhanced reality in left-sided colonic resections. Surg Endosc. 2021;35:4321–31. https://doi.org/10.1007/s00464-020-07922-9.
183. Al-Taher M, Pruimboom T, Schols RM, et al. Influence of intraoperative vasopressor use on indocyanine green fluorescence angiography: first evaluation in an experimental model. Sci Rep. 2021;11:9650. https://doi.org/10.1038/s41598-021-89223-2.
184. Polom K, Murawa D, Rho YS, Nowaczyk P, Hünerbein M, Murawa P. Current trends and emerging future of indocyanine green usage in surgery and oncology. Cancer. 2011;117(21):4812–22. https://doi.org/10.1002/cncr.26087.
185. Marano A, Priora F, Lenti LM, Ravazzoni F, Quarati R, Spinoglio G. Application of fluorescence in robotic general surgery: review of the literature and state of the art. World J Surg. 2013;37(12):2800–11. https://doi.org/10.1007/s00268-013-2066-x.
186. Osterkamp JTF, Patel MQ, Steyn E, Svendsen LB, Forgan T, Achiam MP. Usability of fluorescence angiography with indocyanine green in the surgical management of penetrating abdominal trauma: a case series. Int J Surg Open. 2021;30:100319. https://doi.org/10.1016/j.ijso.2021.02.001.
187. Ugur M, Akkucuk S, Koca YS, Oruc C, Aydogan A. Missed injuries in patients with abdominal gunshot trauma: risk factors and mortality rates. Eur Surg. 2016;48(6):347–51. https://doi.org/10.1007/s10353-016-0411-7.
188. Muckart DJJ, Thomson SR. Undetected injuries: a preventable cause of increased morbidity and mortality. Am J Surg. 1991;162(5):457–60. https://doi.org/10.1016/0002-9610(91)90260-K.
189. Kärkkäinen JM, Acosta S. Acute mesenteric ischemia (part I)—incidence, etiologies, and how to improve early diagnosis. Best Pract Res Clin Gastroenterol. 2017;31(1):15–25. https://doi.org/10.1016/j.bpg.2016.10.018.
190. Ahmed T, Pai MV, Mallik E, et al. Applications of indocyanine green in surgery: a single center case series. Ann Med Surg. 2022;77 https://doi.org/10.1016/j.amsu.2022.103602.

191. Törnqvist B, Waage A, Zheng Z, Ye W, Nilsson M. Severity of acute cholecystitis and risk of iatrogenic bile duct injury during cholecystectomy, a population-based case–control study. World J Surg. 2016;40(5):1060–7. https://doi.org/10.1007/s00268-015-3365-1.
192. Jansen S, Doerner J, Macher-Heidrich S, Zirngibl H, Ambe PC. Outcome of acute perforated cholecystitis: a register study of over 5000 cases from a quality control database in Germany. Surg Endosc. 2017;31(4):1896–900. https://doi.org/10.1007/s00464-016-5190-5.
193. Ren T, Tacey M, Peart LM, Kang YC, Hodgson R. A predictive tool for choledocholithiasis in patients undergoing emergency cholecystectomy. J Laparoendosc Adv Surg Tech. 2023;33(3):263–8. https://doi.org/10.1089/lap.2022.0384.

Managing Difficult Cholecystectomies and Hepatobiliary Procedures with AI

15

Marcello Di Martino, Simone Famularo,
Marco Nicolazzi, Emanuele Tessitore,
and Matteo Donadon

15.1 AI in the Medical and Surgical Field with Special Regard to Cholecystectomies and HPB Surgery

The long journey towards the development of the current concept of Artificial Intelligence (AI) began with Alan Turing defining intelligent behavior in a machine as the ability to achieve human-level performance in cognitive tasks [1]. Since then, AI has made enormous progress, becoming integrated into our daily routines. In the medical field, AI can be categorized into two main subtypes: virtual and physical [2].

The virtual aspect ranges from applications such as handling substantial volumes of data and unveiling complex patterns or trends to providing guidance in diagnosis or treatment decisions.

To this purpose, AI comprises various approaches and methodologies, including machine learning (ML) methods, which involve the ability of computers to identify patterns and make predictions that improve continuously. Some of the most common ML algorithms include artificial neural networks (ANN) and decision tree algorithms. A further evolution of this technology is deep learning (DL), which involves hierarchical representations of data over different layers, also known as deep neural networks, allowing for more sophisticated decision-making. One of the most commonly used algorithms in DL is the convolutional neural network. When

M. Di Martino (✉) · M. Nicolazzi · E. Tessitore · M. Donadon (✉)
Department of Health Sciences, University of Piemonte Orientale, Novara, Italy

Division of Surgery, University Maggiore Hospital della Carità, Novara, Italy
e-mail: marcello.dimartino@uniupo.it; matteo.donadon@uniupo.it

S. Famularo
Hepatobiliary Surgery Unit, Foundation University Hospital 'Agostino Gemelli' IRCCS, Rome, Italy

IRCAD, Research Institute Against Cancer of the Digestive System, 1 Place de l'Hôpital, Strasbourg, France

B. De Simone et al. (eds.), *New Technologies, Precision Medicine, and AI in Emergency General Surgery*, Hot Topics in Acute Care Surgery and Trauma,
https://doi.org/10.1007/978-3-032-09357-8_15

data is widely spread, classic models often struggle to establish clear and reproducible patterns necessary for making accurate predictions. The modelling derived from ML and DL algorithms allows for the establishment of non-parametric associations that could be difficult to capture with traditional models [3]. Clinical applications of these methods include the analysis of specific characteristics of patients or diagnostic tests to increase their precision. AI has the potential to create predictive frameworks that are more efficient at identifying data characteristics and connections that may be unseen by humans, establishing novel associations between clinical parameters and surgical endpoints [4]. Similarly, radiomics is a field of medical imaging that aims to extract a large number of quantitative features from images and provide accurate predictions [5]. Additionally, visual AI applies algorithms to analyze and interpret visual data, allowing the identification of anatomical structures and landmarks, augmenting surgeons' decision-making processes, and supporting safer surgery [6]. Finally, precision medicine is a continuously expanding field based on the analysis of large amounts of patient-level data, such as clinical characteristics, biomarkers (e.g., the mutational status of tumors on surgical specimens or liquid biopsies), and other pre- or intra-operative data, to predict individual patient outcomes and tailor treatment plans [7, 8] (Fig. 15.1).

The physical aspect deals with tools for building personalised prostheses or assisting in performing surgeries. Virtual reality (VR) is defined as a computer-generated simulation of a three-dimensional environment that can be interacted with by a person using special equipment, such as a helmet with a screen inside. Augmented reality (AR) is a technology that overlays digital information on real-world elements, such as popular video games, where digital creatures appear in the real world. Mixed reality (MR) brings together real-world and digital elements: physical and virtual objects may co-exist in MR environments, and subjects can interact in real-time with both elements. The term "extended reality" (XR) has recently emerged as an umbrella term that encompasses all AR, VR, and MR applications (Fig. 15.2) [9].

In the surgical field, and especially in the hepato-pancreato-biliary (HPB) field [6], the main areas where AI has made or is making a significant contribution are:

- Preoperative evaluation of clinical cases, which includes patient selection for treatment allocation, radiomics, and preoperative modelling. AI-based software can help evaluate undetermined lesions, refine the accuracy of preoperative

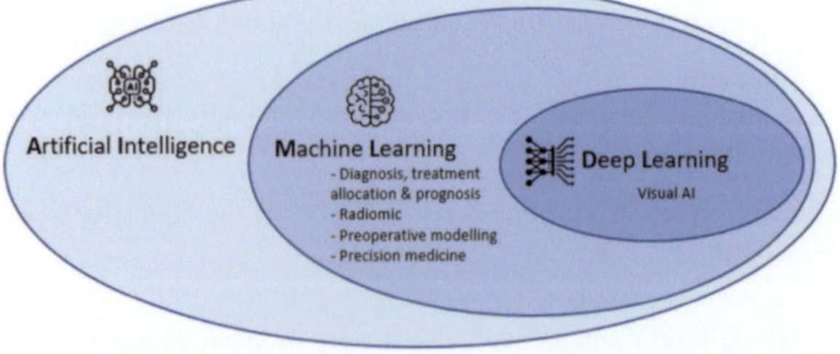

Fig. 15.1 Clinical applications of AI by machine learning and deep learning in the medical field

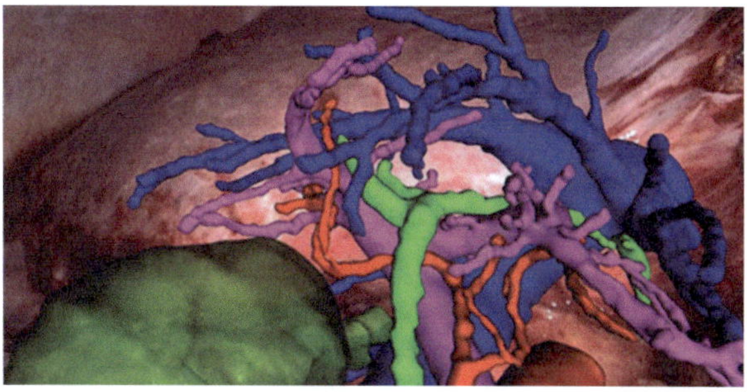

Fig. 15.2 Examples of clinical application of AR: AR visualization of a 3D liver model with the liver surface not displayed to allow a clearer view of blood vessels and bile ducts. (Reproduced from the open access publication by Schneider et al. [10])

imaging, improve the precision of treatment allocation strategies, and predict the prognosis for specific groups of patients [11].

- Intraoperative support with visual AI and surgical navigation methods. AI tools aim to assist the surgeon, especially in the context of challenging cholecystectomy or liver resections, by providing instruments for intraoperative support to decrease the likelihood of intraoperative injuries by identifying dangerous dissection zones, anatomical structures, or landmarks [12, 13].
- Postoperative outcome predictions promoting personalized treatment allocation strategies. AI, through the analysis of complex amounts of data, including genomic data from tissue samples, circulating cells, proteins, and nucleic acids, is making important contributions in the field of precision medicine by predicting oncological prognosis for specific groups of patients [14].

15.2 AI Applications for Preoperative Evaluation

The ability of ML to uncover associations that traditional models might miss, thereby creating novel predictive frameworks, opens new perspectives in the surgical field, potentially leading to improved patient outcomes [15]. An example is the model developed by Famularo et al. [11], which determined the optimal allocation of patients to a neoadjuvant approach rather than upfront surgery in cases of colorectal liver metastases. This model relied solely on clinical parameters. While previous literature primarily considered tumor burden and the timing of presentation as decisive factors for treatment approach, the model identified additional variables that significantly increased the efficacy of patient allocation. These variables included gender, CEA levels, primary tumor localization, and planned R1 vascular surgery—factors not previously recognized as predictors. The model demonstrated an accuracy rate of 88.6% and revealed that upfront surgery was appropriately administered in only 22% of cases. This finding highlights the power of ML models not only in their computational sophistication but also in their ability to recognize non-linear and non-parametric patterns in simple, dichotomized clinical variables.

The application of AI in diagnosis and clinical decision-making in elective and urgent HPB surgery is rapidly evolving. Regarding liver lesions, the preoperative diagnosis of certain hepatic lesions, such as adenomas with a higher risk of malignancy or hepatocellular carcinomas (especially in patients with chronic liver disease), remains challenging. A certain percentage of these patients will undergo liver biopsy, which is not always conclusive. Radiomics can aid in diagnosing malignant and high-risk lesions and predicting prognosis. Ying et al. [16] recently published the results of the Liver Artificial Intelligence Diagnosis System (LiAIDS), a fully automated diagnostic system based on a diverse sample of 12,610 patients from 18 hospitals. LiAIDS can identify potential focal liver lesions (FLL) and classify them into seven common types: malignant lesions, including hepatocellular carcinoma, intrahepatic cholangiocarcinoma, and liver metastases, or benign, such as focal nodular hyperplasia, hemangioma, adenoma, and cysts (Fig. 15.3). LiAIDS outperformed junior radiologists and matched senior radiologists in diagnosing FLL. Additionally, it improved the diagnostic accuracy of all radiologists.

Similarly, evaluating pancreatic cystic lesions at risk of malignancy follows this pattern. Although numerous guidelines describe precise morphological and biochemical criteria to select high-risk patients for surgical resection, these are not always accurate in everyday clinical practice. Watson et al. [17] used DL techniques based on computed tomography (CT) to predict the presence of adenocarcinoma or intraductal papillary mucinous neoplasm (IPMN) with high-grade dysplasia in resected pancreatic cystic lesions. A DL model was trained and tested, and its performance was compared with the Fukuoka guidelines criteria for selecting high-risk IPMN for surgical resection. The DL model outperformed the Fukuoka guidelines criteria: it would have avoided one missed malignancy and one unnecessary operation. Another relevant clinical challenge is the preoperative diagnosis of concurrent common bile duct (CBD) stones in patients undergoing cholecystectomy. Vukicevic et al. [18] exploited AI's ability and trained an ML algorithm to predict the likelihood of CBD stones in patients undergoing cholecystectomy. The model accounted for values of total bilirubin, alanine

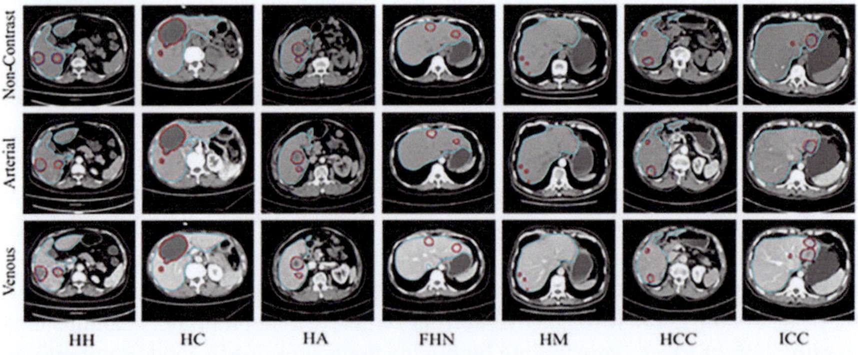

Fig. 15.3 Application of AI in the identification of various lesion types (green line: contours of liver predicted by the AI system; red line: contours of liver lesions predicted by the AI system; blue line: contours of liver lesions labelled by doctors). HH hepatic hemangioma, HC hepatic cyst, HA hepatic adenoma, FNH focal nodular hyperplasia, HM: hepatic metastasis, HCC hepatocellular carcinoma, ICC intrahepatic cholangiocarcinoma. (Reproduced from the open access publication by Ying et al. [16])

aminotransferase, common bile duct diameter, number of stones, size of the smallest calculus, and clinical settings (biliary colic, acute cholecystitis, or pancreatitis). It showed excellent accuracy in predicting concomitant CBD stones in patients undergoing cholecystectomy, with an area under the curve of 0.884, superior to the multivariable logistic regression model, which was 0.787. Finally, surgical emergencies represent another area where challenging and quick decisions can significantly modify patients' outcomes, and AI can offer sound decision-making support. The Predictive Optimal Trees in Emergency Surgery Risk (POTTER) and the Trauma Outcome Predictor (TOP) are examples of AI decision-making support tools designed to assist physicians in emergency settings [19]. Both models examined the American College of Surgeons National Surgical Quality Improvement Program data and trained ML algorithms to predict postoperative mortality and morbidity, showing good accuracy in diagnosis and outcome predictions. However, while there is some enthusiasm about AI's potential, divergent opinions and beliefs still exist in the surgical community regarding AI's role in emergency settings [12, 20]. In conclusion, these findings highlight the potential of AI models to support clinicians in the decision-making process, especially in challenging scenarios where precise and timely diagnosis can radically change the therapeutic approach for patients.

Another relevant clinical application of AI includes radiomics and preoperative surgical planning.

Radiomics is a technique used to extract detailed information from medical images. The process begins by identifying and segmenting a specific area of interest within the body, called the volume of interest (VOI). This VOI is represented as a stack of flat, like slices of a 3D object. Within this volume, smaller sections called regions of interest (ROIs) are selected from 2D images. By analyzing the pixel values within these ROIs, radiomics can provide a detailed texture analysis of the tissues, revealing new information that might not be visible to the naked eye. For example, a recent study by Ingwersen et al. [21] developed a tool called the radiomics preoperative Radiomic Fistula Risk Score (RAD-FRS). The study included two sets of data: a development set and a validation set. In the development set, CT scans from 118 patients were analyzed with the VOI representing the pancreatic remnant (Fig. 15.4). Radiomic features were then extracted, and four ML classifiers were used to develop the final RAD-FRS. The model included three radiomic features: one gray-level dependence matrix feature related to pancreatic texture and two 3D shape-based features related to the volume and thickness of the pancreatic remnant. In the training set, the RAD-FRS had an AUC of 0.90, with a sensitivity of 1.00, specificity of 0.67, positive predictive value (PPV) of 0.71, and negative predictive value (NPV) of 1.00. The validation set confirmed the predictive power of the model with an AUC of 0.81, sensitivity of 0.96, specificity of 0.66, PPV of 0.64, and NPV of 0.96. These results suggest that radiomic models, such as the RAD-FRS, can effectively predict the risk of developing a pancreatic fistula or other complications after surgery.

Surgical planning can also be improved through 3D reconstruction models, allowing for a more precise evaluation of the surgical resectability of tumors and

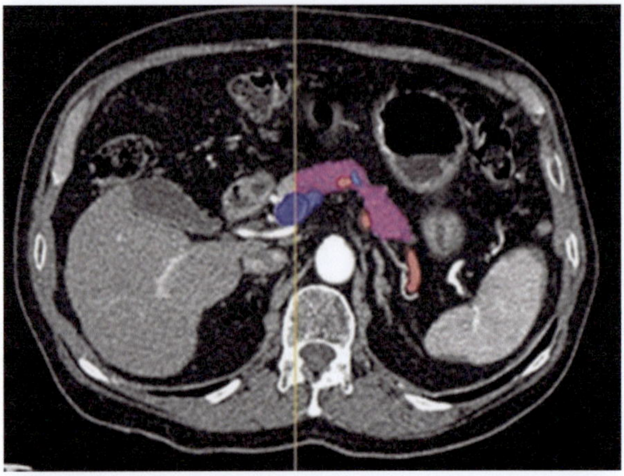

Fig. 15.4 Example of clinical application of radiomic: segmentation of pancreatic remnant to develop the RAD-FRS. (Reproduced from the open access publication by Ingwersen et al. [21])

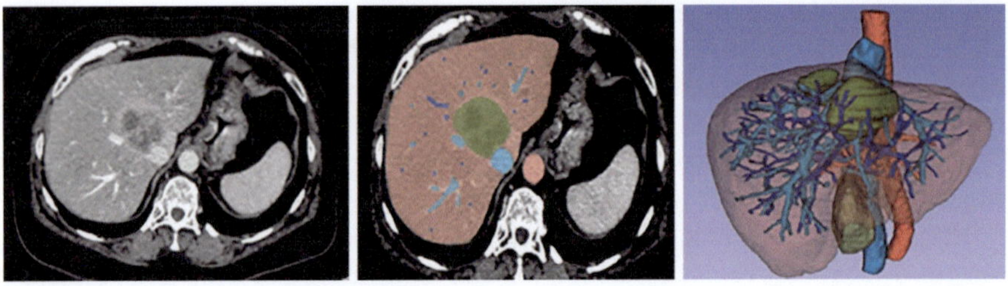

Fig. 15.5 Examples of 3D reconstruction models. Baseline CT image (left); segmented image (middle) where green; final 3D rendering (right) demonstrating corresponding anatomical structures

their anatomical relationships with adjacent structures [14]. Recent literature has highlighted that patient-specific 3D liver models may enhance the comprehension of patients' liver anatomy and thereby provide a useful preoperative planning and intraoperative guidance tool for liver resection [22]. Fang et al. [23] compared 3D visualization systems with traditional preoperative diagnostic systems in patients with pancreatic and periampullary tumors. They demonstrated that the diagnostic accuracy for resectability was 100%, and it was superior to CT. Additionally, 3D visualization techniques are also used to perform virtual liver resection (VLR) before actual surgery to assess the resectability of the lesion and calculate the future liver remnant (Fig. 15.5). A study by Mise et al. [24] compared outcomes of liver resections between patients in whom a VLR was performed and those without. Among HCC patients, portal territory-oriented resection was conducted more often in the VLR group than in the non-VLR group, and the 5-year disease-free survival rate for localized HCC was higher in the VLR group than in the non-VLR group (37.2% vs 23.9%; $P = 0.04$). Despite being an evolving field, 3D models seem to allow for a more precise evaluation of the surgical resectability of tumors and their anatomical relationships with adjacent structures.

15.3 AI Applications for Intraoperative Support

Several tools and instruments have been developed to enhance surgeons' performance and patient safety, potentially decreasing the risk of human errors.

Fluorescence-guided surgery has paved the way for AI-related research in intraoperative support. This technique is based on the ability of indocyanine green (ICG) to emit a fluorescent signal when excited by near-infrared (NIR) light. Over recent decades, NIR imaging has rapidly gained popularity due to ICG's ability to perfuse tissues and its biliary elimination properties [25]. Currently, it is used in surgical procedures for various purposes, such as:

(a) Identification of Anatomical Structures and Regions: During cholecystectomies, ICG allows real-time visualization and identification of extrahepatic biliary structures without the use of intraoperative cholangiography. This enables more precise identification of anatomical details and variants, particularly in difficult cholecystectomies [26]. Additionally, ICG-guided resection of liver lesions with real-time fluorescence guidance is particularly useful for anatomical liver resections [27].
(b) Lymph Node Identification and Mapping in Cancer Surgery: ICG-NIR imaging can identify sentinel lymph nodes, allowing surgeons to resect them [28].
(c) Perfusion of Surgical Anastomoses: This represents a promising optical imaging technique to reduce anastomotic leaks [29].

In recent years, advanced intraoperative optical imaging modalities have emerged, extending the surgeon's visual perception beyond the capabilities of the naked eye. Visual AI aims to enhance the relevance of ICG-NIR-guided surgery by potentially enabling landmark detection and phase recognition, thereby assisting surgeons with intraoperative decision-making. Several approaches based on DL models have been utilized [6, 30–33].

Hyperspectral imaging is a non-invasive technology that detects the relative reflectance of light, combining photography with spectroscopy to precisely identify characteristic tissue signatures. Initially developed for remote sensing, HSI has been successfully applied to various fields, such as military operations, environmental monitoring, geology, agriculture, and global change research. HSI offers several key advantages over other intraoperative imaging modalities because it utilizes contrast-free spectral cameras with many spectral bands. Combining HSI with DL can enhance the identification of characteristic tissue signatures, enabling automatic tissue recognition during surgery [34–37]. Madani et al. [38] combined the principles of HSI and semantic segmentation, which involve assigning a class label to every pixel of an image, and created the GoNoGoNet model. This model, supported by a DL algorithm, was able to delineate anatomical structures in surgical images and identify safe and dangerous anatomical areas, defined as GoZone and No-GoZone. When the model was applied in clinical practice, it demonstrated a 94% accuracy for No-GoZone and 90% for the GoZone. Those findings demonstrated the potential of AI in identifying safe and dangerous dissection zones, which

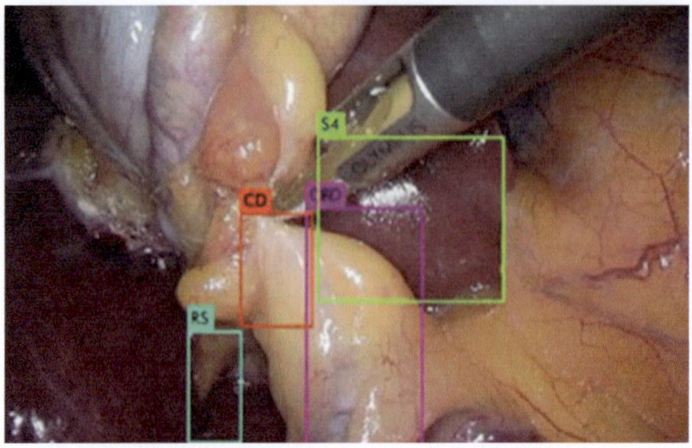

Fig. 15.6 Visual AI model showing bounding boxes for anatomical landmark. CD: cystic duct; CBD: common bile duct; S4: lower edge of the left medial segment; RS Rouviere's sulcus. (Reproduced from the open access publication by Tokuyasu et al. [41])

could enhance surgeons' performance and improve real-time decision-making. A recent study assessed the validity of GoNoGoNet [39]: surgeons and trainees performing laparoscopic cholecystectomy interacted with the AI platform and completed a survey to evaluate the educational value, usability, and design of the platform. The majority agreed or strongly agreed that the AI tool was an effective adjunct to surgical training (81%; neutral = 10%), providing real-time feedback (70%; neutral = 20%), postoperative feedback (73%; neutral = 27%), and capable of improving surgeon confidence (67%; neutral = 29%).

Alternatively, the You Only Look Once algorithm (YOLO) is a real-time object detection algorithm developed by J. Redmon and A. Farhadi in 2015 [40] that uses DL algorithms to predict the bounding boxes and class probabilities of objects in input images. Tokuyasu et al. [41] utilized the YOLOv3 technology to identify four landmarks: the cystic duct, CBD, lower edge of the left medial liver segment, and Rouviere's sulcus (Fig. 15.6). Their pilot study demonstrated that the YOLOv3 model accurately identified landmarks, with 22 out of 23 laparoscopic cholecystectomy videos showing concordance upon human verification.

Incorporating AR with visual AI allows the synchronization of 3D-reconstructed images with real-time surgery, representing a safer and more reliable surgical navigation method. From the early days of projecting liver models onto patients' surfaces to locate a better puncture point to today's assistance in performing liver resection or transplantation, AR has shown relevant possible advantages in surgery. Ntourakis et al. [42] reported in a pilot study that a 3D virtual anatomical model superimposed onto the operative field enhanced the detection of missing colorectal liver metastases after chemotherapy and guided their resection, resulting in a margin-negative resection status without any local recurrence. Nevertheless, the applications of these tools in the clinical practice are still very limited.

15.4 AI Tools and Postoperative Outcome Prediction

The ability to process and analyze vast amounts of data quickly and accurately means that ML can offer personalized treatment recommendations based on a comprehensive analysis of patient data. This represents a significant shift from the one-size-fits-all approach to a more tailored and precise methodology, enhancing patient care and outcomes [43]. An example showing the potential of this technology is an ML prediction model based on an Italian registry of patients with hepatocellular carcinoma (HERCOLES) and an external Japanese cohort [4]. The model was used to predict the risk of recurrence after liver resection for patients with hepatocellular carcinoma. It included variables such as treatment, age, cirrhosis, number and size of recurrent nodules, bilobar presentation, and extrahepatic spread and demonstrated a high predictive ability with AUC values for 3-year survival after resection of 0.805. Prediction models based on the analysis of complex amounts of data, including not only clinical but also genomic data from tissue samples, circulating cells, proteins, and nucleic acids, have the potential to make important contributions in the field of precision medicine.

15.5 Limitations

In clinical practice, the techniques described above still have very selective applications and are used in a limited number of centers and patients. None of the aforementioned applications are used routinely; instead, they still represent research projects and experimental models in the development phase. The main limitations that still exist, not only in clinical but also in experimental settings, include small sample sizes often collected from a single center; lack of collaboration and transparency; lack of external validation, resulting in poor generalizability of the currently available results.

15.6 Conclusions

In conclusion, the integration of AI into clinical practice is proving to be a transformative approach with the potential to revolutionize the diagnosis and treatment of complex and challenging gallbladder and HPB diseases. It could allow a more accurate preoperative evaluation of clinical cases, supporting the decision-making process, improving preoperative planning, and aiding intraoperative strategies. Additionally, based on the analysis of large amounts of data at an individual level, it could significantly boost the impact of precision medicine. Despite its potential, AI models still need to be further improved, validated, and integrated into treatment algorithms in real-life scenarios.

References

1. Ramesh AN, Kambhampati C, Monson JR, Drew PJ. Artificial intelligence in medicine. Ann R Coll Surg Engl. 2004;86(5):334–8.
2. Boutros C, Singh V, Ocuin L, Marks JM, Hashimoto DA. Artificial intelligence in hepatopancreaticobiliary surgery – promises and perils. Artif Intell Surg. 2022;2(4):213–23.
3. Martinino A, Aloulou M, Chatterjee S, Scarano Pereira JP, Singhal S, Patel T, et al. Artificial intelligence in the diagnosis of hepatocellular carcinoma: a systematic review. J Clin Med. 2022;11(21):6368.

4. Famularo S, Donadon M, Cipriani F, Fazio F, Ardito F, Iaria M, et al. Machine learning predictive model to guide treatment allocation for recurrent hepatocellular carcinoma after surgery. JAMA Surg. 2023;158(2):192–202.
5. Cannella R, Santinha J, Bèaufrere A, Ronot M, Sartoris R, Cauchy F, et al. Performances and variability of CT radiomics for the prediction of microvascular invasion and survival in patients with HCC: a matter of chance or standardisation? Eur Radiol. 2023;33(11):7618–28.
6. Mascagni P, Alapatt D, Sestini L, Altieri MS, Madani A, Watanabe Y, et al. Computer vision in surgery: from potential to clinical value. NPJ Digit Med. 2022;5(1):163.
7. Søreide K, Ismail W, Roalsø M, Ghotbi J, Zaharia C. Early diagnosis of pancreatic cancer: clinical premonitions, timely precursor detection and increased curative-intent surgery. Cancer Control. 2023;30:10732748231154711.
8. Podda M, Di Martino M, Ielpo B, Catena F, Coccolini F, Pata F, et al. The 2023 MANCTRA acute biliary pancreatitis care bundle: a joint effort between human knowledge and artificial intelligence (ChatGPT) to optimize the Care of Patients with Acute Biliary Pancreatitis in Western countries. Ann Surg. 2024;279(2):203–12.
9. Andrews C, Southworth MK, Silva JNA, Silva JR. Extended reality in medical practice. Curr Treat Options Cardiovasc Med. 2019;21(4):18.
10. Schneider C, Thompson S, Totz J, Song Y, Allam M, Sodergren MH, et al. Comparison of manual and semi-automatic registration in augmented reality image-guided liver surgery: a clinical feasibility study. Surg Endosc. 2020;34(10):4702–11.
11. Famularo S, Milana F, Cimino M, Franchi E, Giuffrida M, Costa G, et al. Upfront surgery versus Neoadjuvant perioperative chemotherapy for Resectable colorectal liver metastases: a machine-learning decision tree to identify the best potential candidates under a parenchyma-sparing policy. Cancer. 2023;15(3):613.
12. Cobianchi L, Piccolo D, Dal Mas F, Agnoletti V, Ansaloni L, Balch J, et al. Surgeons' perspectives on artificial intelligence to support clinical decision-making in trauma and emergency contexts: results from an international survey. World J Emerg Surg. 2023;18(1):1.
13. Ward TM, Hashimoto DA, Ban Y, Rosman G, Meireles OR. Artificial intelligence prediction of cholecystectomy operative course from automated identification of gallbladder inflammation. Surg Endosc. 2022;36(9):6832–40.
14. Bari H, Wadhwani S, Dasari BVM. Role of artificial intelligence in hepatobiliary and pancreatic surgery. World J Gastrointest Surg. 2021;13(1):7–18.
15. Perez M, Palnaes Hansen C, Burdio F, Sanchez-Velazquez P, Giuliani A, Lancellotti F, et al. A machine learning predictive model for recurrence of resected distal cholangiocarcinoma: development and validation of predictive model using artificial intelligence. Eur J Surg Oncol. 2024;50(7):108375.
16. Ying H, Liu X, Zhang M, Ren Y, Zhen S, Wang X, et al. A multicenter clinical AI system study for detection and diagnosis of focal liver lesions. Nat Commun. 2024;15(1):1131.
17. Watson MD, Lyman WB, Passeri MJ, Murphy KJ, Sarantou JP, Iannitti DA, et al. Use of artificial intelligence deep learning to determine the malignant potential of pancreatic cystic neoplasms with preoperative computed tomography imaging. Am Surg. 2021;87(4):602–7.
18. Vukicevic AM, Stojadinovic M, Radovic M, Djordjevic M, Cirkovic BA, Pejovic T, et al. Automated development of artificial neural networks for clinical purposes: application for predicting the outcome of choledocholithiasis surgery. Comput Biol Med. 2016;75:80–9.
19. Bertsimas D, Dunn J, Velmahos GC, Kaafarani HMA. Surgical risk is not linear: derivation and validation of a novel, user-friendly, and machine-learning-based predictive OpTimal trees in emergency surgery risk (POTTER) calculator. Ann Surg. 2018;268(4):574–83.
20. De Simone B, Abu-Zidan FM, Gumbs AA, Chouillard E, Di Saverio S, Sartelli M, et al. Knowledge, attitude, and practice of artificial intelligence in emergency and trauma surgery, the ARIES project: an international web-based survey. World J Emerg Surg. 2022;17(1):10.
21. Ingwersen EW, Bereska JI, Balduzzi A, Janssen BV, Besselink MG, Kazemier G, et al. Radiomics preoperative-Fistula Risk Score (RAD-FRS) for pancreatoduodenectomy: development and external validation. BJS Open. 2023;7(5):zrad100.

22. Rossi T, Williams A, Sun Z. Three-dimensional printed liver models for surgical planning and intraoperative guidance of liver cancer resection: a systematic review. Appl Sci. 2023;13(19):10757.
23. Fang CH, Tian J, Zhang P, Yee YY, Zhong SZ. Application of digital medical technology in hepatopancreatobiliary surgery: 20 years' retrospective review and prospect. Zhonghua wai ke za zhi [Chin J Surg]. 2021;59(10):807–11.
24. Mise Y, Hasegawa K, Satou S, Shindoh J, Miki K, Akamatsu N, et al. How has virtual hepatectomy changed the practice of liver surgery?: experience of 1194 virtual hepatectomy before liver resection and living donor liver transplantation. Ann Surg. 2018;268(1):127–33.
25. Schmidt EL, Ou Z, Ximendes E, Cui H, Keck CHC, Jaque D, et al. Near-infrared II fluorescence imaging. Nat Rev Methods Primers. 2024;4(1):23.
26. Cassinotti E, Al-Taher M, Antoniou SA, Arezzo A, Baldari L, Boni L, et al. European Association for Endoscopic Surgery (EAES) consensus on Indocyanine Green (ICG) fluorescence-guided surgery. Surg Endosc. 2023;37(3):1629–48.
27. Felli E, Ishizawa T, Cherkaoui Z, Diana M, Tripon S, Baumert TF, et al. Laparoscopic anatomical liver resection for malignancies using positive or negative staining technique with intraoperative indocyanine green-fluorescence imaging. HPB (Oxford). 2021;23(11):1647–55.
28. Grischke EM, Röhm C, Hahn M, Helms G, Brucker S, Wallwiener D. ICG fluorescence technique for the detection of sentinel lymph nodes in breast cancer: results of a prospective open-label clinical trial. Geburtshilfe Frauenheilkd. 2015;75(9):935–40.
29. Morales-Conde S, Alarcon I, Yang T, Licardie E, Camacho V, Aguilar Del Castillo F, et al. Fluorescence angiography with indocyanine green (ICG) to evaluate anastomosis in colorectal surgery: where does it have more value? Surg Endosc. 2020;34(9):3897–907.
30. Golany T, Aides A, Freedman D, Rabani N, Liu Y, Rivlin E, et al. Artificial intelligence for phase recognition in complex laparoscopic cholecystectomy. Surg Endosc. 2022;36(12):9215–23.
31. Laplante S, Namazi B, Kiani P, Hashimoto DA, Alseidi A, Pasten M, et al. Validation of an artificial intelligence platform for the guidance of safe laparoscopic cholecystectomy. Surg Endosc. 2023;37(3):2260–8.
32. Nakanuma H, Endo Y, Fujinaga A, Kawamura M, Kawasaki T, Masuda T, et al. An intraoperative artificial intelligence system identifying anatomical landmarks for laparoscopic cholecystectomy: a prospective clinical feasibility trial (J-SUMMIT-C-01). Surg Endosc. 2023;37(3):1933–42.
33. Hegde SR, Namazi B, Iyengar N, Cao S, Desir A, Marques C, et al. Automated segmentation of phases, steps, and tasks in laparoscopic cholecystectomy using deep learning. Surg Endosc. 2024;38(1):158–70.
34. Bannone E, Collins T, Esposito A, Cinelli L, De Pastena M, Pessaux P, et al. Surgical optomics: hyperspectral imaging and deep learning towards precision intraoperative automatic tissue recognition-results from the EX-MACHYNA trial. Surg Endosc. 2024;38:3758.
35. Mascagni P, Longo F, Barberio M, Seeliger B, Agnus V, Saccomandi P, et al. New intraoperative imaging technologies: innovating the surgeon's eye toward surgical precision. J Surg Oncol. 2018;118(2):265–82.
36. Barberio M, Benedicenti S, Pizzicannella M, Felli E, Collins T, Jansen-Winkeln B, et al. Intraoperative guidance using hyperspectral imaging: a review for surgeons. Diagnostics (Basel, Switzerland). 2021;11:11.
37. Felli E, Cinelli L, Bannone E, Giannone F, Muttillo EM, Barberio M, et al. Hyperspectral imaging in major Hepatectomies: preliminary results from the Ex-Machyna Trial. Cancer. 2022;14(22):5591.
38. Madani A, Namazi B, Altieri MS, Hashimoto DA, Rivera AM, Pucher PH, et al. Artificial intelligence for intraoperative guidance: using semantic segmentation to identify surgical anatomy during laparoscopic cholecystectomy. Ann Surg. 2022;276(2):363–9.
39. Hameed MS, Laplante S, Masino C, Khalid MU, Zhang H, Protserov S, et al. What is the educational value and clinical utility of artificial intelligence for intraoperative and postoperative video analysis? A survey of surgeons and trainees. Surg Endosc. 2023;37(12):9453–60.

40. YOLOv3: an incremental improvement. Available at: https://pjreddie.com/media/files/papers/YOLOv3.pdf. Accessed 20 June 2024.
41. Tokuyasu T, Iwashita Y, Matsunobu Y, Kamiyama T, Ishikake M, Sakaguchi S, et al. Development of an artificial intelligence system using deep learning to indicate anatomical landmarks during laparoscopic cholecystectomy. Surg Endosc. 2021;35(4):1651–8.
42. Ntourakis D, Memeo R, Soler L, Marescaux J, Mutter D, Pessaux P. Augmented reality guidance for the resection of missing colorectal liver metastases: an initial experience. World J Surg. 2016;40(2):419–26.
43. Simpson AL, Peoples J, Creasy JM, Fichtinger G, Gangai N, Keshavamurthy KN, et al. Preoperative CT and survival data for patients undergoing resection of colorectal liver metastases. Scientific Data. 2024;11(1):172.

Artificial Intelligence–Assisted Imaging, Computer-Vision, and Robotic Tools for Small Bowel and Colorectal Surgery

16

Georgios Peros and Ioannis I. Lazaridis

Abbreviations

3D	Three-Dimensional
AdaBoost	Adaptive Boosting
ADR	Adenoma Detection Rate
AI	Artificial Intelligence
CD	Crohn's Disease
CRC	Colorectal Cancer
CRS	Colorectal Surgery
CT	Computed Tomography
CV	Computer Vision
DRS	Diffuse Reflectance Spectroscopy
IBD	Inflammatory Bowel Disease
ICG	Indocyanine Green
Intra-op	Intraoperative
ML	Machine Learning
MRI	Magnetic Resonance Imaging
POI	Postoperative Ileus
Post-op	Postoperative
Pre-op	Preoperative
RTI	Real-Time Imaging
STAR	Smart Tissue Autonomous Robot
UC	Ulcerative Colitis
XGBoost	eXtreme Gradient Boosting

G. Peros (✉)
Department of Surgery, Clinic St. Anna, Luzern, Switzerland

I. I. Lazaridis
Department of Surgery, Limmattal Hospital, Zurich-Schlieren, Switzerland

B. De Simone et al. (eds.), *New Technologies, Precision Medicine, and AI in Emergency General Surgery*, Hot Topics in Acute Care Surgery and Trauma,
https://doi.org/10.1007/978-3-032-09357-8_16

16.1 Introduction

Small bowel and colorectal surgeries encompass a broad spectrum of conditions, including Crohn's disease, ulcerative colitis, colorectal cancer, diverticulitis, and small bowel obstructions. These disorders often present with complications such as fistulas, strictures, adhesions, or tumors, which can make surgical identification and dissection particularly demanding. Surgeons must carefully distinguish between diseased and healthy tissue, preserve critical anatomical structures such as major blood vessels and nerves, and minimize trauma to surrounding areas to enhance patient recovery and reduce postoperative complications.

Recent advancements in artificial intelligence (AI) and computer vision (CV) have revolutionized surgical practice, offering innovative solutions to enhance precision, efficiency, and safety, particularly in small bowel and colorectal procedures. These surgeries pose unique challenges due to the complex and variable anatomy, the dynamic nature of intraoperative conditions, and the necessity for meticulous tissue differentiation. AI-driven tools, including machine learning algorithms, real-time imaging enhancements, and robotic-assisted surgery, have significantly improved surgeons' ability to navigate these intricacies with heightened accuracy.

AI applications in surgery extend across multiple phases of patient care. In preoperative planning, AI can analyze imaging data to provide detailed insights into disease extent, helping surgeons strategize their approach. During surgery, real-time AI-powered guidance can aid in tissue classification, margin identification, and decision support, reducing the risk of errors. Postoperatively, AI can assist in monitoring patient recovery, predicting complications, and optimizing follow-up care [1]. These advancements collectively contribute to improved surgical outcomes, reduced operative times, and enhanced patient safety, highlighting the growing role of AI in modern colorectal and small bowel surgery. In Table 16.1 are shown the key points discussed in this chapter.

Table 16.1 AI in small bowel and colorectal surgery

Section	Key points
Introduction	AI and computer vision (CV) enhance precision, efficiency, and safety in colorectal and small bowel surgery. Applications span preoperative planning, intraoperative assistance, and postoperative monitoring
Preoperative Planning	AI analyzes imaging data (MRI, CT, endoscopy) to improve surgical planning. 3D modeling aids in vascular reconstructions and lymph node mapping, particularly in oncologic surgeries
IBD management	AI enhances lesion detection and classification in endoscopy, improving diagnosis and personalized treatment of Crohn's disease and ulcerative colitis. Deep learning models analyze histological features and predict immune cell patterns
Colorectal Cancer (CRC) Management	AI improves polyp detection in colonoscopy, enhances lymph node metastasis prediction, and assists in CRC staging. AI models improve metastatic lesion identification and patient outcome predictions

(continued)

Table 16.1 (continued)

Section	Key points
Intraoperative AI applications	AI-integrated robotic platforms enhance precision. Optical sensing technologies (e.g., DRS) distinguish cancerous from normal tissues. AI-driven fluorescence imaging optimizes perfusion assessment. Machine learning enhances robotic surgery techniques
Postoperative and follow-up	AI predicts complications like postoperative ileus and anastomotic leaks. Deep learning refines adjuvant therapy selection post-surgery, improving patient outcomes
Discussion and future perspectives	AI is revolutionizing colorectal surgery, but challenges remain: regulatory approval, data biases, ethical concerns, and surgeon-AI collaboration. Future advancements may include real-time AI integration, autonomous robotic systems, and AI-driven postoperative monitoring

16.2 Preoperative Planning

AI and computer vision are increasingly critical in preoperative planning. AI algorithms can analyze medical data, such as patient records and diagnostic findings, as well as medical imaging (e.g., MRI, CT scans, endoscopy), identifying patterns that may be difficult for humans to detect—such as the precise spread of a tumor or the presence of a fistula that might be obscured by conventional imaging techniques. This information enables more personalized surgical approaches and helps predict potential complications. Additionally, AI can generate highly detailed 3D models from CT scans, offering a level of precision in imaging that was previously unattainable, ultimately leading to more effective surgical planning [2].

The use of highly detailed 3D models generated from CT scans has revolutionized both preoperative planning and intraoperative guidance, enabling surgeons to avoid unnecessary tissue damage and minimize complications. These models are particularly valuable for vascular reconstructions, which play a crucial role in planning procedures such as right [3] and left [4] colectomies. By using advanced imaging techniques, surgeons can accurately map vascular structures, reducing the risk of inadvertent vascular injury and optimizing lymph node harvest. This precision is especially critical in oncologic surgeries, where thorough lymph node retrieval is often necessary for accurate staging and improved patient outcomes.

16.2.1 Inflammatory Bowel Disease

AI and CV are transforming the diagnosis of inflammatory bowel disease (IBD) by enhancing the detection, classification, and assessment of lesions in endoscopic imaging. These technologies can process vast amounts of visual data at a level of precision that could surpass human capability, enabling early and more accurate identification of lesions associated with IBD, such as ulcerations, inflammation, and mucosal abnormalities [5]. AI algorithms trained on extensive endoscopic datasets can identify subtle patterns indicative of disease severity and progression, improving diagnostic accuracy and consistency [6, 7]. Furthermore, computer vision models can be integrated into real-time endoscopy systems, providing gastroenterologists with immediate feedback during procedures and facilitating prompt clinical decision-making. This fusion of AI and computer vision not only accelerates diagnosis but also enhances personalized treatment planning by offering insights into disease characteristics, thereby supporting improved patient outcomes in IBD management. Deep learning models can be trained to identify key histological features of both Crohn's disease and ulcerative colitis using endoscopic labels. These models have demonstrated high accuracy in distinguishing between different disease types, normal and lesional tissues, and varying levels of disease severity.

Moreover, AI-driven visual attention maps help interpret the models' findings, revealing strong associations between predictions and inflammatory histopathological features. AI can also predict and analyze immune cell populations, such as plasma cells, providing valuable insights into disease pathology [8]. By improving diagnostic precision and aiding in patient stratification, these advancements have the potential to enhance clinical decision-making and the effectiveness of clinical trials.

16.2.2 Colorectal Cancer

Analog to the IBD, AI is evolving colorectal cancer (CRC) management by enhancing screening, diagnosis, and treatment. In colonoscopy, AI systems improve polyp detection and characterization, addressing limitations in current practices and leading to better patient outcomes. These advancements enable gastroenterologists to identify and assess polyps with accuracy comparable to expert interventionalists, reducing reliance on pathological evaluations and guiding appropriate resection techniques or referrals for complex procedures. Furthermore, AI-assisted techniques in routine screening represent a pivotal step in declining incidence rates of this malignancy [9, 10].

In fact, in a recent multicenter randomized controlled trial, it was shown that AI has significantly enhanced colonoscopy procedures by improving adenoma detection rates (ADR) in both symptomatic and asymptomatic patients [11]. This improvement is crucial, as higher ADRs are associated with a reduced risk of colorectal cancer. By integrating AI into colonoscopy, healthcare providers can achieve more accurate and efficient screenings, ultimately leading to better patient outcomes.

AI is also changing the CRC management in the detection and characterization of metastasis. AI models have demonstrated the potential to predict lymph node metastasis more accurately in rectal and colorectal cancer, enhancing preoperative staging and guiding treatment decisions [12]. By analyzing complex datasets, including imaging studies and genetic profiles, AI can identify patterns indicative of metastatic spread, enabling early intervention and personalized treatment strategies. Furthermore, AI enhances diagnostic accuracy by interpreting imaging modalities such as CT and MRI scans with greater precision, facilitating early detection of metastatic spread. In post-treatment scenarios, AI models can estimate recurrence risks, allowing for tailored surveillance and timely interventions. The integration of AI into CRC management signifies a transformative approach, offering clinicians advanced tools to combat metastasis more effectively.

There are also applications in the management of distal lesions. AI analyses can assist clinicians in all phases of colorectal liver metastases' natural history, from predicting their occurrence to increasing diagnostic accuracy and estimating recurrence risk after treatment and patient outcome. By leveraging machine learning algorithms, AI can predict the likelihood of metastasis by analyzing complex datasets, including genetic profiles and imaging studies. This predictive capability enables personalized treatment strategies, potentially improving patient outcomes. Furthermore, AI enhances diagnostic accuracy by interpreting imaging modalities such as CT and MRI scans with greater precision, facilitating early detection of metastatic spread. In follow-up, AI models can estimate recurrence risks, allowing for tailored surveillance and timely interventions. The integration of AI into CRC management signifies a transformative approach, offering clinicians advanced tools to combat metastasis more effectively [13].

16.3 Intraoperative

AI is increasingly being integrated into surgical procedures, particularly through robotic platforms, to enhance precision and outcomes. While AI has established a presence in general surgery, its application in colorectal surgery is still evolving. A promising development is the use of optical sensing technologies, such as diffuse reflectance spectroscopy (DRS), to differentiate tumor tissue from healthy tissue during surgery. Studies have demonstrated that DRS can effectively distinguish between cancerous and normal tissues in real-time, offering high sensitivity and specificity [14, 15]. This capability is crucial for ensuring complete tumor removal while preserving healthy tissue, thereby improving surgical outcomes. The integration of AI with DRS and robotic platforms holds significant potential for advancing colorectal cancer surgery by providing surgeons with enhanced tools for intraoperative decision-making.

Another notable development is the AI-based real-time microcirculation analysis system for laparoscopic procedures. This system utilizes indocyanine green (ICG) fluorescence imaging to assess tissue perfusion during surgery, providing surgeons with immediate feedback on blood flow and tissue viability (Fig. 16.1). By integrating AI algorithms, the system can analyze fluorescence patterns to predict anastomotic outcomes, thereby reducing the risk of complications such as anastomotic leaks [16, 17]. This advancement underscores AI's potential to improve surgical precision and patient safety in colorectal operations.

Robotic surgery is already transforming the field and will continue to evolve with the integration of AI. While its full adoption in colorectal surgery is still in progress and accompanied by ethical considerations, the combination of AI and robotic technology represents one of the most promising and dynamic areas of surgical research (Fig. 16.2).

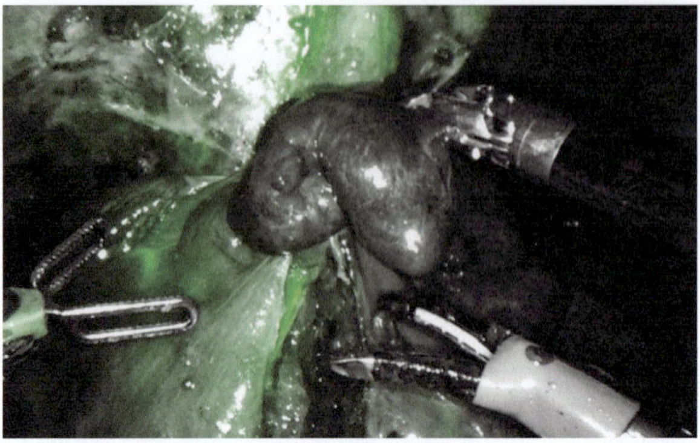

Fig. 16.1 Assessment of bowel perfusion using the da Vinci Firefly® fluorescence imaging system. Future integration of artificial intelligence and advanced imaging modalities may enable real time, automated perfusion analysis, improving intraoperative decision-making and patient outcomes

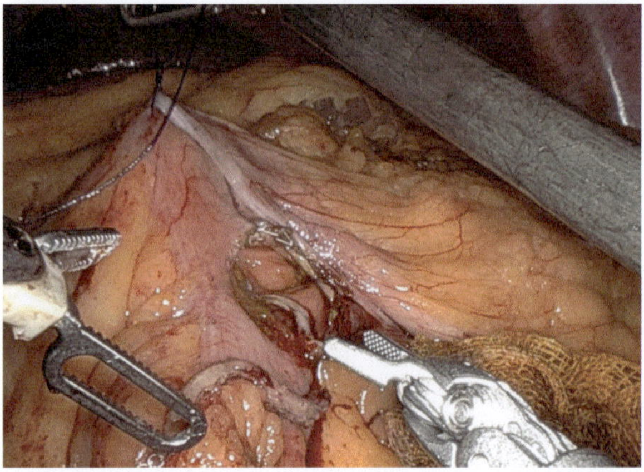

Fig. 16.2 Intraoperative view of the surgical field during anastomosis using the da Vinci Xi® Surgical System. Note the positioning of the fourth robotic arm, which may be subject to future automation to enhance surgical efficiency and precision

Current applications of AI in robotic surgery, though often still in the experimental phase, are showing great potential across various areas. Machine learning and autonomous camera guidance are emerging as valuable tools, enhancing surgical precision [18]. Tactile and surgical feedback systems have already been tested and integrated, improving the surgeon's ability to assess tissue properties [19, 20]. Perhaps the most groundbreaking advancement is autonomous surgery [21], with models like the Smart Tissue Autonomous Robot (STAR) [22], developed at Johns Hopkins University, demonstrating significant progress. These innovations are poised to play a crucial role in improving intraoperative outcomes in colorectal surgery in the near future.

In treatment, AI contributes to the development of robotic surgery and novel computer-assisted methods, ushering in a new era of precision medicine. Machine learning models have the potential to contribute to individual-based cancer care and transform the future of medicine. As healthcare rapidly moves toward personalized approaches, AI's role in CRC management exemplifies its potential to revolutionize patient care.

16.4 Postoperative and Follow-Up

In the postoperative phase of colorectal surgery, AI is increasingly being used to predict and manage complications, ultimately improving patient outcomes. Machine learning models have demonstrated exceptional accuracy in forecasting postoperative ileus (POI), a common complication, by analyzing patient-specific factors such as age, body mass index, and comorbidities. Notably, models like AdaBoost and XGBoost have achieved accuracy rates of 94.2% and 85.2%, respectively, in predicting POI [23].

Beyond POI prediction, AI algorithms play a crucial role in assessing the risk of other postoperative complications, enabling early intervention and personalized patient management. For instance, AI can be utilized to calculate the likelihood of an anastomotic leak [24], providing surgeons with valuable insights for timely clinical decision-making. Additionally, AI has proven effective in histopathology by distinguishing healthy tissue from tumor tissue, enhancing diagnostic precision [14]. Deep learning models are also being applied after primary colorectal resection to refine the selection of adjuvant therapies, ensuring more tailored and effective treatment strategies [25]. With its expanding role, AI is poised to revolutionize postoperative care in colorectal surgery, optimizing recovery and long-term patient outcomes.

16.5 Discussion and Future Perspectives

The integration of AI and CV into small bowel and colorectal surgery represents a paradigm shift in surgical precision, decision-making, and patient outcomes. As demonstrated across multiple domains—ranging from preoperative planning to intraoperative assistance and postoperative management—AI-driven technologies are enhancing the accuracy, efficiency, and safety of colorectal procedures. Machine learning algorithms, computer vision, and robotic platforms are transforming both diagnostics and therapeutic approaches, allowing for personalized surgical planning, real-time intraoperative guidance, and improved postoperative monitoring.

Despite the numerous advantages, several challenges must be addressed before AI can be fully integrated into routine surgical practice. One significant barrier is the need for widespread validation and regulatory approval of AI-driven models. Many current AI applications are developed using specific datasets, which raises concerns regarding their generalizability across diverse patient populations and healthcare settings. To mitigate biases and ensure reliability, robust multicenter trials and standardized evaluation protocols must be established. Additionally, the ethical considerations surrounding AI in surgery, including issues of liability, data privacy, and decision-making autonomy, require comprehensive regulatory frameworks and guidelines.

The future of AI in colorectal surgery will likely see advancements in real-time data integration and autonomous surgical systems. The combination of AI with wearable health monitoring devices and electronic health records could facilitate continuous postoperative surveillance, enabling earlier detection of complications and personalized recovery pathways. Moreover, AI-powered robotic surgery is expected to evolve further, potentially leading to increased automation in colorectal procedures while maintaining surgeon oversight. Innovations in AI-driven optical sensing and fluorescence-guided surgery may further refine intraoperative decision-making, ensuring optimal oncological and functional outcomes.

Interdisciplinary collaboration between surgeons, engineers, data scientists, and policymakers will be crucial in shaping the responsible development and implementation of AI in colorectal surgery. By addressing technical, ethical, and logistical challenges, AI has the potential to revolutionize the field, improving surgical precision, patient safety, and long-term outcomes. With ongoing research and technological advancements, AI-driven surgical innovations are poised to become an indispensable component of modern colorectal surgery, bridging the gap between cutting-edge technology and clinical excellence.

References

1. Spinelli A, Carrano FM, Laino ME, et al. Artificial intelligence in colorectal surgery: an AI-powered systematic review. Tech Coloproctol. 2023;27(8):615–29. https://doi.org/10.1007/s10151-023-02772-8.
2. Takeuchi M, Kitagawa Y. Artificial intelligence and surgery. Ann Gastroenterol Surg. 2024;8(1):4–5. https://doi.org/10.1002/ags3.12766.
3. Romano G, Di Buono G, Galia M, et al. Role of preoperative CT angiography with multimodality imaging reconstruction to perform laparoscopic Complete Mesocolic Excision (CME) and Central Vascular Ligation (CVL) in right-sided colon cancer: is it really useful? A prospective clinical study. Eur J Surg Oncol J Eur Soc Surg Oncol Br Assoc Surg Oncol. 2023;49(1):209–16. https://doi.org/10.1016/j.ejso.2022.08.007.
4. Efetov SK, Zubayraeva AA, Serednyakova DV, Mozharov RN, Saltovets RR, Koziy AY. Vascular-oriented D3 lymph node dissection with left colic artery preservation for distal sigmoid colon cancer: a variety of techniques. Tech Coloproctol. 2024;28(1):119. https://doi.org/10.1007/s10151-024-03003-4.
5. Xie W, Hu J, Liang P, et al. Deep learning-based lesion detection and severity grading of small-bowel Crohn's disease ulcers on double-balloon endoscopy images. Gastrointest Endosc. 2024;99(5):767–777.e5. https://doi.org/10.1016/j.gie.2023.11.059.
6. Jiang X, Luo X, Nan Q, Ye Y, Miao Y, Miao J. Application of deep learning in the diagnosis and evaluation of ulcerative colitis disease severity. Ther Adv Gastroenterol. 2023;16:17562848231215580. https://doi.org/10.1177/17562848231215579.
7. Ahmad HA, East JE, Panaccione R, et al. Artificial intelligence in inflammatory bowel disease endoscopy: implications for clinical trials. J Crohns Colitis. 2023;17(8):1342–53. https://doi.org/10.1093/ecco-jcc/jjad029.
8. Furlanello C, Bussola N, Merzi N, et al. The development of artificial intelligence in the histological diagnosis of inflammatory bowel disease (IBD-AI). Dig Liver Dis. 2025;57(1):184–9. https://doi.org/10.1016/j.dld.2024.05.033.
9. Young E, Edwards L, Singh R. The role of artificial intelligence in colorectal cancer screening: lesion detection and lesion characterization. Cancers (Basel). 2023;15(21) https://doi.org/10.3390/cancers15215126.
10. Mitsala A, Tsalikidis C, Pitiakoudis M, Simopoulos C, Tsaroucha AK. Artificial intelligence in colorectal cancer screening, diagnosis and treatment. A new era. Curr Oncol. 2021;28(3):1581–607. https://doi.org/10.3390/curroncol28030149.

11. Xu H, Tang RSY, Lam TYT, et al. Artificial intelligence-assisted colonoscopy for colorectal cancer screening: a multicenter randomized controlled trial. Clin Gastroenterol Hepatol. 2023;21(2):337–346.e3. https://doi.org/10.1016/j.cgh.2022.07.006.
12. Bedrikovetski S, Dudi-Venkata NN, Kroon HM, et al. Artificial intelligence for pre-operative lymph node staging in colorectal cancer: a systematic review and meta-analysis. BMC Cancer. 2021;21(1):1058. https://doi.org/10.1186/s12885-021-08773-w.
13. Rompianesi G, Pegoraro F, Ceresa CD, Montalti R, Troisi RI. Artificial intelligence in the diagnosis and management of colorectal cancer liver metastases. World J Gastroenterol. 2022;28(1):108–22. https://doi.org/10.3748/wjg.v28.i1.108.
14. Baltussen EJM, Brouwer de Koning SG, Sanders J, et al. Using diffuse reflectance spectroscopy to distinguish tumor tissue from fibrosis in rectal cancer patients as a guide to surgery. Lasers Surg Med. 2020;52(7):604–11. https://doi.org/10.1002/lsm.23196.
15. Baltussen EJM, Brouwer de Koning SG, Sanders J, et al. Tissue diagnosis during colorectal cancer surgery using optical sensing: an in vivo study. J Transl Med. 2019;17(1):333. https://doi.org/10.1186/s12967-019-2083-0.
16. Cahill RA, O'Shea DF, Khan MF, et al. Artificial intelligence indocyanine green (ICG) perfusion for colorectal cancer intra-operative tissue classification. Br J Surg. 2021;108(1):5–9. https://doi.org/10.1093/bjs/znaa004.
17. Park S-H, Park H-M, Baek K-R, Ahn H-M, Lee IY, Son GM. Artificial intelligence based real-time microcirculation analysis system for laparoscopic colorectal surgery. World J Gastroenterol. 2020;26(44):6945–62. https://doi.org/10.3748/wjg.v26.i44.6945.
18. Wagner M, Bihlmaier A, Kenngott HG, et al. A learning robot for cognitive camera control in minimally invasive surgery. Surg Endosc. 2021;35(9):5365–74. https://doi.org/10.1007/s00464-021-08509-8.
19. Alip SL, Kim J, Rha KH, Han WK. Future platforms of robotic surgery. Urol Clin North Am. 2022;49(1):23–38. https://doi.org/10.1016/j.ucl.2021.07.008.
20. Knudsen JE, Ghaffar U, Ma R, Hung AJ. Clinical applications of artificial intelligence in robotic surgery. J Robot Surg. 2024;18(1):102. https://doi.org/10.1007/s11701-024-01867-0.
21. Saeidi H, Opfermann JD, Kam M, et al. Autonomous robotic laparoscopic surgery for intestinal anastomosis. Sci Robot. 2022;7(62):eabj2908. https://doi.org/10.1126/scirobotics.abj2908.
22. Shademan A, Decker RS, Opfermann JD, Leonard S, Krieger A, Kim PCW. Supervised autonomous robotic soft tissue surgery. Sci Transl Med. 2016;8(337):337ra64. https://doi.org/10.1126/scitranslmed.aad9398.
23. Qiu H, Ding S, Liu J, Wang L, Wang X. Applications of artificial intelligence in screening, diagnosis, treatment, and prognosis of colorectal cancer. Curr Oncol. 2022;29(3):1773–95. https://doi.org/10.3390/curroncol29030146.
24. Adams K, Papagrigoriadis S. Creation of an effective colorectal anastomotic leak early detection tool using an artificial neural network. Int J Color Dis. 2014;29(4):437–43. https://doi.org/10.1007/s00384-013-1812-8.
25. Skrede O-J, De Raedt S, Kleppe A, et al. Deep learning for prediction of colorectal cancer outcome: a discovery and validation study. Lancet. 2020;395(10221):350–60. https://doi.org/10.1016/S0140-6736(19)32998-8.

AI-Powered Rehabilitation and Monitoring Systems for Orthopedic Trauma Patients

17

Kyros R. Ipaktchi and Sean E. Higinbotham

17.1 Introduction

Orthopedic trauma rehabilitation often requires precise, prolonged, and closely monitored regimens to ensure optimal recovery. Traditional rehabilitation approaches can face challenges such as limited continuous monitoring and feedback. Patients often only receive guidance during scheduled therapy sessions, leaving them without continuous feedback between appointments [1]. This can lead to slower progress or injury if exercises are done incorrectly at home. Conventional rehabilitation is guided by established and standardized protocols, which may not cater effectively to individual patients' needs [2, 3]. Each patient has a unique recovery trajectory based on injury type, physical condition, and personal lifestyle, and finding an individual treatment plan may be challenging. Likewise, following through with prescribed exercises at home can be difficult for patients.

The lack of real-time guidance or feedback often leads to decreased motivation and lower adherence to rehabilitation routines [4]. The often spaced-out rehabilitation appointments may cause delays in recognizing rehabilitation issues and complications such as persistent joint stiffness, improper healing, or overuse injuries. The high time demands for healthcare providers in rehabilitation and the need for patients to travel frequently to appointments can pose significant logistical and financial burdens. These challenges may result in inconsistent or suboptimal care [5]. Finally, rehabilitation can vary widely based on the therapist's expertise and available resources, instead of objective, data-driven metrics guiding therapy. This,

K. R. Ipaktchi (✉)
Department of Orthopedic Surgery, Denver Health Medical Center, Denver, CO, USA

Orthopedic and Plastic Surgery, University of Colorado, Aurora, CO, USA
e-mail: kyros.ipaktchi@dhha.org

S. E. Higinbotham
Department of Orthopedic Surgery, Denver Health Medical Center, Denver, CO, USA

B. De Simone et al. (eds.), *New Technologies, Precision Medicine, and AI in Emergency General Surgery*, Hot Topics in Acute Care Surgery and Trauma,
https://doi.org/10.1007/978-3-032-09357-8_17

together with a lack of sophisticated data collection and analysis tools, makes it challenging to track a patient's progress or predict future outcomes accurately.

Artificial intelligence (AI) may address many of these challenges of traditional therapy and rehabilitation approaches. AI has begun transforming this field by providing advanced rehabilitation and monitoring systems that offer personalized care, real-time feedback, and predictive insights. These systems represent a significant leap forward, enhancing patient outcomes and healthcare delivery efficiency [6].

17.2 Possible Applications of AI in Orthopedic Trauma Rehabilitation

The unique capabilities of AI can analyze a patient's injury specifics, medical history, and physical abilities and develop a highly individualized rehabilitation protocol. Using advanced algorithms, AI systems assess the type and severity of the injury through medical imaging and information from electronic health records, such as past injuries, surgeries, and underlying conditions. These systems can incorporate data from wearable devices that track real-time metrics like range of motion, muscle engagement, and gait, enabling a dynamic understanding of the patient's current physical state. By synthesizing this information, AI can recommend tailored exercises, adjust therapy intensity, and predict recovery timelines specific to the patient's unique profile. This personalized approach ensures that patients progress optimally, minimizes re-injury risk, and enhances overall recovery by continuously adapting to the patient's evolving needs.

AI can predict recovery timelines and identify potential complications in orthopedic trauma patients by analyzing patient data and identifying patterns associated with different recovery outcomes. Machine learning models trained on historical patient data, including injury type, patient demographics, treatment approaches, and rehabilitation progress, can generate predictive insights on the likely recovery duration for new patients and flag any warning signs that could indicate complications such as joint stiffness, muscle atrophy, or delayed healing. For example, IBM Watson Health has developed AI systems that leverage electronic health records and clinical data to assist healthcare providers in predicting patient outcomes, including recovery timelines, for conditions such as musculoskeletal injuries [7]. The system combines patient-specific data with broader clinical insights to provide recommendations and alert clinicians to potential adverse events, enabling them to adjust treatment plans proactively. Such technologies support more informed decision-making and foster a proactive approach to rehabilitation, possibly addressing complications before they escalate.

Virtual and Augmented Reality (VR/AR) technologies transform rehabilitation and offer immersive, guided physical therapy experiences. This can be of particular benefit to home-based rehab programs. AI-driven VR/AR platforms can simulate interactive, real-world environments, guide patients through prescribed exercises with real-time feedback, and track movement accuracy and routine adherence [8]. For instance, XRHealth offers a VR platform for physical therapy that includes

AI-based analytics, enabling clinicians to monitor patient progress remotely and adjust therapy based on data insights [9]. AI-powered mobile apps that use augmented reality to track a patient's movements via smartphone cameras can offer feedback to ensure correct form and engagement [10]. These technologies enhance patient motivation and engagement through gamified, interactive exercises and provide clinicians with valuable insights into recovery progress, allowing for timely adjustments in therapy and ultimately improving patient outcomes in remote settings.

17.3 Monitoring Systems for Orthopedic Trauma Recovery

AI-powered wearables advance orthopedic rehabilitation by continuously tracking motion, muscle engagement, and joint angles, offering patients and clinicians real-time feedback for adequate recovery. For example, smart knee braces integrate AI algorithms to monitor knee joint angles and movement patterns, which they relay to patients and therapists through an app, allowing adjustments to exercises and alerting users to improper movement that could hinder recovery [11]. Similarly, software-enhanced intelligent compression sleeves that embed sensors to track muscle activity and engagement in the upper limbs can track swelling [12]. By analyzing muscle exertion and joint movement in real time, the sleeve provides feedback to help patients maintain proper form and prevent overexertion; this can be especially useful for those rehabilitating remotely. These AI-enhanced wearables offer a personalized approach to recovery, allowing for data-driven progress tracking and tailored feedback that adapts to the patient's unique rehabilitation needs.

AI-driven Remote Patient Monitoring (RPM) systems are revolutionizing orthopedic rehabilitation and enabling continuous tracking of patient recovery progress and early detection of potential issues [13]. Wearable sensors that track motion and add physiologic data and vital signs can better understand patients' functional status [14]. The option to assess orthopedic patients' heart rate variability, respiratory rate, and activity levels to gauge recovery status and identify irregular patterns indicative of complications like infection, inflammation, or delayed healing. AI algorithms can continuously learn from patient-specific data, creating personalized baselines and alerting healthcare providers if deviations occur, prompting timely intervention. This proactive approach ensures that potential issues are addressed early, reducing the need for emergency visits and allowing clinicians to make data-informed adjustments to rehabilitation protocols, ultimately supporting a smoother recovery process for patients.

Computer vision can play a transformative role in motion analysis for orthopedic rehabilitation. It enables precise evaluation of exercise style, gait patterns, and biomechanics, which assists therapists in fine-tuning exercises to optimize recovery. Systems that use embedded cameras and computer vision technology can analyze a user's movements during exercises, offering real-time feedback on motion patterns to ensure accuracy and prevent strain or injury [15]. This is especially valuable for patients performing at-home exercises without direct supervision. Advanced tracking systems that employ computer vision and AI for comprehensive motion analysis can be used in rehabilitation and fine-tuning training regimens in athletes [16]. These systems can assess joint load, symmetry, and range of motion, providing therapists with insights to customize and adjust therapy routines based on objective, quantitative metrics. This approach may enable a more responsive and adaptive rehabilitation process, reducing the risk of improper movement and enhancing the quality of patient outcomes.

17.4 Benefits of AI-Powered Rehabilitation Systems

AI-driven tools enhance patient engagement and compliance in orthopedic rehabilitation by making the process more interactive, personalized, multilingual, and thus accessible while also helping to reduce healthcare costs. Patient compliance and adherence can wane in rehabilitation [17]. AI-backed real-time feedback can motivate patients to stay consistent by making each session feel customized and achievable. This approach has increased patient adherence, as patients receive guidance that adjusts to their progress and needs, even outside traditional clinical settings. Remote Patient Monitoring (RPM) reduces the need for frequent in-person check-ups by enabling clinicians to track recovery and address issues before they escalate remotely. This offers convenience to patients and significantly cuts down on associated travel and appointment costs, ultimately making quality rehabilitation accessible at a lower cost for both healthcare providers and patients.

Data-driven insights from comprehensive patient databases offer significant long-term benefits for refining treatment approaches in orthopedic rehabilitation. For example, the MIMIC-IV database [18], widely used in healthcare research, contains detailed patient records, including demographics, diagnoses, treatments, and recovery outcomes, which can be invaluable in shaping evidence-based rehabilitation protocols. By analyzing trends in this data type, clinicians and researchers can identify which rehabilitation techniques yield the best outcomes for specific injuries, patient demographics, and comorbidities. Such databases help improve the accuracy of predictive models, enable earlier intervention for complications, and lead to more effective, individualized rehabilitation plans, ultimately enhancing patient recovery and long-term health outcomes.

17.5 Challenges and Limitations

Data privacy and security are critical when handling and sharing sensitive health data. This is especially important as AI-powered rehabilitation systems increasingly rely on extensive patient data to deliver personalized care. Protecting this information is challenging due to the risks of unauthorized access, data theft, or accidental exposure, which can compromise patient privacy and trust. A notable example of a recent data breach and ransomware attack on a cloud service used by nonprofits and healthcare institutions exposed this vulnerability [19]. The incident highlighted vulnerabilities in third-party data handling and raised concerns about healthcare data security practices, and underscored the critical need for robust security protocols, such as encryption, secure access controls, and continuous monitoring. Protecting sensitive health data from breaches and ensuring compliance is the mandate of national regulations like the Health Insurance Portability and Accountability Act (HIPAA) in the U.S. and the 2018 implemented strict General Data Protection Regulation (GDPR) in the EU. There are important differences in acceptance rates of cloud-based patient data storage across countries, which can add barriers to roll out AI-driven technologies in healthcare [20].

In addition to data security concerns, there are important ethical considerations regarding AI in healthcare to consider. There is a risk of a possible over-reliance on technology, undermining the human-centered aspects of care. With AI taking on roles in diagnostics, treatment planning, and even direct patient interaction, there is a growing concern that patients could feel alienated or overlooked as human contact diminishes. Ethical guidelines emphasize that while AI can enhance decision-making and efficiency, it should not replace the empathy, trust, and nuanced judgment that healthcare professionals provide [21]. For example, black-box AI algorithms—whose decision-making processes are not easily interpretable—pose a challenge when transparency is essential for patient trust and understanding [22]. Recent studies challenge the notion that large language models will improve diagnostic decision-making by clinicians [23]. Patient care relies not just on data patterns but on individual patient contexts, which clinicians are uniquely equipped to interpret effectively.

While machine learning algorithms may appear omnipotent to the consumer, technical limitations still exist in AI-powered rehabilitation systems stemming from algorithmic and hardware constraints, affecting these solutions' accuracy, reliability, and usability. Current AI algorithms, particularly in machine learning and neural networks, often require extensive datasets for precise predictions and guidance. However, in healthcare, obtaining large, high-quality datasets that are diverse and representative is challenging, resulting in models that may not adequately represent different patient groups. In addition to challenges in patient literacy and the ability to utilize and finance machine learning devices, AI-driven healthcare heavily depends on the quality of the used datasets, which may open the door to bias in health provision.

Also, the hardware side, such as wearable devices, is central to many AI-driven rehabilitation systems and faces limitations regarding battery life, processing power, and sensor accuracy. For instance, smartwatches [24], while capable of monitoring basic metrics such as heart rate and activity levels, may lack the sensor accuracy needed to reliably track complex biomechanics or muscle engagement for in-depth orthopedic assessments. These constraints limit its application for detailed rehabilitation monitoring and real-time feedback on form and posture, which are essential in physical therapy. Such limitations highlight the need for continued advancement in AI model interpretation and wearable technology capabilities to support effective, data-driven rehabilitation.

Finally, algorithmic and autonomous reacting machine learning networks will challenge our current healthcare liability concepts. These technological advances must stimulate legislative and regulatory review to assess the need for future legal reforms [25].

17.6 Future Directions and Innovations

Integrating robotics with AI in rehabilitation holds promising potential to enhance patient recovery, such as robotic devices that assist with repetitive exercises and precision training. Robotic exoskeletons are increasingly used to aid upper and lower limb rehabilitation, particularly for stroke recovery. These devices can adaptively respond to a patient's motor function, providing appropriate assistance or resistance based on real-time sensor feedback [26]. This approach may help ensure that each session is tailored to the patient's current capabilities and enhance the effectiveness of rehabilitation [27].

Recent work demonstrated that combining robotics with brain-computer interfaces (BCIs) and other assistive technologies can allow patients with severe motor impairments to regain control over movements, sometimes even improving their neuroplasticity over time [28].

Ongoing research in AI-enhanced imaging diagnostics aims to improve the tracking of healing progress by refining algorithms to detect subtle changes in tissue recovery and bone regeneration. Advanced deep learning models are being developed to enhance precision in segmenting and analyzing images from MRI, CT, and other imaging modalities, enabling clinicians to track detailed aspects of healing, such as scar tissue formation, joint mobility, and bone density improvements. These models are designed to analyze progressive changes in scans over time, offering a clearer view of how effectively a patient responds to treatment.

One area of focus is using convolutional neural networks (CNNs) to assess MRI images for musculoskeletal recovery [29] and scan segmentation for 3D structure visualizations [30]. CNNs can automatically detect and measure small structural changes in tissues, helping to guide rehabilitation protocols and adjust interventions as needed. Additionally, AI models integrated into CT imaging are being trained to monitor micro-fracture repair, providing real time, data-driven insights that can inform clinicians on the readiness for increased physical load or further intervention [31].

17.7 Conclusion

Integrating AI into orthopedic rehabilitation and monitoring presents a transformative opportunity to enhance patient care through personalized, data-driven approaches. AI-powered tools like wearable sensors, computer vision, and predictive analytics provide patients and clinicians with real-time feedback, accurate progress tracking, and insights that facilitate tailored rehabilitation plans. These advancements may improve patient engagement and adherence to recovery protocols and allow for timely interventions to reduce the risk of complications, potentially lowering healthcare costs and expanding access to remote care. Autonomous monitoring and AI-driven robotic assistance further highlight AI's potential to make rehabilitation more efficient, adaptive, and effective.

Realizing these benefits will depend on continued research and development to address current limitations. Issues such as data privacy, the need for extensive and diverse datasets, and technical constraints in wearable and robotic hardware must be overcome to ensure AI-driven systems are safe, reliable, and equitable for all patients.

As AI technology evolves, maintaining a balance between automation and the human aspect of care will also be essential to uphold the empathy and individual attention that underpin successful recovery. By advancing research in these areas, the healthcare sector may position itself to better harness AI's potential, ultimately making orthopedic rehabilitation more responsive, personalized, and accessible.

References

1. LaMarca A, Tse I, Keysor J. Rehabilitation technologies for chronic conditions: will we sink or swim? Healthcare (Basel). 2023;11:2751. https://doi.org/10.3390/healthcare11202751.
2. Lee BG, Cho NS, Rhee YG. Effect of two rehabilitation protocols on range of motion and healing rates after arthroscopic rotator cuff repair: aggressive versus limited early passive exercises. Arthroscopy. 2012;28:34–42. https://doi.org/10.1016/j.arthro.2011.07.012.
3. Järvinen TAH, Järvinen TLN, Kääriäinen M, et al. Muscle injuries: optimising recovery. Best Pract Res Clin Rheumatol. 2007;21:317–31. https://doi.org/10.1016/j.berh.2006.12.004.
4. Skov CD, Lindberg-Larsen M, Wiil UK, et al. Impact of motivational feedback on levels of physical activity and quality of life by activity monitoring following knee arthroplasty surgery-protocol for a randomized controlled trial nested in a prospective cohort (Knee-Activity). BMC Musculoskelet Disord. 2024;25:778. https://doi.org/10.1186/s12891-024-07878-0.
5. Hamilton DF, Beard DJ, Barker KL, et al. Targeting rehabilitation to improve outcomes after total knee arthroplasty in patients at risk of poor outcomes: randomised controlled trial. BMJ. 2020;371:m3576. https://doi.org/10.1136/bmj.m3576.
6. Klemt C, Uzosike AC, Esposito JG, et al. The utility of machine learning algorithms for the prediction of patient-reported outcome measures following primary hip and knee total joint arthroplasty. Arch Orthop Trauma Surg. 2023;143:2235–45. https://doi.org/10.1007/s00402-022-04526-x.
7. Tafat W, Budka M, McDonald D, Wainwright TW. Artificial intelligence in orthopaedic surgery: a comprehensive review of current innovations and future directions. Comput Struct Biotechnol Rep. 2024;1:100006. https://doi.org/10.1016/j.csbr.2024.100006.
8. Berton A, Longo UG, Candela V, et al. Virtual reality, augmented reality, gamification, and Telerehabilitation: psychological impact on orthopedic patients' rehabilitation. J Clin Med. 2020;9:2567. https://doi.org/10.3390/jcm9082567.
9. Morimoto T, Kobayashi T, Hirata H, et al. XR (Extended reality: virtual reality, augmented reality, mixed reality) Technology in Spine Medicine: status quo and quo Vadis. J Clin Med. 2022;11:470. https://doi.org/10.3390/jcm11020470.
10. Spielmanns M, Gloeckl R, Jarosch I, et al. Using a smartphone application maintains physical activity following pulmonary rehabilitation in patients with COPD: a randomised controlled trial. Thorax. 2023;78:442–50. https://doi.org/10.1136/thoraxjnl-2021-218338.

11. Bellitti P, Borghetti M, Lopomo NF, et al. Smart brace for static and dynamic knee laxity measurement. Sensors (Basel). 2022;22:5815. https://doi.org/10.3390/s22155815.
12. Mavroidis C, Nikitczuk J, Weinberg B, et al. Smart portable rehabilitation devices. J Neuroeng Rehabil. 2005;2:18. https://doi.org/10.1186/1743-0003-2-18.
13. Ramkumar PN, Haeberle HS, Ramanathan D, et al. Remote patient monitoring using Mobile health for Total knee arthroplasty: validation of a wearable and machine learning-based surveillance platform. J Arthroplast. 2019;34:2253–9. https://doi.org/10.1016/j.arth.2019.05.021.
14. Prigent G, Aminian K, Rodrigues T, et al. Indirect estimation of breathing rate from heart rate monitoring system during running. Sensors (Basel). 2021;21:5651. https://doi.org/10.3390/s21165651.
15. Obukhov A, Volkov A, Pchelintsev A, et al. Examination of the accuracy of movement tracking Systems for Monitoring Exercise for musculoskeletal rehabilitation. Sensors (Basel). 2023;23:8058. https://doi.org/10.3390/s23198058.
16. Philipp NM, Fry AC, Mosier EM, et al. Biological reliability of a movement analysis assessment using a markerless motion capture system. Front Sports Act Living. 2024;6:1417965. https://doi.org/10.3389/fspor.2024.1417965.
17. Jack K, McLean S, Moffett JK, Gardiner E. Barriers to treatment adherence in physiotherapy outpatient clinics: a systematic review. Man Ther. 2010;15:220–8. https://doi.org/10.1016/j.math.2009.12.004.
18. Johnson AEW, Bulgarelli L, Shen L, et al. MIMIC-IV, a freely accessible electronic health record dataset. Sci Data. 2023;10:1. https://doi.org/10.1038/s41597-022-01899-x.
19. Raina MacIntyre C, Engells TE, Scotch M, et al. Converging and emerging threats to health security. Environ Syst Decis. 2018;38:198–207. https://doi.org/10.1007/s10669-017-9667-0.
20. Schmidt J, Schutte NM, Buttigieg S, et al. Mapping the regulatory landscape for artificial intelligence in health within the European Union. NPJ Digit Med. 2024;7:229. https://doi.org/10.1038/s41746-024-01221-6.
21. Elendu C, Amaechi DC, Elendu TC, et al. Ethical implications of AI and robotics in healthcare: a review. Medicine (Baltimore). 2023;102:e36671. https://doi.org/10.1097/MD.0000000000036671.
22. Karim MR, Islam T, Shajalal M, et al. Explainable AI for bioinformatics: methods, tools and applications. Brief Bioinform. 2023;24:bbad236. https://doi.org/10.1093/bib/bbad236.
23. Goh E, Gallo R, Hom J, et al. Large language model influence on diagnostic reasoning: a randomized clinical trial. JAMA Netw Open. 2024;7:e2440969. https://doi.org/10.1001/jamanetworkopen.2024.40969.
24. Miller DJ, Sargent C, Roach GD. A validation of six wearable devices for estimating sleep, heart rate and heart rate variability in healthy adults. Sensors (Basel). 2022;22:6317. https://doi.org/10.3390/s22166317.
25. Haupt CE, Marks M. AI-generated medical advice-GPT and beyond. JAMA. 2023;329:1349–50. https://doi.org/10.1001/jama.2023.5321.
26. Vélez-Guerrero MA, Callejas-Cuervo M, Mazzoleni S. Artificial intelligence-based wearable robotic exoskeletons for upper limb rehabilitation: a review. Sensors (Basel). 2021;21:2146. https://doi.org/10.3390/s21062146.
27. Calafiore D, Negrini F, Tottoli N, et al. Efficacy of robotic exoskeleton for gait rehabilitation in patients with subacute stroke: a systematic review. Eur J Phys Rehabil Med. 2022;58:1–8. https://doi.org/10.23736/S1973-9087.21.06846-5.
28. Mulpuri RP, Konda N, Gadde ST, et al. Artificial intelligence and machine learning in Neuroregeneration: a systematic review. Cureus. 2024;16:e61400. https://doi.org/10.7759/cureus.61400.
29. Kim-Wang SY, Bradley PX, Cutcliffe HC, et al. Auto-segmentation of the tibia and femur from knee MR images via deep learning and its application to cartilage strain and recovery. J Biomech. 2023;149:111473. https://doi.org/10.1016/j.jbiomech.2023.111473.

30. Burton W, Myers C, Rullkoetter P. Semi-supervised learning for automatic segmentation of the knee from MRI with convolutional neural networks. Comput Methods Prog Biomed. 2020;189:105328. https://doi.org/10.1016/j.cmpb.2020.105328.
31. Dankelman LHM, Schilstra S, IJpma FFA, et al. Artificial intelligence fracture recognition on computed tomography: review of literature and recommendations. Eur J Trauma Emerg Surg. 2023;49:681–91. https://doi.org/10.1007/s00068-022-02128-1.

Monitoring Patients in the Intensive Care Unit in the Era of AI

18

Guido Gambetti, Alessandra Morelli, and Vanni Agnoletti

Abbreviations

AI	Artificial intelligence
BPS	Behavioral pain scale
CDSS	Computer-assisted decision support systems
CPOT	Critical care pain observation tool
DT	Decision tree
EHR	Electronic health records
EMPICU	Early mortality prediction for intensive care unit patients
eICU-CRD	electronic intensive care unit collaborative research database
ICU	Intensive care unit
KNN	K-nearest neighbor
LLM	Language learning model
LOS	Length of stay
LR	Logistic regression
LSTM	Long short-term memory
MIMIC	Medical information mart for intensive care
ML	Machine learning
MLP	Multilayer perception
NB	Naive Bayes
PART	Projective adaptive resonance theory
RF	Random forest
SAPS	Simplified acute physiology score
SIRS	Systemic inflammatory response syndrome
SVM	Support vector machines

G. Gambetti (✉) · A. Morelli · V. Agnoletti
Anesthesia and Intensive Care Unit, Bufalini Hospital, AUSL Romagna, Cesena, Italy
e-mail: guido.gambetti@auslromagna.it

B. De Simone et al. (eds.), *New Technologies, Precision Medicine, and AI in Emergency General Surgery*, Hot Topics in Acute Care Surgery and Trauma,
https://doi.org/10.1007/978-3-032-09357-8_18

SOFA	Sequential organ failure assessment
XGBoost	Extreme gradient boosting

18.1 Introduction

Comprehensive monitoring of physiological parameters and vital signs is essential not only to optimize the daily care of critically ill patients and their safety but also to ensure their survival and long-term outcomes.

The extremely dynamic course of diseases encountered in the intensive care unit (ICU) environment, coupled with the changing nature of patients who present an increasing tendency to have polymorbid backgrounds, highlights the pivotal role of technology to aid in the management of a growing amount and complexity of data.

Continuous multiparametric monitoring is, in fact, essential to timely intercept the moments in which the application of a therapeutic maneuver or tailoring of a drug can be lifesaving or can significantly alter the disease course and outcome.

On the other hand, doctors and nurses are facing higher occupational pressure and heavier workloads, making it more difficult to discern heavy loads of information, alarms, and data derived from patient records, monitors, and machines—which sometimes are useful but other times not [1].

Artificial intelligence (AI), by definition, helps to perform tasks which usually are accomplished by human intelligence—i.e., reasoning, discovering patterns, generalizing, and learning from past experience [2]. Applied to the intensive care environment, it enables the prompt identification and resolution of issues in inpatient management, enhances operational efficiency, minimizes human error, optimizes the allocation of personnel, and improves the use and oversight of tools and equipment [1].

In this chapter, we will describe the main applications of AI in the complex setting of the ICU, exploring its potential for the future and also the ethical concerns which invariably—as it happens with every new technology—it has led to raise.

18.2 Outcome: Length of Stay, Mortality, Complications, and Risk Stratification

The first and the most extensively studied application of AI in the ICU environment is outcome prediction. Despite the availability of several scoring systems—i.e., the National Early Warning Score (NEWS), the Sequential Organ Failure Assessment (SOFA), the Acute Physiologic Assessment and Chronic Health Evaluation II (APACHE-II), the Simplified Acute Physiology Score II (SAPS-II), and so on—forecasting outcome in critically ill patients can still be troublesome.

Already in 2016, Calvert et al. developed an algorithm *AutoTriage* for predicting early (the first 12 h) ICU mortality with considerable accuracy (AUROC 0.88) by extracting only eight clinical variables from patients' EHR. In their model, subscores were produced by discrete clinical variables and also by combining them in groups of two or three. The overall mortality risk score was then obtained by the weighted combination of the several subscores [3].

One year later, Awad et al. conducted an ambitious study introducing a new machine learning (ML)-based framework predicting very early (6 h after admission) ICU mortality. Their tool called Early Mortality Prediction for Intensive Care Unit patients (EMPICU) employed the ensemble learning Random Forest (RF), the predictive Decision Trees (DT), the probabilistic Naive Bayes (NB), and the rule-based Projective Adaptive Resonance Theory (PART) models to the MIMIC-II database, specifically focusing on medical ICU, surgical ICU, and cardiac surgery recovery unit (CSRU) patients. The standard and well-known scoring systems were outperformed not only in terms of AUROC but also in terms of time (6 h vs. $>=48$ h after admission) [4].

Another milestone study was published in 2019 by Kim et al., who specifically focused on adverse events' prediction such as cardiac arrest and respiratory failure in ICU patients. Using a tool called Feasible Artificial Intelligence with Simple Trajectories for Predicting Adverse Catastrophic Events (FAST-PACE), they extracted physiological data from the EHR of 29.181 patients to construct an AI model able to forecast the onset of cardiac arrest of respiratory failure from 1 h to 6 h prior its occurrence. Results were impressive: the model showed an AUROC of 0.886 for cardiac arrest and 0.869 for respiratory failure 6 h before the effective presentation [5].

More recently, the COVID-19 pandemic granted a great amount of electronic patient data—and at the same time a great disproportion between personnel availability and workload, which is one of the main issues AI is designed to solve—to fuel several studies focused on outcome prediction of large and specific cohorts of patients.

One of the first studies specifically designed for this purpose combined several clinical and laboratory variables to predict hospital length of stay (LOS) and mortality risk. Among the initial diagnoses, intubation, the need for ventilation support, the use of specific medications commonly used during COVID pandemic (i.e., anti-inflammatory and anticoagulant drugs, antivirals, azithromycin, vitamin C), and lab tests such as platelet count and D-dimer have been combined both though multivariate analysis and a decision tree (DT) algorithm to build two specific predictive models. The first showed satisfying performance for LOS prediction, having a coefficient of determination, R^2, of 49.8% and a median absolute deviation of 2.85 days. The second DT-based model, specifically designed to predict COVID-19-related risk of death also demonstrated excellent performance with sensitivity and specificity of 96.5 and 87.8%, respectively, and overall accuracy of 96% [6].

18.3 Pain Monitoring

Pain monitoring in the ICU is crucial for both postoperative patients and those admitted for acute conditions, as it enables prompt and optimal pain management, enhances recovery, and improves overall patient outcomes.

While patient self-reporting is surely the most accurate way to assess this parameter, it may not always be performed—i.e., in a sedated or delirious patient.

At the same time, the most common tools, such as the Behavioral Pain Scale (BPS) and Critical Care Pain Observation Tool (CPOT), have several other limitations, as they are performed only in an intermittent manner and can suffer from interobserver variability.

For this reason, in 2021, Kobayashi et al. performed an observational study to evaluate the ability of three different machine learning methods in predicting pain through the analysis of vital signs, sedation level, and the age group. Among the three models, namely random forest (RF), support vector machine (SVM), and logistic regression (LR), the first achieved the best performance with an AUROC of 0.853 for predicting a CPOT $\geq$3 [7].

Such an objective, continuous, and semi-automatic evaluation of pain in ICU patients could therefore be hampered by individual variability in vital signs.

This consideration led the same authors to replicate a similar study in 2023, trying to incorporate deviations from baseline parameters in an RF model to improve pain visualization using ML techniques. This led to an increase in the AUROC for the same outcome to 0.903 [8].

Neurophysiology-based methods can be an interesting and complementary alternative. The use of AI algorithms to process electroencephalography signals, vital parameter derivatives (i.e., heart rate variability), and electrodermal activities has led to promising results. However, they suffer limitations in terms of current applicability, specificity, and reliability [9].

Lastly, pervasive sensing technology has also been tested. The Intelligent Intensive Care Unit (I2CU) is one of the clearest examples of how multiple modalities, such as the analysis of depth and RGB images, can be used to diagnose pain in critically ill patients. In the I2CU DL models and computer vision are used to detect patients' faces and to classify facial and behavioral signs of pain such as grimacing or frowning [10].

18.4 Mechanical Ventilation

Mechanical ventilation is one of the most common interventions in ICU patients and for almost 70 years has been a dynamic focus of research for both clinicians and engineers.

One of the main branches of interest is the identification of patient-ventilator asynchronies, which could be detected by machine learning methods.

In 2008, Chen et al. developed an algorithm which, through the analysis of the morphological changes of the pressure and flow curves, could identify ineffective efforts with high sensitivity and specificity (>90%) [11].

Four years later, Blanch et al. developed a tool—later commercialized as Better Care®—which compared the actual flow tracing to a theoretical exponential expiratory curve, being able to detect ineffective efforts with comparable performance [12].

The identification of other types of asynchronies, such as double triggering and flow asynchrony, was the scope of the later works which employed ML classifiers and multialgorithm analytic platforms [13, 14].

RF, naive Bayes, and AdaBoost have been also used by Sottile et al. to determine the presence of double triggering, flow-limited, and ineffective triggering with an area under the curve (AUC) >0.89 [15].

Similarly, an RF classifier was employed by Gholami et al. to accurately detect the presence of secondary asynchronies with high sensitivity (89%) [16].

A much more complex area of research is the use of AI to guide weaning from mechanical ventilation.

Prasad et al. first used reinforcement learning algorithms to develop a decision support tool using available patient information to predict time-to-extubation readiness and to recommend a personalized regimen of sedation and ventilatory support. Of note, their tool was also able to predict the need for reintubation [17].

Similarly, the algorithm developed by Parreco et al. forecasted the need for prolonged ventilation and the need for tracheostomy with an AUC of 0.82 [18].

The more recent study of Liu et al. aimed to develop an AI digital dashboard to assist clinicians in weaning management and decisions regarding extubation time and readiness.

A total of 45 features were used to build two-stage predictive models, the try-weaning stage, and the weaning MV stage, by the implementation of seven different ML algorithms including LR, RF, SVM, KNN, lightGBM, XGBoost, and multi-layer perception (MLP). The algorithms with the better performance were then used to build a dashboard for assisting clinical decision making, thereby shortening patients' intubation time by 21 h. Although it may not seem such a large number, it could make a difference in those settings—as it was the COVID-19 pandemic—characterized by a significant disparity between the demand for and the actual availability of mechanical ventilators [19].

18.5 Hemodynamic Monitoring

By continuously assessing parameters such as cardiac output and blood pressure, clinicians can tailor treatments effectively and in a timely manner, thereby improving patient outcomes.

In 2021, Kashou et al. used an AI-augmented ECG (AI-ECG) algorithm to accurately predict left ventricular systolic dysfunction in cardiac ICU patients, with and without atrial fibrillation [20].

The model was also employed by Jentzer et al. for risk stratification, proving that the AI-ECG could effectively reflect the presence of underlying subclinical myocardial disease [21].

AI-based arrhythmia detection and classification on single, 3-, and 12-lead ECG have been tested with success in several recent trials with the intent to predict all-cause mortality. Deep neural networks (DNN) proved to be useful not only in outcome forecasting but also in detecting electrolyte derangements which could be a cause of future arrhythmias [22, 23].

As previously mentioned, the prognostic value of AI algorithms in cardiovascular monitoring and disease has also been underlined by the FAST-PACE model, an AI tool able to predict the occurrence of catastrophic events—i.e., cardiac arrest—up to 6 h before its onset with an AUROC of 0.886 [5].

Similarly, Vedonske et al. used an RF-based algorithm to forecast rehospitalization for congestive heart failure by the analysis of demographical information and data regarding the initial diagnosis and the surgical or interventional procedures [24].

18.6 Delirium

Although delirium is a very common condition encountered in the ICU, both in the postoperative period and as a complication of acute diseases, it is also extremely underdiagnosed [25].

This is especially true in the older patients, despite available information in hospital medical records and validated bedside tools (i.e., 4As test or the CAM-ICU tool) [26].

Moreover, the core of delirium management is centered upon prevention, through the early identification and correction of modifiable risk factors.

An increasing number of studies show how these risk factors can be easily detected through the use of AI-based algorithms [27, 28].

For example, Zhang et al. recently developed an ML model for early prediction of delirium onset in septic patients. By analyzing large patient databases such as the MIMIC-IV and the eICU-CRD with advanced ML tools—i.e., logistic regression techniques, support vector machines, decision trees, random forest, and extreme gradient boosting—they showed how delirium can be diagnosed earlier and with superior performance compared to standard methods. This was especially true for the extreme gradient boosting (XGBoost) model [29].

Similarly, a study by Ren et al. also applied an AI-derived tool—the MySurgery AI system—to the MIMIC-IV and eICU-CRD databases with the aim of constructing delirium-prediction models. Again, the XGBoost model showed the best performance in postoperative complications and delirium prediction. With this, surgeons responsible for postoperative patient care could be early notified and plan proper adjustments in the treatment path [30].

It must be noted that the XGBoost algorithm is completely an open-source model which can be trained through supervised learning to employ decision tree ensembles, and at the same time incorporating regularization techniques to enhance performance. However, although its effectiveness and efficiency, it requires significant computational resources and meticulous tuning [31].

Another interesting study examined the feasibility of the application of the so-called pervasive sensing technology and AI for autonomous and granular monitoring in the ICU with the aim of identifying delirious patients and the peculiarities of their environment.

With the use of wearable sensors, cameras, and light and sound probes, the group performed face detection, face recognition, facial action unit detection, head pose detection, facial expression recognition, posture recognition, extremity movement analysis, sound pressure level detection, light level detection, and visitation frequency detection. Despite the wide range of variables assessed, the estimated cost of the system was less than $300 per ICU room, which is relatively low compared to the daily cost of thousands of dollars per patient [32].

Finally, the application of large language models (LLM)—which usually comprise millions to billions of parameters—to structured electronic health records (EHR) has been recently explored. At the moment, the only LLM-based delirium forecasting tool for ICU HER is the DeLLirium model developed by Rashidi et al. It has been specifically validated to use the HER data available in the first 24 h of ICU admission for early delirium development prediction [33].

18.7 Infection Management

Infection management in the ICU is a discipline which usually requires a great amount of data to be integrated, along with the urgent need for timely and adequate treatment. For this reason, data scientists and physicians are also exploring the application of ML algorithms to this field. Of note, it must be stated how they could lead to potential benefits not only to individual patients—in terms of outcome amelioration—but also to the overall community through improvement of antimicrobial stewardship.

Several studies have been conducted to develop AI models with the aim of forecasting several types of infections commonly encountered in the ICU environment.

In 2018, Parreco et al., by integrating six illness severity scores and comorbidities, created predictive models for CLABSI using different AI tools such as LR, gradient boost trees, and deep learning—the latter method representing the base of the classifier with the highest predictive performance [34].

Another work by Giang et al. explored the ML-based analysis of EHR to predict VAP diagnosis during the ICU stay. In their study, five different ML models were trained to forecast VAP, with the best performance obtained by the XGBoost-based tool (AUROC 0.854) [35].

Moreover ML algorithms have also been useful in the interpretation of diagnostic procedures such as chest X-rays, potentially enhancing early VAP diagnosis [36].

Finally, new diagnostic approaches are also being explored. For example, Chen et al. tested the combination of electronic nose sensor signals with ML for identification of VAP, attaining good diagnostic accuracy [37].

Multidrug-resistant pathogen colonization and infection have also been a topic of interest for potential AI applications in critical care. Since routine MDR laboratory tests usually take 48 h or more, several algorithms have been proposed for identifying patients at the highest risk.

Mora-Jiménez et al. employed three feature selection strategies on EHR, identifying 24 significant features which could be integrated by appropriate AI models to predict MDR colonization/infection development [38].

RF algorithms were also successfully used by Tacconelli et al. to estimate the impact of antibiotic exposure on intestinal colonization with ESBL-producing Gram-negative bacteria (ESBL-GNB) [39].

Infectious states, however, can be often difficult to distinguish from systemic inflammation without infection. For this reason, Lamping et al. used an RF-based ML approach using eight available clinical and laboratory parameters which outperformed the available biomarkers in their ability to discriminate infectious versus non-infectious conditions in a pediatric critically ill patients [40].

Another diagnostic dilemma can be the identification of bacterial superinfection when another source of inflammation is already in place. Clear examples have been the frequent development of bacterial coinfections seen in intensive care patients during the COVID-19 pandemic. As a consequence, Rawson et al. developed ML models based on routine blood test values which in their preliminary study showed promising results, with an AUROC of 0.96 for diagnosing bacterial infection [41].

Timely interruption of inappropriate or unnecessary antibiotic therapy is also an important issue in critical care. Different ML models have been tested for this purpose, most of them relying on clinical parameters, laboratory values, bedside tests results, and prescribed drugs. As an example, the model constructed by Eickelberg et al., using a set of patients suspected of having community-acquired bacterial infections on the MIMIC-III dataset, reached an AUROC of 0.8 and negative predictive values of >93% in the identification of patients at low risk of actually having an infection in place [42].

18.8 Sepsis

Timely identification and prediction of sepsis enable early initiation of appropriate therapy, thereby leading to improved outcomes. However, being a highly heterogeneous syndrome, sepsis can be subtle in the early phase and can often lie undetected until the development of advanced stages.

AI algorithms have demonstrated better performance in diagnosing sepsis compared to standard tools, which often depend on time-consuming lab analyses and have poor predictive accuracy.

It must be noted that, when the well-known SIRS criteria, SAPS-II, and SOFA scores were tested on a large cohort of more than 22,000 ICU patients, they reached AUCs of 0.609, 0.700, and 0.725 respectively for sepsis identification at the time of onset [43].

Research groups that employed AI models for sepsis forecasting have proven far better results. In 2008 a pilot study employed neural network analysis to analyze cytokine and chemokine data to predict sepsis onset in ICU patients, proving an accuracy of 83% in sepsis prediction from 1 to 4 days in advance before onset [44].

The Artificial Intelligence Sepsis Expert algorithm, later developed by Nemati et al., was able to extract high-resolution vital time series and data from large EHR, calculating a set of 65 variables on an hourly basis, and selecting the most significant for sepsis prediction at different time intervals. It finally showed an AUROC in the range of 0.83–0.85 in the ability to predict sepsis onset 4–12 h in advance [45].

One year later, another AI tool specifically designed for early identification of sepsis and septic shock was developed by Fagerström et al. The so-called LiSep

Long Short-Term Memory (LSTM) neural network, after proper training on the MIMIC database, proved excellent results, with an AUROC of 0.8306 and a median of 40 h between septic shock prediction and effective onset [46].

Similarly, the AI algorithm later created by Yuan et al., through the application of the XGBoost tool to a set of preselected features extracted from real-time data, proved to outperform the SOFA score in sepsis diagnosis with an accuracy greater than 80% [47]. AI algorithms with natural language processing capability have also been tested. The Sepsis Early Risk Assessment tool is able to extract data from clinical journals and EHR, accurately predicting sepsis development from 12 h to 2 days in advance and outperforming physicians' and standard scoring methods [48].

The most recent algorithm designed for sepsis forecasting is the NAVOY® Sepsis, which is also the first prediction tool validated against the Sepsis-3 criteria. It processes 4 h of input for routinely collected vitals, blood gas, and lab values to accurately predict sepsis development 3 h in advance, with satisfying performance [49].

18.9 Nutritional Support

The strong link between critical care patients' nutritional status and outcome is well known and extensively documented in literature. Improper or unbalanced dietary intake could, in fact, have an impact on ventilatory weaning, infection rates, length of ICU and in-hospital stay, readmission rate, and mortality [50].

The ability of AI technologies to integrate multiple data sources to reflect patients' changing needs could be useful when applied to more accurate tailoring of nutritional interventions [51].

For this reason, in 2023, Wang et al. aimed to develop an ML algorithm to tailor clinical nutrition in the intensive care environment. Particularly, their aim was the identification of critical care patients in need of early EN initiation. For this reason, patient information from more than 50,000 EHR for the MIMIC-IV database were collected. This large amount of data was used to test six different ML models, with the XGBoost having the best performance [52].

Computer-assisted decision support systems (CDSS) have also been used to estimate the caloric intake and needs of a mixed cohort of critically ill hematology patients, proving the capability to increase caloric and protein goal compliance by more than 50% compared to the cohort with unmonitored nutritional care. However, a reflection in terms of decreased in-hospital mortality, ICU-acquired infection rate, and LOS was not observed [53].

Finally, red-green-blue (RGB) image analysis has also been used. An interesting study by Papathanail et al. employed an AI-based tool to receive input images of the meals before and after their consumption.

By that, the system was able to estimate the volume of each food component before and after consumption, calculating the energy intake and macronutrient intake for every meal with the aim of early identification of patients at highest risk of malnutrition [54].

18.10 Limitations

The judicious application of AI technologies can be useful in the management of the great amount of information that intensivists must deal with. ML algorithms have proved their utility in analyzing EHR, real-time parameters, and diagnostic test results for outcome prediction and timely identification of patients at risk, or disease development and deterioration.

However, some considerations are needed. Although AI can improve the monitoring and management of patients in the complex reality of the ICU environment, there are still significant challenges in terms of reliability, accountability, and integration with traditional clinical practices.

For example, AI heavily relies on the quality and completeness of the data collected from electronic registers or sensors which could be incomplete, inconsistent, or inaccurate—i.e., due to sensor artifacts or missing data. Therefore, in such cases, the reliability of AI-based decisions may be compromised. Moreover, significant and advanced processing power is needed when dealing with unstructured data such as clinical journals or extended diagnostic reports whose analysis could be helpful in diagnosing or forecasting a condition.

Another significant limitation is the sense of suspicion with which physicians and nurses could experience toward very complex AI tools which make diagnoses or therapeutic decisions in a way that is not clearly and verbally justified, but is just code-based—the so-called black box effect [55, 56].

In this sense, it is even more difficult for clinicians to identify when and how AI is suggesting a wrong diagnosis or recommending an incorrect treatment.

Significant is also the technical expertise required for the update and maintenance of very complex AI-based technologies and machines. If such systems are not constantly ameliorated by integrating updated clinical data or revised in view of eventual medical breakthroughs they can quickly become obsolete or even potentially misleading.

Since ICU patient monitoring implies the collection of large amounts of sensitive personal and medical information, meticulous compliance of data privacy regulations is mandatory. At the same time, the implementation of reliable data protection systems must be encouraged and adopted, to prevent unauthorized access from harming patients' privacy.

Training is therefore mandatory to grant efficient interaction and integration between personnel and AI. On the one hand, this avoids excessive mistrust in potentially useful tools which may be perceived as a threat for professional independence. On the other hand, this prevents AI-based results or data are not judiciously assessed through the lens of clinical interpretation, thereby leading the operators to entirely and uncritically rely on this kind of information [57].

Clinical judgment is in fact mandatory, not only for the complexity of intensive care medicine, but also for the multifaceted nature of critically ill patients. Each patient has their own condition, medical history, physiologic reserve, and response to treatments. Although in most of the cases AI-based decisions ground on a large amount of data from different patients, they may not always be capable of taking such a sophisticated variability into account. This can be true especially for highly compromised patients or when unexpected events take place—i.e., in emergency scenarios—for which some systems may not have been designed for.

When an AI-based technology makes an interpretation mistake or provides a misleading instruction, the question arises as to whose fault it is. Again, it must be highlighted how clinicians must never fully delegate machines for therapeutic decisions or blindly trust on AI-derived data. However, this is still an issue to be clarified at the regulatory level [58].

Finally, as it is common in every field and particularly in healthcare, innovative technology requires a large amount of funding. This could lead to disparities between hospitals or regions with inadequate resources to implement such advanced tools on a large scale.

18.11 Conclusion

Experienced intensivists are skilled at quickly analyzing a large amount of clinical data to make diagnoses and treatment decisions. However, in today's data-heavy ICU environment, managing the overwhelming flow of information, much of which is irrelevant, is a significant challenge. AI technology can help address this information overload. ML algorithms have already shown promise in predicting ICU outcomes and identifying at-risk populations through the analysis of EHR, enabling physicians to timely titrate therapies or guide clinical decisions.

A more ambitious goal is the development of intelligent monitoring systems capable of continuously assessing critical illness with higher accuracy. Such technology could lead to the creation of a semi-autonomous ICU, where machines take over many tasks currently handled by humans. Yet, the full potential of AI in the ICU will be realized only when it becomes a trusted clinical tool, helping intensivists focus on the human aspects of care while managing data in a more effective manner. While there will be challenges and ethical issues, AI's role in ICU care is expected to rise; therefore, it is essential for healthcare professionals to embrace and understand this technology for the benefit of their patients. However, the use of AI in the care of critically ill patients must be approached cautiously, with a proper balance between automation and human oversight. AI should be viewed as a supportive tool rather than a replacement for medical staff, and its implementation requires careful consideration of ethical, legal, and technical implications.

In summary, while AI can enhance patient monitoring and management in the ICU, there are still significant challenges related to reliability, accountability, and integration with traditional clinical practices. A balance between technology and human supervision remains essential to ensure patient safety and treatment effectiveness.

References

1. Mao Z, Liu C, Li Q, Cui Y, Zhou F. Intelligent intensive care unit: current and future trends. Intensive Care Res. 2023;3(2):182–8. https://doi.org/10.1007/s44231-023-00036-5.
2. Copeland B. Artificial Intelligence. Encyclopedia Britannica. 2024. https://www.britannica.com/technology/artificial-intelligence.

3. Calvert J, Mao Q, Hoffman JL, Jay M, Desautels T, Mohamadlou H, et al. Using electronic health record collected clinical variables to predict medical intensive care unit mortality. Ann Med Surg. 2016;11:52–7. https://doi.org/10.1016/j.amsu.2016.09.002.
4. Awad A, Bader-El-Den M, McNicholas J, Briggs J. Early hospital mortality prediction of intensive care unit patients using an ensemble learning approach. Int J Med Inform. 2017;108:185–95.
5. Kim J, Chae M, Chang HJ, Kim YA, Park E. Predicting cardiac arrest and respiratory failure using feasible artificial intelligence with simple trajectories of patient data. J Clin Med. 2019;8(9):1336.
6. Mahboub B, Bataineh MT, Al Alshraideh H, Hamoudi R, Salameh L, Shamayleh A. Prediction of COVID-19 hospital length of stay and risk of death using artificial intelligence-based modeling. Front Med. 2021;8:592336.
7. Kobayashi N, Shiga T, Ikumi S, Watanabe K, Murakami H, Yamauchi M. Semi-automated tracking of pain in critical care patients using artificial intelligence: a retrospective observational study. Sci Rep. 2021;11(1):1–7. https://doi.org/10.1038/s41598-021-84714-8.
8. Kobayashi N, Watanabe K, Murakami H, Yamauchi M. Continuous visualization and validation of pain in critically ill patients using artificial intelligence: a retrospective observational study. Sci Rep. 2023;13(1):1–8. https://doi.org/10.1038/s41598-023-44970-2.
9. Cascella M, Schiavo D, Cuomo A, Ottaiano A, Perri F, Patrone R, et al. Artificial intelligence for automatic pain assessment: research methods and perspectives. Pain Res Manag. 2023;2023:6018736.
10. Nerella S, Guan Z, Siegel S, Zhang J, Khezeli K, Bihorac A, et al. AI-enhanced intensive care unit: revolutionizing patient care with pervasive sensing. 2023. Available from: http://arxiv.org/abs/2303.06252
11. Chen C-W, Lin W-C, Hsu C-H, Cheng K-S, Lo C-S. Detecting ineffective triggering in the expiratory phase in mechanically ventilated patients based on airway flow and pressure deflection: feasibility of using a computer algorithm. Crit Care Med. 2008;36(2):455–61.
12. Blanch L, Sales B, Montanya J, Lucangelo U, Garcia-Esquirol O, Villagra A, et al. Validation of the Better Care® system to detect ineffective efforts during expiration in mechanically ventilated patients: a pilot study. Intensive Care Med. 2012;38(5):772–80.
13. Adams JY, Lieng MK, Kuhn BT, Rehm GB, Guo EC, Taylor SL, et al. Development and validation of a multi-algorithm analytic platform to detect off-target mechanical ventilation. Sci Rep. 2017;7(1):14980.
14. Rehm GB, Han J, Kuhn BT, Delplanque J-P, Anderson NR, Adams JY, et al. Creation of a robust and generalizable machine learning classifier for patient ventilator asynchrony. Methods Inf Med. 2018;57(4):208–19.
15. Sottile PD, Albers D, Higgins C, Mckeehan J, Moss MM. The association between ventilator Dyssynchrony, delivered tidal volume, and sedation using a novel automated ventilator Dyssynchrony detection algorithm. Crit Care Med. 2018;46(2):e151–7.
16. Gholami B, Phan TS, Haddad WM, Cason A, Mullis J, Price L, et al. Replicating human expertise of mechanical ventilation waveform analysis in detecting patient-ventilator cycling asynchrony using machine learning. Comput Biol Med. 2018;97:137–44.
17. Prasad N, Cheng LF, Chivers C, Draugelis M, Engelhardt BE. A reinforcement learning approach to weaning of mechanical ventilation in intensive care units. In: Uncertain artificial intelligence – Proceedings of the 33rd conference, UAI 2017; 2017.
18. Parreco J, Hidalgo A, Parks JJ, Kozol R, Rattan R. Using artificial intelligence to predict prolonged mechanical ventilation and tracheostomy placement. J Surg Res. 2018;228:179–87.
19. Liu C-F, Hung C-M, Ko S-C, Cheng K-C, Chao C-M, Sung M-I, et al. An artificial intelligence system to predict the optimal timing for mechanical ventilation weaning for intensive care unit patients: a two-stage prediction approach. Front Med. 2022;9:935366.
20. Kashou AH, Noseworthy PA, Lopez-Jimenez F, Attia ZI, Kapa S, Friedman PA, et al. The effect of cardiac rhythm on artificial intelligence-enabled ECG evaluation of left ventricular ejection fraction prediction in cardiac intensive care unit patients. Int J Cardiol. 2021;339:54–5.

21. Jentzer JC, Kashou AH, Lopez-Jimenez F, Attia ZI, Kapa S, Friedman PA, et al. Mortality risk stratification using artificial intelligence-augmented electrocardiogram in cardiac intensive care unit patients. Eur Heart J Acute Cardiovasc Care. 2021;10(5):532–41.
22. Raghunath S, Ulloa Cerna AE, Jing L, van Maanen DP, Stough J, Hartzel DN, et al. Prediction of mortality from 12-lead electrocardiogram voltage data using a deep neural network. Nat Med. 2020;26(6):886–91.
23. Medvedofsky D, Mor-Avi V, Amzulescu M, Fernández-Golfín C, Hinojar R, Monaghan MJ, et al. Three-dimensional echocardiographic quantification of the left-heart chambers using an automated adaptive analytics algorithm: multicentre validation study. Eur Heart J. 2018;19(1):47–58.
24. Vedomske M, Brown D, Harrison J. Random Forests on Ubiquitous Data for Heart Failure 30-Day Readmissions Prediction. In: Proceedings – 2013 12th international conference on machine learning and applications, ICMLA 2013, vol. 2; 2013. p. 415–21.
25. Da Silva Baptista Faria R, Moreno RP. Delirium na unidade de cuidados intensivos: uma realidade subdiagnosticada. Rev Bras Ter Intensiva. 2013;25(2):137–47.
26. Titlestad I, Haugarvoll K, Solvang SEH, Norekvål TM, Skogseth RE, Andreassen OA, et al. Delirium is frequently underdiagnosed among older hospitalised patients despite available information in hospital medical records. Age Ageing. 2024;53(2):1–8.
27. Ocagli H, Bottigliengo D, Lorenzoni G, Azzolina D, Acar AS, Sorgato S, et al. A machine learning approach for investigating delirium as a multifactorial syndrome. Int J Environ Res Public Health. 2021;18(13):7105.
28. Othman MI, Nashwan AJ, Abujaber AA, Khatib MY. Artificial intelligence applications in the intensive care unit for sepsis-associated encephalopathy and delirium: a narrative review. Avicenna. 2024;2023(2):1–10.
29. Zhang Y, Hu J, Hua T, Zhang J, Zhang Z, Yang M. Development of a machine learning-based prediction model for sepsis-associated delirium in the intensive care unit. Sci Rep. 2023;13(1):1–12. https://doi.org/10.1038/s41598-023-38650-4.
30. Ren Y, Loftus TJ, Datta S, Ruppert MM, Guan Z, Miao S, et al. Performance of a machine learning algorithm using electronic health record data to predict postoperative complications and report on a Mobile platform. JAMA Netw Open. 2022;5(5):e2211973.
31. Bentéjac C, Csörgő A, Martínez-Muñoz G. A comparative analysis of gradient boosting algorithms. Artif Intell Rev. 2021;54:1937.
32. Davoudi A, Malhotra KR, Shickel B, Siegel S, Williams S, Ruppert M, et al. Intelligent ICU for autonomous patient monitoring using pervasive sensing and deep learning. Sci Rep. 2019;9(1):8020.
33. Contreras M, Kapoor S, Zhang J, Davidson A, Ren Y. DeLLiriuM: a large language model for delirium prediction in the ICU using structured EHR. Res Sq. 2025;77:1–16.
34. Parreco JP, Hidalgo AE, Badilla AD, Ilyas O, Rattan R. Predicting central line-associated bloodstream infections and mortality using supervised machine learning. J Crit Care. 2018;45:156–62.
35. Giang C, Calvert J, Rahmani K, Barnes G, Siefkas A, Green-Saxena A, et al. Predicting ventilator-associated pneumonia with machine learning. Medicine (Baltimore). 2021;100(23):e26246.
36. Hwang EJ, Park S, Jin K-N, Kim JI, Choi SY, Lee JH, et al. Development and validation of a deep learning-based automated detection algorithm for major thoracic diseases on chest radiographs. JAMA Netw Open. 2019;2(3):e191095.
37. Chen CY, Lin WC, Yang HY. Diagnosis of ventilator-associated pneumonia using electronic nose sensor array signals: solutions to improve the application of machine learning in respiratory research. Respir Res. 2020;21(1):1–12.
38. Mora-Jiménez I, Tarancón-Rey J, Álvarez-Rodríguez J, Soguero-Ruiz C. Artificial intelligence to get insights of multi-drug resistance risk factors during the first 48 hours from ICU admission. Antibiot (Basel, Switzerland). 2021;10(3):239.
39. Tacconelli E, Górska A, De Angelis G, Lammens C, Restuccia G, Schrenzel J, et al. Estimating the association between antibiotic exposure and colonization with extended-spectrum

β-lactamase-producing Gram-negative bacteria using machine learning methods: a multicentre, prospective cohort study. Clin Microbiol Infect. 2020;26(1):87–94.
40. Lamping F, Jack T, Rübsamen N, Sasse M, Beerbaum P, Mikolajczyk RT, et al. Development and validation of a diagnostic model for early differentiation of sepsis and non-infectious SIRS in critically ill children – a data-driven approach using machine-learning algorithms. BMC Pediatr. 2018;18(1):1–11.
41. Rawson TM, Hernandez B, Wilson RC, Ming D, Herrero P, Ranganathan N, et al. Supervised machine learning to support the diagnosis of bacterial infection in the context of COVID-19. JAC-Antimicrobial Resist. 2021;3(1):2–5.
42. Eickelberg G, Sanchez-Pinto LN, Luo Y. Predictive modeling of bacterial infections and antibiotic therapy needs in critically ill adults. J Biomed Inform. 2020;109:103540.
43. Desautels T, Calvert J, Hoffman J, Jay M, Kerem Y, Shieh L, et al. Prediction of sepsis in the intensive care unit with minimal electronic health record data: a machine learning approach. JMIR Med Inform. 2016;4(3):e28.
44. Lukaszewski RA, Yates AM, Jackson MC, Swingler K, Scherer JM, Simpson AJ, Sadler P, McQuillan P, Titball RW, Brooks TJG, Pearce MJ. Presymptomatic prediction of sepsis in intensive care unit patients. Clin Vaccine Immunol. 2008;15(7):1089–94. https://doi.org/10.1128/CVI.00486-07.
45. Nemati S, Holder A, Razmi F, Stanley MD, Clifford GD, Buchman TG. An interpretable machine learning model for accurate prediction of sepsis in the ICU. Crit Care Med. 2018;46(4):547–53.
46. Fagerström J, Bång M, Wilhelms D, Chew MS. LiSep LSTM: a machine learning algorithm for early detection of septic shock. Sci Rep. 2019;9(1):1–8.
47. Yuan K-C, Tsai L-W, Lee K-H, Cheng Y-W, Hsu S-C, Lo Y-S, et al. The development an artificial intelligence algorithm for early sepsis diagnosis in the intensive care unit. Int J Med Inform. 2020;141:104176.
48. Goh KH, Wang L, Yeow AYK, Poh H, Li K, Yeow JJL, et al. Artificial intelligence in sepsis early prediction and diagnosis using unstructured data in healthcare. Nat Commun. 2021;12(1):711.
49. Persson I, Macura A, Becedas D, Sjövall F. Early prediction of sepsis in intensive care patients using the machine learning algorithm NAVOY® Sepsis, a prospective randomized clinical validation study. J Crit Care. 2024;80:154400.
50. Ferrie S, Weiss NB, Chau HY, Torkel S, Stepniewski ME. Association of Subjective Global Assessment with outcomes in the intensive care unit: a retrospective cohort study. Nutr Diet. 2022;79(5):572–81.
51. Kittrell HD, Shaikh A, Adintori PA, McCarthy P, Kohli-Seth R, Nadkarni GN, et al. Role of artificial intelligence in critical care nutrition support and research. Nutr Clin Pract. 2024;39(5):1069–80.
52. Wang Y-X, Li X-L, Zhang L-H, Li H-N, Liu X-M, Song W, et al. Machine learning algorithms assist early evaluation of enteral nutrition in ICU patients. Front Nutr. 2023;10:1060398.
53. Ettori F, Henin A, Zemmour C, Chow-Chine L, Sannini A, Bisbal M, et al. Impact of a computer-assisted decision support system (CDSS) on nutrition management in critically ill hematology patients: the NUTCHOCO study (nutritional care in hematology oncologic patients and critical outcome). Ann Intensive Care. 2019;9(1):53.
54. Papathanail I, Brühlmann J, Vasiloglou MF, Stathopoulou T, Exadaktylos AK, Stanga Z, et al. Evaluation of a novel artificial intelligence system to monitor and assess energy and macronutrient intake in hospitalised older patients. Nutrients. 2021;13(12):4539.
55. Filho LACB. Artificial intelligence: what should an intensivist have in mind in the beginning of the new era? Anaesth Pain Intensive Care. 2021;25(1):8–12.
56. Yoon JH, Pinsky MR, Clermont G. Artificial intelligence in critical care medicine. Crit Care. 2022;26(1):75.
57. Schulz CM, Endsley MR, Kochs EF, Gelb AW, Wagner KJ. Situation awareness in anesthesia: concept and research. Anesthesiology. 2013;118(3):729–42.
58. Schulz CM, Burden A, Posner KL, Mincer SL, Steadman R, Wagner KJ, et al. Frequency and type of situational awareness errors contributing to death and brain damage: a closed claims analysis. Anesthesiology. 2017;127(2):326–37.

A Short Review on Artificial Intelligence in MCIs—Current and Future Applications

19

Emmanouil Pikoulis, Dimitrios Papakostantinou, and Nikolaos Pararas

19.1 Transforming MCIs Through AI

Artificial intelligence (AI) has already demonstrated potential in revolutionizing telemedicine by improving diagnostic accuracy, decision-making, and predictive analytics. Through the analysis of diverse data sources such as medical imaging, patient records, and vital signs, AI contributes significantly to clinical processes [2, 22, 58, 64]. It can establish personalized care treatment, provide procedural guidance, and aid in increased remote evaluations of patients, leading to a more streamlined and compassionate approach to effective and accessible care [23, 72].

The frequency and intensity of natural disasters, which include strong storms and heavy precipitation, have caused significant damage in both developed and underdeveloped countries and have been significantly raised by the continuous consequences of global climate change and rapid urbanization [8, 45]. Mass casualty incidents (MCIs), whether caused by man-made catastrophes like terrorist attacks or shootings or natural disasters, also provide challenging circumstances that require careful judgment. These events entail more complicated levels of decision-making, ongoing threats to safety and security, extended efforts in triage and transport, prolonged injuries needing immediate attention, and heightened sensitivity to responders' abilities and inter-agency cooperation [69]. In emergency and disaster medicine, when effective resource management and quick decision-making are crucial, MCIs present some of the most challenging obstacles in healthcare provision. Research shows that the likelihood of surviving serious injuries drastically decreases between 12 and 24 h after a disaster

E. Pikoulis (✉) · D. Papakostantinou · N. Pararas
3d Surgical Department NKUA, Attikon University Hospital, Athens, Greece
e-mail: mpikoul@med.uoa.gr

B. De Simone et al. (eds.), *New Technologies, Precision Medicine, and AI in Emergency General Surgery*, Hot Topics in Acute Care Surgery and Trauma,
https://doi.org/10.1007/978-3-032-09357-8_19

[45]. An immediate and efficient trauma response is essential for preserving lives during such events [70].

Emergency medical service (EMS) systems, operating under MCI conditions, face numerous challenges, including medical coordination, rescue operations, and limited accessibility [2, 12, 46]. A fundamental principle in the effective management of MCIs is triage [65, 66]. Triage plays a crucial role in prehospital emergency care, involving the precise evaluation of patients' injuries or life-threatening conditions [14]. This process helps prioritize patients for treatment and transport to the appropriate medical facilities, ultimately enhancing their chances of survival and overall quality of life [30].

Commonly used triage methods in prehospital settings include Simple Triage and Rapid Treatment (START), modified Simple Triage and Rapid Treatment (mSTART), Field Triage Score (FTS), Amberg-Schwandorf Algorithm for Primary Triage (ASAV), and Sort, Assess, Life-saving, Interventions, Treatment, and Transportation (SALT) [13, 28, 38, 30]. However, these triage methods may not be effective in hazardous environments [56].

Within this context, AI emerges as a transformative innovation for MCI response, offering significant potential in enhancing triage accuracy, clinical decision-making, and resource allocation [63]. By employing advanced risk assessment methodologies, artificial intelligence (AI) systems play a critical role in the detection and classification of victims [34, 20]. These frameworks incorporate technologies such as computer vision (CV), natural language processing (NLP), and machine learning (ML) to assess injury severity and forecast patient outcomes [17, 20]. Consequently, AI contributes significantly to prediction and triage optimization. Deep learning systems, particularly those incorporating computer vision, show great potential in complementing traditional triage protocols [50]. Intelligent victim identification in disaster scenarios, for instance, primarily depends on computer vision. These technologies enable automated systems to extract meaningful insights from imagery captured in disaster zones, thereby supporting rapid and accurate identification of victims [37]. By analyzing extensive volumes of both visual and textual information, AI can also identify subtle signs of life-threatening conditions that may be overlooked by human responders [40, 20]. This is realized by enabling early identification of warning signs through the analysis of images captured by drones or body cameras worn by emergency teams [50]. These approaches hold the potential to reduce casualty rates by ensuring that critical patients receive immediate attention, which is particularly vital when the number of victims overwhelms available resources [34, 63].

MCIs are defined by their sudden onset and the high volume of casualties that exceed the capacity of local response systems [47, 48]. In circumstances characterized by chaos and time urgency, the ability of AI to analyze real-time data improves the speed and accuracy of initial assessments [40, 41]. This level of detailed analysis is especially crucial, given that rapid and accurate decision-making is vital to increasing survival rates in MCIs [34, 63]. Consequently, AI-powered triage has surfaced as a breakthrough innovation that redefines emergency response protocols in both natural and man-made disasters [17, 63].

The integration of AI into emergency medicine, characterized by its demanding organizational dynamics and the necessity for swift and accurate clinical decisions, presents considerable opportunities for technological innovation. Integrating AI in this domain can enhance prioritization of patients, support clinical decision-making, improve operational efficiency, and strengthen early warning capabilities [43, 57]. While AI tools have already demonstrated success in emergency departments, their application in prehospital emergency care remains mostly experimental, calling for further prospective validation [18].

19.2 Current and Future Applications of AI in MCIs

In recent years, there has been a growing interest in researching and developing technological tools to aid first responders (FRs) in sudden onset disasters and MCIs. AI systems based on reinforcement learning algorithms help optimize real-time allocation of medical resources and routing strategies, adapting dynamically to evolving MCI scenarios [2]. Such planning can reduce patient waiting times and improve outcomes. Additionally, continuous monitoring platforms enhance the precision of critical patient tracking and enable early detection of clinical deterioration [50]. Simultaneously, the emergence of generative AI opens new possibilities for processing and synthesizing large volumes of information in real time, providing executive summaries and adaptations of protocols that are useful for healthcare teams deployed on-site [62]. The synergy between AI and other emerging technologies, such as the Internet of Things (IoT) and advanced sensor networks, further enhances mass casualty management. While AI algorithms rapidly predict and assess patient conditions, connected devices can relay real-time physiological data to central command centers, ensuring that every casualty receives timely and appropriate care [39, 54].

The increasing frequency of MCIs underscores the need for advanced health monitoring and electronic triage (E-triage) systems, where machine learning (ML) algorithms can offer substantial advantages. Recent research demonstrates that AI, machine learning (ML), and deep learning (DL) models can outperform traditional triage systems in predicting patient outcomes, such as mortality and hospital admissions [6, 17].

A notable study by Lu et al. [49], for instance, proposed an intelligent triage system that integrated unmanned aerial vehicles (UAVs), artificial intelligence (AI), and 5G technology to support rapid on-site assessment during MCIs. This system employed two AI algorithms: OpenPose, which enabled real-time analysis of human body posture by detecting key anatomical points to evaluate individuals' conditions, and You Only Look Once (YOLO), an object detection model used to locate and identify people within the UAV's visual field, thereby assisting in recognizing injured individuals and their postures. The combined application of these models facilitated an effective and responsive triage framework for emergency scenarios.

An AI application by Jin et al. [39] uses deep neural network (DNN) algorithms (an architecture capable of capturing complex, non-linear relationships in high-dimensional data) that aim to predict vital signs and optimize treatment protocols for hemorrhagic casualties in order to improve clinical outcomes under resource-limited conditions. Researchers generated synthetic vital-sign data using a cardio-respiratory (CR) model that modeled various hemorrhage scenarios. Then, a gated recurrent unit (GRU) model was trained using this data to forecast the time-series evolution of systolic blood pressure (SBP) and heart rate (HR) over the course of fluid resuscitation. The authors compared their model to the vampire program of the Department of Defense, a recommendation for fluid resuscitation, and concluded that their trained AI model was used to maximize fluid distribution. The authors also investigated the capacity of the AI model to identify non-compressible bleeding, a crucial issue in trauma care.

In a study by Kim et al. [42], researchers developed a data-driven artificial intelligence model aimed at enabling remote triage in prehospital settings during MCIs. The intent of this model was to allow for a classification system that would enable survival prediction without input from medical professionals, which would allow for faster communication during triage. To improve prediction accuracy, the study introduced a novel consciousness index as an alternative to conventional medical evaluation criteria. The study tested different machine learning algorithms—logistic regression, random forest, and deep neural networks. Among them, the deep neural network (DNN) demonstrated the best performance, achieving an area under the curve (AUC) of 0.89, significantly surpassing traditional scoring methods such as the revised trauma score (RTS).

An innovative AI-driven framework is also proposed by Olivia et al. [54]. Their model integrates quality-of-service-aware routing protocols with casualty triage prediction mechanisms. Essentially, it leverages wearable body sensor technology for real-time transmission of vital signs (e.g., heart rate, oxygen levels), prediction of clinical severity, and optimal allocation of medical resources. The system uses a quality-of-service (QoS)-aware, load-sensitive routing protocol, which is designed to ensure timely and efficient delivery of high-priority medical data in congested or unstable ad hoc network environments, thereby outperforming conventional protocols like AODV in emergency scenarios. A backpropagation neural network (a type of machine learning model that learns by adjusting its weights based on prediction errors), trained using the MIMIC-II ICU dataset and qSOFA scoring (a quick clinical tool used to assess the severity of illness), enables early forecasting of deteriorating clinical conditions. Moreover, a genetic algorithm (an optimization technique inspired by natural selection) combined with queuing theory (a mathematical model to manage waiting lines) helps allocate resources separately for critical and non-critical patients based on predicted severity transitions, leading to improved throughput (faster data processing) and a reduction in queue length for severe cases. Simulation results showed 95% prediction accuracy and demonstrated effective prioritization and resource optimization. While current validation was based on MIMIC-II data, future work includes real-time deployment in collaboration with emergency response agencies. According to Olivia et al. [54], optimization can be made through ensemble and deep learning models for better prediction accuracy and by refining the resource allocation algorithm to consider factors such as casualty severity, geography, and facility availability.

In the context of MCI management training, the incorporation of AI-powered immersive virtual reality (VR) platforms has significantly impacted the effectiveness of training simulations. Traditional training approaches for MCI preparedness generally fall into three main categories: (1) full-scale live simulations using manikins or actors in temporary, staged environments; (2) tabletop exercises that function similarly to board games; and (3) didactic lectures or presentations that may be supplemented by case-based discussions centered on victim care strategies [69]. In a study by Way et al. [69], a VR-based simulator for MCIs that integrates AI capabilities to provide adaptive training for first responders in areas such as triage and emergency communication was assessed. Generative AI also stands out in the training field, where generative pretrained transformer (GPT) models are being used to create realistic, personalized virtual simulations for training in triage and initial stabilization. These systems offer immediate feedback and support remote, collaborative learning through adaptive clinical cases—particularly valuable for MCIs, where real-life training opportunities are limited [35].

19.2.1 The NIGHTINGALE Project

In line with this innovative trend, the European Union (EU) financed the project NIGHTINGALE, which stands for "Novel Integrated Toolkit for Enhanced Prehospital Life Support and Triage in Challenging and Large Emergencies." The aim of the project is to render first responders more ready and effective via multidisciplinary organizational synergy and technological integration that allows for triaging, prehospital life support, damage control measures, and prehospital processes in the event of an MCI.

The NIGHTINGALE toolkit incorporates a variety of tools, services, and applications for field triage during an MCI, better management of resources, and interagency collaboration [52, 71]. Thus, many AI tools and machine learning projects were situated within the project for additional decision support and predictive abilities in the field that would otherwise improve MCI efforts at the prehospital level. Therefore, these AI-supported efforts focus on real-time triage of the patients, ease of resource allocation for agencies, and casualty prognosis for better field treatment options and chances of survival. Yet the development of such tools faced significant obstacles within the NIGHTINGALE creation process as well, due to the scarce availability of prehospital MCI patient data on which to train the AIs and ML projects according to General Data Protection Regulation (GDPR) requirements. Ultimately, NIGHTINGALE engineers had to rely on hospital data sets to a certain degree [24], which aid in simulating results but do not accurately reflect what happens to patients in the prehospital setting or what occurs to those patients after treatment and subsequent hospital admission.

Effective AI training requires rigorous processes of data collection, preprocessing, validation, and evaluation, steps that are critical to enabling models to recognize patterns, reduce errors, and generalize across varied emergency scenarios [59]. Yet such a comprehensive and controlled collection of data is difficult to achieve in the prehospital environment [21]. These difficulties are especially acute during MCIs, where available resources are overwhelmed and prioritization naturally shifts toward immediate life-saving actions, often at the expense of structured data recording [60]. Therefore, anticipated data—patient names and ages, nature of the incident, past medical history, vital signs, and reaction to any treatment—are unavailable or incomplete. Even when patients are continuously monitored, for example, in mobile intensive care settings, this data is often not stored, as it is not considered necessary for immediate interventions. The absence of curated, high-fidelity data ultimately constrains the development of strong AI models and limits the potential impact of AI on improving emergency outcomes [16].

To address these challenges, the NIGHTINGALE project focused on integrating continuous monitoring of casualties' vital signs, alongside demographic information, patient details, and treatment data [52]. One notable advancement is the use of integrated sensors and applications, such as wearable devices, that continuously monitor and transmit vital signs to a central storage system. Additionally, the project aims to develop a system that enables data interoperability, allowing seamless access, querying, and retrieval of data from different sources [71]. Therefore, when information is received from multi-sensor and application sources, it must be standardized and normalized so that any AI can access and employ it. Standardization allows the systems to operate without concerns about format or structure, ensuring interoperability and enabling efficient use of diverse datasets for decision-making [10].

In the same fashion, Lamine et al. [29] argue that the adoption of advanced technologies in managing prehospital MCIs is significantly hindered by the absence of a cohesive, cross-disciplinary framework for developing and implementing key performance indicators (KPIs). Drawing on qualitative focus group insights from medical professionals and technology developers involved in the NIGHTINGALE project, the study uncovered major discrepancies in how KPIs are interpreted and applied. These differences are particularly noticeable in the debate over whether KPIs should primarily assess the effectiveness of first responders or be used to evaluate the functionality of technological innovations. The findings suggest that without the creation of a shared language and collaborative development processes, the full potential of tools like AI-based decision support, wearable tech, and integrated communication platforms remains unrealized, making it difficult to objectively evaluate and enhance MCI response performance.

19.2.2 AI-Driven Disaster Management Applications

Disaster management in MCIs is one of the most critical areas where technology, especially AI and machine learning (ML), is creating new response and recovery mechanisms for various disasters, both natural and man-made. These innovations are revolutionizing how governments, humanitarian organizations, and communities manage disaster situations. Recent studies emphasize the use of AI combined with social media analytics to gather real-time data and improve communication in disaster-affected areas [44]. The application of AI within smart city infrastructure has also been useful in creating a resilient urban environment for the purpose of limiting disasters [25], while big data analytics has shown significant value in forecasting and reducing the impact of disasters by processing vast amounts of geospatial and weather-related data. It can also aid in planning optimal evacuation routes and managing traffic during emergencies to minimize casualties and enhance safety [11].

Incorporation of artificial intelligence (AI) tools into mass casualty incident (MCI) management has also led to the creation of innovative communication platforms designed to enable swift, secure, and efficient information exchange among emergency response teams [55, 63]. Aboualola et al. [4] explored how the integration of artificial intelligence and edge technologies with social media is being utilized in disaster management. The study emphasized that AI plays a crucial role in enabling real-time data processing to support decision-making, while social media serves as a key tool for spreading information during emergencies. In addition, social media analytics have been used to track public sentiment, identify emerging needs, and foster community engagement during disasters [7]. Also, AI-enabled communication platforms have significantly enhanced the coordination and information sharing among healthcare providers, emergency responders, and government agencies, improving response efforts and ensuring the swift dissemination of vital information to affected populations [27]. Table 19.1 summarizes key AI applications and their outcomes across various disaster types, showcasing the impact of real-time AI implementation on disaster response and management efforts.

Table 19.1 Summary of Real-time AI impact assessment in disaster management

Disaster type	AI application	Impact	Study
Hurricane	AI for prediction and impact analysis	Reduced false alarms by 30%, improved evacuation routes by 20%	Aboualola et al. [4]
Flood	AI-driven early warning systems	Early alerts improved by 25%, reducing casualties by 15%	Abid et al. [3]
Earthquake	Seismic data analysis using machine learning	Enhanced prediction accuracy by 40%	Waghmare et al. [67]
Wildfires	Drone surveillance with AI processing	Reduced damage assessment time by 35%	Ahmed et al. [9]
Flood	Social media analytics	50% faster community response time	Nunavath and Goodwin [53]
Urban disaster	IoT and edge computing	Real-time decision-making, reduced response time by 20%	Murata et al. [51]
General disaster	AI-enhanced UAVs for damage mapping	Increased mapping speed by 60%, aiding faster recovery	Inoguchi et al. [36]
Fire	UAVs with AI for fire control	Improved fire containment rate by 30%	Ahmed et al. [9]
Flood	Machine learning for traffic management	Optimized evacuation traffic flow, reducing congestion by 40%	Aved et al. [11]

(continued)

Table 19.1 (continued)

Disaster type	AI application	Impact	Study
Earthquake	Machine learning for structural integrity assessment	Early structural damage predictions improved by 25%	Wagner and Roopaei [68]
Hurricane	AI-assisted communication systems	Improved coordination among 15% more relief agencies	Aboualola et al. [4]
Flood	Edge decision-making systems	Decreased emergency response time by 50%	Wagner and Roopaei [68]
Wildfires	AI-based risk assessment tools	Early warnings improved by 35%	Ahmed et al. [9]
Fire	Automated incident detection systems	Reduced initial response delays by 20%	Ghadge [32]
General disaster	AI-based predictive analytics	10% overall improvement in disaster preparedness	Elvas et al. [25]

Table adapted from Kumar [44]

19.3 Responsible AI Deployment

The implementation of AI in prehospital care offers significant promise to enhance first responders' effectiveness; however, it also introduces challenges associated with model development, particularly the acquisition and curation of high-quality, relevant, and diverse datasets [33]. The challenge is both the volume and quality of acquired data, as high-quality data is crucial to avoid "garbage in, garbage out" issues [15]. For instance, if AI systems don't accurately match patient data with treatment details, prediction accuracy suffers. Trauma cases add complexity, needing diverse data to handle rare but critical situations like severe abdominal injuries or pregnant women with high intracranial pressure. AI must "learn" from a broad data pool, including trauma mechanisms, field care quality, and treatment timelines. Therefore, practices such as data curation, preprocessing, and filtering are essential for effective AI models in different clinical scenarios [16, 33].

In addition to the non-standardized data collection methods, the lack of interoperability between various systems poses difficulties in the integration and scalability of AI solutions across different stakeholders and regions [5]. Simultaneously, ethical frameworks should prioritize algorithmic transparency and explainability as well as ensure that AI systems are accountable, respect patient autonomy, and adhere to the core principles of justice and beneficence [2, 19]. Furthermore, data privacy and security considerations are increasingly important in protecting sensitive health information and ensuring compliance with existing regulations such as the European General Data Protection Regulation (GDPR) [31]. Compliance with these frameworks involves implementing secure protocols for the storage, transmission, and processing of data as a way to prevent unauthorized access, while also promoting equitable access to technology [1]. These ethical and regulatory imperatives are present in the European Parliament's Artificial Intelligence Act, passed in March 2024, which sets out clear standards for responsible AI development and deployment [26].

The incorporation of AI tools into mass casualty incident (MCI) management is at an early stage. The urgent need for prospective validation studies is continuously underscored by the limited real-world case studies available to assess AI tools' effectiveness in high-pressure, real-time scenarios [18]. Further research and development are necessary to make these tools fully operational, including clinical validation to ensure they can assist first responders and gather critical data without adding complexity or delaying patient care [61]. At the same time, specific regulatory guidelines are required to address issues such as data privacy, result interpretability, and legal responsibility to support widespread implementation [60].

Several recommendations emerge in an effort to address the current gaps in data and enhance the integration of AI technologies in prehospital care. First, transfer learning can address data scarcity by utilizing large, pretrained AI models that can be adapted using smaller, domain-specific datasets. With this approach, the need for vast amounts of data, a challenge in emergency settings where data collection is often restricted, is eliminated. Secondly, the advancement of user-friendly technologies that allow first responders to capture crucial patient and situational data with minimal disruption to their life-saving tasks is recommended [16]. Moreover, sensor-based systems and reliable speech-to-text tools can help streamline the data capture process by ensuring comprehensive records even in environments of MCIs. Standardizing these protocols will help build datasets that not only improve AI models but also support post-incident evaluations. Lastly, the development of advanced emergency technologies requires sustained collaboration between healthcare institutions, research organizations, industry leaders, and policymakers. Fostering these synergies is essential for the long-term success of these initiatives [29].

Current evidence on AI in MCIs largely originates from simulations, though there are some pioneering implementations in coordinating centers that use predictive algorithms for resource management. However, real-world application still requires further validation [50]. Long-term engagement will ensure that technologies evolve to meet operational needs, contribute to the expansion of datasets, and improve the adaptability of AI solutions to the dynamic demands of emergency care in MCIs. Moreover, it is important to consider that their integration into existing systems should be gradual and carefully adapted to current operational protocols in order to avoid disrupting established workflows. By leveraging these recommendations, the path to more effective, AI-driven MCI management can be realized.

References

1. Abbasgholizadeh Rahimi S, Shrivastava R, Brown-Johnson A, Caidor P, Davies C, Idrissi Janati A, et al. EDAI framework for integrating equity, diversity, and inclusion throughout the lifecycle of AI to improve health and oral health care: qualitative study. J Med Internet Res. 2024;26:e63356. https://doi.org/10.2196/63356.
2. Abdul S, Adeghe EP, Adegoke BO, Adegoke AA, Udedeh EH. AI-enhanced healthcare management during natural disasters: conceptual insights. Eng Sci Technol J. 2024;5(5):1794–816. https://doi.org/10.51594/estj.v5i5.1155.

3. Abid SK, Chan SW, Sulaiman N, Bhatti U, Nazir U. Present and future of artificial intelligence in disaster management. In: 2023 international conference on engineering management of communication and technology (EMCTECH); 2023. p. 1–7. https://doi.org/10.1109/EMCTECH58502.2023.10296991.
4. Aboualola M, Abualsaud K, Khattab T, Zorba N, Hassanein HS. Edge technologies for disaster management: A survey of social media and artificial intelligence integration. IEEE Access. 2023;11:73782–802. https://doi.org/10.1109/ACCESS.2023.3293035.
5. Adama HE, Popoola OA, Okeke CD, Akinoso AE. Theoretical frameworks supporting IT and business strategy alignment for sustained competitive advantage. Int J Manag Entrep Res. 2024;6(4):1273–87. https://doi.org/10.51594/ijmer.v6i4.1058. Fair East Publishers. Retrieved from http://www.fepbl.com/index.php/ijmer.
6. Adebayo O, Bhuiyan ZA, Ahmed Z. Exploring the effectiveness of artificial intelligence, machine learning, and deep learning in trauma triage: A systematic review and meta-analysis. Digit Health. 2023;9:20552076231205736. https://doi.org/10.1177/20552076231205736.
7. Adeghe EP, Okolo CA, Ojeyinka OT. A review of the use of machine learning in predictive analytics for patient health outcomes in pharmacy practice. Open Access Res J Life Sci. 2024; https://doi.org/10.53022/oarjls.2024.7.1.0026.
8. Ahmad J, Ahmad MM, Su ZH, Rana IA, Rehman A, Sadia H. A systematic analysis of worldwide disasters, epidemics, and pandemics associated mortality of 210 countries for 15 years (2001-2015). Int J Disaster Risk Reduct. 2022;76:103001. https://doi.org/10.1016/j.ijdrr.2022.103001.
9. Ahmed H, Bakr M, Talib MA, Abbas S, Nasir Q. Unmanned aerial vehicles (UAVs) and artificial intelligence (AI) in fire related disaster recovery: analytical survey study. In: 2022 International Conference on Business Analytics for Technology and Security (ICBATS); 2022. p. 1–6. https://doi.org/10.1109/ICBATS54253.2022.9759056.
10. Andersen G, MoldStud Research Team. Importance of data standardization in healthcare analytics for accurate insights. MoldStud; 2024. https://moldstud.com/articles/p-importance-of-data-standardization-in-healthcare-analytics.
11. Aved A, Ho A, Hua K, Hoang L, Hamza-Lup G. A mobile computing approach to automatic traffic evacuation management. In: 2006 IEEE intelligent transportation systems conference; 2006. p. 85–90. https://doi.org/10.1109/ITSC.2006.1706723.
12. Berben SAA, Vloet LCM, Lischer F, Pieters M, de Cock J. Medical coordination rescue members' and ambulance nurses' perspectives on a new model for mass casualty and disaster management and a novel terror attack mitigation approach in The Netherlands: A qualitative study. Prehosp Disaster Med. 2021;36(5):519–25. https://doi.org/10.1017/S1049023X21000790.
13. Bhalla MC, Frey J, Rider C, Nord M, Hegerhorst M. Simple triage algorithm and rapid treatment and Sort, assess, lifesaving, interventions, treatment, and transportation mass casualty triage methods for sensitivity, specificity, and predictive values. Am J Emerg Med. 2015;33(11):1687–91. https://doi.org/10.1016/j.ajem.2015.08.021.
14. Bhaumik S, Hannun M, Dymond C, DeSanto K, Barrett W, Wallis LA, et al. Prehospital triage tools across the world: A scoping review of the published literature. Scand J Trauma Resusc Emerg Med. 2022;30(1):32. https://doi.org/10.1186/s13049-022-01019-z.
15. Castelvecchi D. Is facial recognition too biased to be let loose? Nature. 2020;587(7834):347–9. https://doi.org/10.1038/d41586-020-03186-4.
16. Caviglia M. Bridging data gaps in emergency care: the nightingale project and the future of ai in mass casualty management. J Med Internet Res. 2025;27:e67318. https://doi.org/10.2196/67318.
17. Chandra R, Lakshmi D. Application of artificial intelligence in disaster management and their challenges, pp 1–27. 2024; https://doi.org/10.4018/979-8-3693-4284-8.ch001.
18. Chee ML, Chee ML, Huang H, Mazzochi K, Taylor K, Wang H, et al. Artificial intelligence and machine learning in pre-hospital emergency care: a systematic scoping review. medRxiv. 2023; https://doi.org/10.1101/2023.04.25.23289087.

19. Chenais G, Lagarde E, Gil-Jardine C. Artificial intelligence in emergency medicine: viewpoint of current applications and foreseeable opportunities and challenges. J Med Internet Res. 2023;25:e40031. https://doi.org/10.2196/40031.
20. Chen W, Fang J. Optimizing AI-driven disaster management through LLMs. Preprints [Preprint]. 2024;2024071446. Available from: https://doi.org/10.20944/preprints202407.1446.v1.
21. Cimino J, Braun C. Clinical research in prehospital care: current and future challenges. Clin Pract. 2023;13(5):1266–85. https://doi.org/10.3390/clinpract13050114.
22. Conforti R. Informatics in emergency medicine: a literature review. Emerg Care Med. 2025;2(1):2. https://doi.org/10.3390/ecm2010002.
23. Davenport T, Kalakota R. The potential for artificial intelligence in healthcare. Future Healthc J. 2019;6(2):94–8. https://doi.org/10.7861/futurehosp.6-2-94.
24. Difino M, Bini R, Reitano E, Faccincani R, Sammartano F, Briani L, et al. Epidemiology of trauma admissions in a level 1 trauma center in Northern Italy: a nine-year study. Updat Surg. 2021;73(5):1963–73. https://doi.org/10.1007/s13304-021-00991-y.Medline:34003478.
25. Elvas LB, Mataloto BM, Martins AL, Ferreira JC. Disaster management in smart cities. Smart Cities. 2021;4(2):819–39. https://doi.org/10.3390/smartcities4020042.
26. European Parliament. Artificial Intelligence Act. 2024.; https://www.europarl.europa.eu/doceo/document/TA-9-2024-0138_EN.pdf.
27. Familoni BT. Cybersecurity challenges in the age of AI: theoretical approaches and practical solutions. Comput Sci IT Res J. 2024;5(3):703–24. https://doi.org/10.51594/csitrj.v5i3.930.
28. Franc JM, Kirkland SW, Wisnesky UD, Campbell S, Rowe BH. METASTART: a systematic review and meta-analysis of the diagnostic accuracy of the simple triage and rapid treatment (START) algorithm for disaster triage. Prehosp Disaster Med. 2022;37(1):106–16. https://doi.org/10.1017/S1049023X2100131X.
29. Lamine H, Markou-Pappas Nikolaos, Ragazzoni L, Caviglia M. Key performance indicators and benchmarks in MCI prehospital response using technological tools: a qualitative study assessing the perception of practitioners and tool developers Abstract European Journal of Trauma and Emergency Surgery. 2024;50(5):2273–79. https://doi.org/10.1007/s00068-024-02627-3.
30. Heller AR, Salvador N, Frank M, Schiffner J, Kipke R, Kleber C. Diagnostic precision of triage algorithms for mass casualty incidents. English version diagnostische güte von vorsichtungsalgorithmen für den massenanfall von verletzten und erkrankten. Englische version der anaesthesist. 2019;68(S1):15–24. https://doi.org/10.1007/s00101-017-0352-y.
31. General Data Protection Regulation. Regulation (EU) 2016/679 of the European Parliament and of the Council of 27 April 2016 on the protection of natural persons with regard to the processing of personal data and on the free movement of such data. 2018.; https://gdpr-info.eu/.
32. Ghadge A. ICT-enabled approach for humanitarian disaster management: a systems perspective. Int J Logist Manag. 2023;34(6):1543–65. https://doi.org/10.1108/IJLM-11-2021-0532.
33. Ghassemi M, Naumann T, Schulam P, Beam AL, Chen IY, Ranganath R, Ossorio PN. Practical guidance on artificial intelligence for healthcare data. Lancet Digit Health. 2019;1(4):e157–9. https://doi.org/10.1016/S2589-7500(19)30084-6.
34. Gupta T, Roy S. Applications of artificial intelligence in disaster management. In: ICCAI 2024: 2024 10th international conference on computing and artificial intelligence; 2024. p. 313–8. https://doi.org/10.1145/3669754.3669802.
35. Gutiérrez Maquilón R, Uhl J, Schrom-Feiertag H, Tscheligi M. Integrating GPT-based AI into virtual patients to facilitate communication training among medical first responders: usability study of mixed reality simulation. JMIR Formative Res. 2024;8:e58623. https://doi.org/10.2196/58623.
36. Inoguchi M, Tamura K, Hamamoto R. Establishment of work-flow for roof damage detection utilizing drones, human and AI based on human-in-the-loop framework. In: 2019 IEEE international conference on big data (Big Data); 2019. p. 4618–23. https://doi.org/10.1109/BigData47090.2019.9006211.

37. Iqbal U, Perez P, Li W, Barthelemy J. How computer vision can facilitate flood management: a systematic review. Int J Disaster Risk Reduct. 2021;53:102030. https://doi.org/10.1016/j.ijdrr.2020.102030.
38. Jain TN, Ragazzoni L, Stryhn H, Stratton SJ, Della Corte F. Comparison of the Sacco triage method versus START triage using a virtual reality scenario in advance care paramedic students. Can J Emerg Med. 2016;18(4):288–92. https://doi.org/10.1017/cem.2015.102.
39. Jin X, Frock A, Nagaraja S, Wallqvist A, Reifman J. Ai algorithm for personalized resource allocation and treatment of hemorrhage casualties. Front Physiol. 2024;15 https://doi.org/10.3389/fphys.2024.1327948.
40. Ruiz-Diaz J, Marroquín-Gutiérrez F, Simancas-Acevedo E, Salgado-Ramírez JC, Trejo-Macotela FR, Ramos-Fernández JC, Tafoya-Rivera EV, Vera U, Morales Cuenca AD, Ruiz-Vanoye JA, Díaz-Parra Ocotlán. Machine and deep learning solutions for achieving the sustainable development goals artificial intelligence applications in emergency response and disaster management igi global. 2025;403–416.
41. Jovičić R, Gostimirović L, Milašinović S. Use of new technologies in the field of protection and rescue during disasters. Int. J. Disaster Risk Manag. [Internet]. 2024 Jun. 28. 2025;6(1):111–22. Available from: https://internationaljournalofdisasterriskmanagement.com/Vol1/article/view/87.
42. Kim D, Kim J, Oh J, Shin SD, Park JO. A data-driven artificial intelligence model for remote triage in the prehospital environment. PLoS One. 2018;13(10):e0206006. https://doi.org/10.1371/journal.pone.0206006.
43. Kirubarajan A, Taher A, Khan S, Masood S. Artificial intelligence in emergency medicine: a scoping review. J Am College Emerg Phys Open. 2020;1(6):1691–702. https://doi.org/10.1002/emp2.12277.
44. Kumar MVKS. Leveraging ai in disaster management: enhancing response and recovery for natural and man-made disasters. Int J Multidiscip Res. 2024;6(2) https://doi.org/10.36948/ijfmr.2024.v06i02.26729.
45. Leaning J, Guha-Sapir D. Natural disasters, armed conflict, and public health. N Engl J Med. 2014;370(8):783–4. https://doi.org/10.1056/NEJMra1109877.
46. Lee C, Walters E, Borger R, Clem K, Fenati G, Kiemeney M, et al. The San Bernardino, California, terror attack: two emergency departments' response. Western J Emerg Med. 2016;17(1):1–7. https://doi.org/10.5811/westjem.2016.1.29720.
47. Lennquist S, editor. Medical response to major incidents and disasters: a practical guide for all medical staff. Springer; 2012. https://doi.org/10.1007/978-3-642-21895-8.
48. Lomaglio L, Ansaloni L, Catena F, Sartelli M, Coccolini F. Mass casualty incident: definitions and current reality. In: Kluger Y, Coccolini F, Catena F, Ansaloni L, editors. WSES handbook of mass casualties incidents management: hot topics in acute care surgery and trauma. Springer; 2020. p. 1–10. https://doi.org/10.1007/978-3-319-92345-1.
49. Lu J, Wang L, Zhang J, Huang Y, Liu S, Li X. Unmanned aerial vehicle based intelligent triage system in mass-casualty incidents using 5G and artificial intelligence. World J Emerg Med. 2023;14(4):273–9. https://doi.org/10.5847/wjem.j.1920-8642.2023.066.
50. Miller S. AI algorithm eases tough task of handling mass casualty events. NoCamels. 2024. Retrieved January 1, 2025, from https://nocamels.com/2024/08/ai-algorithm-eases-tough-task-of-handling-mass-casualty-event/.
51. Murata KT, Kikuta K, Nagatsuma T, Imanaka H, Pavarangkoon P. International deployment of visual IoT for disaster mitigation. In: 2023 33rd international telecommunication networks and applications conference (ITNAC); 2023. p. 228–33. https://doi.org/10.1109/ITNAC59571.2023.10368538.
52. NIGHTINGALE. 2025. https://www.nightingale-triage.eu.
53. Nunavath V, Goodwin M. The use of artificial intelligence in disaster management—A systematic literature review. In: 2019 international conference on information and communication Technologies for Disaster Management (ICT-DM); 2019. p. 1–8. https://doi.org/10.1109/ICT-DM47966.2019.9032935.

54. Olivia D, Attigeri G, Saxena A. Optimization model for mass casualty management system using qos-aware routing protocol and casualty triage prediction. Int J Inf Technol. 2024; https://doi.org/10.1007/s41870-024-02052-0.
55. Ouaissa M, Ouaissa M, Himer S, Boulouard Z. AI and IOT integration for natural disaster management. IGI-Global; 2024. p. 1–16. https://doi.org/10.4018/979-8-3693-3896-4.ch001.
56. Pepper M, Archer F, Moloney J. Triage in complex, coordinated terrorist attacks. Prehosp Disaster Med. 2019;34(4):442–8. https://doi.org/10.1017/S1049023X1900459X.
57. Piliuk K, Tomforde S. Artificial intelligence in emergency medicine: a systematic literature review. Int J Med Inform. 2023;180:105274. https://doi.org/10.1016/j.ijmedinf.2023.105274.
58. Rajkomar A, Oren E, Chen K, Dai AM, Hajaj N, Hardt M, et al. Scalable and accurate deep learning with electronic health records. NPJ Digit Med. 2019;2(1):1–10. https://doi.org/10.1038/s41746-018-0029-1.
59. Ranjbar A, Ravn J. Data quality in healthcare for the purpose of artificial intelligence: a case study on ECG digitalization. Stud Health Technol Inform. 2023;305:471–4. https://doi.org/10.3233/SHTI230534.
60. Režek P, Žvanut B. Enhancing crisis response efficiency through ICT: a Delphi study on operational and decision-making improvements in mass casualty incidents. SSRN. 2024; https://doi.org/10.2139/ssrn.5050475.
61. Romero Olóriz C. Artificial intelligence in mass casualty incidents: current status and future perspectives. Emergencias. 2025;37:159. https://doi.org/10.55633/s3me/018.2025.
62. Sezgin E, Kocaballi AB. The era of generalist conversational AI to support public health communications. J Med Internet Res. 2024;21:69007. https://doi.org/10.2196/69007.
63. Tahernejad A, Sahebi A, Salehi Sahl Abadi A, Safari M. Application of artificial intelligence in triage in emergencies and disasters: a systematic review. BMC Public Health. 2024; https://doi.org/10.1186/s12889-024-20447-3.
64. Topol EJ. High-performance medicine: the convergence of human and artificial intelligence. Nat Med. 2019;25(1):44–56. https://doi.org/10.1038/s41591-018-0300-7.
65. Vassallo J, Smith J. Major incident triage and the evaluation of the triage Sort as a secondary triage method. Emerg Med J. 2019;36(5):281–6. https://doi.org/10.1136/emermed-2018-207986.
66. Vassallo J, Smith JE, Bruijns SR, Wallis LA. Major incident triage: a consensus-based definition of the essential life-saving interventions during the definitive care phase of a major incident. Injury. 2016;47(9):1898–902.
67. Waghmare G, Kumar S, Udhayakumar R, Mannar RR, Singh R, Rawat N. Utilizing social media platforms for artificial intelligence-based detection and developing effective communications in disaster-affected areas. In: 2023 3rd International Conference on Advance Computing and Innovative Technologies in Engineering (ICACITE); 2023. p. 501–4. https://doi.org/10.1109/ICACITE57410.2023.10182484.
68. Wagner J, Roopaei M. Edge based decision making in disaster response systems. In: 2020 10th annual computing and communication workshop and conference (CCWC); 2020. p. 0469–73. https://doi.org/10.1109/CCWC47524.2020.9031219.
69. Way DP, Panchal AR, Price AR, Berezina-Blackburn V, Patterson J, McGrath J., …, Kman N. Learner evaluation of an immersive virtual reality mass casualty incident simulator for triage training. 2024. https://doi.org/10.21203/rs.3.rs-3914970/v1.
70. Yafe E, Walker BB, Amram O, Schuurman N, Randall E, Friger M, Peleg K. Volunteer first responders for optimizing management of mass casualty incidents. Disaster Med Public Health Prep. 2019;13(2):287–94. https://doi.org/10.1017/dmp.2018.56.
71. Yánez Benítez C, Tilsed J, Weinstein ES, Caviglia M, Herman S, Montán C, et al. Education, training, and technological innovation, key components of the ESTES-NIGHTINGALE project cooperation for mass casualty incident preparedness in Europe. Eur J Trauma Emerg Surg. 2023;49(2):653–9. https://doi.org/10.1007/s00068-022-02198-1.
72. Zou K, Lü M, Peng Y, Tang X. Artificial intelligence-based model for lymph node metastases detection in bladder cancer. Lancet Oncol. 2023;24(6):e232. https://doi.org/10.1016/S1470-2045(23)00152-3.

20 3D Printing in Orthopedic Trauma Surgery

Jonas Neijhoft, Johannes Frank, and Ingo Marzi

20.1 Introduction

Orthopedic trauma surgery has consistently evolved with technological advancements, deriving substantial benefits from each wave of industrial innovation. The development of steam-powered mechanical manufacturing in the nineteenth century was a foundational period for the production of more evolved surgical tools, while the late twentieth century saw exponential growth with the advent of mass-produced implants and diagnostic devices made possible by X-ray imaging and the evolving processing power of computers.

Today, another pivotal era is shaped by the further digitalization and introduction of 3D printing technologies, which are improving the field of orthopedic and trauma surgery. 3D printing itself is not actually that new, as it was invented by Charles Hull, who is generally considered the inventor, in the 1980s. It is advancing surgical precision and patient-specific care by providing tools for visualization, customization, and improved surgical planning.

The technique of 3D printing, also known as additive manufacturing, allows the layer-by-layer creation of three-dimensional objects from digital models. In orthopedics, 3D printing has rapidly transitioned from experimental phases to practical applications, allowing surgeons to create patient-specific models, surgical guides, and even implants, often still restricted by medical device laws. Key advancements in this field, including biocompatible materials, software for imaging and modeling, and high-resolution printers, are paving the way for precision in preoperative

J. Neijhoft · J. Frank · I. Marzi (✉)
Department of Trauma Surgery and Orthopedics, University Hospital, Goethe University Frankfurt, Frankfurt/Main, Germany
e-mail: Neijhoft@med.uni-frankfurt.de; j.frank@trauma.uni-frankfurt.de; marzi@trauma.uni-frankfurt.de

B. De Simone et al. (eds.), *New Technologies, Precision Medicine, and AI in Emergency General Surgery*, Hot Topics in Acute Care Surgery and Trauma,
https://doi.org/10.1007/978-3-032-09357-8_20

planning and real-time intraoperative guidance, as well as therapeutic advancements for unsolved problems like long bone defects.

20.2 Overview of the Current and Potential Uses of 3D Printing

20.2.1 3D Analysis and Surgical Planning

One application of 3D printing in orthopedic surgery is the conversion of detailed CT and MRI data into physical (and digital) models that represent complex anatomical structures, enabling precise preoperative planning. For this process, high-resolution imaging scans are obtained in Digital Imaging and Communications in Medicine (DICOM) format. These DICOM images are processed through medical image segmentation software to isolate the relevant bone structures and produce 3D digital surface models.

The models can then be manipulated using computer-aided design (CAD) tools to visualize fracture morphology, assess bone defects, and simulate surgical maneuvers. These tools are valuable not only for preoperative planning but also for patient education, allowing patients to see and understand their injuries, thus improving informed consent.

20.2.2 Preoperative Planning and Intraoperative Guidance

During the preoperative planning phase, 3D models and virtual simulations allow for precise mapping of fracture patterns and surgical steps, enhancing the surgeon's readiness. Moreover, patient-specific 3D-printed surgical guides can be sterilized and used intraoperatively to ensure that preoperative plans are accurately implemented.

The integration of 3D planning into surgeries is particularly transformative in complex procedures, such as acetabular fracture fixation and osteotomies, where alignment and angulation are crucial for successful outcomes. By utilizing 3D-printed models intraoperatively, surgeons can confidently apply planned strategies with greater accuracy, improving outcomes and reducing the need for intraoperative adjustments.

20.2.3 Customized Surgical Tools

Another use case of 3D printing is the ability to produce patient-specific surgical tools, including cutting guides, drilling guides, and reduction devices. These tools are designed based on the patient's unique anatomy, enhancing surgical accuracy.

These tools can be provided by different companies or produced in the hospital itself (called in-house production), which benefits from different advantages: In the case an external company provides the guides, the surgeon is still responsible for checking the result. The segmentation of the CT data, fracture reduction if necessary, digital creation of the guides, 3D printing, and sterilization can be handled entirely by the company, which is less time-consuming for the hospital. In many cases, such a procedure is certified for certain fracture localizations. The disadvantages are, on the one hand, the high costs, which are usually not covered by special cost revenues, and on the other hand, the lack of opportunity to be fully involved as a surgeon in every step of the design process.

Studies indicate that patient-specific guides reduce operative time and improve alignment outcomes. For instance, cutting guides tailored to the contour of the femur in total knee arthroplasty facilitate precise osteotomies, leading to better implant positioning and reduced intraoperative adjustments [1].

20.2.4 Customized Implants

Custom implants, made possible by 3D printing, are particularly beneficial in situations where conventional implants may not fit due to unique anatomical constraints or extensive bone loss, such as in revision surgeries. For instance, in distal radius fractures, customized implants have been shown to provide more consistent correction of deformities compared to standard plates.

20.2.5 Biocompatible Scaffolds for Bone Regeneration

The advent of 3D-printed biocompatible scaffolds represents a breakthrough in the treatment of long bone defects and trauma. These scaffolds, made from materials such as *β-tricalcium phosphate (β-TCP)*, *bioglass*, *hydroxyapatite*, and other bioresorbable materials, provide structural support while facilitating new bone formation. Over time, these scaffolds should be resorbed and replaced by the patient's own bone, potentially eliminating the need for secondary surgeries and preventing weakening of the healed bone [2].

20.2.6 Educational Tools for Training and Simulation

3D-printed models serve as highly valuable educational tools in trauma and orthopedic training, offering tactile and visual aids for students and residents to understand complex anatomical structures. This is particularly important for rare or complex cases where hands-on training opportunities may be limited [3, 4].

20.3 3D Printing Techniques

20.3.1 Fused Filament Fabrication (FFF)/Fused Deposition Modeling (FDM)

Fused deposition modeling (FDM) is one of the most accessible and widely used 3D printing techniques, primarily known for its use in prototyping. FDM printers extrude thermoplastic filaments through a heated nozzle, layer by layer, to create 3D structures. Filaments such as polylactic acid (PLA), acrylonitrile butadiene styrene (ABS), and polyether ether ketone (PEEK) are commonly used due to their thermoplastic properties and also have wide application in the medical field:

It is frequently used to produce scaffolds in tissue engineering or anatomical models for educational purposes. These models provide tactile, hands-on training for medical students and residents, particularly for understanding complex anatomical structures [2, 5, 6].

Advantages

- *Cost-Effective*: FDM is one of the most economical 3D printing techniques, making it accessible for smaller healthcare facilities and research labs.
- *Versatility*: A wide range of thermoplastic materials can be used, providing flexibility for various applications, including surgical guides and anatomical models.
- *Ease of Use*: FDM printers are user-friendly and suitable for rapid prototyping.

Disadvantages

- *Limited Resolution and Accuracy*: FDM printing has lower resolution and surface quality than other techniques, which can limit its use for highly detailed medical models.
- *Material Limitations*: Only certain thermoplastics can be used by the majority of printers, and many of them are not biocompatible, so they are not suitable for long-term implants.

This printing technique should be correctly named fused filament fabrication (FFF), as the wording fused deposition modeling (FDM) originally was used only for the printers from Stratasys. As nowadays the label FDM is widely used for all filament-based printing processes, it will be used in this article as well.

20.3.2 Stereolithography (SLA)

Stereolithography (SLA) uses a laser to cure liquid photopolymer resin into solid layers. The laser traces the design onto a resin-filled tank, and each layer is cured before the next one is added. This process is known for its high resolution and detail, making it suitable for intricate designs. SLA is highly valuable for creating detailed surfaces and models, which are essential for preoperative planning and surgical rehearsals. Another application is the printing of guides for intraoperative use, due to different sterilization options like autoclaving [1].

Advantages

- *High Resolution*: SLA provides superior surface finish and intricate details, essential for complex models and surgical guides.
- *Biocompatibility*: Many biocompatible resins are available, making SLA suitable for creating temporary implants and surgical tools.

- *Speed*: SLA can produce models relatively quickly, especially for small, detailed items.

Disadvantages
- *Cost*: SLA requires expensive resins and machinery, making it less accessible than FDM.
- *Material Brittleness*: The photopolymer resin can be brittle, limiting its durability, especially for load-bearing applications.
- *Post-Processing*: SLA prints often require washing and post-curing, which adds time and complexity to the process.

20.3.3 Selective Laser Sintering (SLS)

Selective laser sintering (SLS) involves a laser that sinters powdered material (typically nylon or other polymers) to form each layer of the model. The unsintered powder supports the object, eliminating the need for additional support structures and allowing for complex designs. SLS is commonly used in creating orthopedic implants and prosthetics due to its strength and ability to produce intricate shapes.

Advantages
- *Strength and Durability*: SLS-printed objects are strong and durable, making them suitable for functional testing and load-bearing applications.
- *No Support Structures Needed*: Since the powder bed supports the model, SLS can produce highly complex and intricate shapes.
- *Versatile Material Options*: SLS is compatible with various biocompatible polymers and metals, expanding its applications in healthcare.

Disadvantages
- *High Cost*: SLS printers and powders are more expensive, and they are typically found in specialized labs and medical centers.
- *Surface Finish*: SLS parts often have a rough surface that requires additional finishing steps, which may not be ideal for detailed anatomical models.
- *Post-Processing Complexity*: The unsintered powder must be carefully removed, adding time and complexity to the process.

20.3.4 Electron Beam Melting (EBM)

EBM uses an electron beam instead of a laser to melt metal powder, layer by layer, to build complex parts. EBM is primarily used in the aerospace and medical fields for parts that require excellent mechanical properties and durability. This technique is particularly suited for producing titanium implants, which are highly biocompatible and durable. Custom orthopedic plates made with EBM often incorporate trabecular or lattice structures that mimic natural bone, improving integration and reducing stress shielding.

Advantages

- Produces implants with high density and excellent mechanical properties, suitable for load-bearing applications.
- Allows for customization of the implant structure to match the patient's bone density and geometry.

Disadvantages

- Requires high vacuum conditions, making the process costly.
- Limited to conductive materials, primarily metals like titanium and cobalt-chrome.

20.3.5 Digital Light Processing (DLP)

Digital light processing (DLP) is similar to SLA but uses a digital light projector instead of a laser to cure the resin. This projector flashes the entire layer pattern at once, resulting in faster printing speeds than SLA while maintaining high resolution. DLP is widely used in the dental industry, where it produces highly detailed and precise models for crowns, bridges, and dentures. In orthopedics, DLP is also being explored for creating surgical guides and other custom-fitted medical devices.

Advantages

- *High Speed*: DLP can cure an entire layer simultaneously, making it faster than SLA for creating detailed models.
- *Fine Details*: DLP provides high resolution and detail, which is crucial for small-scale, complex parts.
- *Biocompatible Resins*: DLP has biocompatible resins suitable for dental applications and some surgical tools.

Disadvantages

- *Expensive Equipment and Materials*: Like SLA, DLP requires costly machines and resins, which may limit its accessibility.
- *Limited Material Choices*: Although there are biocompatible options, DLP has fewer material options than other methods, which can be limiting for specific applications.

20.3.6 Binder Jetting

Description

Binder jetting is a powder-based process where a binding agent selectively adheres to the powder layer by layer. This technique is particularly versatile, as it can work with metals, ceramics, and polymers. After printing, the model may need additional processing, such as sintering, for strength. Binder jetting is often used in making metal-based surgical instruments and custom implants, including orthopedic implants. It also has potential applications in bioprinting, where ceramic materials can be used to fabricate bone-like structures [7, 8].

Advantages

- *Material Variety*: Binder jetting can work with a wide range of materials, including metals and ceramics, which are ideal for bone and dental implants.
- *Low Material Waste*: The powder-based system results in minimal material waste.
- *Good for Large Models*: Binder jetting can produce larger models more cost-effectively than techniques like SLA or DLP.

Disadvantages

- *Lower Mechanical Strength*: Parts produced with binder jetting often require post-processing to achieve structural integrity.
- *Limited Biocompatibility*: While the range of materials is broad, not all are biocompatible without extensive post-processing.

20.3.7 Conclusion

Each 3D printing technique offers distinct advantages and disadvantages, making them suitable for different medical applications. FDM and SLA are generally more accessible for creating anatomical models and educational tools, while SLS and DLP provide the precision and durability required for medical implants and prosthetics. Binder jetting stands out for its ability to print with metals and ceramics, valuable for complex surgical instruments and custom implants. As 3D printing technology continues to advance, the ability to tailor techniques to specific medical needs promises a future of increasingly personalized healthcare solutions.

20.4 In-depth Applications

20.4.1 Custom Plate and Implant Design

3D printing has revolutionized custom implant and plate design in both research and industrial settings. The ability to create patient-specific, anatomically accurate implants enhances surgical outcomes and opens new possibilities in complex reconstructive procedures. With ongoing advancements in materials, imaging integration, and printing technologies, the future of 3D printing in custom orthopedic solutions holds immense potential for improved patient care and personalized medicine. The most common 3D printing techniques used in medical and industrial applications for designing custom plates and implants include selective laser sintering (SLS), electron beam melting (EBM), and stereolithography (SLA). Each method has unique advantages depending on the intended application, from rapid prototyping to creating highly durable end-use parts.

20.4.1.1 Patient-Specific Implants (PSI)

Patient-specific implants are customized implants designed based on an individual patient's anatomy, typically derived from medical imaging data. PSIs are especially beneficial in cases involving complex fractures, bone deformities, and reconstructive surgeries where off-the-shelf implants may not suffice. The process of creating a PSI involves generating a 3D model of the implant based on the patient's CT or MRI data. The digital model is then printed, for example, using metal materials like titanium for durability.

Advantages

- Improves the fit and function of the implant, leading to better surgical outcomes.
- Minimizes the risk of implant-related complications, such as implant loosening and bone resorption.

Disadvantages

- Higher production cost due to customization requirements.
- Requires advanced imaging and modeling expertise, which may not be widely available.

20.4.1.2 Rapid Prototyping and Design Iteration

Rapid prototyping with 3D printing enables engineers and surgeons to quickly iterate on plate and implant designs, testing different shapes, sizes, and features to optimize functionality and patient outcomes. In the research and development phase, engineers can test various configurations of plates and screws to optimize mechanical stability. Rapid prototyping also allows researchers to create anatomically accurate bone models to test implant and medical device designs.

Advantages

- Speeds up the development process by allowing multiple design iterations in a short time.
- Reduces material waste by enabling testing with less expensive materials before final production.

Disadvantages

- Prototyping materials often differ from the final product materials, which may limit the accuracy of mechanical testing.
- Requires specialized expertise to analyze and refine design changes based on prototype performance.

20.4.1.3 Customized Surgical Guides

Customized surgical guides created through 3D printing are tools that guide surgeons during implant placement, ensuring precise alignment and positioning. These guides are tailored to the patient's anatomy and allow for minimally invasive procedures, leading to shorter recovery times. Like PSIs, custom guides are designed based on imaging data, often using SLA or SLS 3D printing. The guides are then sterilized and used intraoperatively, where they fit directly onto the patient's bone [1].

Advantages

- Increases the accuracy of implant positioning, critical for outcomes in knee, hip, and spinal surgeries.
- Reduces operative time and radiation exposure by providing a clear guide for screw and plate placement.

Disadvantages

- Requires extensive preoperative planning and imaging data processing.
- Costly and time-intensive for complex cases requiring extensive customization.

20.4.2 Future Directions and Challenges

As 3D printing technology continues to evolve, it is likely to expand its applications in industrial and medical settings. Future developments are expected to include bioactive and biodegradable materials for PSIs, integrated sensors within implants for real-time monitoring, and further automation in the design and production processes. However, challenges remain, particularly in regulatory approval for custom implants and ensuring consistency and safety in implant production.

Key Challenges

- *Regulatory Approval*: Custom implants require stringent testing and certification to ensure they meet safety and efficacy standards, which can prolong time to market.
- *Cost and Scalability*: Producing PSIs and custom plates can be costly, and scalability remains an issue for widespread clinical adoption.
- *Technical Expertise*: Effective use of 3D printing for implants requires a high level of expertise in biomedical engineering, material science, and medical imaging, making it challenging for general adoption.

20.5 Bioprinting in Medical Applications

Bioprinting is a specialized field of 3D printing dedicated to fabricating biological tissues and structures through layer-by-layer deposition of bioinks. Unlike conventional 3D printing, bioprinting involves complex, biocompatible materials that can form different and living tissues. This technology holds immense promise for regenerative medicine, allowing for the development of tissues and organs that can potentially replace damaged or diseased human tissues. Bioprinting is evolving quickly, with applications in drug testing, tissue engineering, and potentially even whole-organ fabrication. This chapter delves into bioprinting techniques, their applications in healthcare, advantages, limitations, and the emerging field's future direction [9–11].

20.5.1 Techniques in Bioprinting

20.5.1.1 Extrusion-Based Bioprinting

Extrusion-based bioprinting is one of the most common techniques for constructing biological tissues. It uses a syringe or nozzle to extrude bioinks in a controlled manner. These bioinks, typically composed of cells embedded within a biocompatible hydrogel matrix, are deposited layer by layer to create 3D structures. The technique allows for high cell density and can handle viscous materials, which are beneficial for replicating tissue structure. Extrusion-based bioprinting is widely used to create cartilage, bone, and skin models, which are helpful in reconstructive surgery and tissue engineering. For instance, engineered cartilage can replace damaged joints in osteoarthritis, and skin tissue models can aid in wound healing and burn treatment [12].

Advantages

- *Scalability*: Extrusion-based systems can produce large tissue constructs, making them ideal for complex organs or tissue models.
- *High Cell Density*: This method can incorporate a large number of cells, which is crucial for replicating the cellular environment of native tissues.
- *Wide Range of Biomaterials*: A broad variety of bioinks can be used, enhancing versatility.

Disadvantages

- *Lower Resolution*: Compared to other bioprinting methods, extrusion bioprinting has a lower resolution, which may limit the ability to create highly intricate tissue structures.
- *Cell Viability*: High pressures required for extrusion may reduce cell viability, particularly in delicate cells.

20.5.1.2 Inkjet Bioprinting

Inkjet bioprinting is a non-contact printing method that uses thermal or piezoelectric mechanisms to deposit droplets of bioink onto a substrate. This technique allows precise control over cell placement and distribution. Inkjet bioprinting is typically faster and more cost-effective than other bioprinting methods, making it suitable for high-throughput applications. Inkjet bioprinting is particularly valuable for developing skin tissue models, useful in wound healing, skin grafts, and drug testing. Additionally, it has potential in creating vascular networks, which are critical for supporting organ structures and ensuring nutrient delivery to cells [13].

Advantages

- *High Speed*: Inkjet bioprinting enables rapid production, making it ideal for mass tissue production.

- *Cost-Effective*: This method is generally more affordable than other bioprinting techniques.
- *High Precision*: Inkjet printers allow precise droplet placement, which improves cell distribution and accuracy.

Disadvantages
- *Limited Viscosity Range*: Inkjet bioprinting is limited to low-viscosity bioinks, which may restrict its ability to replicate the structural integrity of certain tissues.
- *Risk of Cell Damage*: The thermal process in some inkjet printers can potentially damage cells, which can affect viability.

20.5.1.3 Laser-Assisted Bioprinting (LAB)
Laser-assisted bioprinting (LAB) uses a laser pulse to create high-resolution patterns by transferring cells from a bioink ribbon to a substrate. This technique does not involve direct contact between the print head and the bioink, making it highly suitable for printing sensitive cells and delicate structures. LAB provides excellent resolution, allowing for the precise placement of cells and biomaterials. LAB is widely used for developing neural and vascular tissues due to its high resolution, which is critical for accurately positioning cells in these delicate structures. Additionally, LAB is useful for creating skin and cartilage tissues, where precision is vital [14].

Advantages
- *High Resolution and Precision*: LAB offers unparalleled precision, allowing for the creation of highly intricate tissue structures.
- *Non-Contact Method*: The non-contact nature reduces the risk of contamination and cell damage.
- *Ability to Work with Various Bioinks*: LAB can handle a wide range of viscosities, enhancing versatility in bioink selection.

Disadvantages
- *Cost and Complexity*: The equipment and expertise required for LAB are costly, limiting its accessibility to specialized labs.
- *Limited Throughput*: LAB is slower than other techniques, making it less suitable for large-scale or high-throughput applications.

20.5.1.4 Stereolithography (SLA) in Bioprinting
Stereolithography (SLA) for bioprinting involves using a focused light source to solidify photosensitive hydrogels, layer by layer, into complex 3D structures. As SLA was primarily used for non-biological materials, it has been adapted for bioprinting by using biocompatible resins and hydrogels. SLA is often employed to create scaffolds that support cell growth for bone and cartilage repair. These scaffolds allow cells to grow and differentiate in three dimensions, closely mimicking the natural environment of these tissues [15].

Advantages

- *High Resolution*: SLA offers high resolution, suitable for printing highly detailed structures, such as vascular networks.
- *Structural Integrity*: This method allows for the creation of strong, stable tissue models.
- *Customizable*: SLA is highly adaptable and can be tailored to create specific structures depending on the type of light-sensitive bioink used.

Disadvantages

- *Limited Bioink Options*: The requirement for photosensitive materials narrows the range of usable bioinks.
- *Potential Cytotoxicity*: Some photoinitiators can be toxic to cells, limiting the viability of SLA for certain applications.

20.5.2 Applications of Bioprinting in Medicine

Bioprinting offers diverse applications, from drug testing and disease modeling to regenerative medicine and organ transplantation.

- *Drug Testing and Disease Modeling*: Bioprinted tissues can replicate human tissues closely, allowing for drug testing without relying on animal models, leading to more accurate results and ethical testing practices.
- *Tissue Engineering and Regenerative Medicine*: Bioprinted constructs, such as skin, cartilage, and bone, are already used in regenerative medicine. Bioprinted skin, for example, is useful for treating burn patients, while cartilage and bone models aid in orthopedic surgery. The ability to print human tissue phantoms reduces the need for animal testing, advancing ethical research practices and thus reducing animal testing.
- *Organ Engineering*: Although fully functional organs remain in development, liver, heart, and kidney models are being explored for transplantation research and testing.

Bioprinting is advancing toward the creation of fully functional, vascularized organs, with significant research underway in areas like artificial hearts, livers, and kidneys. Innovations in bioink development, bioprinter design, and tissue maturation processes will further expand the applications of bioprinting, moving the field closer to its goal of creating transplantable organs. Moreover, bioprinting is likely to play a crucial role in personalized medicine, allowing for custom-made tissues and organs that match the patient's genetic and anatomical characteristics.

20.5.3 Challenges and Limitations

- *Cell Viability and Functionality*: Ensuring cells survive the bioprinting process and maintain their natural functions is challenging and requires optimized bio-inks and printing conditions.
- *Vascularization*: For bioprinted tissues to survive long-term, they need a blood supply, which remains a significant technical challenge.
- *Regulatory and Ethical Issues*: The field of bioprinting faces regulatory hurdles, especially for constructs intended for human implantation, and raises ethical questions about the creation of human tissues and organs.

20.6 3D-Printed Scaffolds for Bone Tissue Engineering

3D printing has revolutionized biomedical research by providing innovative methods to create complex structures that can mimic natural tissues, which is especially valuable in regenerative medicine and tissue engineering. Scaffolds serve as support structures that promote cell growth and tissue regeneration for treating injuries, diseases, and degenerative conditions.

20.6.1 Principles of Scaffold Design

Scaffold design in tissue engineering involves creating a three-dimensional matrix that provides support for cells to grow, proliferate, and form tissues. Key characteristics that make a scaffold effective include biocompatibility, porosity, mechanical strength, and resorbability:

1. *Biocompatibility*: Scaffolds must support cell attachment, growth, and differentiation without causing adverse reactions. This requires choosing materials that are safe and can integrate with surrounding tissues.
2. *Porosity and Pore Size*: The scaffold's pore structure is essential for nutrient and oxygen diffusion and waste removal. Ideally, scaffolds have interconnected pores to allow for vascularization and tissue ingrowth, with pore sizes tailored to specific cell types.
3. *Mechanical Strength*: Scaffolds must have sufficient strength to support the tissue they are intended to replace or regenerate. This is particularly critical in load-bearing applications such as bone regeneration.
4. *Resorbability*: Scaffolds are often designed to resorb over time as the new tissue forms, with the degradation rate matched to the rate of tissue regeneration. This minimizes the need for scaffold removal surgery.

5. *Surface Topography*: Scaffold surfaces are designed to mimic the extracellular matrix (ECM) structure, often by including micro- or nanoscale features that promote cell adhesion and tissue growth.

20.6.2 Materials for Tissue Engineering

Choosing the right material for scaffold design is essential to match the requirements of the target tissue. Common materials include biodegradable polymers, ceramics, and metal composites, each offering distinct advantages for specific tissue engineering applications. Scaffold designs are likely to focus on integrating biomimetic and bioactive materials that promote tissue regeneration. Additionally, the development of 4D printing, which enables scaffolds to change shape or properties over time, is a promising avenue for creating dynamic tissue engineering solutions.

20.6.2.1 Biodegradable Polymers

Polymers like PLA, PCL, and poly(lactic-co-glycolic acid) (PLGA) are commonly used for creating scaffolds in tissue engineering. These materials are favorable due to their biocompatibility and gradual degradation, which allows new tissue to replace the scaffold over time.

Advantages

- Biocompatible and partially resorbable by the body.
- Suitable for applications in soft tissue and non-load-bearing bone applications.

Disadvantages

- Lower mechanical strength, unsuitable for load-bearing applications.
- Limited compatibility with certain 3D printing methods like SLS.

20.6.2.2 Bioceramics

Bioceramics such as hydroxyapatite (HA) and tricalcium phosphate (TCP) closely resemble the mineral composition of bone, making them ideal for bone tissue engineering. These materials are often combined with polymers in composite scaffolds to enhance mechanical properties.

Advantages

- High biocompatibility and osteoconductivity, promoting bone growth.
- Suitable for load-bearing applications in combination with polymers.

Disadvantages

- Brittle and prone to fracture without reinforcement.
- Limited by some 3D printing techniques due to high melting points.

20.6.2.3 Metal-Based Scaffolds

Metallic materials like titanium and magnesium alloys provide high mechanical strength, making them suitable for load-bearing scaffolds in bone tissue engineering. Metal scaffolds are often created using techniques like SLS or electron beam melting (EBM).

Advantages

- Excellent mechanical properties suitable for orthopedic applications.
- High biocompatibility and ability to support bone cell growth.

Disadvantages

- Non-biodegradable, which may require surgical removal.
- Limited compatibility with soft tissue engineering.

20.7 Medical 3D-Printing in Space—Medical Applications Beyond Earth

The concept of 3D bioprinting in space is a groundbreaking frontier in both space exploration and medical science. Conducting printing in microgravity environments opens up new possibilities for understanding human biology, developing unique treatments, and advancing regenerative medicine. This technology, developed in response to the constraints of long-duration space missions, also has potential for on-Earth applications. Bioprinting in space addresses the challenge of maintaining astronaut health, potentially creates models for tissue repair and organ transplantation, and supports space-specific biomedical research.

20.7.1 Why Bioprinting in Space?

Bioprinting in space is driven by the unique characteristics of microgravity, which present advantages that cannot be achieved on Earth. In microgravity, cells and biomaterials can be deposited in three dimensions more freely without the force of gravity affecting their structure. This makes it possible to print more complex and stable 3D cellular structures, such as tissues and organoids, that can mimic human biology more accurately. The potential benefits are twofold: improving medical care for astronauts on long-duration missions and creating models that offer insights into human health and disease progression in microgravity [16, 17].

20.7.2 Techniques and Equipment for Bioprinting in Space

Several bioprinting technologies have been adapted for use in space, with notable advancements in extrusion-based and laser-assisted bioprinting. Space-based bioprinters require special adaptations to operate in a zero-gravity environment, including stability features to control bioink flow and mechanisms to manage tissue shape and structure without gravity's support.

20.7.2.1 Extrusion-Based Bioprinting in Microgravity

Extrusion-based bioprinters, such as the Russian-developed Organ.Aut bioprinter, are modified for space use to enable stable extrusion of bioinks in a microgravity environment. For example, the Organ.Aut bioprinter successfully printed thyroid gland tissue using human cells on the International Space Station (ISS) in 2018 [18]. This landmark experiment demonstrated that complex tissue structures could be printed and retained in space, offering potential for printing other vital structures, such as vascularized heart tissues and bone-like structures.

20.7.2.2 Magnetic Levitation Bioprinting

Magnetic levitation Bioprinting uses magnetic fields to assemble cells and materials into 3D shapes without physical scaffolding. In microgravity, magnetic fields provide a way to position and hold cells in place, forming tissue structures that are otherwise challenging to maintain in weightless conditions.

This technique has been explored for creating blood vessels and tubular structures in space. Using magnetic nanoparticles, cells can be assembled into tissue-like configurations that could aid in studying vascular and organ development.

20.7.3 Medical and Biological Applications of Space Bioprinting

Bone and Cartilage Regeneration

Bone density loss is a major health concern for astronauts on long missions. Bioprinting bone and cartilage tissues in space could enable in situ repair for injuries. Using biocompatible materials such as hydroxyapatite and cellular scaffolds, researchers are exploring the bioprinting of bone tissues in microgravity. These tissues could support cell growth and differentiation, potentially providing regenerative solutions for bone injuries sustained during space missions [19].

Heart and Vascular Tissues

Cardiovascular health is crucial for astronauts, as microgravity impacts cardiovascular function. Bioprinting heart and vascular tissues in space provides a way to study these changes in a controlled environment, supporting heart health research. Techniques such as magnetic levitation are used to create vascular networks that can sustain nutrient diffusion, enabling long-term cell viability. These models are valuable for testing treatments for cardiovascular conditions, potentially benefiting space and Earth-based medicine [20].

Skin and Soft Tissue Models for Wound Healing
Astronauts face unique risks for skin injuries in space, which can be challenging to treat due to limited resources. Bioprinting skin models could offer a solution for rapid wound healing and repair. Bioprinters on the ISS have been used to develop layers of skin tissue. These bioprinted skin models incorporate cell-laden bioinks with growth factors, which can promote wound healing and tissue regeneration [16, 21].

20.7.4 Future Directions and Implications

The future of bioprinting in space is promising, with advances aimed at creating more complex tissues and potentially transplantable organs. Some key directions include:

- *Organ Development*: With advancements in bioprinting, the possibility of creating whole organs in space for human transplantation may become a reality. The unique conditions in microgravity could allow for complex tissue growth and vascularization not achievable on Earth.
- *Long-Duration Space Missions*: As missions to Mars and beyond are planned, bioprinting could serve as an essential medical tool, providing an on-demand solution for tissue repair, drug production, and personalized medicine.
- *Cross-Over to Earth Medicine*: Insights gained from bioprinting in space could improve 3D bioprinting practices on Earth, especially for complex tissues that are difficult to replicate in a gravitational environment. Additionally, space-based research could advance understanding in fields like oncology, as certain cancers behave differently in microgravity.

20.8 Conclusion

The integration of 3D printing technology into the medical field marks a significant advancement in how healthcare providers approach patient treatment and surgical procedures. From initial explorations into the applications of 3D printing in orthopedic surgery to more specialized uses in tissue engineering and scaffold design, the evolution of this technology has fostered innovation and improved patient outcomes. 3D printing has transformed numerous aspects of medical practice. By enabling the production of patient-specific models, tools, and implants, it has bridged the gap between digital planning and physical execution. Surgeons can visualize complex anatomical structures in three dimensions, allowing for improved preoperative planning, intraoperative guidance, and postoperative assessments. This capability not only enhances surgical precision but also minimizes the time spent in the operating room, ultimately improving recovery times and patient satisfaction.

Future developments in medical 3D printing are expected to focus on advances in material science, improved biocompatibility and degradability, and the integration of complementary technologies such as artificial intelligence and machine learning to optimize design and manufacturing processes. These advances are likely to further support personalized medical solutions and expand the applicability of 3D printing in resource-limited or remote settings.

Research into 3D printing in space highlights its potential for addressing healthcare needs in isolated environments. This exploration paves the way for future applications in remote areas on Earth, where access to conventional medical resources may be limited.

References

1. Assink N, Reininga IHF, ten Duis K, Doornberg JN, Hoekstra H, Kraeima J, et al. Does 3D-assisted surgery of tibial plateau fractures improve surgical and patient outcome? A systematic review of 1074 patients. Eur J Trauma Emerg Surg. 2022;48:1737–49. https://doi.org/10.1007/s00068-021-01773-2.
2. Hutmacher DW. Scaffolds in tissue engineering bone and cartilage. Biomaterials. 2000;21:2529–43. https://doi.org/10.1016/s0142-9612(00)00121-6.
3. Weidert S, Andress S, Suero E, Becker C, Hartel M, Behle M, Willy C. 3D-Druck in der unfallchirurgischen Fort- und Weiterbildung: Möglichkeiten und Anwendungsbereiche. [3D printing in orthopedic and trauma surgery education and training: possibilities and fields of application]. Unfallchirurg. 2019;122:444–51. https://doi.org/10.1007/s00113-019-0650-8.
4. Neijhoft J, Henrich D, Mörs K, Marzi I, Janko M. Visualization of complicated fractures by 3D-printed models for teaching and surgery: hands-on transitional fractures of the ankle. Eur J Trauma Emerg Surg. 2022;48:3923–31. https://doi.org/10.1007/s00068-022-01879-1.
5. Neijhoft J, Sterz J, Rüsseler M, Britz V, Bepler L, Freund V, et al. Evaluation of a 3D-printed hands-on radius fracture model during teaching courses. Eur J Trauma Emerg Surg. 2024;50:49–57. https://doi.org/10.1007/s00068-023-02327-4.
6. Ford S, Minshall T. Invited review article: where and how 3D printing is used in teaching and education. Addit Manuf. 2019;25:131–50. https://doi.org/10.1016/j.addma.2018.10.028.
7. Bandyopadhyay A, Mitra I, Bose S. 3D printing for bone regeneration. Curr Osteoporos Rep. 2020;18:505–14. https://doi.org/10.1007/s11914-020-00606-2.
8. Lee G, Carrillo M, McKittrick J, Martin DG, Olevsky EA. Fabrication of ceramic bone scaffolds by solvent jetting 3D printing and sintering: towards load-bearing applications. Addit Manuf. 2020;33:101107. https://doi.org/10.1016/j.addma.2020.101107.
9. Stanco D, Urbán P, Tirendi S, Ciardelli G, Barrero J. 3D bioprinting for orthopaedic applications: current advances, challenges and regulatory considerations. Bioprinting. 2020;20:None. https://doi.org/10.1016/j.bprint.2020.e00103.
10. Kilian D, Ahlfeld T, Akkineni AR, Bernhardt A, Gelinsky M, Lode A. 3D bioprinting of osteochondral tissue substitutes - in vitro-chondrogenesis in multi-layered mineralized constructs. Sci Rep. 2020;10:8277. https://doi.org/10.1038/s41598-020-65050-9.
11. Blaeser A, Duarte Campos DF, Fischer H. 3D bioprinting of cell-laden hydrogels for advanced tissue engineering. Curr Opin Biomed Eng. 2017;2:58–66. https://doi.org/10.1016/j.cobme.2017.04.003.
12. Murphy SV, Atala A. 3D bioprinting of tissues and organs. Nat Biotechnol. 2014;32:773–85. https://doi.org/10.1038/nbt.2958.
13. Xu T, Jin J, Gregory C, Hickman JJJJ, Boland T. Inkjet printing of viable mammalian cells. Biomaterials. 2005;26:93–9. https://doi.org/10.1016/j.biomaterials.2004.04.011.
14. Guillotin B, Guillemot F. Cell patterning technologies for organotypic tissue fabrication. Trends Biotechnol. 2011;29:183–90. https://doi.org/10.1016/j.tibtech.2010.12.008.

15. Melchels FPW, Feijen J, Grijpma DW. A review on stereolithography and its applications in biomedical engineering. Biomaterials. 2010;31:6121–30. https://doi.org/10.1016/j.biomaterials.2010.04.050.
16. van Ombergen A, Chalupa-Gantner F, Chansoria P, Colosimo BM, Costantini M, Domingos M, et al. 3D bioprinting in microgravity: opportunities, challenges, and possible applications in space. Adv Healthc Mater. 2023;12:e2300443. https://doi.org/10.1002/adhm.202300443.
17. Cubo-Mateo N, Gelinsky M. Wound and skin healing in space: the 3D bioprinting perspective. Front Bioeng Biotechnol. 2021;9:720217. https://doi.org/10.3389/fbioe.2021.720217.
18. Parfenov VA, Petrov SV, Pereira FDAS, Levin AA, Koudan EV, Nezhurina EK, et al. Scaffold-free, label-free, and nozzle-free magnetic levitational bioassembler for rapid formative biofabrication of 3D tissues and organs. Int J Bioprint. 2020;6:304. https://doi.org/10.18063/ijb.v6i3.304.
19. Kang H-W, Lee SJ, Ko IK, Kengla C, Yoo JJ, Atala A. A 3D bioprinting system to produce human-scale tissue constructs with structural integrity. Nat Biotechnol. 2016;34:312–9. https://doi.org/10.1038/nbt.3413.
20. Zhang YS, Yue K, Aleman J, Moghaddam KM, Bakht SM, Yang J, et al. 3D bioprinting for tissue and organ fabrication. Ann Biomed Eng. 2017;45:148–63. https://doi.org/10.1007/s10439-016-1612-8.
21. Kolesky DB, Truby RL, Gladman AS, Busbee TA, Homan KA, Lewis JA. 3D bioprinting of vascularized, heterogeneous cell-laden tissue constructs. Adv Mater. 2014;26:3124–30. https://doi.org/10.1002/adma.201305506.

21 Artificial Intelligence in Bleeding Control and Other Advanced Gastrointestinal Procedures

Giulia Gibiino, Matteo Secco, Luigi Tuccillo, Chiara Coluccio, Carlo Fabbri, and Cecilia Binda

21.1 Introduction

Digestive bleeding is one of the most common conditions encountered by endoscopists during urgent endoscopies. Non-variceal upper gastrointestinal bleeding (NVUGIB) has an incidence of 61–78 cases per 100,000 persons in the United States with a mortality ranging between 2% and 10% meanwhile lower gastrointestinal bleeding (GIB) has an estimated incidence of 33–87 cases per 100,000 persons and accounts for around 3% of emergency surgical referrals [1, 2]. Whether in an emergency setting or following an interventional procedure, identifying and subsequently treating the source of bleeding can be challenging even for expert endoscopists. Furthermore, various types of interference often manifest in endoscopic images, ranging from organic substances like digestive fluid, food remnants, and bodily fluids to technical challenges leading to image blurring or distortions [3].

Efforts are underway to create new devices assisted with artificial intelligence (AI) and computer vision algorithms aimed at aiding physicians through automated bleeding detection methods. Nevertheless, the endeavor remains undeniably demanding.

Methods for identifying bleeding during endoscopic examination encompass computer vision techniques using comprehensive feature descriptors, traditional machine learning (ML) approaches employing established classifiers, and deep learning methodologies, which rely solely on neural network training for feature extraction and classification [3].

Among these, image-enhanced endoscopy (IEE), including chromoendoscopy, narrow-band imaging (NBI), blue laser imaging, the I-scan, and other systems, is remarkably improving the quality of endoscopy [4].

G. Gibiino · M. Secco · L. Tuccillo · C. Coluccio · C. Fabbri · C. Binda (✉)
Gastroenterology and Digestive Endoscopy Unit, Forlì-Cesena Hospitals, AUSL Romagna, Forlì-Cesena, Italy

B. De Simone et al. (eds.), *New Technologies, Precision Medicine, and AI in Emergency General Surgery*, Hot Topics in Acute Care Surgery and Trauma,
https://doi.org/10.1007/978-3-032-09357-8_21

In addition to bleeding detection, artificial intelligence in endoscopy is being applied to a wide range of standard and advanced procedures. Its use has become a routine in most endoscopy units for improving adenoma detection rate and classification of polyps. In the future, artificial intelligence is further expected to become a customary practice tool to assist endoscopists in performing advanced procedures ranging from granting a better definition of the dissection plane when performing submucosal dissection to helping endoscopists in performing the correct diagnosis during endoscopic ultrasonography (EUS) or endoscopic retrograde cholangiopancreatography (ERCP) [5–8].

21.2 Artificial Intelligence–Assisted Bleeding Detection Methods

A broad array of methods for identifying bleeding have been developed using traditional computer vision techniques. Such methods rely on feature descriptors derived from image analysis and statistical metrics. These descriptors are tailored to identify characteristics of the target objects and present them as feature vectors. Subsequently, these vectors are categorized using basic machine learning techniques like support vector machine (SVM) classifiers or shallow neural networks [3].

21.2.1 Classical Computer Vision Techniques

In traditional computer vision methodologies, significant emphasis is placed on feature descriptors. When it comes to detecting endoscopic bleeding, most techniques concentrate on analyzing the color features of the images [3, 9]. Texture, contours, and segmentation methods are less frequently employed for this purpose. Feature descriptors typically involve intricate mathematical transformations that capture specific image statistics, constituting low-level image attributes. Classical methods have achieved reasonable success in endoscopic bleeding detection, particularly when only limited endoscopic image datasets were available [9].

A notable advantage of classical approaches is their ability to develop algorithms even with small image collections. However, classical methods encounter various challenges. Crafting feature descriptors manually is typically laborious and time-intensive. Ensuring the suitability of low-level features with the distinctive visual characteristics of the detected object poses a significant challenge and requires individual solutions for each new object.

Several methods have been developed in the last decades, some of them applied to other purposes such as tumor detection, bleeding detection for wireless capsule endoscopy [10, 11], and intestinal bowel diseases [12].

The high computational complexity involved in feature evaluation, coupled with the characteristics of common classifiers, complicates human verification of intermediate results and the overall process. Consequently, pinpointing the reasons behind incorrect predictions made by the system becomes challenging, hindering the integration of new features to enhance algorithm accuracy.

21.2.2 Classical Machine Learning Approaches

Diverse techniques for analyzing endoscopic images have emerged, rooted in classical machine learning algorithms [3].

These methods prioritize the utilization of classification techniques to streamline their training process.

Among them, the Bayesian classifier has been proposed by Wang and Yang [13], while Yeh et al. used SVM feature elimination, OneR, and RELIEF algorithms to select features for bleeding detection analysis in wireless capsule endoscopy [14].

21.2.3 Deep Learning Approaches

Deep learning represents a contemporary domain within machine learning that focuses on training intricate neural network models using extensive datasets [3].

These networks, inspired by the structure and functionality of the human brain, consist of interconnected layers of artificial neurons organized into networks, learning to discern patterns and make decisions.

Prominent neural network architectures include convolutional neural networks (CNNs), recurrent neural networks (RNNs), and transformers. The advent of deep learning models, particularly convolutional neural networks, presented a fundamentally different approach to computer vision tasks.

Neural networks now handle feature extraction, learning features directly from images, thereby eliminating the need for manual design and implementation. This yields a streamlined and elegant approach where all processing steps, from feature extraction to classification, are carried out by a unified mechanism in the guise of a neural network [3].

Various neural network architectures that consequently improved the accuracy for multiple computer vision tasks have been developed over the last years.

Most of them are based on existing CNN architectures [15, 16] and their direct utilization for training on an endoscopic dataset of annotated blood images. Some of the approaches acknowledge the problem of a limited training data size, which is addressed by applying a transfer learning technique, typically using models trained on the ImageNet dataset [17].

Before examining the applications of artificial intelligence in endoscopic bleeding detection, a focus must be put on recently developed techniques such as red dichromatic imaging (RDI) which are of extreme importance in bleeding control and are already part of the clinical practice of most endoscopic units.

21.3 Red Dichromatic Imaging

Red dichromatic imaging (RDI) is a recently developed technique that employs longer wavelength lights (520–550, 595–610, and 620–640 nm). These wavelengths possess minimal light scattering properties, a departure from narrow-band imaging. RDI aims to heighten the visibility of deep-seated blood vessels and regions of bleeding. It is integrated into the latest Olympus endoscopy system, the EVIS X1, as an advanced iteration of the original optical-digital method. By enhancing the discernibility of deep blood vessels, it enables a more precise assessment of esophageal varices and the extent of inflammation in ulcerative colitis. Simplified identification of bleeding sources streamlines hemostasis, expediting procedures like endoscopic submucosal dissection (ESD) and peroral endoscopic myotomy, as well as the management of gastrointestinal bleeding from peptic ulcers or colon diverticula [4].

RDI offers three distinct observation modes tailored to specific purposes: enhancing visibility of thick blood vessels in deep tissues (mode 1), deeper vessels (mode 2), and both superficial and deep vessels (mode 3). These versatile modalities enable its application in various stages of hemostatic treatment during bleeding and in the preventative phase of submucosal dissections. Moreover, this technique proves valuable for assessing vascular patterns in chronic intestinal diseases [18].

To initiate the assessment of vessel visibility using RDI, an initial study was undertaken to evaluate the feasibility. This study compared the visibility of blood vessels through static endoscopic images of healthy human mucosa and submucosa [19].

In this study, the visibility scores obtained from a prototype of RDI were markedly superior to those from WLI for all participants. These findings facilitated the straightforward identification of vessels and aided in avoiding vessel-related complications during procedures like endoscopic mucosal resection and endoscopic submucosal dissection (ESD) when performing submucosal injections [4, 19].

The ease of use of this technique and the amazing results are the reasons for its increasing use in the treatment and prophylaxis of digestive bleeding.

21.4 Clinical Prediction Models

Accurately stratifying the risk of patients with gastrointestinal bleeding (GIB) upon initial presentation can enhance the efficiency of triage and optimize the allocation of hospital resources. An ideal risk stratification tool should possess high positive and negative predictive values, enabling the discharge of low-risk patients for outpatient follow-up and facilitating early endoscopy for those with high-risk indicators. Implementing such a model within a healthcare system could potentially reduce costs while improving clinical outcomes like overall mortality and hospital length of stay [20].

Machine learning (ML) involves computers analyzing vast datasets to identify useful patterns and associations, leveraging their substantial processing capacity.

ML can uncover novel relationships between variables, enhancing the prediction of clinical outcomes beyond traditional linear and logistic regression models.

However, ML models are susceptible to misleading inputs, necessitating mechanisms to verify the accuracy and reliability of clinical data. This underscores the importance of curated and structured inputs, along with standardized definitions for low- and high-risk outcomes of upper and lower GIB. Developing GIB-specific quality metrics derived from guidelines could aid in standardization and ensure the reliability of data used in ML algorithms [20, 21].

All available clinical models use standard statistical analyses to identify predictors and most assign fixed weights based on the original dataset used to derive a score; the most commonly used are the Glasgow-Blatchford (GBS), admission-Rockall score, and AIMS65 which synthesize clinical, hemodynamic, and initial laboratory variables to help guide patient triage [22, 23]. Several new artificial intelligence-based tools have been developed during the last years and their sensitivity and specificity are under investigation to be compared with other scoring systems.

Past research on machine learning models in upper gastrointestinal bleeding (UGIB) has been constrained by small sample sizes, uniform patient groups, and the absence of validation from external sources. For instance, the most extensive examination of machine learning in UGIB involved 2380 patients. It demonstrated that a neural network model outperformed the complete Rockall score (comprising endoscopic observations) in predicting 30-day mortality, albeit solely through internal validation. However, this study lacked external validation and did not evaluate more clinically significant pre-endoscopic clinical risk scores or the crucial composite outcome [24].

Regarding mortality prediction, alternative machine learning (ML) models show a tendency toward superior performance compared to clinical risk scores. However, to the best of our knowledge only three studies have directly compared ML models to clinical risk scores specifically tailored for evaluating risk in gastrointestinal bleeding. Among these studies, only one study compared ML models to a pre-endoscopic clinical risk score, which serves as the appropriate benchmark for risk assessment in gastrointestinal bleeding [25, 26].

Recently, Shung et al. [27] provided a gradient-boosting ML model derived from a large international multicenter cohort predicting the composite outcome of transfusion, hemostatic intervention, or death better than the commonly used clinical risk scores, achieving the same sensitivity of GBS score with higher specificity.

While still evolving, ML technology shows significant promise. Future advancements will rely on establishing standardized and reliable data elements, along with prospective testing in large-scale trials. The integration of ML into clinical practice hinges on a broader understanding and acceptance of its role in healthcare delivery. Collaborative efforts between healthcare groups and systems, with a focus on meaningful clinical outcomes, hold the potential to positively impact patient management and care delivery [20, 28].

Since recent research has shown that only 30% of physician providers in the United States have ever used a score in caring for patients with acute upper gastrointestinal bleeding and it is reasonable to think that usage of scoring system is as low for patients with lower gastrointestinal bleeding we can expect that machine learning models based scores will become in the years to come an important tool to stratify and manage patients affected by gastrointestinal bleeding [29, 30].

21.5 Artificial Intelligence and Bleeding Classification

Peptic ulcer bleeding (PUB) is considered the most common cause of upper gastrointestinal bleeding with a potential risk of death for patients [31–33].

Different classifications have been proposed over the years to accurately classify and stratify the risk of bleeding and rebleeding linked to peptic ulcer. The most widely used is the Forrest classification because of its simplicity of use and predictive value to detect recurrent bleeding [34]. One of the limits of this classification is the interobserver and intraobserver variations which can limit its efficacy and predictive value in clinical practice.

A recent study by He et al. [35] showed that a real-time deep convolutional neural network system showed good diagnostic performance, which was slightly superior to that of senior endoscopists, in the assessment of Forrest classification for PUB when analyzing videos of peptic ulcers.

Even if this analysis was performed on videos of PUB and so its value in real patients must be still confirmed by prospective studies, its application in the future could enhance and assist junior endoscopists in making the correct classification of PUB with consequent benefits on treatment and recurrence of bleeding linked to this condition.

21.6 Artificial Intelligence and Endoscopic Submucosal Dissection

Endoscopic submucosal dissection (ESD) is the procedure of choice for removing early-stage gastrointestinal cancers. A major challenge during ESD is managing bleeding, which can obscure visibility and complicate the procedure. Red dichromatic imaging (RDI) has emerged as a promising technology to enhance visibility and improve hemostasis [36]. Even so, ESD remains a demanding technique since it is extremely time demanding and the definition of the best dissection plane can be challenging even for an endoscopist familiar with this technique.

A recent study by Furube et al. [7] showed that the artificial intelligence-based system is accurate in recognition of esophageal ESD phases (marking, injection, incision, dissection, etc.). Authors highlight the fact that this AI system could improve endoscopy room efficiency by displaying the remaining time and phase transition timing, thereby helping medical staff prepare the next instrument or patient. Moreover, this system is useful to estimate the endoscopist's skill and learning curve [7].

21.7 Artificial Intelligence in Prediction of Adverse Events During Endoscopic Retrograde Cholangiopancreatography

One of the most common adverse events of ERCP is post-ERCP pancreatitis (PEP), which occurs at a frequency of 3–10%, with a mortality rate of 0.7% [37, 38].

There is no universally accepted scoring system for prediction of PEP. Takahashi and al [39]. recently published a prediction model based on machine learning algorithm using 10 features which are known risk factors for PEP. This model stratifies patients in three groups (low, intermediate, and high risk of PEP) and has shown statistically significant accuracy in predicting patients at risk of PEP.

21.8 Artificial Intelligence in Diagnosis of Biliary Strictures

AI is revolutionizing the medical field, and its application in diagnosing malignant biliary strictures (MBS) is a promising development. Malignant biliary stricture is the narrowing of the bile ducts caused by cancer or benign conditions, and their accurate diagnosis is crucial for an effective treatment. Traditional diagnostic methods, such as endoscopic retrograde cholangiopancreatography (ERCP) with brush cytology and forceps biopsy, often yield inconclusive results. Cholangioscopy, a procedure that allows direct visualization of the bile ducts, increased endoscopists' potential to perform the correct diagnosis and achieve adequate histologic sampling. AI, particularly through deep learning techniques, offers a novel approach to enhance diagnostic accuracy and efficiency.

The use of convolutional neural networks (CNNs) in cholangioscopy represents a significant advancement. In a study conducted by Marya et al., a CNN was developed and tested to identify malignant features in cholangioscopy images. The CNN was trained using a vast dataset of cholangioscopy images annotated by experts, and its performance was compared to traditional ERCP-based sampling techniques. The results were remarkable: the CNN demonstrated an accuracy of 90.6%, significantly higher than the 62.5% and 60.9% accuracy of brush cytology and forceps biopsy, respectively [40].

Cholangioscopy has always held potential due to its direct visualization capability. However, its effectiveness was hampered by the subjective nature of image interpretation and interobserver variability. AI mitigates these issues by providing consistent and objective analysis of cholangioscopy images. The study highlighted that AI could identify specific cholangioscopic features associated with malignancy, such as frond-like mucosa or papillary projections, with a higher degree of accuracy than human observers [40–42].

Despite these promising results, the application of AI in this field is not without challenges. The CNN developed by Marya et al. was trained on data from a single center, which raises questions about its generalizability. In addition, the annotations used for training were provided by a single expert, potentially introducing bias. To address these limitations, further research involving multicenter studies and diverse datasets is necessary to validate and refine the AI models [40, 41].

The integration of AI with cholangioscopy also opens up possibilities for real-time analysis during procedures. This could transform clinical practice by providing immediate diagnostic feedback, potentially leading to quicker decision-making and treatment initiation. However, this also raises important questions about the role of AI in clinical decision-making. If AI-based diagnoses are more accurate than traditional tissue-based methods, it challenges the paradigm of relying on histological confirmation for treatment decisions [41, 42].

In conclusion, AI-assisted cholangioscopy represents a significant leap forward in the diagnosis of malignant biliary strictures. By leveraging the power of deep learning, it offers a more accurate, efficient, and potentially real-time diagnostic tool compared to traditional methods. While challenges remain in terms of validation and clinical integration, the groundwork laid by current studies suggests a future where AI becomes an indispensable part of endoscopic practice. The ongoing evolution of AI technology and its application in medical diagnostics holds great promise for improving patient outcomes and transforming healthcare delivery.

21.9 Conclusions

Artificial intelligence is progressively transforming gastrointestinal endoscopy, with particular impact on bleeding control, risk stratification, and complex therapeutic procedures. As illustrated throughout this chapter, AI-based systems—ranging from computer vision–assisted bleeding detection and advanced imaging modalities to predictive models and procedural guidance—have the potential to enhance diagnostic accuracy, procedural safety, and clinical efficiency. Several of these applications, such as image-enhanced endoscopy and red dichromatic imaging, are already integrated into routine practice, while others remain in active development and evaluation. Despite promising results, the widespread clinical adoption of AI in endoscopy faces important challenges. These include the need for high-quality and representative datasets, external and prospective validation, model interpretability, and seamless integration into existing workflows. In addition, variability in endoscopic technique, operator expertise, and clinical context underscores the importance of positioning AI as a decision-support tool rather than a replacement for clinical judgment. Future progress will depend on multidisciplinary collaboration between endoscopists, surgeons, data scientists, engineers, and industry partners, as well as on structured training programs that promote AI literacy among clinicians. With careful validation, ethical oversight, and user-centered implementation, artificial intelligence has the potential to become a reliable adjunct in the management of gastrointestinal bleeding and other advanced endoscopic procedures, ultimately improving patient outcomes and procedural safety.

References

1. Mullady DK, Wang AY, Waschke KA. AGA clinical practice update on endoscopic therapies for non-variceal upper gastrointestinal bleeding: expert review. Gastroenterology. 2020;159:1120–8. https://doi.org/10.1053/j.gastro.2020.05.095.
2. Oakland K, Chadwick G, East JE, Guy R, Humphries A, Jairath V, McPherson S, Metzner M, Morris AJ, Murphy MF, Tham T, Uberoi R, Veitch AM, Wheeler J, Regan C, Hoare J. Diagnosis and management of acute lower gastrointestinal bleeding: guidelines from the British Society of Gastroenterology. Gut. 2019;68:776–89. https://doi.org/10.1136/gutjnl-2018-317807.
3. Brzeski A, Dziubich T, Krawczyk H. Visual features for improving endoscopic bleeding detection using convolutional neural networks. Sensors (Basel). 2023;23:9717. https://doi.org/10.3390/s23249717.
4. Uraoka T, Igarashi M. Development and clinical usefulness of a unique red dichromatic imaging technology in gastrointestinal endoscopy: a narrative review. Ther Adv Gastroenterol. 2022;15:17562848221118302. https://doi.org/10.1177/17562848221118302.
5. Koleth G, Emmanue J, Spadaccini M, Mascagni P, Khalaf K, Mori Y, Antonelli G, Maselli R, Carrara S, Galtieri PA, Pellegatta G, Fugazza A, Anderloni A, Selvaggio C, Bretthauer M, Aghemo A, Spinelli A, Savevski V, Sharma P, Hassan C, Repici A. Artificial intelligence in gastroenterology: where are we heading? Endosc Int Open. 2022;10:E1474–80. https://doi.org/10.1055/a-1907-6569.
6. Artificial intelligence implementation in pancreaticobiliary endoscopy - PubMed. https://pubmed.ncbi.nlm.nih.gov/35639864/. Accessed 30 May 2024.
7. Furube T, Takeuchi M, Kawakubo H, Maeda Y, Matsuda S, Fukuda K, Nakamura R, Kato M, Yahagi N, Kitagawa Y. Automated artificial intelligence-based phase-recognition system for esophageal endoscopic submucosal dissection (with video). Gastrointest Endosc. 2024;99:830–8. https://doi.org/10.1016/j.gie.2023.12.037.
8. Xiao Y, Song Z, Zou S, You Y, Cui J, Wang S, Ku C, Wu X, Xue X, Han W, Zhou W. Artificial intelligence assisted topographic mapping system for endoscopic submucosal dissection specimens. Front Med (Lausanne). 2022;9:822731. https://doi.org/10.3389/fmed.2022.822731.
9. Karkanis S, Magoulas GD, Theofanous N. Image recognition and neuronal networks: intelligent systems for the improvement of imaging information. Minim Invasive Ther Allied Technol. 2000;9:225–30. https://doi.org/10.1080/13645700009169652.
10. Li B, Meng MQ-H. Computer-aided detection of bleeding regions for capsule endoscopy images. IEEE Trans Biomed Eng. 2009;56:1032–9. https://doi.org/10.1109/TBME.2008.2010526.
11. Giritharan B, Yuan X, Liu J, Buckles B, Oh J, Tang SJ. Bleeding detection from capsule endoscopy videos. Annu Int Conf IEEE Eng Med Biol Soc. 2008;2008:4780–3. https://doi.org/10.1109/IEMBS.2008.4650282.
12. Kumar R, Zhao Q, Seshamani S, Mullin G, Hager G, Dassopoulos T. Assessment of Crohn's disease lesions in wireless capsule endoscopy images. IEEE Trans Biomed Eng. 2012;59:355–62. https://doi.org/10.1109/TBME.2011.2172438.
13. Wang B, Yang D. Computer-assisted diagnosis of digestive endoscopic images based on Bayesian theory. In: 2009 international conference on information engineering and computer science; 2009. p. 1–4.
14. Yeh J-Y, Wu T-H, Tsai W-J. Bleeding and ulcer detection using wireless capsule endoscopy images. J Softw Eng Appl. 2014;07:422. https://doi.org/10.4236/jsea.2014.75039.
15. He K, Zhang X, Ren S, Sun J. Deep residual learning for image recognition. In: 2016 IEEE conference on Computer Vision and Pattern Recognition (CVPR); 2016. p. 770–8.
16. Szegedy C, Vanhoucke V, Ioffe S, Shlens J, Wojna Z. Rethinking the inception architecture for computer vision. In: 2016 IEEE conference on computer vision and pattern recognition (CVPR); 2016. p. 2818–26.
17. Krizhevsky A, Sutskever I, Hinton GE. ImageNet classification with deep convolutional neural networks. In: Advances in neural information processing systems. Curran Associates, Inc.; 2012.

18. Hirai Y, Fujimoto A, Matsutani N, Murakami S, Nakajima Y, Miyanaga R, Nakazato Y, Watanabe K, Kikuchi M, Yahagi N. Evaluation of the visibility of bleeding points using red dichromatic imaging in endoscopic hemostasis for acute GI bleeding (with video). Gastrointest Endosc. 2022;95:692–700.e3. https://doi.org/10.1016/j.gie.2021.10.031.
19. Yahagi N, Fujimoto A, Horii J, Uraoka T, Shimoda M, Takabayashi K, Nisizawa T, Goto O, Ochiai Y, Maehata T, Nakayama A, Kato M, Hosoe N, Naganuma M. Dual red imaging: a novel endoscopic imaging technology visualizing thick blood vessels in the gastrointestinal wall. Endosc Int Open. 2019;7:E1632–E1635. https://doi.org/10.1055/a-0749-0075.
20. Sengupta N, Leiman DA. Improving acute GI bleeding management through artificial intelligence: unnatural selection? Dig Dis Sci. 2019;64:2061–4. https://doi.org/10.1007/s10620-019-05698-0.
21. Stanley AJ, Laine L. Management of acute upper gastrointestinal bleeding. BMJ. 2019;364:l536. https://doi.org/10.1136/bmj.l536.
22. Laine L, Barkun AN, Saltzman JR, Martel M, Leontiadis GI. ACG clinical guideline: upper gastrointestinal and ulcer bleeding. Am J Gastroenterol. 2021;116:899–917. https://doi.org/10.14309/ajg.0000000000001245.
23. Stanley AJ, Laine L, Dalton HR, Ngu JH, Schultz M, Abazi R, Zakko L, Thornton S, Wilkinson K, CJL K, Murray IA, Laursen SB, International Gastrointestinal Bleeding Consortium. Comparison of risk scoring systems for patients presenting with upper gastrointestinal bleeding: international multicentre prospective study. BMJ. 2017;356:i6432. https://doi.org/10.1136/bmj.i6432.
24. Rotondano G, Cipolletta L, Grossi E, Koch M, Intraligi M, Buscema M, Marmo R, Italian Registry on Upper Gastrointestinal Bleeding (Progetto Nazionale Emorragie Digestive). Artificial neural networks accurately predict mortality in patients with nonvariceal upper GI bleeding. Gastrointest Endosc. 2011;73:218–26., 226.e1–2. https://doi.org/10.1016/j.gie.2010.10.006.
25. Lee HH, Park JM, Han S, Park SM, Kim HY, Oh JH, Kim CW, Yoon SK, Choi M-G. A simplified prognostic model to predict mortality in patients with acute variceal bleeding. Dig Liver Dis. 2018;50:247–53. https://doi.org/10.1016/j.dld.2017.11.006.
26. Lyles T, Elliott A, Rockey DC. A risk scoring system to predict in-hospital mortality in patients with cirrhosis presenting with upper gastrointestinal bleeding. J Clin Gastroenterol. 2014;48:712–20. https://doi.org/10.1097/MCG.0000000000000014.
27. Shung DL, Au B, Taylor RA, Tay JK, Laursen SB, Stanley AJ, Dalton HR, Ngu J, Schultz M, Laine L. Validation of a machine learning model that outperforms clinical risk scoring systems for upper gastrointestinal bleeding. Gastroenterology. 2020;158:160–7. https://doi.org/10.1053/j.gastro.2019.09.009.
28. Topol EJ. High-performance medicine: the convergence of human and artificial intelligence. Nat Med. 2019;25:44–56. https://doi.org/10.1038/s41591-018-0300-7.
29. Liang PS, Saltzman JR. A national survey on the initial management of upper gastrointestinal bleeding. J Clin Gastroenterol. 2014;48:e93–8. https://doi.org/10.1097/MCG.0000000000000095.
30. Shung DL. Advancing care for acute gastrointestinal bleeding using artificial intelligence. J Gastroenterol Hepatol. 2021;36:273–8. https://doi.org/10.1111/jgh.15372.
31. Gralnek IM, Stanley AJ, Morris AJ, Camus M, Lau J, Lanas A, Laursen SB, Radaelli F, Papanikolaou IS, Cúrdia Gonçalves T, Dinis-Ribeiro M, Awadie H, Braun G, de Groot N, Udd M, Sanchez-Yague A, Neeman Z, van Hooft JE. Endoscopic diagnosis and management of nonvariceal upper gastrointestinal hemorrhage (NVUGIH): European Society of Gastrointestinal Endoscopy (ESGE) Guideline - Update 2021. Endoscopy. 2021;53:300–32. https://doi.org/10.1055/a-1369-5274.
32. Kate V, Sureshkumar S, Gurushankari B, Kalayarasan R. Acute upper non-variceal and lower gastrointestinal bleeding. J Gastrointest Surg. 2022;26:932–49. https://doi.org/10.1007/s11605-022-05258-4.

33. Chang-Chien CS, Wu CS, Chen PC, Lin DY, Chu CM, Fang KM, Sheen IS, Liaw YF. Different implications of stigmata of recent hemorrhage in gastric and duodenal ulcers. Dig Dis Sci. 1988;33:400–4. https://doi.org/10.1007/BF01536021.
34. de Groot NL, van Oijen MGH, Kessels K, Hemmink M, Weusten BLAM, Timmer R, Hazen WL, van Lelyveld N, Vermeijden RR, Curvers WL, Baak BC, Verburg R, Bosman JH, de Wijkerslooth LRH, de Rooij J, Venneman NG, Pennings M, van Hee K, Scheffer BCH, van Eijk RL, Meiland R, Siersema PD, Bredenoord AJ. Reassessment of the predictive value of the Forrest classification for peptic ulcer rebleeding and mortality: can classification be simplified? Endoscopy. 2014;46:46–52. https://doi.org/10.1055/s-0033-1344884.
35. He X-J, Wang X-L, Su T-K, Yao L-J, Zheng J, Wen X-D, Xu Q-W, Huang Q-R, Chen L-B, Chen C-X, Lin H-F, Chen Y-Q, Hu Y-X, Zhang K-H, Jiang C-S, Liu G, Li D-Z, Li D-L, Wen W. Artificial intelligence-assisted system for the assessment of Forrest classification of peptic ulcer bleeding: a multicenter diagnostic study. Endoscopy. 2024;56:334–42. https://doi.org/10.1055/a-2252-4874.
36. Mori Y, Iwatsubo T, Hakoda A, Kameishi S, Takayama K, Sasaki S, Koshiba R, Nishida S, Harada S, Tanaka H, Sugawara N, Ota K, Kawaguchi S, Kojima Y, Takeuchi T, Higuchi K, Nishikawa H. Red dichromatic imaging improves the recognition of bleeding points during endoscopic submucosal dissection. Dig Dis Sci. 2024;69:216–27. https://doi.org/10.1007/s10620-023-08145-3.
37. ASGE Standards of Practice Committee, Chandrasekhara V, Khashab MA, Muthusamy VR, Acosta RD, Agrawal D, Bruining DH, Eloubeidi MA, Fanelli RD, Faulx AL, Gurudu SR, Kothari S, Lightdale JR, Qumseya BJ, Shaukat A, Wang A, Wani SB, Yang J, DeWitt JM. Adverse events associated with ERCP. Gastrointest Endosc. 2017;85:32–47. https://doi.org/10.1016/j.gie.2016.06.051.
38. Dumonceau J-M, Kapral C, Aabakken L, Papanikolaou IS, Tringali A, Vanbiervliet G, Beyna T, Dinis-Ribeiro M, Hritz I, Mariani A, Paspatis G, Radaelli F, Lakhtakia S, Veitch AM, van Hooft JE. ERCP-related adverse events: European Society of Gastrointestinal Endoscopy (ESGE) guideline. Endoscopy. 2020;52:127–49. https://doi.org/10.1055/a-1075-4080.
39. Takahashi H, Ohno E, Furukawa T, Yamao K, Ishikawa T, Mizutani Y, Iida T, Shiratori Y, Oyama S, Koyama J, Mori K, Hayashi Y, Oda M, Suzuki T, Kawashima H. Artificial intelligence in a prediction model for postendoscopic retrograde cholangiopancreatography pancreatitis. Dig Endosc. 2024;36:463–72. https://doi.org/10.1111/den.14622.
40. Marya NB, Powers PD, Petersen BT, Law R, Storm A, Abusaleh RR, Rau P, Stead C, Levy MJ, Martin J, Vargas EJ, Abu Dayyeh BK, Chandrasekhara V. Identification of patients with malignant biliary strictures using a cholangioscopy-based deep learning artificial intelligence (with video). Gastrointest Endosc. 2023;97:268–278.e1. https://doi.org/10.1016/j.gie.2022.08.021.
41. Diehl DL. Artificial intelligence-assisted cholangioscopy of malignant biliary strictures: changing the paradigm? Gastrointest Endosc. 2023;97:279–81. https://doi.org/10.1016/j.gie.2022.10.021.
42. Saraiva MM, Ribeiro T, Ferreira JPS, Boas FV, Afonso J, Santos AL, Parente MPL, Jorge RN, Pereira P, Macedo G. Artificial intelligence for automatic diagnosis of biliary stricture malignancy status in single-operator cholangioscopy: a pilot study. Gastrointest Endosc. 2022;95:339–48. https://doi.org/10.1016/j.gie.2021.08.027.

Part IV

The Operating Theatre of the Future

Advancements in Emergency Surgery Through AI-Powered Hybrid Operating Rooms

22

Aishwarya Boini, S. Vincent Grasso, Elie Chouillard, and Andrew A. Gumbs

22.1 Introduction

22.1.1 Definition of Emergency Surgery and Its Importance in Healthcare

In the field of emergency surgery, where time can often be a distinction between life and death, the Hybrid Operating Room (OR) emerges as a paradigm shift. This chapter discusses the significance and functionality of the Hybrid OR in emergency surgery settings. We highlight its tremendous impact on the care of the acute patient by evaluating its integration of innovative technology such as artificial intelligence (AI) with surgical expertise. To appreciate the significance of the Hybrid OR in emergency surgery, it is essential to understand the nature of emergency surgical interventions. To do this, we must understand what surgery means nowadays: specifically, it follows traditional surgical methods such as open and minimally invasive techniques (e.g., laparoscopy, thoracoscopic, arthroscopic, and robotic-assisted), and also incorporates other interventional techniques such as endoscopic surgery

A. Boini
Davao Medical School Foundation, Davao City, Philippines

S. V. Grasso
Department of Electrical & Computer Engineering, University of New Mexico, Albuquerque, NM, USA

E. Chouillard
American Hospital of Paris, Paris, France

A. A. Gumbs (✉)
Department of General-, Visceral-, Vascular and Transplantation Surgery, University of Magdeburg, Magdeburg, Germany

Service de Chirurgie Digestive Minimale Invasive, Hôpital Antoine Béclère, Assistance Publique-Hôpitaux de Paris, Clamart, France

B. De Simone et al. (eds.), *New Technologies, Precision Medicine, and AI in Emergency General Surgery*, Hot Topics in Acute Care Surgery and Trauma,
https://doi.org/10.1007/978-3-032-09357-8_22

(e.g., natural orifice transluminal endoscopic surgery) and percutaneous surgery (e.g., interventional radiology and cardiology).

Emergency surgery is the emergency procedure/intervention required to treat acute issues or life-threatening conditions in which tissues, organs, and limbs have been damaged. These conditions may be the result of acute illness, trauma, acute disease, acute exacerbation of chronic disease, or complications from medical procedures. Areas of specialty for emergency surgeons include: abdominal surgery, thoracic surgery, vascular surgery, and soft tissue surgery. Many of these procedures can be performed on the same day [1].

Acute care surgery (ACS) in the United States has been evolving since 2008 to include trauma, critical care, and emergency surgery. In the United Kingdom, there has been an increasing emphasis on emergency general surgery (EGS) within the wider field of general surgery in the last decade. This is in line with the global challenge of delivering high-quality care to emergency surgical patients, especially after traffic accidents around the world, with trauma being a leading cause of death in individuals up to 40 years old in the United States alone [2].

22.2 Fundamentals of Hybrid Operating Rooms

22.2.1 Definition and Concept of Hybrid Operating Rooms

Hybrid Operating Rooms (ORs) represent a significant advancement in surgical facilities, integrating advanced imaging capabilities seamlessly with fully equipped OR suites. The term "operating room" was first used in 1846 by a dentist performing surgery under anesthesia in a library in the United States. Operating rooms began with basic setups in 1846 and evolved over time from decentralized, centralized, nonclean environments to the digitally integrated, Hybrid operating rooms we know today.

The Hybrid OR was developed in 1996 by a British academic, Angelini, and was first introduced in Monaco. The Hybrid OR combines surgical, endoscopic, and interventional therapy with imaging functions in one space. This cutting-edge approach reduces patient movement during the procedure and allows real-time visualization of surgical information via various imaging devices. Hybrid ORs improve efficiency and enable smart medicine practices within modern healthcare settings [3].

By definition, a Hybrid OR combines advanced imaging capabilities, such as angiography and fluoroscopic imaging, with the functionalities of a conventional operating room (e.g., endoscopic and robotic-assisted surgery) (Fig. 22.1). Originally, Hybrid ORs were designed to support complex cardiovascular procedures, such as percutaneous coronary interventions (PCI) or minimally invasive coronary artery bypass grafting. With the development of advanced medical technologies and the innovative procedures they enable, for example, the transcatheter valve replacement (TVR), Hybrid ORs have evolved into versatile spaces that can support a wide variety of surgical interventions.

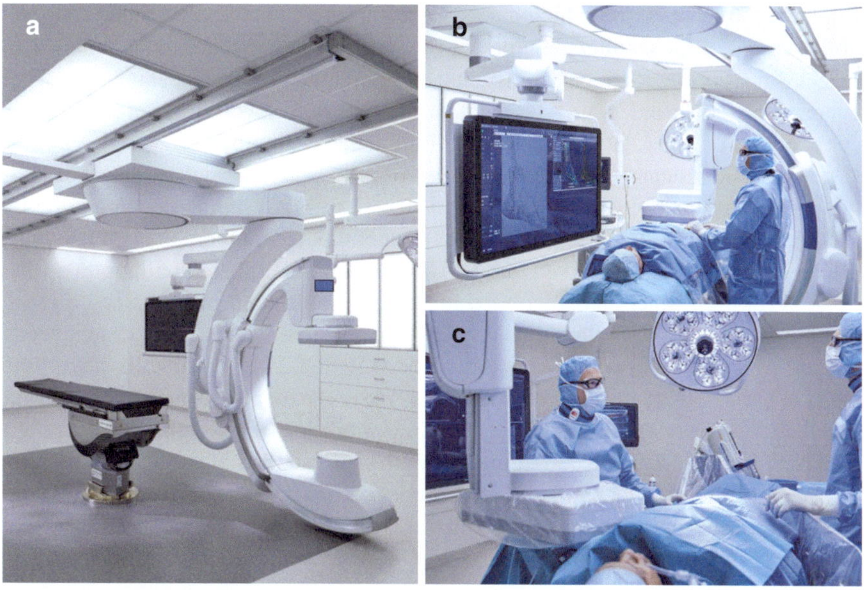

Fig. 22.1 State-of-the-Hybrid OR at the American Hospital of Paris, (**a**) C-arm for intra-operative fluoroscopy, (**b**) enhanced angiography of the lower limb, and (**c**) doctors utilizing intraoperative ultrasound and protected with lead lined protective shields so that intraoperative fluoroscopy is permitted

Hybrid ORs provide surgeons with real-time intraoperative imaging guidance that allows for accurate visualization and intervention during the procedure. The technical setup of a Hybrid OR requires careful consideration, especially when it comes to radiation safety. To ensure the safety of patients and medical staff, stringent safety protocols must be implemented, such as lead-lined walls and protective aprons, as well as regular radiation exposure monitoring. The layout and equipment selection also play an important role in optimizing functionality. Features, such as high-quality fluoroscopy systems and radiolucent operational tables, and strategically positioned monitors enhance procedural efficiency and safety in these advanced surgical environments [4].

22.2.2 Components and Infrastructure Requirements

There are several key steps in the OR planning process. The first step is determining the layout. This involves the optimal positioning of the patient table with the overall system based upon an optimal workflow. The second step is collaboration. Clear communication between stakeholders is essential, and a team approach that involves customers and vendors. The third step is equipment planning. Choosing the right OR tables is key, and making sure that they are easy to position, ergonomically designed, and have efficient cable management is fundamental. Space requirements emphasize at least 70 m^2, which meets radiation safety standards. Vendor cooperation is essential for seamless equipment integration. Best practices include visits to successful Hybrid ORs (e.g., for insights) and implementing glass cabinets (e.g., for material location efficiency). Along with a comprehensive workflow definition, vendor cooperation is essential for successful implementation [5].

Hybrid ORs integrate surgical and invasive procedures through a variety of configurations, from single functional composites, like digital subtraction angiography (DSA), magnetic resonance imaging (MRI), or computed tomography (CT), to multifunctional configurations like DSA + MRI or DSA + CT. These configurations can be single or multifunctional; increased functionality correlates with increased space requirements, so careful planning is required to consider hospital department needs and patient volume, as well as operational data (Table 22.1). Hybrid ORs streamline medical processes, consolidate procedures, reduce patient secondary injury, and accelerate recovery. As they grow, they allow seamless medical transitions between facilities, facilitated by telecommunication advances such as 5G.

Spatial utilization entails two main models: shared machine rooms or shared operating rooms with equipment rooms and auxiliary spaces. Cost-saving measures include sharing expensive equipment between operating rooms, with layouts accommodating equipment specifications and flexible space for future advancements like intelligent surgical robots. Examples demonstrate varied spatial arrangements, such as shared control rooms, thereby enhancing functional partitioning and serving as references for hospital transformations. Maximizing space usage involves leveraging the axial network of the frame and reserving flexible space for adaptability [3].

22.2.3 Advantages of Hybrid ORs in Emergency Surgery

- Integrated Management: Diverse resources and expertise to improve coordination in an emergency response and improve response times.
- Resource Sharing: Efficient sharing of various resources, including humans, equipment, vehicles, and facilities, optimizes resource utilization, and strengthens emergency response.
- Flexibility and Adaptability: Hybrid systems provide a flexible structure that can be adapted to different emergency scenarios, can be scaled as needed, and support efficient communication between medical teams and emergency response teams [6].
- Reduced Time to Intervention: These state-of-the-art facilities can potentially expedite the time it takes to treat an injury and provide life-saving care, especially in cases of serious trauma that necessitate a combination of invasive and noninvasive procedures.
- Improved Patient Outcomes: Hybrid ORs provide early access to surgical and non-surgical radiological interventions, which can be especially helpful in complex cases such as noncompressible torso hemorrhage or severe pelvic and thoraco-abdominal injuries [7].

Table 22.1 Equipment and layout recommendations for a hybrid OR in addition to surgical suite [46]

No.	Equipment and layout recommendations	Additional details
1	High-quality fluoroscopy with flat-panel imaging in a lead-lined room	Ensures precise imaging during procedures
2	Integration of modalities: biplane system, C-arm CT, integrated ultrasound, electromagnetic navigation systems (optional)	Enhances diagnostic and interventional capabilities
3	Control area for radiologic technicians, with a direct view of the surgical field	Facilitates real-time imaging adjustments and collaboration between radiology and surgical teams
4	Radiolucent operating table made of nonmetallic carbon fiber, integrated with the imaging system to prevent collisions; features a floating tabletop with multidirectional tilt	Enables flexible patient positioning and accurate catheter maneuvering
5	Adequate room size (800–1000 square feet or more) to accommodate equipment for various medical teams; careful equipment positioning for swift conversion to conventional surgery	Ensures sufficient space for seamless workflow and equipment accessibility
6	Ceiling-mounted monitors for simultaneous visualization by surgical, anesthesia, and intervention teams, displaying angiography, echocardiography, and hemodynamic monitoring images	Facilitates real-time collaboration and decision-making among multidisciplinary teams
7	Circulating heating, ventilation, and laminar airflow suitable for conventional surgical operations	Maintains a sterile and comfortable environment for surgical procedures
8	Adequate high-output lighting for surgical interventions	Provides optimal illumination for precision surgical procedures
9	Additional requirements: power receptacles, gas and suction outlets, hot/cold water outlets for cardiopulmonary bypass	Supports the functionality of anesthesia and cardiopulmonary bypass equipment
10	Essential equipment: high-definition displays, oxygen analyzer, suction, oxygen supply, defibrillator/resuscitation cart, echocardiographic equipment, anesthesia and cardiopulmonary bypass equipment, syringe pumps, radiation protection, blood warmers, blood bank access, point-of-care laboratory monitoring, and crash carts for emergencies	Ensures readiness for various medical emergencies and procedures
11	Complete sterile environment for procedures	Maintains a sterile environment to minimize the risk of infections and complications during surgical interventions

- Increased Success Rates: Studies have shown that the use of Hybrid ORs could significantly increase success rates for various surgical procedures. This can lead to better outcomes for patients undergoing surgeries in these advanced facilities.
- Decreased Surgical Duration: Hybrid ORs can reduce surgical duration compared to conventional ORs, which can lead to cost savings, lower anesthesia exposure for the patient, and better workflow for the healthcare provider.
- Reduced Mortality and Complications: Patients treated in Hybrid ORs have experienced reduced rates of mortality and complications. This is a crucial benefit that can enhance patient safety and overall surgical outcomes.
- Expanded Range of Procedures: While cardiac, vascular, and neurosurgeries have been common in Hybrid OR suites, Hybrid ORs can also be used to perform a wider range of procedures, such as orthopedic and gynecological surgeries, allowing healthcare facilities to meet the needs of a wider range of patients. This can help to streamline the surgical process and improve patient outcomes.
- Efficient and Safe Procedures: Hybrid ORs contribute to efficient and safe procedures, potentially leading to decreased recovery times and a reduced need for additional interventions. This can benefit both patients and healthcare providers by streamlining the surgical process and improving patient outcomes [8].

22.2.4 Disadvantages of Hybrid ORs in Emergency Surgery

- Cost Considerations: The initial setup and ongoing maintenance of Hybrid OR suites can be costly. Healthcare facilities need to carefully assess the financial implications of integrating this advanced technology into their infrastructure.
- Facility Planning: Retrofitting existing ORs or building new Hybrid OR suites requires careful facility planning to ensure optimal layout, equipment placement, and workflow efficiency. Proper design considerations are essential to maximize the benefits of Hybrid ORs.
- Radiation Safety: Radiation safety is a critical consideration in Hybrid ORs, both for patients and healthcare providers. Implementing measures to minimize radiation exposure and ensuring staff are trained in radiation safety protocols are essential for safe operations.
- Anesthetic Care Challenges: Anesthetic-related safety issues, such as lower equipment reliability and inaccessibility of the patient and airway, can pose challenges in Hybrid OR settings. Healthcare providers need to address these issues to ensure patient safety during procedures.
- Staff Training and Expertise: Healthcare professionals working in Hybrid OR suites may require specialized training to effectively utilize the advanced technology and equipment available. Ongoing education and training programs are essential to ensure staff competency and patient safety.
- Operational Efficiency: Hybrid ORs may face operational challenges, such as scheduling conflicts and underutilization due to the specific requirements of certain procedures. Healthcare facilities need to optimize operational processes to maximize the efficiency and utilization of Hybrid OR suites.

- Patient and Provider Experiences: Patient and provider experiences in Hybrid ORs should be carefully monitored and evaluated to ensure that the integration of advanced technology enhances overall care delivery. Feedback from stakeholders can help identify areas for improvement and optimize the use of Hybrid OR suites [8].
- Limited Availability: Hybrid ORs may have limited availability due to the specialized equipment and personnel required, which can lead to delays in accessing the facility for emergency surgeries.
- Complex Workflow: Running a Hybrid OR for emergency surgeries can be challenging due to the coordination required between various personnel such as surgeons, anesthesiologists, and interventional radiology staff, leading to potential delays and complications in patient care.
- Manpower Requirements: Maintaining on-call manpower for performing interventional radiology procedures in the Hybrid OR can be demanding, especially in emergency situations where immediate access to skilled personnel is crucial.
- Low Patient Volume: In some cases, the low number of patients requiring emergency surgeries or interventional radiology procedures in a Hybrid OR each month may not justify the resources and staffing needed to operate the facility efficiently [9].

22.3 Types of Emergency Surgeries

22.3.1 Trauma Surgery

22.3.1.1 Overview of Trauma Surgery and Its Challenges

Traumatic injuries cause more than five million deaths worldwide every year, accounting for around 9% of global mortality. Between 1999 and 2015, in the United States, unintentional injury and homicide accounted for more than half of the years of life lost before the age of 70, demonstrating the significant impact of trauma mortality. Hemorrhage is the leading cause of trauma death, accounting for about 40% of all traumatic deaths and more than 80% of deaths in the operating room [10].

Trauma surgery is the surgical treatment of patients who have been injured by external trauma. It includes acute surgical care of traumatic injuries to different anatomical regions, including the abdominal, urological, thoracic areas, vasculature, and soft tissues, as well as skeletal structures. Trauma surgeons are responsible for responding to life-altering injuries and coordinating multidisciplinary care to improve patient outcomes [2].

Trauma and acute care surgery often involve complex patient presentations, sometimes involving multiple traumatic injuries, or acute surgical conditions requiring rapid and accurate evaluation and management. Time is of the essence as these surgeries often require immediate intervention to avoid further complications or to save the patient's life. Coordination among multidisciplinary teams is critical, as communication and collaboration between surgeons, anesthetists, nurses, and other healthcare professionals is necessary to maximize patient outcomes. Due to limited resources, such as equipment, personnel, or facilities, timely and appropriate care can be difficult to provide in some settings. Due to the high-stress environment, the surgical team must remain focused and make rapid decisions under pressure.

Postoperative complications, including infections, bleeding, and organ dysfunction, present a significant risk to patients and require careful postoperative monitoring and care. Surgeons may be faced with ethical dilemmas as to how to balance patient autonomy with the urgency of life-saving interventions. These challenges highlight the need for specialized training and expertise to effectively manage trauma and acute care cases [11].

22.3.1.2 Role of Artificial Intelligence in Trauma Assessment and Decision-Making

The use of artificial intelligence (AI) in surgery marks a paradigm shift in the surgical field, leveraging cutting-edge technologies such as machine learning (ML), deep learning (DL), and computer vision (CV) to enhance surgical practices and patient results. AI provides significant advances in preoperative risk detection and intraoperative video analytics, enabling personalized risk evaluation, real-time support for decision-making, and phase recognition throughout procedures.

However, challenges such as data labeling, regulatory requirements, and the requirement for clear standards remain. Surgeons play a critical role in the adoption of AI technology, collaborating with engineering and data scientists, providing education to stakeholders, and advocating for responsible adoption to promote patient safety and the advancement of surgical care [12]. It is essential to use AI in a responsible and ethical way, with proper data governance and patient safety considerations in the deployment process.

Ethical and governance considerations include transparency and quality standards, as well as strong data governance legislation and frameworks. The future landscape for AI in surgery will include autonomous AI systems that will consult with patients, recommend diagnoses and treatment plans, and provide empathy-based interactions [13]. Artificial intelligence technologies, such as machine learning and computer vision, have the capability to improve clinical decision-making in emergency surgery and trauma care, resulting in better patient outcomes. They also play a critical role in anticipating and minimizing human error in critical circumstances, supporting surgeons in various surgical procedures [14].

AI tools used in surgery can be classified based on their autonomy levels, ranging from full human control to full automation, each with its unique implications for surgical decision-making [15]. There are several factors to be considered for the implementation of autonomous actions using AI in surgery, such as the reluctance of laparoscopic surgeons to adopt robotic telemanipulation technology, concerns about AI's continuous learning requirements, and the complexity of fully autonomous surgical machines, among others.

AI can help in decision-making, navigation, and object recognition, improving surgical outcomes, reducing errors, and optimizing techniques. By incorporating AI into surgery, surgeons can more accurately manipulate and navigate surgical tools, potentially resulting in shorter operation times, quicker recovery, and improved safety for patients and healthcare providers alike. AI-driven technologies also enable complex surgical tasks, leading to advances in minimally invasive techniques and personalized medicine [16].

Using machine learning and AI, trauma centers can predict patient flow by looking at past data and identifying trends that can be used to predict future patient volume and level of acuity. Machine learning algorithms can use various predictors, such as weather, traffic, and location, to train their algorithms to make predictions about how many and how severe trauma cases are expected at any given time. With this predictive capability, trauma centers can adjust staffing levels, allocate resources more efficiently, optimize bed management to provide timely and effective treatment for incoming patients, identify areas of process improvement, enhance patient care, reduce costs, and foresee outcomes support clinical decision-making within trauma centers [17].

22.3.1.3 Integration of Hybrid OR in Trauma Surgery

The implementation of a Trauma Hybrid Operating Room (THOR) at a level-1 trauma center has significantly improved the management of abdominopelvic trauma patients. Patients requiring surgery and invasive radiology procedures were included in the THOR protocol. Multiple bleeding control interventions could be performed in one location without the need for patient transport, which resulted in shorter procedural time and lower mortality rates. The addition of trauma staff during this period also improved endovascular procedure capabilities, resulting in improved patient outcomes [18].

Hybrid ORs offer the potential for faster bleeding control while allowing for simultaneous operative exploration. However, dedicated ORs for trauma patients are rare in the United States and are often occupied by nontrauma cases. In a study of a Hybrid operating room for trauma patients (Loftus et al. 2015), the Hybrid OR was housed in a former angiography unit adjacent to the ER. The OR provided immediate access for trauma surgeons to perform resuscitative endovascular balloon occlusion of the aorta (REBOA) and other catheter-based surgical interventions while interventional radiology and vascular surgeons performed diagnostic and therapeutic angiographic interventions in the OR.

The Hybrid OR model resulted in faster bleeding control and fewer transfusion requirements. The Hybrid cohort also had fewer infectious complications and a shorter mechanical ventilation duration compared to the traditional care group, as well as a lower rate of severe complications. The overall conclusion of the study was that the Hybrid OR model has the potential to improve trauma patient outcomes and streamline care delivery [10].

22.3.2 Cardiovascular Emergencies

22.3.2.1 Common Cardiovascular Emergencies Requiring Surgical Intervention

Emergency surgery is a common practice in cardiovascular units for conditions like acute coronary syndrome, endocarditis, valvular diseases, trauma, acute aortic dissection, embolisms, and Leriche syndrome. The most frequent issues necessitating emergency intervention were thoracic aortic aneurysms, coronary artery disease, abdominal aortic aneurysms (with or without rupture), peripheral vascular problems, and others. Emergency repairs for thoracic and abdominal aortic aneurysms constituted a significant portion, alongside procedures for acute coronary ischemia, valvular, and congenital heart diseases [19].

22.3.2.2 Role of AI in Cardiothoracic Surgery

AI plays a critical role in improving various aspects of cardiac surgery at various stages (Table 22.2). In the preoperative stage, AI helps predict individual death risks for patients with congenital heart failure, automates administrative procedures, and provides personalized risk assessment for conditions such as acute heart failure.

During surgery, AI continuously monitors team performance, provides real-time assessments through systems such as the OR Black Box, and analyzes surgeon techniques objectively using computer vision. AI predicts risks such as intraoperative

Table 22.2 Application of AI in cardiothoracic surgical planning [47]

Application	Description
AI in cardiothoracic surgery	
Surgical decision-making	Integrating patient data, anatomy, and disease factors to aid in informed surgical decisions
Predictive modeling	Providing predictive models to guide surgical teams, reducing risks and ensuring safer surgeries
Risk prediction	Utilizing machine learning algorithms to predict intrahospital mortality post-cardiac procedures
Surgical technique improvement	Facilitating advancements like remote-controlled robotic surgery, enhancing safety and precision
Surgical data science (SDS)	
Data capture and organization	Capturing and organizing vast amounts of surgical data to support comprehensive analysis
Modeling data	Leveraging machine learning techniques to extract valuable insights and aid in predictive modeling
Supporting surgical decision-making	Providing predictive models and risk assessments based on collected data, supporting surgeons in decision-making
Improving quality of care	Optimizing surgical coordination, mitigating errors, and enhancing patient safety and healthcare quality
Performance assessment	Assessing physician competence, evaluating intraoperative performance, and predicting complications
Automation and standardization	Automating and standardizing performance assessment to ensure objective evaluations of surgical performance

hypoxemia and provides accurate estimates of surgery duration to optimize resource utilization. Postoperative, AI facilitates individual risk assessments for complications, predicts outcomes like the need for intraoperative care (IC) or ventilator support, and integrates intraoperative information to predict complications such as acute kidney injury. These advances highlight AI's fundamental importance in improving safety, effectiveness, and overall patient outcomes throughout the whole spectrum of cardiac surgery [20].

Artificial intelligence (AI) and Extended Reality (XR) modalities are revolutionizing cardiothoracic surgery at every step of patient care. Preoperatively, XR allows for detailed anatomical visualization that aids in tumor location and surgical planning. Intraoperatively, XR improves precision and spatial perception. Postoperatively, XR enhances pain management, rehabilitation, and patient education to improve overall care. These applications demonstrate the versatility and effectiveness of XR in improving surgical outcomes from preoperative planning to postoperative recovery. As we leverage the power of artificial Intelligence (AI), ethical considerations and patient privacy must be addressed to ensure its proper integration in clinical practice. While challenges remain, we can look forward to more efficient, more effective, and more patient-centric care in the future [21].

22.3.2.3 Integration of Hybrid OR in Cardiovascular Surgeries

The evolution of cardiovascular surgery from traditional open procedures to minimally invasive techniques has significantly transformed patient care. Minimally invasive approaches offer reduced trauma, smaller incisions, and lower infection risks, resulting in faster recoveries and improved outcomes. However, they also pose challenges such as the need for specialized training and advanced equipment, such as a biplane system used in interventional radiology and surgery, consisting of two X-ray sources and detectors positioned at right angles. It provides real-time, high-quality, three-dimensional imaging of the patient's anatomy, enhancing visualization and guidance during complex procedures. In thoracic instrumentation, the use of a biplane fluoroscopy system in a Hybrid operating room allows for better visualization of the mid and upper thoracic spine compared to traditional C-arm fluoroscopy machines [22].

The advancement of Hybrid surgical rooms represents a significant milestone, seamlessly integrating surgical sterility with advanced imaging capabilities. These Hybrid environments enable a wide range of minimally invasive and open surgical procedures to be performed in a single space, with careful considerations for design and planning [23]. A Hybrid cardiac procedure blends surgical and catheter-based interventions to address complex cardiac issues.

These procedures can be planned or unplanned, with the goal of enhancing overall treatment feasibility and reducing risks. Planned Hybrids involve collaborative decision-making by interventional cardiologists and cardiac surgeons, aiming to optimize patient outcomes. Examples include revascularization with a left internal mammary artery (LIMA) to the left anterior descending artery (LAD) combined with percutaneous coronary intervention (PCI) for other vessels. Unplanned Hybrids occur when unexpected outcomes arise during scheduled procedures, necessitating additional therapy, such as PCI following failed grafts post-coronary artery bypass grafting (CABG). While the frequency of Hybrid interventions has decreased with advances in surgical techniques, they remain valuable for certain cases, especially those involving complex pathologies or previous surgeries [24].

Examples of Hybrid procedures include Hybrid coronary revascularization (CABG/PCI), minimally invasive valve surgery combined with PCI to coronary lesions (valve/PCI), Hybrid endomyocardial/epicardial atrial fibrillation procedures, and Hybrid aortic arch debranching combined with endovascular grafting for thoracic aortic procedures. The key requirement in all of these approaches is the need for collaboration between specialists to ensure the success of Hybrid programs [25].

22.3.3 Neurosurgery

22.3.3.1 Overview of Neurosurgical Emergencies

Neurosurgical emergencies encompass a range of critical conditions requiring urgent operative management. These emergencies can be categorized based on the level of urgency and threat to life and organ function. Immediate life-threatening conditions, such as intracranial events with a risk of "coning" and acute extradural hematomas, demand immediate surgical intervention to prevent catastrophic outcomes.

Life-threatening situations include subdural and intracerebral hematomas, penetrating injuries, and postoperative deteriorations, requiring urgent surgical attention to mitigate further harm. Organ-threatening conditions, like spinal cord compression, intracranial tumors causing raised intracranial pressure, and skull fractures, jeopardize organ function and mandate prompt surgical management to prevent irreversible damage. Emergent but noncritical conditions, such as cerebral abscesses and ruptured meningomyeloceles, necessitate urgent surgical intervention to prevent complications.

In addition, nonemergent yet urgent conditions like hydrocephalus and aneurysms require timely surgical treatment to prevent deterioration. Overall, the classification of neurosurgical emergencies guides clinicians in prioritizing interventions to optimize patient outcomes and prevent irreversible neurological damage [26, 27].

22.3.3.2 Application of AI in Neurosurgical Planning

Artificial intelligence (AI) has revolutionized neurosurgery across pre-, intra-, and postoperative phases. In the preoperative stage, AI assists in diagnosis, patient selection, and decision-making. During surgery, it enhances surgical performance and reduces errors. In postoperative care, AI predicts prognosis, identifies complications, and aids in tracking patient data for better recovery. AI algorithms analyze large datasets, predict surgical complications, and assist in disease diagnosis and classification.

For instance, AI accurately segments tumors, predicts disease progression, and improves biopsy diagnosis in real-time. Telemedicine, coupled with AI, facilitates remote monitoring and follow-up care, especially in geographically restricted areas. Despite challenges, AI holds immense potential in transforming neurosurgical practice, offering personalized care and optimizing patient outcomes [28]. Applications of artificial intelligence (AI) in neurosurgery across three key areas: tumor classification, spine surgery, and epilepsy management. In tumor classification, AI facilitates neuroimaging analysis for accurate diagnosis, predicts surgical outcomes, and develops survival calculators for patients with glioblastoma multiforme (GBM). However, challenges such as data completeness and prospective validation must be addressed. In spine surgery, AI predicts adverse events, opioid prescription practices, and delayed discharge, emphasizing the need for comprehensive data and prospective validation. Moreover, AI enhances epilepsy management by predicting seizure outcomes after surgery and improving disease diagnosis [29].

22.3.3.3 Integration of Hybrid OR in Neurosurgical Surgeries

The design and operation of a neurosurgical Hybrid operating room (NHOR) involve meticulous consideration of various factors to ensure optimal functionality and patient care. NHORs integrate neuroendovascular and open surgical capabilities, necessitating careful planning of room geometry, equipment placement, and adherence to established operating room standards. Layout optimization is crucial to prioritize safety and efficiency, facilitating smooth patient transitions between different stations while minimizing crowding. Equipment versatility, including features like radiolucent and floating tabletops and mobile biplane monitors, enhances precision and flexibility during procedures.

Design configurations should be assessed for trade-offs, considering factors like table rotation and imaging plane positioning [30]. Technologies commonly used in Hybrid operating rooms for neurosurgery procedures include surgical navigation or surgical robots in spine surgery, indocyanine green video angiography (ICGV), and intraoperative angiography in cerebrovascular surgery, and other technologies such as surgical navigation, ultrasound, intraoperative MRI, EEG, and augmented reality for optimal planning of minimally invasive craniotomy. These technologies are employed to enhance surgical precision, provide real-time imaging, and improve patient safety during neurosurgical procedures [31].

The study on functional outcome in patients with severe traumatic brain injury demonstrated significantly improved functional outcomes in patients with severe traumatic brain injury (TBI) by reducing unfavorable outcomes and shortening the time to CT examination and emergency intracranial surgery. Timely treatment of severe TBI is crucial, and the Hybrid ER system enables immediate CT examination and neurosurgical interventions without the need for patient transfers. This results in better long-term functional outcomes for patients with severe TBI. The novel trauma workflow utilizing the Hybrid ER system has shown promising results in enhancing patient care and outcomes, particularly in cases of isolated TBI [32].

22.3.4 Abdominal Emergencies

22.3.4.1 Overview of Abdominal Emergencies

Acute abdominal conditions encompass a diverse array of emergent surgical situations, each requiring prompt intervention to mitigate potentially life-threatening complications. From the incarceration and strangulation of inguinal hernias to the inflammatory cascade of appendicitis, these conditions demand immediate attention to prevent further tissue damage or systemic infection. Intestinal obstructions, whether caused by adhesions, hernias, or tumors, necessitate urgent surgical decompression to restore intestinal flow and prevent bowel ischemia.

Similarly, complications of peptic ulcers, such as perforation or bleeding, pose imminent risks of peritonitis or hemorrhage, necessitating swift surgical intervention. Bleeding from esophageal varices, pelvic infections with abscess formation, and perforated typhoid ulcers further exemplify the spectrum of acute abdominal emergencies that mandate surgical management to safeguard patient well-being. Furthermore, conditions affecting the hepatobiliary system, respiratory tract, urinary system, and musculoskeletal system underscore the broad scope of surgical emergencies that may present with abdominal manifestations, demanding timely diagnosis and intervention to optimize outcomes and mitigate morbidity and mortality [33].

22.3.4.2 Application of AI in the Surgical Planning of Abdominal Emergencies

The clinical applications of artificial intelligence (AI) in acute abdominal imaging are diverse and impactful, offering a range of benefits to both patients and healthcare providers in surgical planning. First, AI-assisted image analysis expedites the diagnostic process for nontraumatic pathologies such as appendicitis, cholecystitis, and bowel obstructions, leading to quicker and more accurate decision-making. Second, AI algorithms based on deep learning show promise in identifying acute bowel pathologies like pneumoperitoneum, bowel perforation, obstruction, and inflammatory conditions with high accuracy.

AI extends to optimizing workflow by assisting in study protocoling, worklist prioritization, and automated triaging of cases, thereby improving patient flow through the emergency department and reducing turnaround times for critical studies. Moreover, AI models provide valuable clinical decision support by offering individualized data beyond current emergency department pathways, aiding in diagnostic and prognostic applications for conditions like ovarian torsion, bowel obstruction, and abdominal trauma [34].

In healthcare, scalability and automation are pivotal for enhancing efficiency and efficacy, particularly in emergency situations such as abdominal emergencies. Scalability in telemedicine enables remote consultations and treatment planning, transcending geographical barriers and reaching a broader patient base. Automation through AI streamlines diagnostic processes by analyzing extensive medical data, aiding healthcare providers in making faster and more accurate assessments. Together, scalability and automation optimize resource utilization, reduce diagnostic delays, and ensure timely access to specialized care, ultimately leading to improved patient management and clinical outcomes [35].

22.3.4.3 Integration of Hybrid OR in Abdominal Surgeries

A case report study demonstrated the versatile applications of the Hybrid operating room (OR) in managing a range of complex abdominal and thoracic conditions. In the first case, acute arterial mesenteric infarction was successfully treated through a combination of interventional radiology procedures and laparotomy, highlighting the Hybrid OR's capability in addressing acute vascular emergencies. The second case showed the use of radiofrequency ablation for liver metastases, emphasizing the role of the Hybrid OR in providing minimally invasive treatment options for metastatic lesions.

In addition, thoracoscopic wedge resection in the Hybrid OR facilitated efficient histopathologic diagnosis of lung tumors, thereby streamlining the diagnostic process and minimizing procedural risks. Lastly, laparoscopic tumor resection aided by endoscopy and CT imaging demonstrated the collaborative nature of procedures performed in the Hybrid OR, enabling comprehensive management of gastrointestinal tumors [36]. Hybrid ORs facilitate minimally invasive techniques in surgery, leading to reduced postoperative pain, shorter recovery times, and increased patient satisfaction. The availability of various imaging modalities, such as CT scans and MRI, further enhances surgical planning and intraoperative guidance, empowering surgeons to perform interventions with unparalleled accuracy. Overall, HORs revolutionize surgical practice by optimizing patient care through comprehensive imaging and precise surgical interventions [37].

22.3.5 Orthopedic Emergencies

22.3.5.1 Overview of Orthopedic Emergencies

Acute orthopedic problems represent a significant portion of emergency department cases, with misdiagnosis posing substantial risks to patients and accounting for a notable portion of malpractice claims in emergency medicine. The challenges lie in recognizing injuries such as closed tendon injuries of the hand, carpal bone injuries, occult fractures around the elbow, femoral neck fractures, posterior shoulder dislocations, epiphyseal plate injuries, fractures of the pubic ramus, patellar tendon ruptures, Lisfranc injuries, compartment syndromes, and multiple injuries [38].

22.3.5.2 Application of AI in Fracture Classification and Surgical Planning

AI plays a pivotal role in revolutionizing the diagnosis and management of orthopedic diseases, osteoporosis, and arthritis. Notably, AI models, including an improved U-Net model, have been successfully employed for grading osteoporosis with an impressive accuracy of 0.81. In arthritis diagnosis, AI techniques such as the VGG-16 network, transfer learning, and the YOLO-v4 algorithm have demonstrated remarkable accuracy, sensitivity, specificity, and precision, enabling precise detection and classification of conditions like hip osteoarthritis and rheumatoid arthritis from medical images.

AI technologies play a critical role in evaluating disease severity, aiding in patient triage for critical cases such as traumatic fractures and joint dislocations. Specifically in osteoporosis diagnosis, AI models analyze bone mineral density data from DXA scans, providing accurate assessments that enhance diagnostic accuracy and efficiency [39]. The application of artificial intelligence (AI) in fracture imaging is broad and multifaceted, typically categorized into four main areas. First, AI is utilized for pathology detection, where algorithms are trained to recognize specific patterns indicative of fractures within medical images like X-rays or CT scans.

Second, segmentation techniques are employed to precisely delineate fracture regions from surrounding tissues or structures, enabling accurate analysis and measurement. In addition, AI plays a crucial role in fracture classification by categorizing fractures based on various criteria such as type, location, or severity, aiding in treatment planning and prognostic assessment. Lastly, AI is used for noninterpretive tasks like image enhancement and artifact correction, improving image quality and facilitating more reliable interpretation by radiologists and clinicians. Through these applications, AI enhances fracture imaging by improving detection accuracy, segmentation precision, classification efficiency, and overall diagnostic quality, thereby contributing to more effective patient care and treatment outcomes [40].

AI has emerged as a transformative tool in orthopedic surgical training, providing new opportunities for performance assessment and individualized feedback. AI systems, including machine learning (ML) and computer vision, can collect data and provide significant insights about surgical performance. For example, an ML system can accurately assess laparoscopic cholecystectomy skills, indicating the potential for AI to provide constructive feedback to surgeons. This technique could be applied to orthopedic training, providing a framework for skill evaluation and development.

Furthermore, integrating AI systems such as the virtual operative assistant into virtual and augmented reality environments allows for objective evaluation rather than relying primarily on traditional apprenticeship-based learning methods, and exhibits successful AI integration into augmented reality, allowing for exact placement of surgical instruments in cadaveric models [41]. AI applications in orthopedics hold promise for optimizing clinical and paraclinical processes, but require evidence-based validation to ensure non-inferior or improved outcomes compared to conventional standards. While AI algorithms, especially deep convolutional neural networks, excel in image recognition and risk prediction, their implementation must be carefully balanced against costs and benefits. Governance and regulatory frameworks must evolve in tandem with technological advancements to ensure safe and ethical utilization of AI in orthopedic practice [42].

22.3.5.3 Integration of Hybrid OR in Orthopedic Trauma Surgeries

Pelvic or acetabular fracture surgeries are ideally managed in orthopedic Hybrid ORs. These included acetabular open reduction and internal fixation surgeries, utilizing both anterior modified ilioinguinal and posterior Kocher-Langenbach approaches. In addition, pelvic procedures such as closed reduction, percutaneous pelvic screw placement,and pelvic external fixation were performed. The use of the Hybrid OR provided advanced imaging capabilities, including 3D fluoroscopy and angiography, facilitating interdisciplinary collaboration for hemorrhage management.

The superior image quality offered by the flat plate C-arm allowed for comprehensive visualization of the pelvis, even in challenging patient cases. Overall, the utilization of the HOR in pelvic and acetabular fracture surgery offers significant advantages in imaging quality and interdisciplinary care [43]. In a study, the authors have included their one-year experience utilizing a Hybrid operating room for orthopedic trauma surgery proved to be successful, with no higher rate of complications compared to conventional operating rooms. The HOR, equipped with 3D fluoroscopic imaging and navigation capabilities, facilitated confident implant placement and appropriate reduction in trauma cases, particularly for spine and pelvis surgeries, both minimally invasive and conventional.

The advanced imaging system provided excellent image quality, with wide field views and large volume 3D fluoroscopic scans, aiding in precise positioning and reducing the need for postoperative CT scans. The interdisciplinary approach, shared among orthopedics, neurosurgery, cardiothoracic surgery, and vascular surgery, allowed efficient utilization of the HOR, with orthopedic trauma utilizing the room for 2 days per week. In some cases, a custom robotic arm integrated into a Hybrid operating room (OR), equipped with an AR surgical navigation system (ARSN), was utilized.

The robot autonomously aligned with planned screw trajectories, assisting surgeons in placing Jamshidi needles in pedicles. Accuracy measurements revealed technical accuracy at bone entry points and angular errors well within clinically acceptable ranges, with statistically superior results compared to ARSN without robotic assistance. Simulated pedicle screw grading demonstrated 100% clinical accuracy [44]. Overall, the use of the Hybrid OR proved to be a useful and safe tool for orthopedic trauma surgery, offering enhanced imaging capabilities and facilitating interdisciplinary collaboration [45].

22.4 Conclusion

Hybrid operating rooms (ORs) provide a unique surgical environment that incorporates modern imaging techniques, sophisticated information technology and telecommunications platforms, evolving AI applications, with a range of surgical modalities. This integration enables a wide range of complex surgical procedures to be performed with greater efficiency, effectiveness, decreased complications, and at a lower cost of delivery. This efficiency also decreases patient anxiety by decreasing unnecessary and time-consuming transportation between multiple clinical locations for testing and related.

From positioning equipment and ensuring radiation safety, to managing clinical workflows effectively, meticulous planning, and patient care, stakeholder communication is essential for the successful implementation of Hybrid ORs. The successful implementation of technological advances including but not limited to the judicious use of AI will continue to reinforce and evolve the importance of the Hybrid OR within the global healthcare delivery marketplace.

References

1. UEMS Section of Surgery. UNION EUROPÉENNE DES MÉDECINS SPÉCIALISTES EUROPEAN UNION OF MEDICAL SPECIALISTS Section of Surgery & European Board of Surgery [Internet]; 2024 [cited 2024 May 1]. Available from: https://uemssurg.org/surgicalspecialties/emergency-surgery/
2. Surlin V. Emergency and trauma surgery, vol. 116. Chirurgia (Romania): Editura Celsius; 2021. p. 643–4.
3. Ai Y, Wu Y, Zhang S. Analysis of key points in the design of hybrid operating room for the future. In: Design for health; 2023. p. 417–26.
4. Zakhary WZA, Ender JK. Chapter 21 - Procedures in the hybrid operating room. In: Kaplan JA, editor. Kaplan's essentials of cardiac anesthesia [Internet]. 2nd ed. Philadelphia: Elsevier; 2018. p. 534–50. Available from: https://www.sciencedirect.com/science/article/pii/B9780323497985000218.
5. Bulitta CJ. Imaging meets surgery - the Hybrid OR. Biomed Tech. 2012;57(SUPPL. 1 TRACK-I):1029–32.
6. Akpınar MN, Koç B, Özşahin B, Uğur B, Akçadağ Z, Demirel A, et al. Comprehensive review of hybrid emergency room systems: benefits, challenges, and future prospects. Eur Arch Med Res. 2023;39(3):134–40.
7. Khoo CY, Liew TYS, Mathur S. Systematic review of the efficacy of a hybrid operating theatre in the management of severe trauma, World Journal of Emergency Surgery, vol. 16. BioMed Central Ltd; 2021.
8. Clark M, Horton J. CADTH horizon scan hybrid operating room suites 2.
9. Jang JY, Oh J, Shim H, Kim S, Jung PY, Kim S, et al. The need for a rapid transfer to a hybrid operating theatre: do we lose benefit with poor efficiency? Injury. 2020;51(9):1987–93.
10. Loftus TJ, Croft CA, Rosenthal MD, Mohr AM, Efron PA, Moore FA, et al. Clinical impact of a dedicated trauma hybrid operating room. J Am Coll Surg. 2021;232(4):560–70.
11. Agolia JP, Forrester JD. In: BMJ Publishing Group, editor. Challenges in trauma and acute care surgery, Trauma Surgery and Acute Care Open, vol. 8; 2023.
12. Hashimoto DA, Ward TM, Meireles OR. The role of artificial intelligence in surgery. Adv Surg [Internet]. 2020;54:89–101. https://doi.org/10.1016/j.yasu.2020.05.010.
13. Guni A, Varma P, Zhang J, Fehervari M, Ashrafian H. Artificial intelligence in surgery: the future is now. Eur Surg Res [Internet]. 2024;65(1):22–39. https://doi.org/10.1159/000536393.
14. De Simone B, Chouillard E, Gumbs AA, Loftus TJ, Kaafarani H, Catena F. Artificial intelligence in surgery: the emergency surgeon's perspective (the ARIES project). Discov Health Sys. 2022;1(1):9.
15. Boini A, Acciuffi S, Croner R, Illanes A, Milone L, Turner B, et al. Scoping review: autonomous endoscopic navigation. Artif Intell Surg [Internet]. 2023;3(4) Available from: https://www.oaepublish.com/articles/ais.2023.36
16. Gumbs AA, Frigerio I, Spolverato G, Croner R, Illanes A, Chouillard E, et al. Artificial intelligence surgery: how do we get to autonomous actions in surgery? Sensors. 2021;21(16)
17. Stonko DP, Guillamondegui OD, Fischer PE, Dennis BM. Artificial intelligence in trauma systems. Surgery (United States). 2021;169(6):1295–9.
18. Prichayudh S, Rajruangrabin J, Sriussadaporn S, Pak-art R, Sriussadaporn S, Kritayakirana K, et al. Trauma Hybrid Operating Room (THOR) shortened procedure time in abdominopelvic trauma patients requiring surgery and interventional radiology procedures. Injury

[Internet]. 2023;54(2):513–8. Available from: https://www.sciencedirect.com/science/article/pii/S0020138322008051
19. Mitrev Z, Anguseva T. Emergencies in cardiovascular surgery. J Cardiothorac Surg [Internet]. 2013;8(1):O2. https://doi.org/10.1186/1749-8090-8-S1-O2.
20. Mumtaz H, Saqib M, Ansar F, Zargar D, Hameed M, Hasan M, et al. The future of cardiothoracic surgery in artificial intelligence. Ann Med Surg [Internet]. 2022;80. Available from: https://journals.lww.com/annals-of-medicine-and-surgery/fulltext/2022/08000/the_future_of_cardiothoracic_surgery_in_artificial.139.aspx
21. Vaidya YP, Shumway SJ. Artificial intelligence: the future of cardiothoracic surgery. J Thorac Cardiovasc Surg [Internet]. 2024; Available from: https://www.sciencedirect.com/science/article/pii/S0022522324003714
22. Nguyen A, Lyon K, Robinson T, Vance AZ. Biplane fluoroscopic-guided percutaneous thoracic instrumentation: a technical note. Cureus. 2020;12:e11939.
23. Kpodonu J. The cardiovascular hybrid surgical room: evolving into the future of cardiovascular surgery [Internet]; 2013. Available from: http://www.cathlabdigest.com
24. Hybrid cardiac procedure: the ultimate cooperation.
25. Byrne JG, Leacche M, Vaughan DE, Zhao DX, Nashville F. Hybrid cardiovascular procedures; 2008.
26. Malan BJ, Chb MB. Emergency presentation of neurosurgical conditions P Semple, MB ChB, FCS (Neurosurg) (SA), vol. 31. CME March; 2013.
27. Kulkarni D. Pattern and categorisation of neurosurgical emergencies. J Neuroanaesth Crit Care. 2017;04(04):S6–8.
28. Mofatteh M. Neurosurgery and artificial intelligence. AIMS Neurosci. 2021;8(4):477–95.
29. Tangsrivimol JA, Schonfeld E, Zhang M, Veeravagu A, Smith TR, Härtl R, et al. Artificial intelligence in neurosurgery: a state-of-the-art review from past to future, Diagnostics, vol. 13. Multidisciplinary Digital Publishing Institute (MDPI); 2023.
30. Aljuboori Z. Optimal design of neurosurgical hybrid operating room, Surgical Neurology International, vol. 12. Scientific Scholar; 2021.
31. Gharios M, El-Hajj VG, Frisk H, Ohlsson M, Omar A, Edström E, et al. The use of hybrid operating rooms in neurosurgery, advantages, disadvantages, and future perspectives: a systematic review, Acta Neurochirurgica, vol. 165. Springer; 2023. p. 2343–58.
32. Kinoshita T, Hayashi M, Yamakawa K, Watanabe A, Yoshimura J, Hamasaki T, et al. Effect of the hybrid emergency room system on functional outcome in patients with severe traumatic brain injury. World Neurosurg. 2018;118:e792–9.
33. McCord C ODBJ et al. GSEmergenciesIDHDPGA et al. editors. DISEASE CONTROL PRIORITIES • THIRD EDITION Essential Surgery [Internet]; 2015 [cited 2024 May 12]. Available from: Chapter 4. Available from: https://www.ncbi.nlm.nih.gov/books/NBK333506/
34. Yao J, Chu LC, Patlas M. Applications of artificial intelligence in acute abdominal imaging. Can Assoc Radiol J [Internet]. 2024; Available from: https://journals.sagepub.com/doi/10.1177/08465371241250197
35. Gorincour G, Monneuse O, Ben Cheikh A, Avondo J, Chaillot PF, Journe C, et al. Management of abdominal emergencies in adults using telemedicine and artificial intelligence. J Visc Surg. 2021;158(3):S26–31.
36. Dietl KH, Novák K, Bothe EM, Schönberger H. New experience with the integrated and hybrid operating room at the Department of General, Visceral and Thoracic surgery. Eur Surg Acta Chir Austriaca. 2016;(48):135–7.
37. Pilz da Cunha G, van Delden OM, Kazemier G, Vahrmeijer AL, Bonjer HJ, Meijerink MR, et al. Hybrid operating room applications for precision hepatobiliary surgery: a narrative review. J Surg Oncol. 2024;129:1265.
38. Noble J, Sankarankutty FM, Orth M. Orthopaedic emergencies: a review1. J R Soc Med. 1981;74:510.
39. Liu P, Zhang J, Liu S, Huo T, He J, Xue M, et al. Application of artificial intelligence technology in the field of orthopedics: a narrative review. Artif Intell Rev. 2024;57(1)

40. Alghaithi A, Al Maskari S. Artificial intelligence application in bone fracture detection, Journal of Musculoskeletal Surgery and Research, vol. 5. Scientific Scholar LLC; 2021. p. 4–9.
41. Lisacek-Kiosoglous AB, Powling AS, Fontalis A, Gabr A, Mazomenos E, Haddad FS. Artificial intelligence in orthopaedic surgery EXPLORING ITS APPLICATIONS, LIMITATIONS, AND FUTURE DIRECTION introduction: artificial intelligence, time for clear nomenclature. Bone Joint Res. 2023;12(7):447–54.
42. Kurmis AP, Ianunzio JR. Artificial intelligence in orthopedic surgery: evolution, current state and future directions, Arthroplasty, vol. 4. BioMed Central Ltd; 2022. p. 9.
43. Davis JA, Movassaghi K, Refaat MI, Lindvall EM. Use of the hybrid operating room for pelvic and acetabular fracture surgery. Injury [Internet]. 2022;53(11):3754–8. Available from: https://www.sciencedirect.com/science/article/pii/S0020138322006659
44. Burström G, Balicki M, Patriciu A, Kyne S, Popovic A, Holthuizen R, et al. Feasibility and accuracy of a robotic guidance system for navigated spine surgery in a hybrid operating room: a cadaver study. Sci Rep. 2020;10(1):7522.
45. Richter PH, Yarboro S, Kraus M, Gebhard F. One year orthopaedic trauma experience using an advanced interdisciplinary hybrid operating room. Injury [Internet]. 2015;46:S129–34. Available from: https://www.sciencedirect.com/science/article/pii/S0020138315300322
46. Zakhary WZA, Ender JK. Procedures in the hybrid operating room. In: Kaplan JA, editor. Kaplan's essentials of cardiac anesthesia [Internet]. 2nd ed. Philadelphia: Elsevier; 2018. p. 534–50. Available from: https://linkinghub.elsevier.com/retrieve/pii/B9780323497985000218.
47. Dias RD, Shah JA, Zenati MA. Artificial intelligence in cardiothoracic surgery, Minerva Cardioangiologica, vol. 68. Edizioni Minerva Medica; 2020. p. 532–8.

Management of Emergency Surgical Flow and Operating Rooms with AI Support

23

Rodolfo Catena and Denise Adaoyibo Okpala

This chapter explores the management of emergency surgical flow and operating rooms with artificial intelligence (AI) support. It describes the role of AI in supporting the diagnostic process. It then describes how to leverage AI to improve the management of the diagnosed patient. It illustrates value stream mapping (VSM) and process mapping and describes an example to explain how to use them. It then describes how AI can support facilities in the emergency surgery context. The last part of the chapter describes how to implement AI.

23.1 How AI Can Contribute to Diagnosis

The importance of prompt and precise response to surgical emergencies cannot be overemphasized. There is the need for timely screening and identification of prevalent, commonly observed, and seldom encountered diseases. Artificial intelligence and machine learning (ML) are crucial in healthcare for analyzing and visualizing diverse data [1], which is required to identify medical conditions, determine optimal treatments, and identify patient-specific disease patterns. This assists medical personnel with rendering appropriate choices, optimizing patient outcomes, and expediting clinical treatment. AI and ML also facilitate communication and coordination among healthcare providers, enhancing patient care.

R. Catena (✉) · D. A. Okpala
Global Business School for Health, University College London, London, UK
e-mail: r.catena@ucl.ac.uk

B. De Simone et al. (eds.), *New Technologies, Precision Medicine, and AI in Emergency General Surgery*, Hot Topics in Acute Care Surgery and Trauma,
https://doi.org/10.1007/978-3-032-09357-8_23

23.1.1 AI-Powered Diagnostic Tools

Machine learning algorithms can analyze large amounts of medical data to improve diagnosis by utilizing various approaches. One approach is to use ML algorithms to retrieve and group data, perform principal component analysis, and identify imaging biomarkers [2]. Machine learning algorithms can detect and predict safety problems, enabling real-time information and predictive analytics to guide clinical decision-making.

AI algorithms analyze large datasets to identify patterns, trends, and relationships, using advanced statistical and machine learning techniques. This process can uncover hidden insights, making predictions and enabling more precise diagnoses in Maguire et al. [24], and ultimately resulting in enhanced patient satisfaction and tailored treatment plans.

Machine learning can improve patient outcomes by analyzing patient data triaging patients according to importance, putting first high-risk situations, minimizing waiting periods, and improving flow of patients [4]. By introducing reliable symptom assessment tools, ML can reduce emergency department visits by assessing symptoms, providing real-time suggestions for diagnosis and treatment, and optimizing resources. AI-powered decision support systems can predict patient demand, optimize therapy selection, and suggest length of stay. This leads to more accurate treatment, reduced waste, and improved patient outcomes.

23.1.2 Image Recognition and Analysis

Artificial Intelligence (AI) is used for measuring and controlling depth of anesthesia (DOA) in operating rooms [21]. Neural networks and fuzzy logic can be used to analyze auditory evoked potentials (AEP) to measure Doppler anesthesia (DOA), with multiresolution wavelet analysis and adaptive network–based fuzzy inference system (ANFIS) classifying AEP-based DOA, ensuring patient anesthetic depth maintenance and accurate data fusion.

The accuracy of diagnostics can be improved with certain AI and result in more tailored therapies by utilizing machine learning algorithms to extract and analyze comprehensive patient information [1]. Deep learning aids clinicians in real-time health risk alerts, reducing diagnostic errors, and identifying imaging biomarkers, improving diagnostic precision, and promoting personalized and population medicine.

AI image analysis can save energy by automating interpretation processes, reducing manual examination and resource use in operating rooms and surgeries. AI-enabled surgical robots improve control, precision, and precision, resulting in reduced hospitalization duration and faster periods of recuperation [28], thereby reducing energy consumption.

23.1.3 Real-Time Data Monitoring in Operating Rooms

The development of patient safety active management (PSAM) system utilizes electronic health records (EHRs) to diagnose damage and its precursors in real time at faster rates than present levels are discovered, and it has the capability to anticipate potential damage [5]. This system helps identify high-risk patients, prioritize care, and implement targeted interventions. Predictive analytics in PSAM aids in resource allocation, improved patient monitoring, and overall patient safety in emergency surgical flow and operating rooms.

The combination of artificial intelligence and microfluidic technology has enabled early intervention and improved patient outcomes by identifying abnormalities or significant changes in patients' situations [22]. AI algorithms are revolutionizing cancer screening, drug-susceptibility testing, and disease diagnosis, enhancing accuracy and efficiency. This real-time monitoring improves surgical outcomes and surgical flow. The integration of AI and microfluidics enhances cost-effective, high-throughput screening.

Real-time monitoring and remote monitoring are crucial for timely interventions, reducing resource consumption, complications, and emergency procedures, thus preventing or minimizing complications [33]. The approach may not only enhance outcomes for patients, but also decreases medical expenses, improves the patient's satisfaction, and minimizes the risk of hospital-acquired infections.

23.1.3.1 Rule-Based Expert System AI

Rule-based fuzzy logic tool is utilized for automatic drug delivery in general anesthesia patients before surgical procedures, utilizing clinician-provided heuristic knowledge to adjust doses [26]. The system, designed by an anesthetist, uses the bispectral index (BIS) to assess a patient's hypnotic state and a fuzzy controller in a closed-loop system to improve the anesthetic procedure. It reduces operating room usage and patient recovery time, outperforming manual administration in accuracy through maintenance.

Traditional rule-based expert systems face constraints like predefined rules and difficulties in managing complex medical situations. Traditional closed-loop strategies struggle with interpatient variability and intuitive patient relationships [26]. Fuzzy logic can help translate clinician expertise into controllers, considering all possible hypnotic state situations during surgery. A fuzzy inference system with intuitive logic rules addresses these challenges. It is important to continuously refine and update the result-based expert system to ensure its effectiveness in clinical practice [8].

23.1.4 Benefits of AI-Assisted Diagnosis

AI has the potential to aid in real-time reaction to pathology, facilitating reactive drug release or therapy. By leveraging AI technology to analyze and interpret medical data, healthcare providers can make more precise and informed decisions, thereby reducing the likelihood of unnecessary surgical interventions [2]. This not only benefits patient outcomes but also contributes to the efficient use of healthcare resources and a reduction in the environmental impact associated with unnecessary medical procedures.

The use of AI technology in evidence-based clinical decision support, detection of adverse events, and prediction of patients at risk for readmission has been further discussed by Johnson et al. [15], who also state that it is beneficial in precision medicine, helping design individualized treatment regimens based on patient traits and medical background, as demonstrated during the COVID-19 pandemic [15]. Precision medicine, utilizing genetic biology, diagnostic imaging, and information technology, enables personalized treatment plans by integrating patient-specific information from various sources [20]. This approach optimizes medication use and minimizes waste.

By incorporating cognitive technology and virtual reality modeling into surgeries and health curriculum, machine learning algorithms can differentiate specialization levels and discover measurable indicators that can be used for teaching contributing to this categorization [27]. A virtual operative assistant uses AI-powered simulations to analyze performance metrics, providing automated feedback to healthcare professionals, enhancing clinical reasoning, non-technical skills, and knowledge progression. They also enhance nursing education by providing a safe environment, improving clinical reasoning, and facilitating active learning [12]. This experience can hone the diagnostic and decision-making capabilities of healthcare professionals working in operating rooms.

AI algorithms can analyze diverse data sources like Electronic Health Records, genetic information, and wearable lifestyle data to offer personalized interventions, while machine learning algorithms help identify patterns and predict models, enabling healthcare providers to tailor interventions based on individual patient profiles, and AI-driven chatbots collect patient information for actionable insights [14]. This incorporation of cognitive computing into clinical decision support systems gives medical practitioners advice and direction in real time as they are diagnosing patients. As AI technologies have the ability to utilize vast amounts of data and to recognize trends, they have the potential to offer enhanced precision, decreased expenses, and time efficiency while reducing human mistakes, revolutionizing individualized healthcare, optimizing drug dosages, establishing standards, offering digital health aides, and facilitating mental healthcare, enhancing patient awareness, and cultivating confidence between patients and clinicians [2]. Hence, these systems can provide evidence-based insights and treatment suggestions to augment the knowledge and experience of healthcare personnel.

AI can support healthcare workers' continuous learning and development through the development of machine learning platforms with several functions for extracting, aggregating, managing, and analyzing medical information, which can support clinicians by efficiently stratifying subjects to understand specific scenarios and optimize decision-making [1], resulting in substantial advancements in attaining the objectives of delivering improved individualized and population healthcare at reduced prices. By providing real-time feedback to healthcare professionals, AI systems help them to evaluate the results of diagnostic tests, and compare them to predetermined benchmarks, thereby helping them to identify areas for improvement and enhance their diagnostic skills [12]. This feedback can contribute to ongoing professional development and the delivery of high-quality patient care.

23.1.5 Challenges and Constraints

Problems arise from navigating incomplete, erroneous, or conflicting data from multiple sources. There is a need for enhanced integration of data currently kept in several systems lacking a standardized data-exchange interface [1]. Also, AI models trained on specific datasets may struggle to adapt to diverse patient populations and healthcare environments, resulting in bias and limitations in their application. This highlights the need for robust AI techniques and models, as well as innovative data annotation methods, to address these challenges and helps guarantee the proper and beneficial integration of AI in medical procedures [2].

Healthcare professionals face possible difficulties while incorporating AI recommendations or findings into their decision-making process or electronic health records. Incorporating AI recommendations or findings may be perceived as an additional task for healthcare professionals [5]. There are also known potential concerns related to the continuous nature of data collection due to regular updates from wearable devices [14]. There are issues about the extent of surveillance and the potential misuse of sensitive health information, as well as issues concerning evolving cyber threats.

Implementing AI-assisted diagnosis may require significant investments in infrastructure, training, and maintenance [2]. These issues can be checkmated by cooperation between law enforcement agencies, medical entities, and experts in AI, to establish guidelines and standards for AI algorithms and their use in clinical decision-making. Such collaboration can help in identifying cost-effective solutions and best practices for implementing AI in healthcare.

23.2 How AI Can Contribute to the Management of the Diagnosed Patient

AI technologies exist and are being developed to support the management of the diagnosed patient. An example of a technology that already exists is natural language processing (NLP). Instead of typing, surgeons can use NLP to automatically transcribe their notes when they interact with patients. Technologies are being developed for intraoperative assistance. For example, in robotic surgery it will be possible to use AI to tie a knot [25]. There is a project to use AI to make laparoscopic cholecystectomy procedures safer [25]. AI might send an alert warning the surgeons about the risk of cutting the common bile duct [25]. To improve our processes for the management of the diagnosed patient, we can consider two tools: value stream mapping (VSM) and process mapping.

23.2.1 Value Stream Mapping (VMS)

This tool displays in its upper part the information flow, in its lower part the patient flow. This tool is part of the Toyota method [3], and it offers a visual perspective on patient flow.

An example can be helpful to understand how to apply this tool (Fig. 23.1).

We can assume that this value stream map represents the journey of an emergency inguinal hernia patient who will not require a transfer to the intensive care unit. This journey starts in the A&E that is represented in Fig. 23.2.

The shape of the symbol in Fig. 23.2 reminds us of the shape of a warehouse. In its original manufacturing applications, Value Stream Mapping was used to illustrate the flow of a product from the supplier's warehouse, which is outside the direct scope of control of the organization drawing the value stream map. In our context, the patient is transferred from the A&E (outside the Emergency Surgery Department) to the Emergency Surgery Department, an arrow documents this transfer[1] (Fig. 23.3).

The next steps in Fig. 23.1 describe the rest of the journey of the patient. After the admission, the patient undergoes the preparation for the operation, a procedure, and he/she is then transferred to a recovery room and discharged to an inpatient ward. We use a rectangle to describe the various steps of the process and the inpatient ward, the place where the patient is discharged and where the value stream map ends. We would use the symbol in Fig. 23.2 if the end of this value stream was outside the direct scope of control of the Emergency Surgery Department.

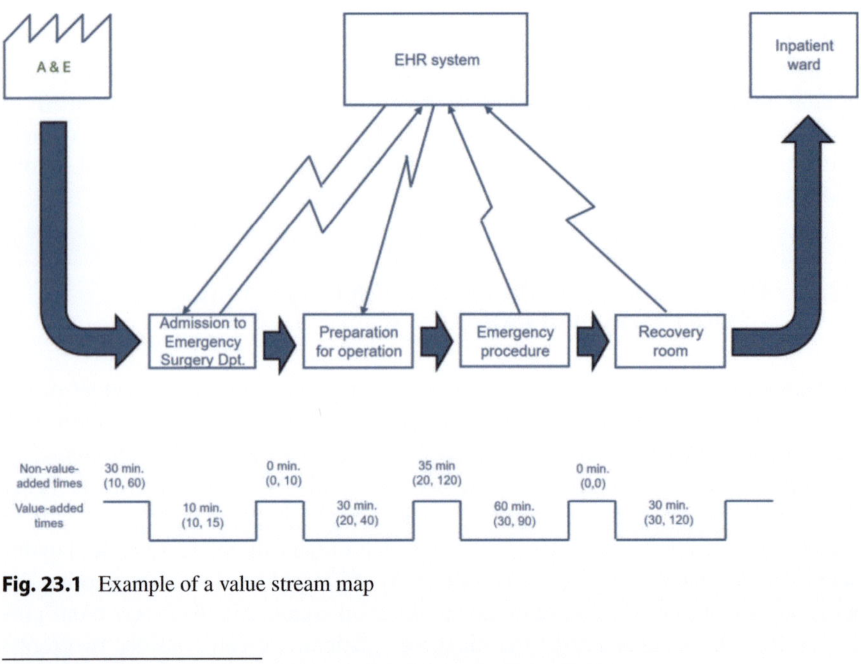

Fig. 23.1 Example of a value stream map

[1] In manufacturing, this arrow would document the transfer of material.

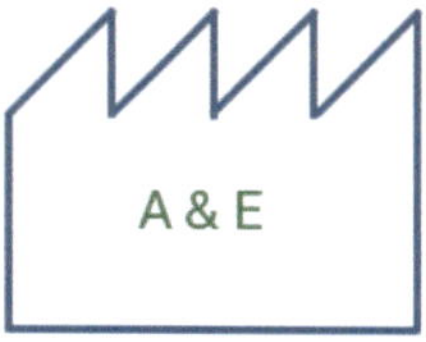

Fig. 23.2 Source of the value stream map (the A&E)

Fig. 23.3 Arrow used to illustrate the transfer of patients

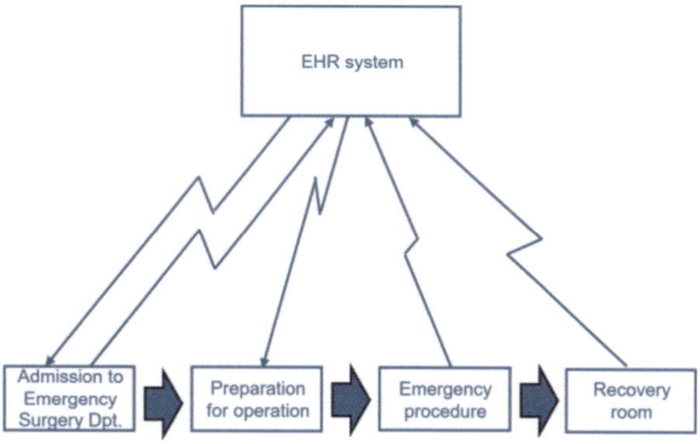

Fig. 23.4 Information flow of the value stream map

The upper part of Fig. 23.1 represents the information flow (Fig. 23.4).

For example, during the admission to the Emergency Surgery Department, the Emergency Surgery Department receives and transmits data to the Electronic Health Records (EHR) system. For example, information on patient is received and updates on state of health are transmitted. The zigzag arrow represents the transmission of an electronic information flow (Fig. 23.5).

A standard arrow is, instead, used to document a paper information flow (Fig. 23.6).

The lower part of Fig. 23.1 displays other relevant information: the timeline of the value stream map [29].

There are three values for each step (Fig. 23.7). While the first value measures the "normal" duration of the step, the values in parentheses display the typical

Fig. 23.5 Electronic information flow

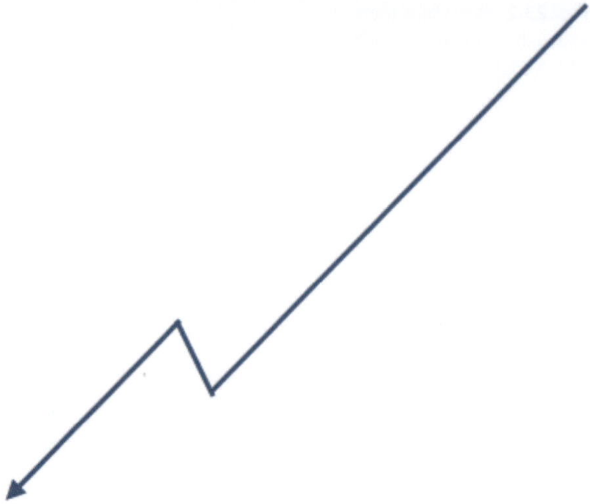

Fig. 23.6 Paper information flow

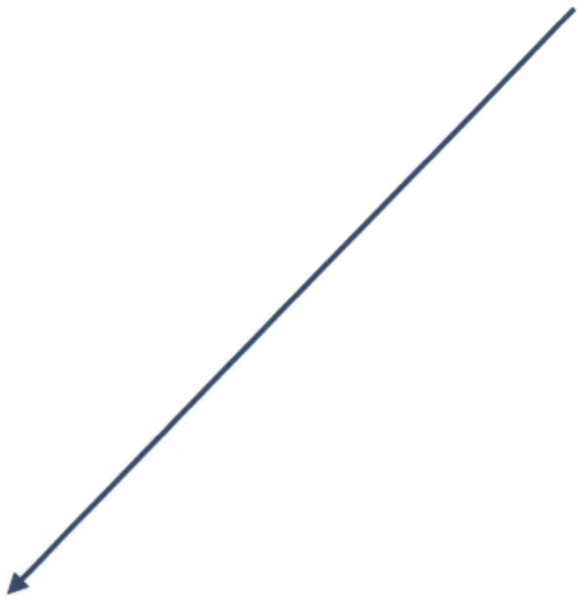

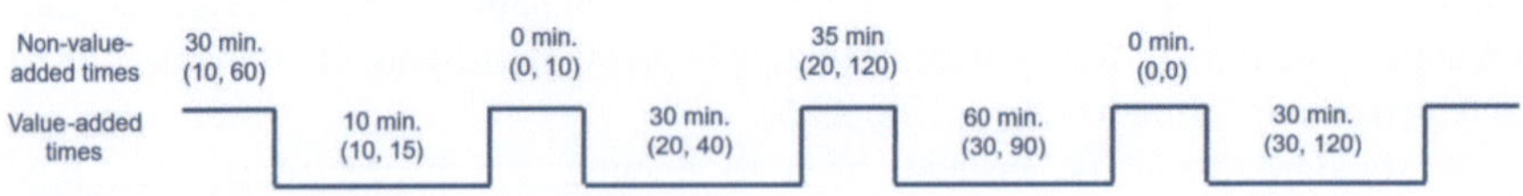

Fig. 23.7 Timeline of the value stream map

duration variability for that step. The timeline displays value-added times (bottom values) and non-value-added times (top values). The value-added time measures the time spent on an activity that adds value to the patient. The non-value-added time measures the waiting time. The lead time measures the time a patient spends in the value stream. In our example, we can calculate for the "normal" durations the following metrics:

Total value-added time = 10 + 30 + 60 + 30 = 130 minutes
Total non-value-added time = 30 + 0 + 35 + 0 = 65 minutes
Lead time = total value-added time + total non-value-added time = 130 + 65 = 195 minutes
Proportion of value-added time = total value-added time/lead time = 130/195 = 67%

The information reported in a value stream map and the data on value- and non-value-added times enable team discussions on how to improve the delivery of care and to consider AI as a tool to improve the management of the diagnosed patient. A meeting can be an opportunity to show a value stream map on a poster and to draw kaizen bursts on it. A kaizen burst is a new idea to improve the management of the diagnosed patient in a value stream map. We represent it with the following symbol (Fig. 23.8):

We include the kaizen burst in the value stream map with the idea we suggest to implement (Fig. 23.9). For example, the idea is to use AI to extract medical history more quickly during the admission.

We have seen how Value Stream Mapping can be used to represent the current state of an Emergency Surgery Department. Another use of Value Stream Mapping is to visualize the future state we are trying to achieve. Value Stream Mapping can become helpful to visualize how the flow of patients will occur in an AI-enabled future.

23.2.2 Process Mapping

Healthcare leaders will need to understand how to integrate AI technologies in their wards. To achieve this goal, it is necessary to understand how healthcare is delivered. This understanding allows us to identify where there are issues to address and to ensure that a technology is integrated seamlessly.

A key tool to understand how healthcare is delivered is the process map. A process map illustrates the key steps that allow us to complete our work. A simple

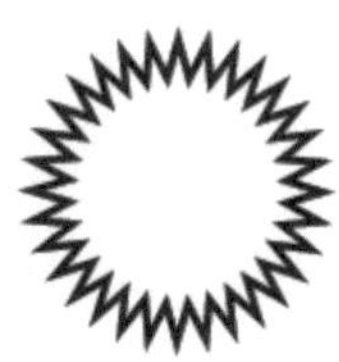

Fig. 23.8 Kaizen burst

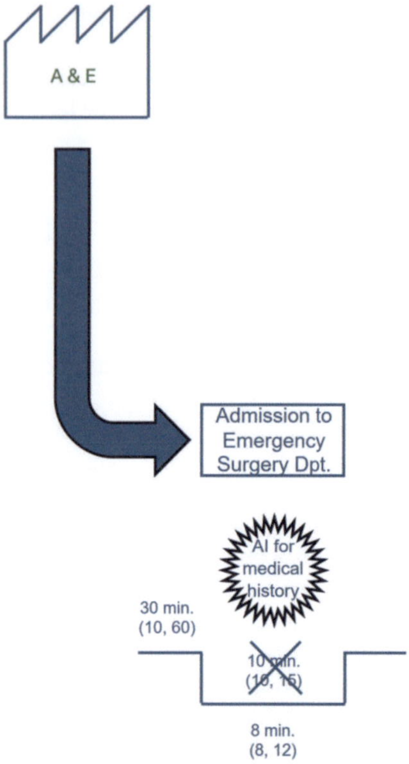

Fig. 23.9 Kaizen burst in Value Stream Mapping

process map can be drawn with just two symbols, a rectangle for the tasks and a diamond for the decision points.

Let's see an example to illustrate how to draw a process map. We want to focus on the interaction of the surgeon with the patient during a follow-up visit. The patient had an emergency gallbladder removal.

From left to right, Fig. 23.10 is telling us the different tasks of the follow-up process. After registration at reception, the patient enters the medical office. The physician, as shown in the third rectangle from the left, assesses symptoms and wound. The diamond following this step represents a decision point. If the recovery has been successful, the physician informs the patient, and the patient leaves the medical office. If the recovery has not been successful, the physician still informs the patient, and if a readmission is required, the patient is readmitted. If a readmission is not required, the physician prescribes a follow-up therapy, and another appointment is booked. After these two steps, the patient leaves the office.

To know how to draw a process map, you can talk with the staff involved in the process, and you can review documentation about the process, and if you are describing the patient journey, you can follow the patient during the delivery of care.

Process maps give you the opportunity to visualize a process and to determine whether there are opportunities to change it. They allow you to understand where to collect data for AI software. You can draw in a process map where you will be

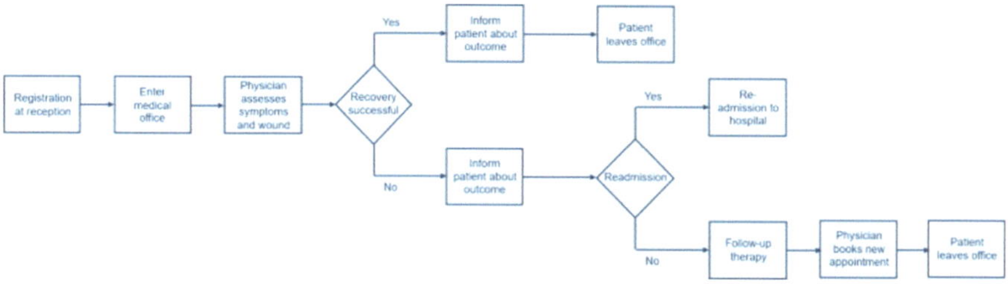

Fig. 23.10 Example of process for follow-up after emergency gallbladder removal

collecting data and you can annotate how. Process maps can describe delivery of care at different levels of detail. Every step in a process map can be described with a subprocess. Every process can become a single step of a higher level process map. In the emergency surgery context, it may be useful to start with high-level process maps to understand the main activities in the department and improve them. More detailed process maps can then be useful to improve the processes that make up these activities.

23.3 How AI Can Contribute to Facilities

The function of healthcare facilities in surgical flows and operating rooms is to provide a well-planned and designed environment that supports the efficient and effective delivery of medical care [7]. The design of healthcare facilities should take into account the specific needs of surgical departments, including workload history and forecasts, descriptions of activities and procedures, and any unique planning considerations. This can help ensure that the operating rooms are designed to meet the specific requirements of surgical procedures and the needs of medical staff. Effective healthcare facilities management and sustainable practices are important in hospitals, as they play a crucial role in ensuring the optimized functioning of healthcare services [19]. These helps ensure patient and staff safety, as well as contribute to a more efficient, cost-effective, and environmentally friendly healthcare facility, hence improving overall outcomes for surgical flows and operating rooms.

23.3.1 Energy Management in Healthcare Facilities

23.3.1.1 Smart Energy Systems

The use of AI- and IOT-based building structures for medical facilities can help lower power expenditure by being employed to optimize the lighting systems [34]. This not only manages the energy consumption and costs, but it also assists in maintaining a comfortable and safe environment in operating rooms by regulating temperature, humidity, and lighting levels based on real-time data and feedback. By integrating energy management systems, healthcare institutions can efficiently monitor and control energy usage, identify areas of inefficiency, and adopt renewable energy sources, thus contributing to greener practices [16]. This can enhance the overall experience for both patients and healthcare professionals, ensuring optimal conditions for surgical procedures. Smart energy systems also contribute to the overall efficiency of surgical flow by predicting and managing energy requirements, ensuring that all equipment and systems are functioning optimally during surgical procedures. This can minimize the risk of disruptions or downtime due to energy-related issues, ultimately improving patient care and safety.

Renewable energy experts are now able to remotely verify the real-time indoor comfort levels and regulate the upgraded HVAC systems of the healthcare facility using IoT and ICT technologies along with cloud-based machine learning algorithms. These upgraded systems are now effectively meeting the required set points through advanced optimization strategies, thanks to the machine learning adaptive algorithms [9]. Temperature variations are less and stabilize when using adaptive and predictive control logics in an automated control system. By enabling remote monitoring and management of HVAC systems, they enhance operational efficiency in medical facilities by enabling facility managers to make changes to settings and solve problems without having to physically be present.

Deep learning methods, including deep neural networks (DNNs) and long short-term memory (LSTM) networks, can be utilized for fault detection and maintenance scheduling in HVAC equipment in healthcare facilities [32]. These are important to optimize energy consumption in buildings, reduce carbon dioxide emissions, and improve building efficiency making a more sustainable environment. Healthcare facilities can make use of cutting-edge cloud computing and big data technologies, which can assist in predictive maintenance by processing data from medical equipment in real time, detecting event patterns, and utilizing predictive analytics methods and machine learning algorithms to forecast infrastructure or device malfunctions [6]. By utilizing cloud computing, IoT, and big data technologies, AI can allow systems to collect data from the many medical equipment utilized in healthcare facilities, enabling early detection of important events and malfunctions in biomedical devices, allowing for timely intervention and maintenance. Through predictive maintenance, healthcare facilities mitigate energy waste in operating by detecting and resolving problems before they worsen, resulting in enhanced energy efficiency and reduced resource consumption [10]. In operating rooms, this is important as it can enable healthcare facilities to track the output of devices and equipment in real time, utilize data to guide choices, and predict maintenance needs, thus contributing to sustainable and uninterrupted healthcare services.

23.3.2 Waste Management in Healthcare Facilities

AI can be used to group waste images into categories such as glass, metal, paper, and clinical waste linked to COVID; this aims to ensure data-driven decisions for recycling within the framework of circular economy and exhibits the capacity to handle the COVID-related clinical waste combined with other waste types [18]. This automated technique for classifying waste improves the circularity, ensuring a positive environmental impact and promoting remanufacturing. This is particularly important in emergency situations where efficient waste management is crucial for maintaining environmental safety, public health, and reduced spread of infection.

AI-furnished robotics can reliably identify items and perform automatic sorting using machine learning through image classification, which lessens the need for human intervention in the management of solid waste while simultaneously recycling certain materials effectively to increase ecological sustainability in the wake of the pandemic [30]. This can lead to a safer and more hygienic environment in emergency surgical flow and operating rooms, reducing the risk of contamination and spread of infectious diseases. Additionally, AI can assist in predicting the amount of advantageous and detrimental materials in waste, which is crucial for efficient waste management in healthcare facilities.

23.3.3 Optimization of Healthcare Supply Management Using AI Technology

Artificial intelligence algorithms assist healthcare supply chain in managing inventories and projecting demand, thereby reducing waste, boosting cost effectiveness, and enabling timely delivery of essential materials [23]. AI algorithms can enhance the healthcare supply chain's logistics, boost the effectiveness of transportation, use less fuel, and emit fewer greenhouse gases, all of which will contribute to the chain's sustainability. AI techniques can be used for demand forecasting and patient health management, allowing healthcare facilities to analyze and compare patient indicators with standard data to provide personalized health services and control for key patients. This can be particularly beneficial in emergency surgical situations where the health status of patients needs to be closely monitored and managed.

AI algorithms have the ability to assess consumption patterns of medical supplies, as well as their expiration dates, and demand forecasts in order to enhance supply levels and reduce wastage in healthcare supply chain management [31]. This is particularly important to ensure the availability of affordable medicines, which is crucial for emergency surgical procedures and patient care. By optimizing the inventory control policies for the hospital pharmacy and point-of-care units, the system can help in maintaining adequate stock of essential medications needed for emergency surgeries and post-operative care. Also, the algorithm's ability to consider uncertain medication demand and demand dependencies among medicines prescribed to patients can lead to improved inventory performance, ensuring that essential medications are readily available for emergency surgical flow and operating rooms. This can help in minimizing stockouts and delays in treatment, ultimately improving the quality of healthcare services provided to patients.

23.3.4 Automated Space Optimization in Hospital Facilities

AI technology can be used for simulation modeling to test design concepts and layout configurations in healthcare facilities, as well as in determining optimal resource locations, staffing methods, and unit sizes and adjacencies [11]. This can lead to better patient flow, shorter wait times, and more efficient use of available resources. AI support in simulation and optimization of layout designs can also help in creating a more patient-centered and efficient environment in emergency surgical flow and operating rooms. AI algorithms used in space optimization are also beneficial for room allocation by identifying patterns and trends in occupancy data, allowing for proactive management of resources. This can help in ensuring that operating rooms are utilized to their full capacity, reducing the risk of underutilization or overbooking.

23.3.5 Telemedicine and Remote Monitoring

AI incorporated into telemedicine can be used to enhance the provision of preventive and customized treatment to individuals with mental health issues, as well as to support isolated patients such as the self-isolated COVID-19 patients seen during the COVID pandemic [13]. Telemedicine can assist in triaging patients in emergency situations, helping healthcare facilities prioritize cases based on severity and urgency. It also allows for remote consultations with specialists, enabling timely and expert input in emergency surgical cases, even if the specialist is not physically present in the facility. By allowing patients to receive healthcare services remotely, telemedicine reduces the need for patients to travel to healthcare facilities, thereby decreasing the carbon footprint associated with transportation.

23.3.6 Challenges and Constraints

A number of challenges can be seen when integrating AI technology into existing healthcare facilities and systems. Some of these include the need for endorsement from regulatory bodies, incorporation into current systems, and adequate uniformity with comparable products and providing sufficient training for medical personnel [17]. These challenges can be reduced by investing in adequate high-quality training programs for clinical personnel to endeavor that they are equipped with the required skills for such technologies. Also, it is essential to work closely with regulating institutions to ensure that AI applications meet all necessary standards and regulations. Furthermore, in order to ensure seamless integration with existing systems, it is important to conduct thorough compatibility assessments and work closely with IT and healthcare professionals to identify any potential challenges and develop effective integration strategies. This may involve customizing AI solutions to meet the specific needs and requirements of each hospital's existing infrastructure.

23.4 How to Implement AI

Projects can support us in implementing AI for the management of the emergency surgical flow and operating rooms. Whereas there are activities that the hospital staff performs on a daily basis, projects have a beginning and an end. A project is how we can introduce a new AI technology or ensure that an existing one meets the objectives of the hospital leadership.

The first step to start a project is the business case. The business case is a presentation on the need for the project in front of the senior leadership of the hospital. If the senior leadership approves the project, resources will be allocated to start the project.

A good business case includes information on the rationale for the project, its benefits, its disbenefits, a financial appraisal, timelines, and risks. A simple tool to complete the financial appraisal is to explain how much time we will need to recoup the investment required for the project. We call this technique the payback period method.

Assume that the hospital is investing $200,000 to implement a new AI technology to improve efficiency that will yield $50,000 in yearly savings. The amount of time to recoup the investment is 4 years. The financial department of the hospital can perform more complex analyses to justify the investment; however, quantifying the amount of time required to recoup the investment provides key information to those who will need to fund the project. Regardless of the size of the investment, they will have an idea on how much time it will take to recover the resources they have allocated.

Once a project is approved, the senior leadership will appoint a project manager to ensure that it will be brought to completion. The choice of the project manager is probably one of the most important decisions that will affect the likelihood your project will be successful. Project managers have the responsibility to ensure the project will progress. A project manager can be a member of the hospital staff with good relational skills. This person needs to use a project plan to ensure that the required tasks will be completed.

A project plan is a document listing all the tasks that need to be completed in a project. You can find in Fig. 23.11 an example of a project plan. Specifically, it includes information on the task, who is responsible to complete that task, and what is the timeline (start date and end date) to complete it. Project plans typically include also an accountable person. The accountable person is the person who will have "to pay" if the task is not completed. The accountable person is often the supervisor of the person who is responsible for the task.

Task	Start Date	End Date	Responsible	Accountable

Fig. 23.11 Example of a project plan

The project manager is in charge of the project plan. The project manager monitors the document and ensures that all tasks are completed on time. A good project manager is proactive with the responsible persons in charge of the different tasks to understand the potential issues with the tasks to complete and what to do to overcome them.

Whereas projects are an effective tool to implement AI, we have mentioned that they need to be approved and resources need to be allocated to them. A question arises on who should be in charge of these approvals. Different organizations manage the approval of change projects in different ways. Typically, the greater the investment, the more senior are the leaders that can release this amount of resources and approve the project. Healthcare staff need to be aware of the pathway they need to follow to access the resources they need for their project.

Another question is who should initiate an AI project in the Emergency General Surgery context. There can be different approaches. Emergency Surgery Departments can identify a member of the staff who will be responsible to identify new AI opportunities. In this case, this person is the initiator of most of the initiatives the department proposes and implements. This approach does not preclude other members of the staff from being able to propose an AI initiative. The member of the staff in charge of AI can support these proposals from colleagues and initiate the process for the release of the resources required.

AI implementation needs to become a criterion to assess the performance of the budget holders who can approve the release of funds and start of a project. The engagement of senior leaders across the organization on the potential of AI is the conditio sine qua non to lead the AI transformation. Including AI implementation in the annual performance reviews across the organization can incentivize the approval of AI projects.

The importance of failure is another aspect to consider when implementing an AI project. Failure is possible when organizations lead innovative initiatives. Hospitals need to acknowledge that initiatives can fail. This acknowledgment, however, should not be an obstacle to start an AI project.

Healthcare organizations need to understand the value of a failure. Whereas organizations often focus on financial losses, in an innovative project, it is essential to appreciate the value of learning. Projects are not only an opportunity to improve performance or increase revenues. They are also an opportunity to learn. And the value of a learning experience can be greater than the cost of a financial loss.

To avoid significant financial losses, hospital leaders need to consider the potential of pilots. Pilots are small projects that minimize the financial investment and maximize the learning return of the project. The use of pilots can be used to successfully explore how to implement AI in the hospital.

The importance of low-hanging fruit should also be considered. Hospital leaders can consider to prioritize projects that are easier to complete successfully. The completion of successful AI projects can further reinforce the engagement of the staff and their willingness to commit to AI.

References

1. Ahmed Z, Mohamed K, Zeeshan S, Dong X. Artificial intelligence with multi-functional machine learning platform development for better healthcare and precision medicine. Database. 2020;2020:baaa010.
2. Cazap E, Magrath I, Kingham TP, Elzawawy A. Structural barriers to diagnosis and treatment of cancer in low-and middle-income countries: the urgent need for scaling up. Journal of Clinical Oncology. 2016;34(1):14–19.
3. Bicheno J, Holweg M. The lean toolbox: a handbook for lean transformation. Picsie Books; 2016.
4. Alowais SA, Alghamdi SS, Alsuhebany N, Alqahtani T, Alshaya AI, Almohareb SN, Aldairem A, Alrashed M, Bin Saleh K, Badreldin HA, Al Yami MS. Revolutionizing healthcare: the role of artificial intelligence in clinical practice. BMC Med Educ. 2023;23(1):689.
5. Classen D, Li M, Miller S, Ladner D. An electronic health record–based real-time analytics program for patient safety surveillance and improvement. Health Aff. 2018;37(11):1805–12.
6. Çoban S, Gökalp MO, Gökalp E, Eren PE, Koçyiğit A. [WiP] Predictive maintenance in healthcare services with big data technologies. In: 2018 IEEE 11th conference on Service-Oriented Computing and Applications (SOCA). IEEE; 2018. p. 93–8.
7. Currie JM. An overview of health care facilities planning. About The Editor. 2004:709.
8. Fan L, Evans DH, Naylor AR. Automated embolus identification using a rule-based expert system. Ultrasound Med Biol. 2001;27(8):1065–77.
9. Frassanito R, Buso T, Aumann S, Toniolo J, Albrici P, Canevari P, Iemmi M, Mapelli F. How IoT and artificial intelligence can improve energy efficiency in hospitals-a North Italian case study. In: E3S web of conferences, vol. 343. EDP Sciences; 2022. p. 02001.
10. Gallab M, Ahidar I, Zrira N, Ngote N. Towards a digital predictive maintenance (DPM): healthcare case study. Procedia Comput Sci. 2024;232:3183–94.
11. Halawa F, Madathil SC, Gittler A, Khasawneh MT. Advancing evidence-based healthcare facility design: a systematic literature review. Health Care Manag Sci. 2020;23:453–80.
12. Harmon J, Pitt V, Summons P, Inder KJ. Use of artificial intelligence and virtual reality within clinical simulation for nursing pain education: a scoping review. Nurse Educ Today. 2021;97:104700.
13. Huang J, Gu SS, Hou L, Wu Y, Wang X, Yu H, Han J. Large language models can self-improve. arXiv preprint arXiv:2210.11610. 2022.
14. Ibeh CV, Elufioye OA, Olorunsogo T, Asuzu OF, Nduubuisi NL, Daraojimba AI. Data analytics in healthcare: a review of patient-centric approaches and healthcare delivery. World J Adv Res Rev. 2024;21(02):1750–60.
15. Johnson KB, Wei WQ, Weeraratne D, Frisse ME, Misulis K, Rhee K, Zhao J, Snowdon JL. Precision medicine, AI, and the future of personalized health care. Clin Transl Sci. 2021;14(1):86–93.
16. Kaur J. Towards a sustainable triad: uniting energy management systems, smart cities, and green healthcare for a greener future. In: Emerging materials, technologies, and solutions for energy harvesting. IGI Global; 2024. p. 258–85.
17. Klumpp M, Hintze M, Immonen M, Ródenas-Rigla F, Pilati F, Aparicio-Martínez F, Çelebi D, Liebig T, Jirstrand M, Urbann O, Hedman M. Artificial intelligence for hospital health care: application cases and answers to challenges in European hospitals. In: Healthcare, vol. 9, no. 8. MDPI; 2021. p. 961.
18. Kumar NM, Mohammed MA, Abdulkareem KH, Damasevicius R, Mostafa SA, Maashi MS, Chopra SS. Artificial intelligence-based solution for sorting COVID related medical waste streams and supporting data-driven decisions for smart circular economy practice. Process Saf Environ Prot. 2021;152:482–94.
19. Lai JH, Hou HC, Chiu BW, Edwards D, Yuen PL, Sing M, Wong P. Importance of hospital facilities management performance indicators: building practitioners' perspectives. J Build Eng. 2022;45:103428.

20. Liefaard MC, Lips EH, Wesseling J, Hylton NM, Lou B, Mansi T, Pusztai L. The way of the future: personalizing treatment plans through technology. Am Soc Clin Oncol Educ Book. 2021;41:12–23.
21. Linkens DA. Intelligent computer-based systems for anaesthesia control in hospital operating rooms. In: Intelligent and adaptive systems in medicine. CRC Press; 2002.
22. Liu L, Bi M, Wang Y, Liu J, Jiang X, Xu Z, Zhang X. Artificial intelligence-powered microfluidics for nanomedicine and materials synthesis. Nanoscale. 2021;13(46):19352–66.
23. Long P, Lu L, Chen Q, Chen Y, Li C, Luo X. Intelligent selection of healthcare supply chain mode–an applied research based on artificial intelligence. Front Public Health. 2023;11:1310016.
24. Maguire R, McCann L, Kotronoulas G, Kearney N, Ream E, Armes J, Patiraki E, Furlong E, Fox P, Gaiger A, McCrone P. Real time remote symptom monitoring during chemotherapy for cancer: European multicentre randomised controlled trial (eSMART). Bmj. 2021;374:n1647.
25. McCartney J. AI is poised to "revolutionize" surgery. American College of Surgeons Bulletin; 2023.
26. Mendez JA, Leon A, Marrero A, Gonzalez-Cava JM, Reboso JA, Estevez JI, Gomez-Gonzalez JF. Improving the anesthetic process by a fuzzy rule based medical decision system. Artif Intell Med. 2018;84:159–70.
27. Mirchi N, Bissonnette V, Yilmaz R, Ledwos N, Winkler-Schwartz A, Del Maestro RF. The virtual operative assistant: an explainable artificial intelligence tool for simulation-based training in surgery and medicine. PLoS One. 2020;15(2):e0229596.
28. Patil S, Shankar H. Transforming healthcare: harnessing the power of AI in the modern era. Int J Multidiscip Sci Arts. 2023;2(1):60–70.
29. Rother M, Shook J. Learning to see VSM to create value and eliminate muda. Lean Enterprise Institute, Cambridge. 2009.
30. Rubab S, Khan MM, Uddin F, Abbas Bangash Y, Taqvi SAA. A study on ai-based waste management strategies for the covid-19 pandemic. ChemBioEng Rev. 2022;9(2):212–26.
31. Saha E, Rathore P. A smart inventory management system with medication demand dependencies in a hospital supply chain: a multi-agent reinforcement learning approach. Comput Ind Eng. 2024;191:110165.
32. Sanzana MR, Maul T, Wong JY, Abdulrazic MOM, Yip CC. Application of deep learning in facility management and maintenance for heating, ventilation, and air conditioning. Autom Constr. 2022;141:104445.
33. Ullah M, Hamayun S, Wahab A, Khan SU, Rehman MU, Haq ZU, Rehman KU, Ullah A, Mehreen A, Awan UA, Qayum M. Smart technologies used as smart tools in the management of cardiovascular disease and their future perspective. Curr Probl Cardiol. 2023;48(11):101922.
34. Vallathan G, Meyyappan S, Rajani T. Healthcare: energy optimization techniques using IoT and machine learning. In: Hybrid intelligent approaches for smart energy: practical applications. Wiley; 2022. p. 279–90.

Part V

Clinical Prediction, Data Management, and Education

24 Virtual Reality, Large Language Models, and Chatbots in Surgical Education and Training

Belinda De Simone, Giovanna Di Meo, Andrey Litvin, and Fausto Catena

Abbreviations

AI	Artificial intelligence
AR	Augmented reality
LLM	Large language model
VR	Visual reality
XR	Extended reality

B. De Simone (✉)
Department of Emergency and General Minimally Invasive Surgery, Level I Trauma Center, Bufalini Hospital, AUSL Romagna, Cesena, Italy

Department of Theoretical and Applied Sciences, eCampus University, Novedrate, Italy

G. Di Meo
Department of Precision and Regenerative Medicine and Ionian Area, University of Bari "Aldo Moro", Bari, Italy

A. Litvin
Department of Surgical Diseases No. 3, Gomel State Medical University, University Clinic, Gomel, Belarus

F. Catena
Department of Medical and Surgical Sciences Alma Mater Studiorum, University of Bologna, Bologna, Italy

Department of General and Emergency Surgery, Level I Trauma Center, Bufalini Hospital, AUSL Romagna, Cesena, Italy

B. De Simone et al. (eds.), *New Technologies, Precision Medicine, and AI in Emergency General Surgery*, Hot Topics in Acute Care Surgery and Trauma,
https://doi.org/10.1007/978-3-032-09357-8_24

24.1 Introduction

Surgical education and training are critical components in developing proficient and safe surgeons. The complexities of surgical procedures require not only theoretical knowledge but also extensive practical skills and decision-making abilities. Traditional surgical training methods often involve a steep learning curve, where novice surgeons practice directly on patients under the supervision of experienced mentors. While this approach has been the cornerstone of surgical education, it presents inherent risks and limitations, including the potential for patient harm and the variable availability of surgical cases [1].

In recent years, virtual reality (VR) and simulation-based training have emerged as innovative solutions to address these challenges. VR offers immersive environments that can replicate real-world surgical scenarios, enabling trainees to practice techniques without the immediate pressures and risks associated with live surgeries. Simulation-based training, which encompasses various modalities including high-fidelity simulators and task trainers, allows learners to engage in repetitive practice of specific skills in a controlled setting. These advanced educational tools not only enhance skill acquisition and knowledge retention but also improve overall surgical performance and patient safety. Research has shown that simulation-based education can lead to better preparedness for real-life surgical situations, ultimately resulting in improved patient outcomes [1, 2].

The use of VR, chatbots, and large language models (LLMs) in surgical education has gained considerable attention from healthcare professionals and researchers worldwide. When effectively integrated into healthcare, these technologies hold the potential to transform medical and surgical care. Research shows that they can assist in diagnosis, problem-solving, disease identification, and treatment planning for complex clinical scenarios.

This chapter aims to provide an overview of VR, simulation, and other AI-based tools in surgical training and education. We will examine the current landscape of these training and learning modalities, highlighting their benefits, applications, and the challenges they face, to guide a successful implementation in practice, as summarized in Table 24.1.

Table 24.1 Applications, benefits, limits, and barriers of virtual reality (VR), AI-based tools, and large language models (LLMs) in surgical education

Technology	Applications and benefits	Limits and barriers
VR	Enhances technical and non-technical skills in a risk-free, immersive environment	High costs and limited access in resource-constrained settings
	Offers unlimited practice opportunities with real-time feedback	Lack of tactile feedback and realism
	Improves performance, confidence, and patient safety through life-like simulations	Cybersickness and physical discomfort affect usability
AI	Assists in clinical decision-making by analyzing patient data and surgical videos	Ethical concerns around data bias and privacy

(continued)

Table 24.1 (continued)

Technology	Applications and benefits	Limits and barriers
	Enables personalized training by tracking individual performance	Requires significant computational resources and expertise
	Facilitates predictive analytics for better surgical planning and risk management	Regulatory and implementation challenges
LLMs	Enhances surgical training by generating accurate notes and personalized curricula	Risk of misinformation (AI hallucinations)
	Supports research and clinical decisions with advanced language processing	Limited ability to assess patient's emotional and physical states
	Assists in presurgical planning and continuous medical education	Dependency on high-quality training data and risk of over-reliance by trainees

24.2 Virtual Reality in Surgical Training: A Modern and Effective Approach

Virtual reality (VR) represents a transformative tool in surgical education, enhancing practitioner training through immersive technology. By creating realistic, interactive three-dimensional environments, VR allows users to explore surgical pathways and anatomical structures safely and cost-effectively, thus facilitating the acquisition of both surgical and nonsurgical skills [3, 4]. The importance of VR was underscored during the COVID-19 pandemic when it enabled remote learning and reduced the need for physical presence in training environments [5, 6].

Medical students consistently report high satisfaction with VR as a learning tool, citing its effectiveness in complementing traditional clinical placements and increasing motivation [7, 8]. By offering a three-dimensional perspective on patient data, VR is an invaluable tool for the future of medical education, improving anatomical understanding and clinical decision-making. As the demand for innovative, flexible, and efficient learning methods grows, the integration of VR in surgical training is expected to expand [9]. Integrating cognitive learning theories with VR applications allows trainees to maximize learning outcomes, making VR indispensable in modern surgical education. Overall, VR bridges the gap between theoretical knowledge and practical skills, providing lasting advantages for continuous professional development in surgical careers [10]. It also facilitates the generation of structured data to develop algorithms that can be used for visual-controlled interventions and further improvement of learning [11, 12].

VR has demonstrated significant potential in improving visual-motor coordination in surgical training by creating an immersive and controlled environment that mimics real-life scenarios. Studies testing objective indicators of hand movement skills and visual-motor coordination have shown that mid-level trainees exhibit smoother hand movements and increased visual concentration [13]. Real-time performance feedback integrated into VR simulators further enhances the learning process by offering practical guidance to novices [14–16]. When implementing surgical training in VR, the simulation can include either some basic tasks that are performed during specific surgeries or full surgical procedures. Simulators that are specialized in specific surgeries, like the LAP Simulator, have already integrated most of the corresponding tasks and require no further configurations to be ready for use. All the images and 3D models contained in the aforementioned simulators are based on computed tomography (CT), magnetic resonance imaging (MRI), and recordings of in vivo procedures. Therefore, to create realistic 3D models of internal organs, a collection of CT scans and MRIs are required. Sampogna et al. [17] described in detail the procedure of recreating 3D reconstructions based on medical imaging.

The devices used for promoting surgical education with the use of VR are mostly expensive [18, 19]. Simulators such as the Lap Sim and Lap Mentor are often combined with some additional head mount displays (HMDs), like HTC Vive 360 or Google VR, to create an immersive and engaging user experience. Most simulation technologies include special controllers (some with haptic feedback) that accurately simulate the use of surgical instruments and a high-resolution display of the virtual environment. The combination of VR, HMDs, and VR simulators promotes immersiveness and enhances the interaction between the participants and the virtual environment [17–19]. However, affordable alternatives, such as Oculus Rift, Meta Quest, HTC Vive, and Pico, provide cost-effective solutions without compromising accuracy, making surgical training more accessible. Devices like the Oculus Rift, priced under $500, allow beginner surgeons to train efficiently at reduced costs, though they often require additional setups, such as computer connections and specialized software [17, 19, 20].

Wearable devices are integral to VR experiences, particularly in metaverse applications and human-machine interfaces (HMIs). These devices, including smart glasses and electronic contact lenses, capture dynamic information such as gestures, eye movements, and body posture. This data enables natural multimodal sensing and enhances tactile perception through haptic feedback [21–24]. For instance, smart glasses equipped with integrated displays are extensively used in virtual reality applications to provide augmented information. In addition, electronic contact lenses have potential applications in checking body fluids. A notable innovation in this domain is GlasSense, a wearable device designed to monitor subtle vibration patterns of the temporalis muscle. This device incorporates two ball load cells mounted on the hinges of 3D-printed glasses, which detect minute forces generated by the temporalis muscle and convert them into electrical signals. The GlasSense system employs a support vector machine algorithm to classify behaviors such as chewing, talking, and winking with high accuracy. By capturing facial movements, this technology enables the translation of emotions and facial expressions into avatar representations within the metaverse, enhancing user interaction and engagement [25–27].

Numerous studies have investigated the impact of VR and augmented reality (AR) on surgical education, reporting promising results. For example, Barré et al. demonstrated the effectiveness of a VR-based scenario for sleeve gastrectomy training. Participants described the simulation, which utilized the HTC Vive, as "realistic and useful for learning surgery." The setup included sensors attached to actual surgical instruments, enabling navigation within a virtual operating room and leading to a measurable reduction in cognitive effort and stress during extended surgical practice [28].

Similarly, Yoganathan et al. demonstrated that 360° video-based training significantly enhanced knot-tying skills, even when used as a stand-alone learning tool [29]. Hooper et al. evaluated VR training for hip arthroplasty using the Oculus Rift CV1. While the impact on medical knowledge was inconclusive, their findings suggested that presurgical VR training could enhance technical skills [30].

Logishetty et al. assessed AR training with the Microsoft HoloLens, reporting comparable outcomes to traditional training for hip arthroplasty, while acknowledging its value as a supplementary tool for surgical education [31]. Peden et al. investigated the use of HMDs, specifically Google Glass, for teaching suture skills to medical students. Their study revealed outcomes similar to those achieved through face-to-face instruction, suggesting that AR-based tools are viable alternatives to traditional methods [32].

Qin et al. compared a variety of extended reality (XR) devices for peg transfer training, concluding that such systems foster immersive and successful learning experiences [33].

Harrington et al. demonstrated that surgeons were more attentive during laparoscopic cholecystectomy training using 360° videos on the Samsung Gear VR. Although information retention was comparable to traditional 2D video training, the immersive experience was deemed beneficial and engaging [34]. Huber et al. examined laparoscopic skill acquisition with an HMD (HTC Vive), reporting that participants found the immersive training feasible and exciting. Accuracy scores were similar between VR and traditional methods, confirming VR's noninferiority in this context [19].

Huang et al. investigated the application of AR simulations for venous catheter insertion, utilizing AR glasses (Brother AirScouter) to provide digital overlays of procedural steps during the intervention. Their study demonstrated the effectiveness of AR head-mounted displays in facilitating skill transfer within operating room settings [35]. Similarly, Rochlen et al. examined the use of AR technology for central venous catheter placement with Google Glass, reporting enhanced skill acquisition and improved procedural focus among participants [36]. Wu et al. evaluated AR-guided ultrasound for central venous access, also employing Google Glass, and concluded that while AR significantly improved procedural focus, users required additional familiarization with the technology to maximize its potential [37].

Moreover, Azimi et al. found that mixed reality using the Microsoft HoloLens improved nursing students' training in needle chest decompression, noting increased training frequency, enthusiasm, and retention of proficiency over time [38].

In emergency scenarios, Ferrandini Price et al. evaluated VR in a simulated mass casualty triage exercise using the Samsung Gear VR. While they acknowledged that VR cannot fully replace clinical simulations, they emphasized its role as a valuable complementary tool in medical training [39].

24.3 Enhancing Surgical Skills and Outcomes with Virtual Reality

In real-life surgical training, the primary challenge for trainees performing a procedure for the first time is the lack of prior experience viewing the operation from the lead surgeon's perspective. VR addresses this gap by offering a fully immersive environment where users can interact through controllers and sensors. Unlike AR, which overlays virtual images onto the real world, VR creates a completely virtual environment, offering a unique platform for learning. Through VR simulations, trainees can practice surgical procedures and refine both technical and nontechnical skills without the risks associated with live surgeries [40, 41]. Metrics used to evaluate VR-based surgical training typically include task completion time, hand usage efficiency, procedural accuracy, incision depth, error rates, damaged or burned vessels, and overall performance scores as measured by systems like Lap Sim. Questionnaires are also administered to assess trainees' perceptions of interaction, concentration, and realism in the simulations [19].

Huber et al. [19] examined VR-based training outcomes (time, number of movements, and path length) during clipping and grasping tasks, and two-handed maneuvers in 4 task-specific performance metrics across medial and lateral dissection, anastomosis, and full-task simulations. Similarly, Sampogna et al. developed evaluation tools to measure simplicity, precision, fidelity, guidance, satisfaction, 3D reconstruction quality, and VR immersiveness [17]. The use of VR provides surgeons with clearer 3D images and visual signals, facilitating faster, more precise hand movements compared to 2D training modalities [42]. Studies have shown that VR-based training improves motor skills, visual perception, and hand-eye coordination, critical components of surgical performance. These improvements include reduced target search times and enhanced response rates [43–45]. Additionally, VR systems with multi-sensory feedback—visual, auditory, and tactile—enhance the realism of surgical simulations, contributing to greater precision in surgical maneuvers [46]. For example, cataract surgery simulations highlight VR's ability to train both dominant and nondominant hands, emphasizing its potential for comprehensive skill development [47, 48].

VR training has also been shown to reduce surgical task durations, improve performance, and decrease cognitive load, ultimately enhancing learning efficiency [15]. Evidence suggests that VR is as effective as traditional box trainers and outperforms video trainers [48, 49]. Gamified platforms, such as the Nintendo® Wii™, have further demonstrated the ability of VR to improve laparoscopic skills, showcasing its potential for enhancing mental processing and surgical agility [31]. Moreover, the prognostic reliability of VR training, as evidenced by improved clinical outcomes, underscores its effectiveness in translating simulated skills into real-world surgical applications [50].

Seymour et al. conducted a prospective randomized, blinded study assessing VR training's ability to reduce errors in laparoscopic cholecystectomy. Sixteen surgical residents performed procedures with attending surgeons blinded to their training status, who scored for eight predefined errors for each procedure minute (interrater reliability of error assessment $r > 0.80$). Results revealed that VR-trained residents completed gallbladder dissections 29% faster; instead, non-VR-trained residents were nine times more likely to fail to make progress transiently and five times more likely to injure the gallbladder or burn nontarget tissue. VR training significantly reduced errors, with VR-trained residents recording an average of 1.19 errors per case compared to 7.38 in the non-VR group ($p < 0.008$) [51]. This study assessed the validity of a VR training tool for laparoscopic cholecystectomy, focusing on the safe and efficient use of electrosurgical instruments and proper tissue positioning with the nondissecting hand. It reported the higher potential of VR to train effectively residents to a high level of objectively measured skill before they operate on patients.

VR training tools provide unlimited practice opportunities, allowing trainees to progress at their own pace while being continuously assessed until proficiency is achieved. Computer-assisted mentoring enhances this approach by offering high-quality guidance without overburdening supervising surgeons. VR logs serve as valuable quality assurance tools, objectively assessing individual technical skills over time. Incorporating VR into surgical education not only enhances performance but also establishes a reproducible, safe, and cost-effective training method. Trainees can practice complex procedures in realistic simulations without posing any risk to patients, thereby improving both competence and confidence. It is important to recognize that surgical training encompasses a broad range of competencies, including cognitive abilities such as anatomical recognition and decision-making. While VR simulations represent just one component of comprehensive skill development, their impact on surgical education is substantial. Evidence demonstrates that VR training significantly enhances the performance of surgical residents, leading to safer and more effective procedures. VR simulations also show great promise in reducing surgical errors by improving the skill levels and preparedness of surgeons. Furthermore, integrating structured communication systems, such as Situation, Background, Assessment, Recommendation (SBAR) and Introduction, Patient/Problem, Assessment, Situation, Safety concerns (IPASS), into VR environments has been associated with increased competence and confidence. This integration helps reduce misunderstandings and enhances decision-making in high-stakes surgical contexts [52].

By offering a reproducible, safe, and cost-effective alternative to traditional training methods, VR enables the rehearsal of complex surgical procedures without exposing patients to unnecessary risks. As such, VR simulations stand out as a critical innovation in modern surgical education [53].

24.4 The Role of the Metaverse in Surgical Training

The metaverse represents a significant advancement in surgical education, offering a unique, immersive learning platform that goes beyond traditional VR interfaces. Unlike conventional screen-based interactions, the metaverse places users directly within a digital environment, enabling real-time interaction and collaboration. By integrating VR, augmented reality (AR), and mixed reality technologies, the metaverse provides highly interactive and interoperable training experiences. A defining feature of the metaverse is its ability to enable real-time interaction among users, creating a sense of presence that enhances learning. Traditional Internet interactions are limited to 2D screens and physical inputs, but the metaverse allows users to effectively "enter" and become part of the Internet.

In the context of surgical education, the metaverse offers immersive environments where trainees can simulate complex surgical procedures, hone their skills, and collaborate with peers and expert mentors. Virtual operating theaters create life-like surgical scenarios, providing participants with realistic practice opportunities. For example, a South Korean study demonstrated how surgical residents used head-mounted displays (HMDs) to access 360° live video coverage of operating rooms at Seoul National University Bundang Hospital, offering a unique first-surgeon perspective for skill development and collaboration [54].

The metaverse also facilitates expert consultation and second opinions during surgical cases through remote connectivity. Surgeons can log in via avatars using HMDs to provide real-time assistance for laparoscopic, robotic, and even open surgeries. In 2017, surgeons in the UK employed Microsoft HoloLens to collaborate with colleagues in India and the United States during a colorectal surgery. In this extended reality (XR) environment, avatars representing remote surgeons had access to imaging and intraoperative views, assisting the operating team [54]. Platforms like Proximie extend this functionality by enabling annotations on a 2D screen, but the metaverse could enhance this by using AR to overlay instructional information directly within the surgeon's field of view [55].

In 2023, the first USA-licensed Metaverse Surgical Hospital was established, integrating physical and virtual healthcare environments. Patients in the physical hospital benefited from the guidance provided by global experts operating as avatars in the metaverse's virtual operating theater. These avatars controlled robotic arms in real-world surgeries, leveraging audiovisual technology and AI for preoperative, intraoperative, and postoperative support. Early successes have encouraged further exploration of cost-effective telementoring applications in real-world surgical practice [56].

Advancements in image recording and interpretation are essential to fully unlock the metaverse's potential. However, its benefits for robotic surgery training and remote surgical collaboration are already evident [56, 57]. The metaverse enables surgeons to perform remote surgeries, engage in telementoring, and provide hands-on training from field hospitals or nearby facilities. By connecting robotic systems to the metaverse, surgeons can collaborate on surgical tasks, leveraging real-time data integration to enhance safety and outcomes.

This virtual environment also facilitates distance education, perioperative planning, and clinical discussions, while addressing issues of medical responsibility through agreements among participating hospitals. Although reliance on low-cost VR applications may initially seem risky, continuous technological advancements are ensuring their reliability for verbal telementoring, case discussions, and image sharing [56, 57]. To fully realize the potential of remote robotic control, connectivity between surgical consoles must be optimized for safety.

The metaverse provides a focused, distraction-free space for exchanging surgical, clinical, and scientific information, including 3D reconstructions for perioperative consultations. Additionally, robotic consoles facilitate remote interventions, reducing procedural costs and increasing affordability.

The metaverse's transformative role in surgical education includes providing trainees with opportunities for independent study, simulations with tutor support, and access to VR resources, videos, images, and conferences [57]. While early VR systems lacked tactile feedback, reducing realism, advancements in force-feedback technology have improved the experience [58]. However, training individuals in VR systems remains time-intensive, potentially impacting overall efficiency [59].

Despite its promise, the metaverse presents challenges. Resource requirements and educator expertise may exacerbate inequalities in healthcare education. Physical and psychological issues such as cybersickness, simulator sickness, cognitive strain, and dizziness also pose limitations [60]. Nonetheless, ongoing technological advancements are steadily enhancing the functionality and applicability of the metaverse in surgical practice [61].

24.5 Chatbots in Surgical Education and Practice

Chatbots powered by advanced AI technologies, such as ChatGPT, are becoming integral to surgical education and clinical practice. Leveraging multilingual models like ChatGPT, these tools enhance surgical training by providing dynamic educational platforms. In educational settings, chatbots simulate patient interactions, allowing medical trainees to practice diagnostic and communication skills in controlled environments. They also generate training materials and virtual patient simulations, creating interactive learning opportunities [62]. However, the content produced by chatbots requires careful oversight to ensure accuracy and address ethical concerns, such as plagiarism and misinformation [62–64].

In clinical practice, chatbots assist in diagnosis and treatment planning by analyzing patient data and medical images, improving decision-making efficiency [64]. For example, ChatGPT demonstrated high accuracy in answering surgical exam questions, such as the Korean General Surgery Board exam, where GPT-4 achieved a remarkable 76.4% accuracy rate. This showcases its ability to process and communicate complex surgical information effectively [65, 66]. Specialized fields, such as plastic surgery, benefit from chatbots that provide general knowledge, refine medical information, and promote evidence-based practices [62]. Furthermore, chatbots can facilitate the development of training materials, such as FAQs on microsurgical procedures, serving as a reliable resource with human oversight [67].

Chatbots also optimize neurosurgery research and patient care by facilitating data collection, conducting surveys, and supporting long-term research and continuing medical education (CME) [67]. Customizable AI models, like ChatGPT API 3.5 Turbo, offer fast and accurate answers to specific medical questions, aiding healthcare professionals in both education and clinical decision-making [62, 66]. In microvascular surgery, tools like FlapBot assist in clinical decision-making by turning observational data into actionable monitoring solutions, potentially rescuing compromised grafts with timely, data-driven interventions [68].

Additionally, chatbots serve as virtual scribes, generating clinical notes and surgical reports, streamlining workflows, and reducing administrative burdens on healthcare professionals [62, 69]. For instance, ChatGPT efficiently creates accurate surgical notes, saving surgeons valuable time that can be redirected to training and patient care [70, 71]. These tools enhance documentation quality, with operative notes receiving high ratings for accuracy and efficiency from both surgeons and patients [65, 72–79].

Despite their advantages, the use of chatbots in healthcare presents challenges. Patient privacy concerns are paramount, as chatbots may inadequately protect sensitive information, potentially leading to privacy breaches [80]. Furthermore, chatbots lack the empathy, intuition, and experience inherent to healthcare professionals, which are crucial for building patient trust and ensuring effective care [81–83]. Over-reliance on chatbots risks diminishing healthcare professionals' communication skills and making interactions impersonal, potentially eroding patient confidence [84]. Additionally, chatbots are susceptible to generating false or misleading information, which could have detrimental effects in medical contexts [85].

Ethical and legal challenges also arise, including copyright infringement and transparency issues in AI-generated content, which could lead to medico-legal complications [86]. Integrating chatbots into existing health systems, such as electronic health records, poses technical and operational challenges, and their effectiveness in fully supporting clinical practice requires further evaluation [87].

While chatbots hold significant potential to enhance communication efficiency, reduce costs, and improve surgical education, they should complement, rather than replace, human interaction to prevent misunderstandings and errors in patient care [88]. Striking a balance between innovation and safeguarding patient trust and data privacy is essential for the ethical and effective implementation of chatbots in healthcare settings.

24.6 Large Language Models in Surgery

Large Language Models (LLMs), such as Generative Pre-Trained Transformers (GPT), are revolutionizing surgical education and practice by enhancing diagnostic accuracy, supporting clinical decision-making, and optimizing educational methodologies [69, 72]. By analyzing large datasets, LLMs can identify patterns, predict outcomes, and propose innovative surgical techniques, making them highly valuable for both research and clinical applications [88]. Their potential to assist in generating scientific manuscripts is noteworthy, but the risk of AI-generated misinformation highlights the importance of careful oversight [89, 90]. While LLMs have shown promising results, their variable responses to repeated queries underline the need for ongoing development to ensure consistent, safe, and reliable performance [66].

LLMs significantly enhance surgical training by demonstrating human-level proficiency in various academic and professional assessments, including board exams and surgical knowledge evaluation [72, 90–92]. In surgical training, LLMs contribute to the creation of personalized curricula and continuous medical education (CME) programs. However, challenges such as algorithmic bias, privacy concerns, and ethical issues related to AI integration must be addressed to ensure responsible implementation in healthcare [93, 94].

LLMs allow for analyzing enormous amounts of patient data, identifying patterns and trends, predicting patient treatment outcomes, and suggesting improvements to surgical techniques, thereby contributing to the development of new, more effective procedures, optimizing surgery procedures, and reducing risks [72, 95]. They can significantly improve presurgical planning, using advanced natural language processing capabilities to analyze and synthesize huge volumes of medical data. These models can help in drawing up detailed and accurate surgical notes needed for preoperative planning by understanding the complexities and features of surgical procedures [96]. In addition, the integration of vision and speech processing in models such as the Language-Vision GPT (LV-GPT) enables enhanced visual response to questions (VQA) tasks in robotic surgery, surpassing other modern VQA models on surgical data sets [95, 97]. Furthermore, LLMs can be integrated into the heuristic frameworks of search algorithms, such as Monte Carlo Tree Search (MCTS), to explore potential different scenarios and support more informed decision-making, which is critical for planning complex surgical tasks [69, 92]. Moreover, embedding LLMs into algorithms or programs can improve their functionality, as demonstrated by their ability to provide more accurate answers to factual questions without any refinement [66]. Using precondition errors to repeat querying and extracting executable corrective actions, LLMs can improve the executability and semantic correctness of surgical plans, ensuring that all necessary prerequisites for surgery are met [66, 90]. Despite their impressive performance, these models show some inconsistencies and variability in responses, highlighting the need for further training to ensure safe and stable results [69]. However, the use of LLMs in surgery involves a number of potential risks that require careful consideration. A serious concern is the problem of "AI hallucinations," where LLMs generate misleading or incorrect information with unreasonable credibility, which can lead to misrepresentation and misinformation in clinical literature [98]. Furthermore, master's programs can perpetuate harmful medical misconceptions based on race, which can lead to biased and unsafe medical practices [90]. The inconsistencies in LLM responses further raise questions about their reliability in a clinical setting [99, 100]. Therefore, the integration of the LLM into preoperative planning can lead to improved efficiency, accuracy, and safety of surgical procedures, provided that their application is carefully managed and complemented by the expertise of specialists [99]. While the cost and potential disadvantages of implementing these models are significant limitations, their undeniable ability to enhance surgical education, training, and continuing medical education (CME) ultimately aims to improve treatment outcomes and patient safety [66]. However, challenges related to data privacy and accountability in AI-generated surgical documentation highlight the need for a cautious and responsible approach to integrating AI in healthcare [91]. The risks of disclosing confidential data and producing harmful outcomes raise serious ethical and security concerns [101, 102]. Additionally, the potential misuse of LLMs for harmful activities, such as creating pandemic pathogens, underscores the necessity of implementing strict safeguards and ethical guidelines [102]. These concerns emphasize the critical importance of developing robust guidelines and regulatory frameworks to ensure the safe, ethical, and responsible application of LLMs in surgery and other medical fields [103, 104].

24.7 Conclusion

The integration of virtual reality, chatbots, and large language models in surgical education and practice offers significant opportunities to transform medical training and patient care. These technologies enhance skill acquisition, minimize surgical errors, and optimize clinical workflows, making them essential components of modern healthcare. However, it is vital to address the challenges and limitations associated with their implementation to fully harness their potential and ensure ethical and effective use. The ongoing development of these tools promises a future in which medical professionals are better equipped, patient outcomes are improved, and healthcare processes are more efficient. Continuous evaluation and regulatory measures will be crucial in balancing innovation with patient safety and ethical considerations.

References

1. Aggarwal R, Ward J, Balasundaram I, Sains P, Athanasiou T, Darzi A. Proving the effectiveness of virtual reality simulation for training in laparoscopic surgery. Ann Surg. 2007;246:771–9. https://doi.org/10.1097/SLA.0b013e3180f61b09.
2. Gurusamy KS, Aggarwal R, Palanivelu L, Davidson BR. Virtual reality training for surgical trainees in laparoscopic surgery. Cochrane database Syst Rev. 2009:CD006575. https://doi.org/10.1002/14651858.CD006575.pub2.
3. Sheik-Ali S, Edgcombe H, Paton C. Next-generation virtual and augmented reality in surgical education: a narrative review. Surg Technol Int. 2019;35:27–35.
4. Agbafe V, Jazayeri HE, Baker N, Cederna PS, Laspro M, Groysman L, Verzella AN, Kimberly LL, Flores RL. The use of virtual reality in surgical training: implications for education, patient safety, and global health equity. Surgeries. 2023;4:635–46. https://doi.org/10.3390/surgeries4040061.
5. Agbafe V, Jazayeri HE, Baker N, Cederna PS. Augmenting medical and surgical education with virtual reality. Plast Reconstr Surg. 2023;152:556e–8e. https://doi.org/10.1097/PRS.0000000000010546.
6. Gandsas A, Dorey T, Park A. Immersive live streaming of surgery using 360-degree video to head-mounted virtual reality devices: a new paradigm in surgical education. Surg Innov. 2023;30:486–92. https://doi.org/10.1177/15533506231165828.
7. Velazquez-Pimentel D, Hurkxkens T, Nehme J. A virtual reality for the digital surgeon BT - digital surgery. In: Atallah S, editor. . Cham: Springer; 2021. p. 183–201.
8. Nassar AK, Al-Manaseer F, Knowlton LM, Tuma F. Virtual reality (VR) as a simulation modality for technical skills acquisition. Ann Med Surg. 2021;71:102945. https://doi.org/10.1016/j.amsu.2021.102945.

9. Kovalchuk O, M.P. B, Okhrei A, I.Y. P, Reshetnik E. Features of using immersive technologies (virtual and augmented reality) in medical education and practice. Morphologia. 2020;14:158–64. https://doi.org/10.26641/1997-9665.2020.3.158-164.
10. Munawar A, Li Z, Kunjam P, Nagururu N, Ding A, Kazanzides P, Looi T, Creighton F, Taylor R, Unberath M. Virtual reality for synergistic surgical training and data generation. In: Computer methods in biomechanics and biomedical engineering: imaging & visualization, vol. 10; 2021. p. 366.
11. Yu P, Pan J, Wang Z, Shen Y, Li J, Hao A, Wang H. Quantitative influence and performance analysis of virtual reality laparoscopic surgical training system. BMC Med Educ. 2022;22:92. https://doi.org/10.1186/s12909-022-03150-y.
12. Hasan LK, Haratian A, Kim M, Bolia IK, Weber AE, Petrigliano FA. Virtual reality in orthopedic surgery training. Adv Med Educ Pract. 2021;12:1295–301. https://doi.org/10.2147/AMEP.S321885.
13. Mutasim A, Batmaz A, Stuerzlinger W. Gaze tracking for eye-hand coordination training systems in virtual reality; 2020.
14. Parham G, Bing EG, Cuevas A, Fisher B, Skinner J, Mwanahamuntu M, Sullivan R. Creating a low-cost virtual reality surgical simulation to increase surgical oncology capacity and capability. Ecancermedicalscience. 2019;13:910. https://doi.org/10.3332/ecancer.2019.910.
15. Feeley A, Feeley I, Mohamed K, Sheehan E. Use of virtual reality simulation in surgical training: a systematic review on predictive validity and current use in surgical curricula. J Surg Simul. 2021; https://doi.org/10.1102/2051-7726.2021.0001.
16. Ntakakis G, Plomariti C, Frantzidis C, Antoniou PE, Bamidis PD, Tsoulfas G. Exploring the use of virtual reality in surgical education. World J Transplant. 2023;13(2):36–43. https://doi.org/10.5500/wjt.v13.i2.36. PMID: 36908307; PMCID: PMC9993190
17. Sampogna G, Pugliese R, Elli M, Vanzulli A, Forgione A. Routine clinical application of virtual reality in abdominal surgery. Minim Invasive Ther Allied Technol. 2017;26:135–43. https://doi.org/10.1080/13645706.2016.1275016.
18. Beyer-Berjot L, Berdah S, Hashimoto DA, Darzi A, Aggarwal R. A virtual reality training curriculum for laparoscopic colorectal surgery. J Surg Educ. 2016;73:932–41. https://doi.org/10.1016/j.jsurg.2016.05.012.
19. Huber T, Paschold M, Hansen C, Wunderling T, Lang H, Kneist W. New dimensions in surgical training: immersive virtual reality laparoscopic simulation exhilarates surgical staff. Surg Endosc. 2017;31:4472–7. https://doi.org/10.1007/s00464-017-5500-6.
20. Martin-Perez B, Bennis H, Lacy AM. Virtual reality simulation for surgery: from video games to transanal total mesorectal excision. Tech Coloproctol. 2018;22:5–6. https://doi.org/10.1007/s10151-017-1738-1.
21. Sandrone S. Medical education in the metaverse. Nat Med. 2022;28:2456–7.
22. Greenbaum D. The virtual worlds of the metaverseThe Metaverse: And How It Will Revolutionize Everything Matthew Ball Liveright, 2022. 352 pp. Science. 2022;377:377. https://doi.org/10.1126/science.add5905.
23. Dwivedi YK, Hughes L, Baabdullah AM, Ribeiro-Navarrete S, Giannakis M, Al-Debei MM, Dennehy D, Metri B, Buhalis D, Cheung CMK, Conboy K, Doyle R, Dubey R, Dutot V, Felix R, Goyal DP, Gustafsson A, Hinsch C, Jebabli I, Janssen M, Kim Y-G, Kim J, Koos S, Kreps D, Kshetri N, Kumar V, Ooi K-B, Papagiannidis S, Pappas IO, Polyviou A, Park S-M, Pandey N, Queiroz MM, Raman R, Rauschnabel PA, Shirish A, Sigala M, Spanaki K, Wei-Han Tan G, Tiwari MK, Viglia G, Wamba SF. Metaverse beyond the hype: multidisciplinary perspectives on emerging challenges, opportunities, and agenda for research, practice and policy. Int J Inf Manag. 2022;66:102542. https://doi.org/10.1016/j.ijinfomgt.2022.102542.
24. Vlake JH, van Bommel J, Riva G, Wiederhold BK, Cipresso P, Rizzo AS, Botella C, Hooft L, Bienvenu OJ, Geerts B, Wils E-J, Gommers D, van Genderen ME. Reporting the early stage clinical evaluation of virtual-reality-based intervention trials: RATE-VR. Nat Med. 2023;29:12–3. https://doi.org/10.1038/s41591-022-02085-7.
25. Kim J, Kim M, Lee M-S, Kim K, Ji S, Kim Y-T, Park J, Na K, Bae K-H, Kyun Kim H, Bien F, Young Lee C, Park J-U. Wearable smart sensor systems integrated on soft contact

lenses for wireless ocular diagnostics. Nat Commun. 2017;8:14997. https://doi.org/10.1038/ncomms14997.
26. Chung J, Chung J, Oh W, Yoo Y, Lee WG, Bang H. A glasses-type wearable device for monitoring the patterns of food intake and facial activity. Sci Rep. 2017;7:41690. https://doi.org/10.1038/srep41690.
27. Lee JH, Kim H, Hwang J-Y, Chung J, Jang T-M, Seo DG, Gao Y, Lee J, Park H, Lee S, Moon HC, Cheng H, Lee S-H, Hwang S-W. 3D printed, customizable, and multifunctional smart electronic eyeglasses for wearable healthcare systems and human-machine interfaces. ACS Appl Mater Interfaces. 2020;12:21424–32. https://doi.org/10.1021/acsami.0c03110.
28. Barré J, Michelet D, Truchot J, Jolivet E, Recanzone T, Stiti S, Tesnière A, Pourcher G. Virtual reality single-port sleeve gastrectomy training decreases physical and mental workload in novice surgeons: an exploratory study. Obes Surg. 2019;29:1309–16. https://doi.org/10.1007/s11695-018-03680-9.
29. Yoganathan S, Finch DA, Parkin E, Pollard J. 360° virtual reality video for the acquisition of knot tying skills: a randomised controlled trial. Int J Surg. 2018;54:24–7. https://doi.org/10.1016/j.ijsu.2018.04.002.
30. Hooper J, Tsiridis E, Feng JE, Schwarzkopf R, Waren D, Long WJ, Poultsides L, Macaulay W. Virtual reality simulation facilitates resident training in total hip arthroplasty: a randomized controlled trial. J Arthroplast. 2019;34:2278–83. https://doi.org/10.1016/j.arth.2019.04.002.
31. Logishetty K, Western L, Morgan R, Iranpour F, Cobb JP, Auvinet E. Can an augmented reality headset improve accuracy of acetabular cup orientation in simulated THA? A randomized trial. Clin Orthop Relat Res. 2019;477:1190–9. https://doi.org/10.1097/CORR.0000000000000542.
32. Peden RG, Mercer R, Tatham AJ. The use of head-mounted display eyeglasses for teaching surgical skills: a prospective randomised study. Int J Surg. 2016;34:169–73. https://doi.org/10.1016/j.ijsu.2016.09.002.
33. Qin Z, Tai Y, Xia C, Peng J, Huang X, Chen Z, Li Q, Shi J. Towards virtual VATS, face, and construct evaluation for peg transfer training of box, VR, AR, and MR trainer. J Healthc Eng. 2019;2019:6813719. https://doi.org/10.1155/2019/6813719.
34. Harrington CM, Kavanagh DO, Wright Ballester G, Wright Ballester A, Dicker P, Traynor O, Hill A, Tierney S. 360° operative videos: a randomised cross-over study evaluating attentiveness and information retention. J Surg Educ. 2018;75:993–1000. https://doi.org/10.1016/j.jsurg.2017.10.010.
35. Huang CY, Thomas JB, Alismail A, Cohen A, Almutairi W, Daher NS, Terry MH, Tan LD. The use of augmented reality glasses in central line simulation: "see one, simulate many, do one competently, and teach everyone". Adv Med Educ Pract. 2018;9:357–63. https://doi.org/10.2147/AMEP.S160704.
36. Rochlen LR, Levine R, Tait AR. First-person point-of-view-augmented reality for central line insertion training: a usability and feasibility study. Simul Healthc. 2017;12:57–62. https://doi.org/10.1097/SIH.0000000000000185.
37. Wu TS, Dameff CJ, Tully JL. Ultrasound-guided central venous access using Google glass. J Emerg Med. 2014;47:668–75. https://doi.org/10.1016/j.jemermed.2014.07.045.
38. Azimi E, Winkler A, Tucker E, Qian L, Doswell J, Navab N, Kazanzides P. Can mixed-reality improve the training of medical procedures? In: 2018 40th annual international conference of the IEEE Engineering in Medicine and Biology Society (EMBC); 2018. p. 4065.
39. Ferrandini Price M, Escribano Tortosa D, Nieto Fernandez-Pacheco A, Perez Alonso N, Cerón Madrigal JJ, Melendreras-Ruiz R, García-Collado ÁJ, Pardo Rios M, Juguera Rodriguez L. Comparative study of a simulated incident with multiple victims and immersive virtual reality. Nurse Educ Today. 2018;71:48–53. https://doi.org/10.1016/j.nedt.2018.09.006.
40. Gin C, Reyna J, Khanal S, Chakrabarti R. Trainee attitudes towards virtual reality simulation to develop microsurgical skills in ophthalmology. Int J Healthc Simul. 2023; https://doi.org/10.54531/tyqn1977.

41. Karimov BN, Makirov TR, Dokuchaeva NY. Innovative technologies in the training of surgeons using virtual interactive training complexes. Int J Innov Res Multidiscip Educ. 2023;02:10.58806/ijirme.2023.v2i4n04.
42. Topalli D, Cagiltay NE. Eye-hand coordination patterns of intermediate and novice surgeons in a simulation-based endoscopic surgery training environment. J Eye Mov Res. 2018;11 https://doi.org/10.16910/jemr.11.6.1.
43. Piedra J, Ojeda-Castelo J, Quero Valenzuela F, Piedra-Fernández J. Virtual environment for the training of the hands in minimally invasive thoracic surgery. In: 2016 8th international conference on games and virtual worlds for serious applications (VS-GAMES); 2016.
44. Batmaz A, De Mathelin M, Dresp B. Effects of 2D and 3D image views on hand movement trajectories in the surgeon's peri-personal space in a computer controlled simulator environment. Cogent Med. 2018;5 https://doi.org/10.1080/2331205X.2018.1426232.
45. Eltanamly RM, Elmekawey H, Youssef MM, Hassan LM. Can virtual reality surgical simulator improve the function of the non-dominant hand in ophthalmic surgeons? Indian J Ophthalmol. 2022;70:1795–9. https://doi.org/10.4103/ijo.IJO_2652_21.
46. Preiss M, Walder A, Kim Y. Haptically enhanced VR surgical training system. Curr Dir Biomed Eng. 2022;8:737–40. https://doi.org/10.1515/cdbme-2022-1188.
47. Mughrabi M, Kaya F, Batmaz A, Aliza A, Stuerzlinger W, Borazan B, Tonyali E, Sarac M. On the effectiveness of virtual eye-hand coordination training with head mounted displays. In: 2023 IEEE conference on virtual reality and 3D user interfaces abstracts and workshops (VRW); 2023.
48. Burger K. The effectiveness of eye-hand coordination training in virtual reality. LSU Doctoral Dissertations; 2023.
49. Karadimos A, Tzes A, Evangeliou N, Dermatas E. Virtual reality simulation of a robotic laparoscopic surgical system. In: 2022 8th international conference on control, decision and information technologies (CoDIT); 2022. p. 1573–9.
50. Wang Z, Lin Y, Chen H, Yuan W. Improved simulation of virtual bone drilling surgery with a voxel-based model. EasyChair Prepr; 2018.
51. Seymour NE, Gallagher AG, Roman SA, O'Brien MK, Bansal VK, Andersen DK, Satava RM. Virtual reality training improves operating room performance: results of a randomized, double-blinded study. Ann Surg. 2002;236:454–8. https://doi.org/10.1097/00000658-200210000-00008.
52. Shah DJ, Nelson T, Sadighi M, Mehta A, Greilich PE, Hamilton EC. Effects of a virtual simulation on student understanding of structured communication in the surgical learning environment. J Am Coll Surg. 2022;235
53. Li H, Sun Y, Song K, Yin C. Establishment of emergency teaching model and optimization of discrete dynamic calculation in complex virtual simulation environment. Math Probl Eng. 2022;2022:1–10. https://doi.org/10.1155/2022/6767237.
54. Koo H. Training of lung cancer surgery through metaverse including extended reality in the smart surgical room in Seoul National University Bundang Hospital. Korea J Educ Eval Health Prof. 2021;18:33. https://doi.org/10.3352/jeehp.2021.18.33.
55. Matwala K, Shakir T, Bhan C, Chand M. The surgical metaverse. Cir Esp. 2024;102(Suppl 1):S61–5. https://doi.org/10.1016/j.cireng.2023.11.009.
56. Ammendola M, Al Ansari M, de'Angelis N, Currò G. The metaverse in surgery: a real life low-cost clinical application for telementoring. Asian J Surg. 2023;46:4972–3.
57. Ammendola M, Memeo R, Al Ansari M. The revolution of metaverse in surgery: a mini-review with video. Updat Surg. 2024;76:1699–703. https://doi.org/10.1007/s13304-024-01960-x.
58. Hari K, Thompson R, Chambless L, Miga M. Development of a mixed reality application to simulate neurosurgical procedures. In: Image-guided procedures, robotic interventions, and modeling; 2023.
59. Riordan E, Yung A, Cheng K, Lim L, Clark J, Rtshiladze M, Ch'ng S. Modeling methods in craniofacial virtual surgical planning. J Craniofac Surg. 2023;34:1191–8. https://doi.org/10.1097/SCS.0000000000009187.

60. Bernardes A, Gardim L, Araújo AAC, Jensen R, Motta RA, de Almeida DM, de Lima RR, Peres HHC. Exploring the metaverse in the education of healthcare students: a scoping review. Rev Lat Am Enfermagem. 2024;32:e4347. https://doi.org/10.1590/1518-8345.7256.4347.
61. Khan RA. Challenges in surgical training- exploring the role of virtual and augmented reality. Health Prof Educ J. 2020;3:9–10. https://doi.org/10.53708/hpej.v3i1.751.
62. Kleebayoon A, Wiwanitkit V, D'Amico RS, White TG, Shah HA, Langer DJ. Neurosurgery. 2023) Letter: I asked a ChatGPT to write an editorial about how we can incorporate Chatbots into neurosurgical research and patient care….;93:e77. https://doi.org/10.1227/neu.0000000000002588.
63. Sue GR. Artificial intelligence for plastic surgeons. Plast Reconstr Surg. 2023;11:e5057. https://doi.org/10.1097/GOX.0000000000005057.
64. Lavadia WT, Sana EA, Salvacion MS. Smart phone chat apps for teaching and assessment in orthopaedic residency training. Malaysian Orthop J. 2023;17:45–60. https://doi.org/10.5704/MOJ.2303.007.
65. Abdelhady AM, Davis CR. Plastic surgery and artificial intelligence: how ChatGPT improved operation note accuracy, time, and education. Mayo Clin Proc Digit Health. 2023;1:299–308. https://doi.org/10.1016/j.mcpdig.2023.06.002.
66. Oh N, Choi G-S, Lee WY. ChatGPT goes to the operating room: evaluating GPT-4 performance and its potential in surgical education and training in the era of large language models. Ann Surg Treat Res. 2023;104:269–73. https://doi.org/10.4174/astr.2023.104.5.269.
67. Manolitsis I, Feretzakis G, Tzelves L, Kalles D, Katsimperis S, Angelopoulos P, Anastasiou A, Koutsouris D, Kosmidis T, Verykios VS, Skolarikos A, Varkarakis I. Training ChatGPT models in assisting urologists in daily practice. Stud Health Technol Inform. 2023;305:576–9. https://doi.org/10.3233/SHTI230562.
68. Seth I, Cox A, Xie Y, Bulloch G, Hunter-Smith DJ, Rozen WM, Ross RJ. Evaluating Chatbot efficacy for answering frequently asked questions in plastic surgery: a ChatGPT case study focused on breast augmentation. Aesthetic Surg J. 2023;43:1126–35. https://doi.org/10.1093/asj/sjad140.
69. Moglia A, Georgiou K, Satava R, Cuschieri A. Large language models in surgical education: do they reach human level on fundamentals of robotic surgery test? (Preprint); 2023.
70. Robinson A, Aggarwal SJ. When precision meets penmanship: ChatGPT and surgery documentation. Cureus. 2023;15:e40546. https://doi.org/10.7759/cureus.40546.
71. Gupta RR, Herzog I, Park JB, Weisberger J, Firouzbakht PK, Ocon VA, Chao J, Lee ES, Mailey BA. Performance of ChatGPT on the plastic surgery Inservice training examination. Aesthetic Surg J. 2023;
72. Beaulieu-Jones B, Shah S, Berrigan M, Marwaha J, Lai S-L, Brat G. Evaluating capabilities of large language models: performance of GPT4 on American Board of Surgery Qualifying Exam Question Banks; 2023.
73. Tian WM, Sergesketter AR, Hollenbeck ST. The role of ChatGPT in microsurgery: assessing content quality and potential applications. J Reconstr Microsurg. 2024;40:e1–2.
74. Dias P, Cardoso M, Guede-Fernandez F, Martins A, Londral A. Remote patient monitoring systems based on conversational agents for health data collection. In: Workshop on scaling-up health-IT; 2022.
75. Kumar K, Govindaraju R, Selvakumar V, Bharathiraja N, Thiagarajan R, Venkateswaralu B. IoT based smart surgical management platform for hospitals to enhance safety in medical treatment. Int J Health Sci (Qassim). 2022:8470–8. https://doi.org/10.53730/ijhs.v6nS4.11084.
76. Singh B, Olds T, Brinsley J, Dumuid D, Virgara R, Matricciani L, Watson A, Szeto K, Eglitis E, Miatke A, Simpson CEM, Vandelanotte C, Maher C. Systematic review and meta-analysis of the effectiveness of chatbots on lifestyle behaviours. npj Digit Med. 2023;6:118. https://doi.org/10.1038/s41746-023-00856-1.
77. Eysenbach G. The role of ChatGPT, generative language models, and artificial intelligence in medical education: a conversation with ChatGPT and a call for papers. JMIR Med Educ. 2023;9:e46885. https://doi.org/10.2196/46885.

78. Ali SR, Dobbs TD, Whitaker IS. Using a ChatBot to support clinical decision-making in free flap monitoring. J Plast Reconstr Aesthet Surg. 2022;75:2387–440.
79. Patnaik SS, Hoffmann U. Comparison of ChatGPT vs. bard to anesthesia-related queries. medRxiv. 2023;
80. Kanter GP, Packel EA. Health care privacy risks of AI Chatbots. JAMA. 2023;330:311–2. https://doi.org/10.1001/jama.2023.9618.
81. Altamimi I, Altamimi A, Alhumimidi AS, Altamimi A, Temsah M-H. Artificial Intelligence (AI) Chatbots in medicine: a supplement, not a substitute. Cureus. 2023;15:e40922.
82. Scerri A, Morin KH. Using chatbots like ChatGPT to support nursing practice. J Clin Nurs. 2023;32:4211–3.
83. Sakakibara K, Shigemi D, Toriumi R, Michihata N, Yasunaga H. Usability, satisfaction, and post-use health problems of a medical Chatbot service providing medicine use recommendations for women during pregnancy and lactation in Japan (preprint); 2023.
84. Dave T, Athaluri SA, Singh S. ChatGPT in medicine: an overview of its applications, advantages, limitations, future prospects, and ethical considerations. Front Artif Intell. 2023;6 https://doi.org/10.3389/frai.2023.1169595.
85. Li J, Dada A, Puladi B, Kleesiek J, Egger J. ChatGPT in healthcare: a taxonomy and systematic review. Comput Methods Prog Biomed. 2024;245:108013. https://doi.org/10.1016/j.cmpb.2024.108013.
86. Calonge D, Medina-Aguerrebere P, Hultberg P, Shah M. Can ChatGPT improve communication in hospitals? El Prof la Inf. 2023;32 https://doi.org/10.3145/epi.2023.mar.19.
87. Xu L, Sanders L, Li K, Chow JCL. Chatbot for health care and oncology applications using artificial intelligence and machine learning: systematic review. JMIR Cancer. 2021;7:e27850. https://doi.org/10.2196/27850.
88. Nagaraj P, Mohammed AS, Muneeswaran V, Akshay KN, Manoj G, Venkata TG. Knowledge based perceptions of Chatbots in healthcare. In: 2023 international conference on computer communication and informatics (ICCCI); 2023. p. 1–6.
89. Palacios JF, Bastidas N. Man, or machine? Artificial intelligence language systems in plastic surgery. Aesthetic Surg J. 2023;43:NP918–23. https://doi.org/10.1093/asj/sjad197.
90. ElHawary H, Gorgy A, Janis JE. Large language models in academic plastic surgery: the way forward. Plast Reconstr Surg. 2023;11:e4949.
91. Lawson McLean A. Artificial intelligence in surgical documentation: a critical review of the role of large language models. Ann Biomed Eng. 2023;51:2641–2.
92. Zhao Z, Lee WS, Hsu D. Large language models as commonsense knowledge for large-scale task planning. ArXiv. 2023:abs/2305.14078.
93. Abd-Alrazaq A, AlSaad R, Alhuwail D, Ahmed A, Healy PM, Latifi S, Aziz S, Damseh R, Alabed Alrazak S, Sheikh J. Large language models in medical education: opportunities, challenges, and future directions. JMIR Med Educ. 2023;9:e48291. https://doi.org/10.2196/48291.
94. Karabacak M, Margetis K. Embracing large language models for medical applications: opportunities and challenges. Cureus. 2023;15:e39305.
95. Seenivasan L, Islam M, Kannan G. SurgicalGPT: end-to-end language-vision GPT for visual question answering in surgery; 2023. p. 281–90.
96. Miller R. A surgical perspective on large language models. Ann Surg. 2023;278:e211–3. https://doi.org/10.1097/SLA.0000000000005896.
97. Schlag I, Sukhbaatar S, Asli C, Yih W, Weston J, Schmidhuber J, Li X. Large language model programs; 2023.
98. Brameier DT, Alnasser AA, Carnino JM, Bhashyam AR, von Keudell AG, Weaver MJ. Artificial intelligence in orthopaedic surgery: can a large language model "write" a believable orthopaedic journal article? J Bone Joint Surg Am. 2023;
99. Raman S, Cohen V, Rosen E, Idrees I, Paulius D, Tellex S. Planning with large language models via corrective re-prompting; 2022.
100. Omiye J, Lester J, Spichak S, Rotemberg V, Daneshjou R. Beyond the hype: large language models propagate race-based medicine; 2023.

101. Janssen BV, Kazemier G, Besselink MG. The use of ChatGPT and other large language models in surgical science. BJS Open. 2023;7 https://doi.org/10.1093/bjsopen/zrad032.
102. Connor M, O'Neill M. Large language models in sport science & medicine: opportunities, risks and considerations; 2023.
103. Ali H, Qadir J, Alam T, Househ M, Shah Z. ChatGPT and large language models in healthcare: opportunities and risks. In: 2023 IEEE international conference on artificial intelligence, blockchain, and internet of things (AIBThings); 2023. p. 1–4.
104. Thirunavukarasu AJ. Large language models will not replace healthcare professionals: curbing popular fears and hype. J R Soc Med. 2023;116:181–2. https://doi.org/10.1177/01410768231173123.

25 Machine Learning Models for Predicting Unplanned Hospital Readmission After Transcatheter Aortic Valve Replacement (TAVR): The Role of Electronic Health Records

Rema Padman, Karmel S. Shehadeh, Ashish Mohanan, and Arman Kilic

25.1 Introduction

Unplanned hospital readmission after initial hospitalization is a worldwide challenge and is associated with poor clinical outcomes, reduced quality of care, and high costs [9, 14, 23]. Early readmissions (within 30 days of discharge), in particular, impose the largest pressure on hospital resources and have generated significant debate [19]. Nearly 20% of Medicare beneficiaries in the United States are readmitted within 30 days after an index hospitalization and are associated with additional healthcare costs exceeding $15 billion [14, 19]. Globally, the 30-day readmission rate is recognized as an essential metric for assessing the quality of care, hospital performance, targets for cost reduction, and the subject of provider payment restrictions [19, 23]. Consequently, identifying the likelihood and

R. Padman (✉)
Heinz College of Information Systems and Public Policy, Carnegie Mellon University, Pittsburgh, PA, USA
e-mail: rpadman@cmu.edu

K. S. Shehadeh
Daniel J. Epstein Department of Industrial and Systems Engineering, University of Southern California, Los Angeles, CA, USA
e-mail: kshehade@usc.edu

A. Mohanan
Heinz College of Information Systems and Public Policy, Carnegie Mellon University, Pittsburgh, PA, USA
e-mail: amohanan@alumni.cmu.edu

A. Kilic
Department of Surgery, Medical University of South Carolina, Charleston, SC, USA
e-mail: kilica@musc.edu

B. De Simone et al. (eds.), *New Technologies, Precision Medicine, and AI in Emergency General Surgery*, Hot Topics in Acute Care Surgery and Trauma,
https://doi.org/10.1007/978-3-032-09357-8_25

predictors of unplanned readmissions is critical for implementing appropriate and timely preventive measures.

Transcatheter aortic valve replacement (TAVR) is the standard treatment option for patients with severe symptomatic aortic valve stenosis (AS) and high surgical risk [9, 18, 23]. The significant pre-existing patient clinical conditions, frailty, comorbidities, and peri- and post-surgery complications in patients currently undergoing TAVR and the reported relatively high rates of peri-procedural complications result in a high likelihood of hospital readmissions in such patients [19–21]. In fact, hospital readmission after TAVR is very common, with 30-day rates ranging from 10% to 21% and 1-year rates as high as 55% [2, 8, 19, 23]. Thus, predicting who is likely to be readmitted and a systematic analysis of the key predictors of readmissions after TAVR can inform preventative strategies for reducing them. However, data and studies on unplanned readmissions after TAVR are scarce, particularly regarding the timing (short-term vs. long-term), specific causes, and predictors of readmission. Moreover, with the increasing availability of detailed surgery data captured in clinical information systems, the potential for applying machine learning (ML) approaches for analyzing and predicting unplanned readmission after TAVR has seen limited investigation [22].

In this paper, using data from a large, multi-hospital health system in the United States, we apply statistical analysis and ML techniques to: (*i*) assess the differences in the baseline characteristics between patients who did and did not experience at least one hospital readmission during the first 30 days (short-term) and 1 year (long-term), respectively, after the index TAVR; (*ii*) predict the likelihood of readmission at the two landmarks; and (*iii*) identify the key predictors of readmission after TAVR for each scenario. To this end, we define hospital readmission within 30 days and 1 year, respectively, as any "*new hospitalization*" with a length of stay of at least 1 day after the index TAVR.

Using transcatheter aortic valve replacement (TAVR) as a representative clinical use case, this chapter explores how machine learning methods applied to large-scale electronic health record (EHR) data can support the prediction of unplanned hospital readmissions in complex perioperative pathways. Analysis of retrospective data from over 1000 TAVR admissions demonstrates that readmission remains a frequent outcome, occurring both in the early post-discharge period and during longer-term follow-up, in line with previously published evidence [15]. By combining advanced feature engineering with multiple machine learning approaches, the study illustrates how clinically meaningful predictors can be extracted from routinely collected EHR data to support outcome risk stratification. The remainder of the chapter is structured as follows: Sect. 25.2 describes the study population, data sources, and machine learning methods; Sect. 25.3 presents the main findings; and Sect. 25.4 discusses the broader implications of these results, with particular attention to the role of EHR quality and data integration in enabling scalable and clinically actionable AI applications.

25.2 Methods

25.2.1 Study Population and Data

This is a retrospective cohort study with 1043 patients who underwent TAVR surgery between 2011 and 2019 at a large, multi-hospital health system in the United States. We extracted 1858 data elements comprising demographic, clinical, preoperative, operative, and postoperative data on these patients from a prospectively maintained cardiac Society for Thoracic Surgery (STS) and STS/Transcatheter Valve Therapy database. The health system's Institutional Review Board (IRB) approved the use and analysis of the data.

Readmission date and primary reasons for hospitalization were recorded after a detailed chart review. We calculated the time to readmission as the time between the hospital discharge date after the index TAVR and the first hospital readmission day. We then labeled each readmission as early (less than 30 days) [15] or late (between 30 days and 1 year) [2]. We excluded 14 patients who died during the index hospitalization and another 14 (43) patients who died within 30 days (1 year) post-discharge.

Figure 25.1 presents the distribution of hospital readmissions at four time periods within a year after the index TAVR and the number of patients in the analysis cohort in each scenario. Of the 1-year analysis cohort, 318 out of 972 patients (32.7%) experienced at least one hospital readmission during the first year after the index TAVR. Of the 318 readmitted patients, 111 out of 1015 patients (10.9% of the 30-day analysis cohort) were readmitted early (i.e., within 30 days), 181 (18%) were readmitted within 90 days, and 242 (24%) were readmitted within 6 months.

25.2.2 Data Preprocessing

The initial dataset included 1858 attributes describing demographic, clinical, preoperative, operative, and postoperative characteristics of patients who underwent

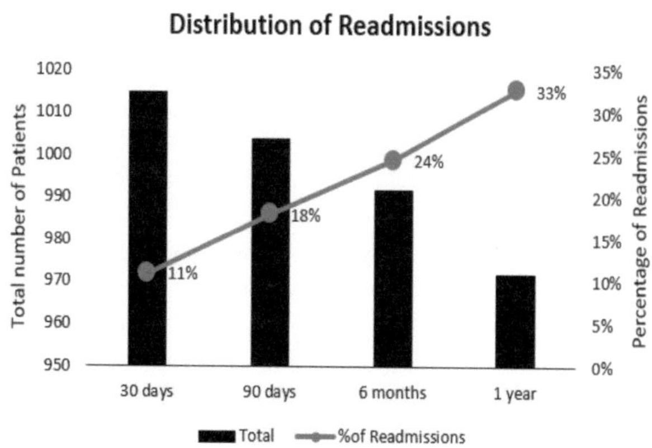

Fig. 25.1 Study cohort, percentage readmitted, and the number of readmissions within a year after TAVR, categorized according to the timing of readmission

TAVR procedure. We constructed 8 additional features that reflect clinical relevance: surgery duration, total time in the operating room, days in hospital after TAVR, estimated glomerular filtration rate (eGFR), change in ejection fraction (EF), change in hemoglobin (Hgb), and change in creatinine. We computed the change in EF, Hgb, and creatinine as the difference between their pre- and postoperative levels. We used the National Kidney Foundation's Chronic Kidney Disease Epidemiology Collaboration CKD-EPI Equation [16] to compute the eGFR.

Data preprocessing eliminated a large number of attributes with a high percentage of missing values or highly correlated (for example, height and weight vs. BMI), resulting in 253 features. To investigate the effect of social determinants on readmission likelihood [6], we added the area deprivation index (ADI) as an additional attribute to our dataset, aggregated at the ZIP code level (https://www.neighborhoodatlas.medicine.wisc.edu/). Including ADI, the final feature set consisted of 254 attributes.

We report baseline characteristics as percentages for categorical features and mean and standard deviation (mean ± SD) for continuous features. We compare the categorical (e.g., NYHA classification), binary (e.g., if the patient suffers from sleep apnea or not), and continuous baseline characteristics of the two cohorts (i.e., readmitted and non-readmitted) using Chi-square test, Fisher's exact test, and *t*-tests, respectively, with Bonferroni correction. In the next section, we summarize the machine learning methods that were evaluated for readmission prediction.

25.2.3 Prediction Models

After preprocessing the raw data, our final dataset consisted of 1015 patients in the 30-day readmission cohort and 972 patients in the 1-year cohort with 254 features about them. To develop a parsimonious model for clinical use and investigate the predictive power of the 254 features, we investigated several ML-based feature selection techniques, specifically, recursive feature elimination with cross-validation, feature importance [3, 12], and Markov Blanket [24]. We used the features with non-zero weights obtained from logistic regression with L-1 regularization (LASSO) in the feature importance approach [12]. The Markov Blanket approach, in particular, often identifies the smallest set of significant features. Specifically, this approach creates a Bayesian network and returns the Markov blanket of the target variable (in our case, Readmit Flag). The Markov Blanket of a random variable Y includes its children, its parents, and the co-parents of its children (see Spirtes et al. [24, 25], and Bai et al. [1] for a thorough discussion of the Markov Blanket approach for feature selection and prediction).

Using the selected features, we applied multiple ML models to predict readmission likelihood at two landmarks, 30 days and 1 year, respectively, based on logistic regression (LASSO and RIDGE) [13], K-nearest neighbors (KNN), decision tree, random forest (RF) [4], AdaBoost, XGBoost [7, 10], support vector machine (SVM), and multi-layer perceptron (MLP) (see [3, 12] for detailed discussions of these methods). For both feature selection and prediction, we considered a train-test split of 80:20 in our analysis. We compared the performance of the prediction models using 5-fold cross-validation, with AUC as the major performance metric [11].

Note that the admitted patients are a small proportion of the analysis cohort in each interval of interest (~11% and ~33% readmitted within 30 days and 1 year, respectively), resulting in highly imbalanced datasets for prediction modeling. Therefore, we applied different sampling techniques to tackle imbalance in the outcome variable (readmitted vs. non-readmitted); specifically, under-sampling, over-sampling, and synthetic minority over-sampling technique [5], with undersampling producing the best results using our data.

25.3 Results

25.3.1 Analysis of 30-Day Readmission

25.3.1.1 Baseline Characteristics

For presentation brevity, Table 25.1 presents only the significant continuous and categorical baseline characteristics identified using the appropriate significance tests out of the 254 variables included in this study. In this table, we observe that, compared to the non-readmitted patients, patients who were readmitted early have

Table 25.1 30-day readmission: significant baseline characteristics

Predictor	Total	Readmitted	Non-readmitted	*p*-value
	$N = 1015$	$N = 111$	$N = 904$	(<0.05)
Change in Creatinine	0 ± 0.5	0.19 ± 0.58	0.02 ± 0.49	0
(Pre-Op vs Post-Op)	0.08 ± 0.05	0.09 ± 0.05	0.07 ± 0.04	0.0002
STS Score				
Peak Post-op Creatinine	1.43 ± 1.25	1.85 ± 1.53	1.38 ± 1.2	0.0002
Days in Hospital	6.03 ± 6.22	8.06 ± 8.66	5.79 ± 5.8	0.0003
Hemoglobin	11.89 ± 1.61	11.38 ± 1.82	11.95 ± 1.57	0.0004
Lowest Intra-op Hematocrit	32.7 ± 4.95	31.14 ± 5.39	32.89 ± 4.86	0.0004
Lowest Intra-op Hemoglobin	10.62 ± 1.65	10.1 ± 1.8	10.68 ± 1.62	0.0005
Total Albumin	3.69 ± 0.45	3.55 ± 0.52	3.7 ± 0.44	0.0007
Hematocrit	35.82 ± 5.42	34.24 ± 5.71	36.01 ± 5.35	0.0011
MELD score	10.65 ± 3.89	11.76 ± 4.54	10.51 ± 3.79	0.0015
Cardiac Arrhythmia	503(49.56%)	70(63.06%)	433(47.9%)	0.0034
Tricuspid Valve Disease	698(68.77%)	91(81.98%)	607(67.15%)	0.0011
Tricuspid Regurgitation				0.0002
−999	26 (2.56%)	2 (1.8%)	24 (2.65%)	
0	12 (1.18%)	1 (0.9%)	11 (1.22%)	
1	260 (25.62%)	15 (13.51%)	245 (27.1%)	
2	396 (39.01%)	46 (41.44%)	350 (38.72%)	
3	203 (20%)	28 (25.23%)	175 (19.36%)	
4	54 (5.32%)	15 (13.51%)	39 (4.31%)	
5	64 (6.31%)	4 (3.6%)	60 (6.64%)	

Note: All continuous features are presented as mean ± standard deviation while bivariate/multivariate characteristics are presented as frequencies (%)

higher creatinine after TAVR (the difference in creatinine before and after TAVR are 0.19 versus 0.02 and peak post-op creatinine levels are 1.85 versus 1.38), higher STS scores at the time of TAVR (0.09 ± 0.05 versus 0.07 ± 0.04), and longer length-of-stay (LoS) in hospital after TAVR (8.06 ± 8.66 versus 5.79 ± 5.8. (Sanchez et al. [23] also report LoS as a predictor of 30-day readmission after TAVR), lower preoperative, intraoperative, and postoperative hemoglobin and hematocrit, higher MELD (model of end-stage liver disease) score (11.76 ± 4.54 versus 10.51 ± 3.79), and lower albumin (3.55 ± 0.52 versus 3.7 ± 0.44). The early readmission group has a higher percentage of patients who have pre-existing conditions such as cardiac arrhythmia (63% versus 48%) and tricuspid valve disease (82% versus 67%).

25.3.1.2 Key Characteristics Using Feature Selection Methods

Table 25.2 presents the reduced lists of important variables identified by LASSO regression and Markov Blanket methods. Of the two methods used for feature selection, the feature importance (using LASSO), and Markov Blanket methods resulted

Table 25.2 30-Day readmission: comparing Markov Blanket vs. LASSO feature selection (highlighted features are common to both methods)

Feature Selection - Markov Blanket

Selected Feature
asmtascaa
Change in Creatinine (Pre-Op vs Post-Op)
Incidence
Pneumonia
Renal Failure
Sleep Apnea
STS Score
Tobacco use
Total Albumin
Tricuspid Valve Disease

Feature Selection - LASSO

Selected Feature
012-Lead EKG Findings
Aortic Valve Regurgitation
Approach
cardref
dcasa
dcliplowstat
dominance
Hemoglobin
Highest Intra-op Glucose
Level mitral insufficiency found
Lipid Lowering
Lowest Intra-op Hemoglobin
Mitral Valve Disease
Other In HospitalPostoperative Event Occurred
PayorGovMcaid
PayorGovMcareFFS
PayorHMO
Primary Coronary Symptom for Surgery
Pulmonic Valve Disease
Readmission to ICU:
STS Score
Tobacco use
Total Albumin
Tricuspid Regurgitation

Table 25.3 30-day readmission: prediction results using the significant features from baseline analysis

Model	Accuracy	Recall	AUC	CI of AUC (95%)
Ridge regression	0.67	0.76	0.72	[0.61, 0.82]
Random forest	0.63	0.68	0.72	[0.63, 0.81]

Table 25.4 30-day readmission: prediction results using feature selection

Feature-selection method	Prediction model	Accuracy	Recall	AUC	CI of AUC (95%)
LASSO	XGBoost	0.61	0.80	0.75	[0.67, 0.82]
Markov Blanket	SVM	0.67	0.60	0.73	[0.62, 0.82]

in the highest ROC-AUC (see Table 25.3). The Markov Blanket methods with greedy search (to maximize cross-validation recall) selected 10 features out of the 254: tricuspid valve disease, sleep apnea, renal failure, incidence, pneumonia, STS score, total albumin, tobacco use, change in creatinine (Pre-Op vs Post-Op), and asmtascaa. The LASSO method identified a larger set of 24 significant features, and both methods identified STS score, tobacco use, and total albumin as significant predictors.

25.3.1.3 Prediction Results

We executed the nine selected prediction models using the two sets of features. The first set included the 13 significant baseline characteristics identified in Table 25.1. The second set included the reduced set of significant features identified by the feature selection methods, specifically LASSO regression and Markov Blanket methods, displayed in Table 25.2. Applying the 9 ML-based models to the data on the significant baseline characteristics, we find that LR-Ridge and RF had the best discrimination between the early readmitted and non-readmitted groups (see Table 25.3), with LR-Ridge predicting the likelihood of early 30-day readmission with 0.67 accuracy and 0.72 AUC. Results from other ML-based models are presented in Tables 25.10 and 25.9 in Appendix A.

Using the set of features identified by Markov Blanket shown in Table 25.4, the SVM model predicted 30-day readmission with an accuracy of 0.67 and an AUC of 0.73. Although the LASSO feature selection method results in a more robust model (better AUC), the Markov Blanket method provides a smaller set of predictors, allowing for a parsimonious and easily interpretable model. Finally, a Shapley value analysis (SHAP) [17] indicates that the most important features for 30-day readmission prediction include tricuspid valve disease, tobacco use, total albumin, change in creatinine, and STS risk score.

25.3.2 Analysis of 1-Year Readmission

25.3.2.1 Baseline Characteristics

Table 25.5 presents the significant continuous and categorical baseline characteristics identified using the statistical tests. We observe that patients who were

Table 25.5 1-year readmission: significant baseline characteristics

Predictor	Total	Readmitted	Non-readmitted	p-value
	$N = 972$	$N = 318$	$N = 654$	
STS score	0.08 ± 0.04	0.08 ± 0.05	0.07 ± 0.04	0.0001
Hemoglobin	11.89 ± 1.63	11.59 ± 1.72	12.04 ± 1.56	0
Hematocrit	35.85 ± 5.44	34.9 ± 5.74	36.32 ± 5.23	0.0001
Total albumin	3.69 ± 0.45	3.6 ± 0.49	3.73 ± 0.43	0
MELD Score	10.61 ± 3.89	11.17 ± 4.1	10.33 ± 3.76	0.0016
L ventricle end-systolic dimension	33.19 ± 9.03	34.41 ± 9.22	32.6 ± 8.88	0.0032
L ventricle end-diastolic dimension	46.09 ± 7.94	47.21 ± 7.84	45.55 ± 7.94	0.0022
Mean gradient	49.5 ± 14.34	46.99 ± 14.28	50.72 ± 14.22	0.0001
Lowest Intra-op Hemoglobin	10.62 ± 1.66	10.39 ± 1.75	10.74 ± 1.61	0.0021
Lowest Intra-op Hematocrit	32.73 ± 4.99	31.97 ± 5.14	33.1 ± 4.88	0.001
Peak Postoperative Creatinine	1.42 ± 1.25	1.59 ± 1.41	1.34 ± 1.16	0.0035
Hemoglobin level prior to discharge	10.07 ± 1.67	9.83 ± 1.65	10.19 ± 1.66	0.0018
Discharge hematocrit	30.26 ± 4.81	29.6 ± 4.79	30.58 ± 4.8	0.0029
Post Op ejection fraction	57.37 ± 12.8	55.69 ± 13.73	58.19 ± 12.25	0.0043
Days in Hosp	5.95 ± 6.1	7.22 ± 7.41	5.33 ± 5.24	0
Inhaled medication or oral bronchodilator therapy	215(22.12%)	88(27.67%)	127(19.42%)	0.005
Immunocompromised present	124(12.76%)	58(18.24%)	66(10.09%)	0.0005
Anticoagulants (Intravenous/ SubQ)	163(16.77%)	73(22.96%)	90(13.76%)	0.0005
Cardiac arrhythmia	478(49.18%)	178(55.97%)	300(45.87%)	0.0033
Other in hospital postoperative	225(23.15%)	92(28.93%)	133(20.34%)	0.0035
Event occurred				
Steroids				0.0013
0	875 (90.02%)	271 (85.22%)	604 (92.35%)	
1	96 (9.88%)	46 (14.47%)	50 (7.65%)	
3	1 (0.1%)	1 (0.31%)	0 (0.0%)	
Admit source				0
1	779 (80.14%)	230 (72.33%)	549 (83.94%)	
2	42 (4.32%)	22 (6.92%)	20 (3.06%)	
3	137 (14.09%)	56 (17.61%)	81 (12.39%)	
4	14 (1.44%)	10 (3.14%)	4 (0.61%)	
Chronic lung disease				0.0045
−9	1 (0.1%)	1 (0.31%)	0 (0.0%)	
0	616 (63.37%)	175 (55.03%)	441 (67.43%)	
2	109 (11.21%)	47 (14.78%)	62 (9.48%)	
3	80 (8.23%)	29 (9.12%)	51 (7.8%)	
4	109 (11.21%)	42 (13.21%)	67 (10.24%)	
5	57 (5.86%)	24 (7.55%)	33 (5.05%)	
Home oxygen				0.0027

(continued)

Table 25.5 (continued)

Predictor	Total	Readmitted	Non-readmitted	*p*-value
0	807 (83.02%)	247 (77.67%)	560 (85.63%)	
1	48 (4.94%)	15 (4.72%)	33 (5.05%)	
3	39 (4.01%)	20 (6.29%)	19 (2.91%)	
4	78 (8.02%)	36 (11.32%)	42 (6.42%)	
Tricuspid regurgitation				0.0033
−999	24 (2.47%)	6 (1.89%)	18 (2.75%)	
0	12 (1.23%)	2 (0.63%)	10 (1.53%)	
1	249 (25.62%)	70 (22.01%)	179 (27.37%)	
2	381 (39.2%)	124 (38.99%)	257 (39.3%)	
3	190 (19.55%)	70 (22.01%)	120 (18.35%)	
4	52 (5.35%)	29 (9.12%)	23 (3.52%)	
5	64 (6.58%)	17 (5.35%)	47 (7.19%)	
Status				0.0003
1	768 (79.01%)	228 (71.7%)	540 (82.57%)	
2	203 (20.88%)	90 (28.3%)	113 (17.28%)	
4	1 (0.1%)	0 (0.0%)	1 (0.15%)	
Level mitral insufficiency found				0.0003
−999	18 (1.85%)	4 (1.26%)	14 (2.14%)	
−8	20 (2.06%)	2 (0.63%)	18 (2.75%)	
0	36 (3.7%)	13 (4.09%)	23 (3.52%)	
1	325 (33.44%)	98 (30.82%)	227 (34.71%)	
2	382 (39.3%)	119 (37.42%)	263 (40.21%)	
3	135 (13.89%)	66 (20.75%)	69 (10.55%)	
4	17 (1.75%)	8 (2.52%)	9 (1.38%)	
5	39 (4.01%)	8 (2.52%)	31 (4.74%)	
dcace				0.0024
0	542 (55.76%)	186 (58.49%)	356 (54.43%)	
1	287 (29.53%)	78 (24.53%)	209 (31.96%)	
3	22 (2.26%)	14 (4.4%)	8 (1.22%)	
4	11 (1.13%)	3 (0.94%)	8 (1.22%)	
5	108 (11.11%)	35 (11.01%)	73 (11.16%)	
6	2 (0.21%)	2 (0.63%)	0 (0.0%)	

Note: All continuous characteristics are presented as mean ± standard deviation while bivariate/multivariate characteristics are presented as frequencies (percentages%)

readmitted within 1 year from index TAVR have higher STS score, lower (preoperative, intraoperative, and discharge) hemoglobin, lower albumin (3.6 ± 0.49 versus 3.73 ± 0.43), higher MELD score (11.17 ± 4.1 versus 10.33 ± 3.76), higher LV end-diastolic dimension (34.41 ± 9.22 versus 32.6 ± 8.88 mm), higher LV end-systolic dimension (47.21 ± 7.84 versus 45.55 ± 7.94), lower postoperative ejection fraction (55.69 ± 13.73 versus 58.19 ± 12.25), and longer LoS after TAVR (7.22 ± 7.41 versus 5.33 ± 5.24). Late readmission group also has a higher percentage of patients who have risk factors and pre-existing conditions such as cardiac arrhythmia (56% versus 46%) and immunocompromised (18% versus 10%).

25.3.2.2 Key Characteristics Using Feature Selection Methods

Table 25.6 shows that LASSO's feature importance method selected 89 features and Markov Blanket selected 11 features. Both methods identified angina class, family

Table 25.6 1-year readmission: comparing Lasso vs. Markov Blanket feature selection (highlighted features are common to both methods)

Feature Selection - LASSO

Selected Features		
012-Lead EKG Findings	Gender	Platelet Count
A1CLevel	Hemoglobin	Pneumonia
ACE or ARB	Home Oxygen	pocint1
Admit Source - Trsnfer/ ED/ Elective Admission	Hypertension	Primary Coronary Symptom for Surgery
ADP Inhibitor	ICU Visit	Primary Coronary Symptom for Surgery
ADP Inhibitor**(includes P2Y12)	imedeaca	Prior Heart failure
Amiodarone	ImmunocompromisedPresent	Prior Myocardial Infarction
anginalclass	Incidence	Pulmonic Valve Disease
Aortic Valve Area	Initial Operative Approach	RaceAsian
Aortic Valve Regurgitation	intraoperative TEE Performed post procedure	RaceNativeAm
Approach:	Level aortic insufficiency found	Readmission to ICU
Beta Blocker	Level mitral insufficiency found	ReIntub
Beta Blocker++	Level pulmonic insufficiency found	Rhythm Disturbance
cancer	Lipid Lowering	Room Air ABG Performed
cardref	llicit Drug Use within One Year	smokcoun
ChronicLung Disease - Mild/Moderate/Severe etc	LV End-Systolic Dimension	stensource
Classification-NYHA	Mean Gradient	Steroids
Number of Days in Hospital	medaplt5days	StressTst
dcace	Mitral Regurgitation	Surg_NonCard
dcamiodarone	Mitral Valve Stenosis	Surgery Duration
dcbeta	Nitrates, intravenous	Surgical Site Complications
dcfactorxa	Number Diseased Vessels	Syncope
dcliplowstat	Other Non-Cardiac Procedure	thaodisease
dcothantiplat	PA Systolic Pressure Measured	Tobacco use
depression	PayorGovMcaid	Total Albumin
Diff_Creat	PayorGovMcare	Tricuspid Regurgitation
Dimensions Available	PayorGovMcareFFS	vdmitet
Discharge location (destination after discharge)	PayorHMO	VSAoDeviceType
dominance	Peak Postoperative Creatinine Level prior to discharge	VTach/VFib
Family History of Premature Coronary Artery Disease	Perfusion Strategy	

Feature Selection - Markov Blanket

Selected Features
Area based Deprivation Index
anginalclass
Family History of Premature Coronary Artery Disease
Gender
ImmunocompromisedPresent
Incidence
LV End-Systolic Dimension
Pneumonia
STS Score
Total Albumin
Tricuspid Valve Disease

Table 25.7 1-year readmission: prediction results using the significant features from baseline analysis

Model	Accuracy	Recall	AUC	CI of AUC (95%)
Ridge regression	0.64	0.68	0.69	[0.61, 0.77]
Random forest	0.61	0.61	0.62	[0.53, 0.71]

Table 25.8 1-year readmission: prediction results using feature selection

Feature selection model	Prediction model	Accuracy	Recall	AUC	CI of AUC (95%)
Lasso	AdaBoost	0.61	0.59	0.66	[0.59, 0.73]
Markov Blanket	Ridge regression	0.58	0.62	0.65	[0.58, 0.72]

history of premature coronary artery disease, gender, immunocompromised, incidence, LV end-systolic dimension, pneumonia, and total albumin as significant predictors of 1-year readmission.

25.3.2.3 Prediction Results

Similar to the 30-day readmission prediction analysis, we compared 1-year readmission predictions using the nine ML models based on significant features from baseline analysis and those identified using the feature selection methods. The top two models for predicting 1-year readmission using baseline features are Ridge Regression (with 0.64 accuracy and 0.69 AUC) and Random Forest (with 0.61 accuracy and 0.62 AUC); see Table 25.7. Results from other ML-based models are presented in Tables 25.10 in Appendix A and 25.11 in Appendix B. Table 25.8 presents the best models for predicting 1-year readmission using feature selection methods. Using features selected by LASSO, AdaBoost provided the best 1-year readmission prediction with 0.61 accuracy, 0.59 recall, and 0.66 AUC, while using features selected by Markov Blanket, ridge regression provided the best 1-year readmission prediction with 0.58 accuracy, 0.62 recall, and 0.65 AUC. Prediction results of other ML models using these 11 features are presented in Table 25.12 in Appendix B. Shapley value analysis indicated that STS risk score, immunocompromised present, left ventricular end - diastolic dimension, total albumin, tricuspid valve disease, and pneumonia are long-term risk factors for 1-year readmission after index TAVR.

25.4 Discussion and Conclusion

Transcatheter aortic valve replacement (TAVR) has emerged as an important therapeutic intervention for both low- and high-surgical-risk patients but with high rates of readmission. This study summarizes the application and comparison of multiple machine learning methods to predict the likelihood of readmission within 30 days and 1 year, respectively, of 1049 patients who had TAVR procedure at multiple hospitals affiliated with a major health system in the United States. Our analysis reports on the performance of nine widely used machine learning models from the literature and the key predictors of the performance after applying multiple feature selection methods to reduce the high dimensionality of the dataset. It is not surprising that the prediction accuracy for the

1-year readmission is lower than the 30-day prediction. As the time from discharge after index TAVR increases, predicting the likelihood of readmission becomes tougher because various factors/variables contribute to late readmission other than the ones recorded at discharge, and these variables are often not documented in the patient record.

25.4.1 Limitations and Future Work

The retrospective study design and single health system data limit the generalizability of the results and insights. While the data is obtained from a large health system with multiple hospitals so that most readmissions are likely to be included, it is possible that a few could have been missed. We did not consider multiple readmissions that some patients in the analysis cohort may have experienced. Future work will assess these limitations and address them using data from multiple institutions.

Machine learning methods show considerable promise in improving readmission prediction performance for TAVR and identifying key predictors that may inform clinicians in designing targeted actions for improving outcomes and quality of care. Beyond the specific clinical context discussed, this example illustrates a broader and highly relevant challenge for the application of artificial intelligence in emergency and acute care surgery: the dependence of advanced predictive models on the quality, completeness, and structure of electronic health record (EHR) data. As demonstrated, the ability of machine learning algorithms to predict outcomes deteriorates when clinically meaningful variables, particularly those related to intraoperative findings, postoperative trajectories, and longitudinal patient follow-up, are inconsistently captured or entirely absent. In emergency surgical settings, where decisions are time-critical and data fragmentation is common, strengthening EHR infrastructures through standardized documentation, interoperability across institutions, and integration of perioperative and post-discharge information is essential. Such efforts are a prerequisite for moving AI applications from retrospective feasibility studies to robust, generalizable, and clinically actionable decision-support tools capable of improving outcomes and quality of care in emergency surgery.

Acknowledgment We sincerely thank the health system that provided access to the dataset analyzed in this study along with the IRB approval.

Appendices

Appendix A: 30-Day Prediction Results

Table 25.9 30-day readmission: prediction results using the significant features from baseline analysis

Model	Accuracy	Recall	AUC
Naïve Bayes	13%	96%	0.69
Logistic	64%	68%	0.65
Logistic—LASSO	64%	64%	0.65
Logistic—RIDGE	**66%**	**76%**	**0.72**
KNN	62%	56%	0.63
SVM	64%	64%	0.65
Decision Tree	65%	44%	0.51
Random Forest	**63%**	**68%**	**0.72**
ADABoost	51%	36%	0.53
XGBoost	64%	68%	0.69
MLP	63%	72%	0.64

Table 25.10 30-day readmission: prediction results using Markov Blanket feature selection

Model	Accuracy	Recall	AUC
Naïve Bayes	15%	96%	0.63
Logistic	69%	60%	0.69
Logistic—LASSO	63%	56%	0.68
Logistic—RIDGE	67%	48%	0.66
KNN	67%	60%	0.67
SVM	**67%**	**60%**	**0.73**
Decision Trees	40%	80%	0.57
Random Forest	67%	60%	0.72
ADABoost	66%	56%	0.67
XGBoost	65%	68%	0.71
MLP	59%	64%	0.65

Appendix B: 1-Year Prediction Results

Table 25.11 1-year readmission: prediction results using the significant features from baseline analysis

Model	Accuracy	Recall	AUC
Naïve Bayes	62%	61%	0.69
Logistic	63%	66%	0.69
Logistic—LASSO	32%	100%	0.50
Logistic—RIDGE	**63%**	**68%**	**0.69**
KNN	55%	53%	0.54
SVM	56%	76%	0.68
Decision Tree	48%	77%	0.61
Random Forest	61%	61%	0.62
ADABoost	58%	60%	0.61
XGBoost	58%	60%	0.62
MLP	48%	79%	0.62

Table 25.12 1-year readmission: prediction results using Markov Blanket feature selection

Model	Accuracy	Recall	AUC
Naïve Bayes	32%	100%	0.61
Logistic	56%	59%	0.63
Logistic—LASSO	32%	100%	0.50
Logistic—RIDGE	**58%**	**62%**	**0.65**
KNN	52%	46%	0.50
SVM	55%	73%	0.64
Decision Trees	52%	70%	0.57
Random Forest	57%	55%	0.60
ADABoost	61%	62%	0.62
XGBoost	57%	67%	0.61
MLP	61%	30%	0.60

References

1. Bai X, Padman R, Ramsey J, Spirtes P, Airoldi E. Tabu search enhanced graphical models for classification in high dimensions. INFORMS J Comput. 2008;20(3):423–37.
2. Bianco V, Kilic A, Gleason TG, Lee JS, Schindler J, Aranda-Michel E, Wang Y, Navid F, Kliner D, Cavalcante JL, Mulukutla SR, Sultan I. Long-term hospital readmissions after surgical vs transcatheter aortic valve replacement. Ann Thorac Surg. 2019 Oct;108(4):1146–52.
3. Bishop CM. Pattern recognition and machine learning. New York: Springer; 2006.
4. Breiman L. Random forests. Mach Learn. 2001;45(1):5–32.
5. Chawla NV, Bowyer KW, Hall LO, Kegelmeyer WP. SMOTE: synthetic minority oversampling technique. J Artif Intell Res. 2002;16:321–57.
6. Chen M, Tan X, Padman R. Social determinants of health in electronic health records and their impact on analysis and risk prediction: a systematic review. J Am Med Inform Assoc. 2020;27(11):1764–73.
7. Chen T, Guestrin C. XGBoost: a scalable tree boosting system. In: Proceedings of the 22nd ACM SIGKDD international conference on knowledge discovery and data mining; 2016. p. 785–94.
8. Elbaz-Greener G, Qiu F, Webb JG, Henning KA, Ko DT, Czarnecki A, Roifman I, Austin PC, Wijeysundera HC. Profiling hospital performance on the basis of readmission after transcatheter aortic valve replacement in Ontario, Canada. J Am Heart Assoc. 2019;8:e012355.
9. Franzone A, Pilgrim T, Arnold N, Heg D, Langhammer B, Piccolo R, Roost E, Praz F, Raber L, Valgimigli M, et al. Rates and predictors of hospital readmission after transcatheter aortic valve implantation. Eur Heart J. 2017;38:2211–7.
10. Friedman JH. Greedy function approximation: a gradient boosting machine. Ann Stat. 2001;29(5):1189–232.
11. Hanley JA, McNeil BJ. The meaning and use of the area under a receiver operating characteristic (ROC) curve. Radiology. 1982;143(1):29–36.
12. Hastie T, Tibshirani R, Friedman J. The elements of statistical learning. New York: Springer; 2009.
13. Hosmer DW Jr, Lemeshow S, Sturdivant RX. Applied logistic regression. 3rd ed. Hoboken: Wiley; 2013.
14. Jencks SF, Williams MV, Coleman EA. Rehospitalizations among patients in the medicare fee-for-service program. N Engl J Med. 2009;360:1418–28.
15. Kolte D, Khera S, Sardar MR, Gheewala N, Gupta T, Chatterjee S, Goldsweig A, Aronow WS, Fonarow GC, Bhatt DL, Greenbaum AB, Gordon PC, Sharaf B, Abbott JD. Thirty-day readmissions after Transcatheter aortic valve replacement in the United States: insights from

the Nationwide readmissions database. Circ Cardiovasc Interv. 2017;10(1):e004472. https://doi.org/10.1161/CIRCINTERVENTIONS.116.004472. PMID: 28034845

16. Levey AS, Stevens LA, et al. A new equation to estimate glomerular filtration rate. Ann Intern Med. 2009;150:604–12.
17. Lundberg S, Lee SI. A unified approach to interpreting model predictions. In: Proceedings of the 31st international conference on neural information processing systems. 2017 Dec Presented at: NeurIPS '17; December 4–9, 2017; Long Beach, CA, USA; 2017. p. 4768–77.
18. van Mourik MS, Geenen LM, Delewi R, Wiegerinck EM, Koch KT, Bouma BJ, Hen-riques JP, de Winter RJ, Baan J, Vis MM. Predicting hospitalisation duration after transcatheter aortic valve implantation. Open Heart. 2017;4:e000549.
19. Nombela-Franco L, del Trigo M, Morrison-Polo G, Veiga G, Jimenez-Quevedo P, Altisent OAJ, Campelo-Parada F, Biagioni C, Puri R, De Larochellière R, et al. Incidence, causes, and predictors of early (30 days) and late unplanned hospital readmissions after transcatheter aortic valve replacement. J Am Coll Cardiol Intv. 2015;8:1748–57.
20. Patel RV, Ravindran M, Manoragavan R, Sriharan A, Wijeysundera HC. Risk factors for hospital readmission post-Transcatheter aortic valve implantation in the contemporary era: a systematic review. CJC Open. 2022;4(9):792–801.
21. Rodés-Cabau J. Transcatheter aortic valve implantation: current and future approaches. Nat Rev Cardiol. 2012;9:15.
22. Russo MJ, Elmariah S, Kaneko T, Daniels DV, Makkar RR, Chikermane SG, Thompson C, Benuzillo J, Clancy S, Pawlikowski A, Lawrence S, Luck J. Machine learning identification of modifiable predictors of patient outcomes after Transcatheter aortic valve replacement. JACC Adv. 2024;3(8):101116. https://doi.org/10.1016/j.jacadv.2024.101116. PMID: 39108421; PMCID: PMC11301356.
23. Sanchez CE, Hermiller JB Jr, Pinto DS, et al. Predictors and risk calculator of early unplanned hospital readmission following contemporary self-expanding transcatheter aortic valve replacement from the STS/ACC TVT Registry. Cardiovasc Revasc Med. 2020;21:263–70. https://doi.org/10.1016/j.carrev.2019.05.032.
24. Spirtes P, Glymour C, Scheines R. Causation, prediction, and search. Boston: MIT Press; 2000.
25. Zeng Y, Luo J, Lin S. Classification using Markov blanket for feature selection, 2009 IEEE International Conference on Granular Computing, Nanchang, China. 2009. pp. 743–7, https://doi.org/10.1109/GRC.2009.5255023.

Big Data Management in the Era of Artificial Intelligence

26

Fikri M. Abu-Zidan and Hani O. Eid

26.1 Introduction

Over the last 50 years, we have seen tremendous development in the methods of data collection, storage, and their statistical modeling. Computers used to be large, having small data storage, and slow data processing. In comparison, handheld small smartphones nowadays quickly process and store large data, including text conversations, images, and videos. Supercomputers can process huge data for statistical modeling that may take a few days to finish, which the human brain is incapable of performing.

Big data are defined as "sets of information that are too large or too complex to handle, analyze or use with standard methods" [1]. These can be numbers, text, audios, images, or videos. The term "*Data model*" refers to "the way data is organized, documented, and defined within a database" [2].

The world became a global interconnected village. Advancements in technology, including multiple sources of high-quality big data and artificial intelligence (AI) tools, have a strong potential to impact our future healthcare. Healthcare providers should be part of this process, understanding its potentials and limitations. We aim in this book chapter to highlight the role of big data and its relationship to artificial intelligence in the future of healthcare.

F. M. Abu-Zidan (✉)
College of Medicine and Health Sciences, United Arab Emirates University, Al-Ain, United Arab Emirates

H. O. Eid
Rescue and Air Ambulance, Abu Dhabi Police Aviation, Abu Dhabi, United Arab Emirates

B. De Simone et al. (eds.), *New Technologies, Precision Medicine, and AI in Emergency General Surgery*, Hot Topics in Acute Care Surgery and Trauma,
https://doi.org/10.1007/978-3-032-09357-8_26

26.2 Data Management

The most important criteria of collected clinical data are authenticity, accuracy, and completeness. These principles are essential for all research projects and all designs, whether a small cohort or a big database analyzed by AI. It is a major misconception to think that having big data will solve all quality assurance concerns when dealing with data. Having big data may even augment a systematic error of data collection like mislabeling or double entry. This had been highlighted in 2009 when the prediction of a flu pandemic had major flaws [3, 4]. Furthermore, electronic health records may contain linguistic errors, unknown abbreviations, and ambiguous notes or data entered in the wrong location [5]. The quality of the outcome of an analysis depends on the accuracy and completeness of the data.

The **F**indable, **A**ccessible, **I**nteroperable, and **R**eusable (FAIR) principles are the pillars of good data and will hight the basic principles of data management. Health data should be **F**indable, **A**ccessible, **I**nteroperable, and **R**eusable *(FAIR)*. Findable indicates that it is easy to find and refind assuring validity and reliability; accessible indicates that when found it can be accessed to collect or check data; interoperable indicates to be easily operated by different parties; while reusable indicates that the same data set can be used for different objectives. Adopting these principles will improve the standards of data management, leading to better standardized approaches for data sharing, which encourages parties to work in harmony, in a win-win situation, which prevents duplication of efforts [6, 7].

Dealing with large data for more than a quarter of a century, we learned that assuring the quality of data is pivotal for the success of any research project. This includes proper planning of an accurate, clear, relevant, simple, and organized data collection protocol that has the minimum dataset. Proper accurate data precoding saves a lot of time. Planning should include practical and theoretical considerations for reducing data entry errors, dealing with missing data, recognizing and deleting double entries, and keeping the data backed up in another safe place having privacy protection [8].

26.3 Artificial Intelligence (AI)

In 1958, Frank Rosenblatt developed a hypothetical statistical modeling system mimicking the nervous system which was called a *perceptron*. This system aimed to answer three questions, which were: (1) how are data about the real world sensed? (2) in what form are data stored to be remembered? and (3) how do stored data affect our recognition? As a sequence, the model could predict learning curves from neurological variables [9]. During the period from 1958 till 1960, Professor John McCarthy developed the LISP program whereby a machine was instructed to exhibit "common sense" in response to these instructions. It was initially developed for the IBM 704 computer but gained quick popularity among AI developers and was adopted by the AI industry [10]. Professor John McCarthy defined AI as "the science and engineering of making intelligent machines, especially intelligent computer programs. It is related to the similar task of using computers to understand human intelligence, but AI does not have to confine itself to methods that are biologically observable" [11]. Mimicking human intelligence, AI uses algorithms to solve problems, which constitute a specific order of computational steps. These algorithms use variables (dimensions) as input data to train the statistical model [12]. AI can be used in the **4P** general medical domains (**P**rediction, **P**articipation, **P**revention, and **P**ersonalized medicine) in many areas, including imaging, error reduction, virtual patient care, patient engagement and compliance, medical research, drug delivery, rehabilitation, administrative applications, and workforce management [13, 14].

Machine learning (ML) refers to "various statistical techniques that allow computers to learn from experience without being explicitly programmed. This learning usually takes the form of changes to how an algorithm works" [15]. Natural language processing refers to "the field of study that focuses on the interactions between human language and computers. It is a computational approach to text analysis" [16]. It reads, understands, and interprets human language using computational language.

Deep learning uses algorithms that process data through multiple layers to produce advanced information from simple input variables [17]. An example of that is the artificial neural networks (ANN) model, which mimics the networks of human neurons. This complex model can analyze nonlinear relationships between different input and output variables. ANN models have a minimum of three layers, including the input layer, the hidden layer(s), and the output layer (Fig. 26.1). The hidden layers can be more than one depending on the structure of the model. You can observe in Fig. 26.1 that each neuron of these layers is not connected with any of the neurons of the same layer but is connected with every neuron of the next layer [12]. *The activation function* is a statistical equation permitting the progress of the output of a neuron to the next neuron and activating it, or alternatively stopping the progress of the output [18, 19]. Neurons receive inputs, which are weighted by the different variables of the model, advancing the learning process between the input and output layers [12]. Backpropagation is pivotal for an accurate AI output. When there is an error in the output, the weights and biases of the analysis are updated by feedback to the neurons to improve the prediction of the model [19]. Computer vision algorithms classify images by analyzing their different parts after training and learning on repeated observations from previous images to reach a radiological diagnosis [20].

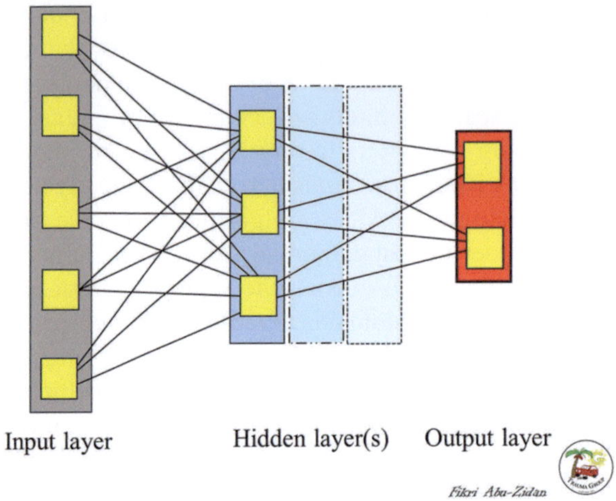

Fig. 26.1 Artificial neural networks mimic human neuron networks. They have at least three layers: (1) input layer, (2) hidden layer(s), and (3) output layer. Each neuron of a layer is connected with every neuron of the following layer but not with any of the neurons of the same layer. (Illustrated by Professor Fikri Abu-Zidan, Department of Surgery, College of Medicine and Health Sciences, United Arab Emirates University)

26.4 Big Data and AI

Sources of big data may include electronic healthcare records, medical images and videos, medical instruments, laboratory data, pharmacy data, patient-reported data, and internet data, including social media and smartphone data [21]. AI-driven diagnostic models using big data are better than traditional statistical models in their sensitivity, specificity, and the area under the receiver operating curve. Furthermore, risk stratification statistical models of the Web and/or mobile versions can help clinicians to make quick critical clinical decisions [22]. AI analysis based on big data can be used for predicting risks and prognosis and classifying patients according to these risks, which may improve the clinical outcome [23]. Data mining explores the relationships and patterns in the big data to predict a risk or outcome of a disease. Big data, which are extracted from social media and advanced sensors, are being utilized to better monitor and respond to disasters [24].

The Emergency Department, like the Intensive Care Unit (ICU), is a critical area where decisions with serious effects may need to be made once, in a very short time, and should be correct for a favorable clinical outcome [14, 23]. The ideal ratio between nurses and patients in the ICU should be one to one. Due to a lack of nurses or the sudden increase in the number of patients, like what occurred during the COVID-19 Pandemic, this ratio can be much less. This will be a real disaster situation where AI may play an important role, especially when the hospital and its communications are preserved. Mao et al. [23] described the future intelligent ICU in which big data, AI, internet of things, robotics, and advanced 5G communication technology can play a major role in the management of critically ill patients. Figure 26.2 shows the structure of this intelligent ICU. Real-time data of patients, like systolic blood pressure, heart rate, and oxygen saturation, can be collected from machines in the ICU to be analyzed by AI models. These models can pick up abnormal findings, give an alarm for the treating nurse, and communicate with the treating intensivist. These real-time critical alarms and decisions should be accurate, use intelligent AI for prediction of risks, and support interaction between the readings of the patient, the nurse, and the intensivist.

The surveillance, epidemiology, and end results program (SEER), which started collecting information on cancer epidemiology in the USA since 1975, is an example of the use of big data and AI in the medical field. SEER covers almost half of the population of the USA. Figure 26.3 shows the publications on machine learning during the period of 2017–2023 that stemmed from SEER. These studies concentrated on prediction of lymph node or distant metastasis and cancer prognosis [25]. The global increase in the elderly population supports the use of big data and AI in diagnosis, decision-making, and outcome prediction of emergency vascular conditions [14]. AI has great potential in the field of medical imaging. There are currently 5 AI radiological projects in the European Union that either use the centralized approach, in which data are collected centrally; the federated approach, in which data are stored at hospitals individually and shared when needed, or a hybrid approach using these two approaches [26].

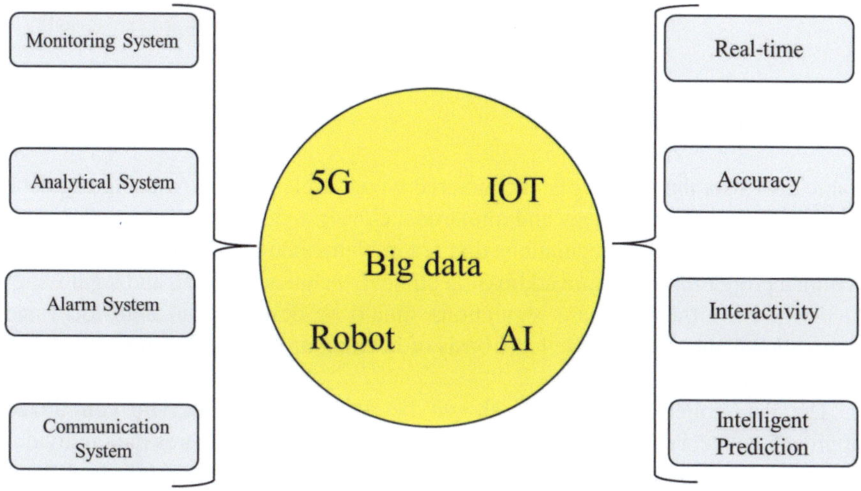

Fig. 26.2 An illustration showing the composition functions of a future intelligent ICU. Retrieved and adapted from Mao et al. [23] which is licensed under a Creative Commons Attribution 4.0 International License, that permits use, sharing, adaptation, distribution and reproduction in any medium or format, as long as appropriate credit to the original author(s) and the source is given

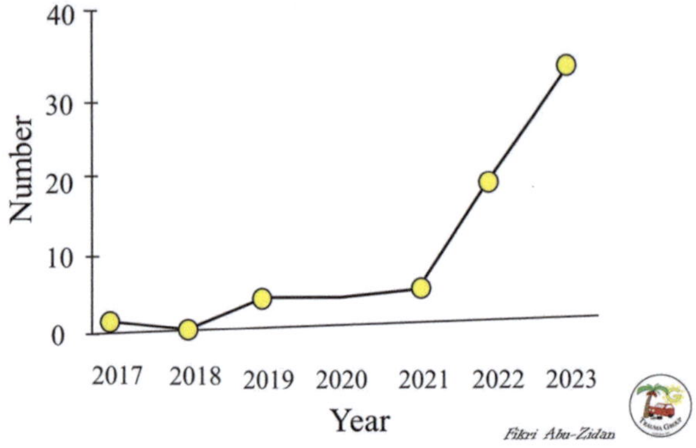

Fig. 26.3 PubMed Publication on cancer research using the SEER database as the source of data and machine learning as the AI method. Publications were located using the Search term: (SEER database [Title/Abstract]) AND (Neoplasms[MeSH Major Topic]) AND (machine learning[Title/Abstract]) as recommended by Li S et al. [25] (Illustrated by Professor Fikri Abu-Zidan, Department of Surgery, College of Medicine and Health Sciences, United Arab Emirates University)

Table 26.1 Challenges of using big data

(1)	Governance and regulations
(2)	Difficult findability
(3)	Lack of accessibility
(4)	Reduced sharing/interoperability
(5)	Unclarity of data ownership
(6)	Data quality
(7)	Technological challenges
(8)	Economical challenges
(9)	Accountability
(10)	Transparency and explainability

26.5 Challenges

Table 26.1 lists the challenges encountered when implementing AI using big data. The challenges are enormous and numerous; *Governance* is one of the major challenges. This needs clear regulations that are implemented by administrative leaders within a proper infrastructure addressing clinical, technical, ethical, and legal issues [13, 14]. Nevertheless, these regulations should be developed in both local and international standards, as the legal basis of health data sharing varies significantly between different countries.

The data-collecting approach should be well thought out. The centralized approach collects data centrally, while the federated approach stores data individually at hospitals, and data can be shared when needed. A hybrid approach of these two approaches can be adopted. Each approach has its own advantages. The centralized approach provides efficiency in processing the data, while the federated approach has better control over data privacy. The hybrid approach seems to be the best one by combining both advantages [26].

The dynamic nature of data collection makes the *findability* of these data more difficult. Furthermore, researchers who own specific data usually spend large budget grants to collect these data and feel ownership of the data. They become protective of their data, which reduces data *accessibility*. Furthermore, the lack of data collection standards reduces the ability of *sharing, reusability,* and *interoperability* of these data. Moreover, trust between data providers is very important for data sharing [6, 26].

Quality of the data is a major issue. Unstructured data are usually heterogeneous and have a lot of noise. *Technical barriers* include the IT structure, speed of transmission, storing ability, security, and IT maintenance. Furthermore, the huge size of the unstructured part of the big data is very challenging to deal with because it needs large storage of data, quick transmission, and efficient processing and analysis to achieve proper on-time decisions.

Economic challenges have a great impact on the development of AI. The majority of private or governmental organizations in developed countries are currently investing heavily in big data and AI, which is reflected in university academic education and research [14]. It is anticipated that economic challenges for adopting and implementing big data and AI will be more in developing countries. Less than 10% of the global research funds are spent in low-resource countries, where more than 90% of diseases occur [27].

Priorities for addressing these challenges vary between developed and developing countries. Economic and technological problems are more obvious in the developing countries, while the huge size of unstructured data to deal with, privacy issues, accountability, and legal issues have more priority in the developed countries.

26.6 Ethical Considerations

Table 26.2 summarizes the ethical and responsible AI principles when using big data [28]. The main four ethical principles, like other medical fields, should be adopted. These are: (1) do no harm (non-maleficence), (2) do good (beneficence), (3) respect the patient's autonomy, and finally (4) fairness and equity between patients, communities, and populations.

The clinical needs and objectives of an AI model should be very clear before developing or using it. Health care providers and patients, by being part of this process, can formulate these objectives and needs. Clinicians who are not aware of AI methods and their limitations may think that AI will replace their jobs. AI is just a tool that supports clinical activities. Clinical judgement, which differentiates between statistical significance and clinical significance and between correlations and cause effects, is essential for the development and adoption of AI [14]. The art of medical care, which includes a mixture of knowledge, ethics, professionalism, competency, sympathetic care, teamwork, and decision-making cannot be simply replaced by a machine [13]. Furthermore, clinical decisions are complex. These decisions are individualized, taking into consideration the disease, the clinical condition, preference, and social circumstances of the patient. AI can evaluate the risk

Table 26.2 Principles of ethical and responsible AI

(1)	Do not harm
(2)	Do good
(3)	Patient's autonomy
(4)	Fairness
(5)	Data privacy
(6)	Data sharing
(7)	Reduction of bias
(8)	Transparency of data
(9)	Validation of AI models
(10)	Clinicians in the loop
(11)	Teamwork
(12)	Responsible AI research

Modified after Walsh et al. [28] which is an open access article distributed under the terms of the Creative Commons Attribution 4.0 International License, which permits unrestricted use, distribution and reproduction in any medium, provided the original author and source are credited

and prognosis of patients, helping the treating physician to explain the facts to the patients or their legal representative to make timely shared decisions.

Medical privacy, security, and confidentiality of patients' data and their communications are major ethical challenges [14, 29]. The permission to access and share patients' data is usually given by a Medical Research Ethics Committee (MREC) after reviewing the research project. The requirements and standards of these MRECs vary significantly between different countries. Nevertheless, there should be a balance between privacy and utility, reflecting the personal and community needs, when giving these permissions. Personal identifiers should be strictly protected unless the patient consents to sharing them. Different techniques have been developed trying to address and protect the patient's privacy. These can be (1) cryptographic techniques that encrypt the data, (2) noncryptographic techniques by adding noise to the data, (3) hybrid techniques of the two previous techniques, and (4) decentralized techniques by storing data in the form of blocks [29]. These tools are costly, might slow the processing of data (either because of the added noise or increased communication demands), may cause failure of an algorithm when supporting multiple parties at the same time, or may reduce the accuracy of an applied AI model [29].

Defining the accountability when using big data and AI is very challenging because there are many stakeholders involved, taking different responsibilities in different parts of the process. This includes regulations, ethical approval, data collection, developing an AI model, investment, marketing, communications, and applications. Clinicians are at the end of this providing chain and will be accountable for their clinical decisions. Accordingly, they should be part of this loop to assure that the end-product will be useful for their patients. Defining the roles and responsibilities of each of these stakeholders is pivotal for a successful adoption of big data and AI in clinical practice. To have a fair accountability, it is very important to educate healthcare providers on the principles of AI. Using big data for the development of AI models should be transparent and easily explainable to the patient. Formal academic-led training can support clinicians to be part of the AI progress and to adopt the principles of transparency so that they can adequately explain the AI models for the patients in a simple, understandable way [28].

26.7 Statistical Limitations

It is a misconception to consider that using big data can overcome the basic principles of data analysis like accuracy, completeness, validity, and proper sampling. Actually, a systematic bias can be augmented by using large numbers. Although big data are a good source for studying relationships, these data should be valid and reliable to produce meaningful results [4]. Table 26.3 shows some of the pitfalls that are encountered in AI modeling.

Blackbox effect of the AI model indicates that the healthcare provider does not know how the model was structured, neither what is being measured, and how was it analyzed (Fig. 26.4). Traditional statistical models can be understood and critically appraised by clinicians. Since the clinicians will be accountable for their decisions, and they must take an informed consent for interventions, they may find difficulties in justifying their decisions when explaining how AI reached it [25].

Algorithm dynamics are the continuous changes of the algorithm either by the IT engineer or the consumer. This will affect the *findability* of the data and its *reliability,* as the results of a model can be difficult to reproduce. Furthermore, the prevalent search terms may be changed, which also affects the findability. *Commercial bias* has a major impact on AI. There is major industrial investment in AI. Accordingly, there can be modifications of the model to support business activities. This will cause disharmony between the model developers and those who provide the service. Furthermore, the web data itself can be modified for commercial or political interests. *Generalizability* of the data is another concern. The AI model tries to find the best model that explains specific data, which may not be generalizable for other populations. This is called overfitting, indicating that the AI model has good results on the study population but poor generalizability [12, 25]. In comparison, underfitting occurs when the model is very simple, having few variables to predict the output, or the model cannot capture the non-linear relationships between the variables. Most AI research studies come from high-income countries. These may not be generalizable for low-income countries. Furthermore, errors in the analysis may have autocorrelation and seasonality effects because the data are continuous and dynamic [4, 12].

Table 26.3 Statistical pitfalls of AI models developed by big data

(1)	Blackbox effect
(2)	Overfitting and underfitting
(3)	Algorithm dynamics
(4)	Disagreement between developers and providers
(5)	Commercial and political bias
(6)	Using prevalent search terms
(7)	Sampling of studied population
(8)	Temporal autocorrelation and seasonality

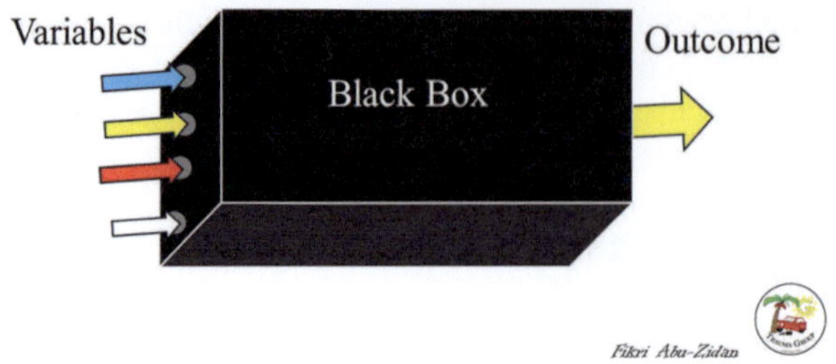

Fig. 26.4 An illustration showing the *Blackbox effect* of the AI model which indicates that the healthcare provider does not know how the model was structured, neither what is being measured, or how was it analysed? (Illustrated by Professor Fikri Abu-Zidan, Department of Surgery, College of Medicine and Health Sciences, United Arab Emirates University)

26.8 The Way Forward

There are multiple anticipated challenges that are expected to be faced when trying to use big data and AI in clinical practice. Despite that, we think that there will be numerous benefits associated with big data and its AI applications. Digital health data changes can be fast with dramatic effects on patients, health care providers, and health care systems. These changes may improve the health care, tailoring it to patient's needs to be precise and personalized [14]. We should be ready for this fast-changing working environment. This may require restructuring our traditional operating systems, having a clear strategic vision and plan, and gaining the needed new skills, including understanding AI and its applications. Restructuring our technological and computational infrastructure while integrating the new AI methods to be accepted and understood by mainstream practicing clinicians so that they can use and control AI in critical decision-making, while being accountable for it. This will be a demanding resource-intense task that needs proper planning, preparation, and collaboration between all stakeholders, including patients, clinicians, health data experts, data engineers, statisticians, epidemiologists, administrators, policy makers, and legislators [23]. This task will be even more difficult in low-resource settings, hindering the adoption of these new technologies.

26.9 Conclusions

The use of big data and artificial intelligence may have a major impact on the way we practice medicine in the future. They can support clinical decision-making in prediction and prognosis, improve alarming in serious conditions, and facilitate communication between patients and health care providers. To achieve that we need proper planning, establishment of effective governance, major changes to the healthcare infrastructure, and gradual changes in the culture of data management. We should thrive for a future health care system that is transparent, ethical, accountable, and sustainable which has high quality and equity of care. The success of digital big data and AI depends on adopting a multidisciplinary teamwork collaborating, learning, and addressing challenges together to improve patients' health care. In this context, effective big data management should be regarded as a foundational element for the responsible and sustainable integration of artificial intelligence into clinical practice.

Take Home Messages

1. Planning for the application of big data is pivotal for its success, including having clear structure and instructions for governance and accountability.
2. Multiple ethical, legal, administrative, technical, and economical challenges should be anticipated while adopting big data and AI.
3. Clinicians should demand to be part of the process of adopting big data and AI and not simply deliver data and apply the models without understanding their limitations.
4. AI education for clinicians can help them explain AI models to their patients and use them properly in clinical practice.
5. Practicing high ethical standards is essential for the success of adoption of big data and AI.

Conflict of Interest All authors declare that they have no conflict of interest.

References

1. Oxford Learner's Dictionaries. https://www.oxfordlearnersdictionaries.com/definition/english/. Accessed 6 Sept 2024.
2. ScyllaDB. Data model. https://www.scylladb.com/glossary/data-model/. Accessed 13 Sept 2024.
3. Ginsberg J, Mohebbi MH, Patel RS, Brammer L, Smolinski MS, Brilliant L. Detecting influenza epidemics using search engine query data. Nature. 2009;457(7232):1012–4.
4. Lazer D, Kennedy R, King G, Vespignani A. Big data. The parable of Google Flu: traps in big data analysis. Science. 2014;343(6176):1203–5.
5. Awrahman BJ, Aziz Fatah C, Hamaamin MY. A review of the role and challenges of Big data in healthcare informatics and analytics. Comput Intell Neurosci. 2022;2022:5317760.
6. Inau ET, Sack J, Waltemath D, Zeleke AA. Initiatives, concepts, and implementation practices of the findable, accessible, interoperable, and reusable data principles in health data stewardship: scoping review. J Med Internet Res. 2023;25:e45013.
7. Kotecha D, Asselbergs FW, Achenbach S, Anker SD, Atar D, Baigent C, Banerjee A, et al. CODE-EHR best-practice framework for the use of structured electronic health-care records in clinical research. Lancet Digit Health. 2022;4(10):e757–64.
8. Abu-Zidan FM. Common pitfalls in research design and its reporting. In: Ceresoli M, Abu-Zidan FM, Staudenmayer KL, Catena F, Coccolini F, editors. Statistics and research methods for acute care and general surgeons. Springer-Verlag; 2022. p. 29–37.
9. Rosenblatt F. The perceptron: a probabilistic model for information storage and organization in the brain. Psychol Rev. 1958;65:386–408.
10. McCarthy J. Recursive functions of symbolic expressions and their computation by machine, Part I. Commun ACM. 1960;3:184–95. https://dl.acm.org/doi/10.1145/367177.367199. Accessed 14 Sept 2024.

11. McCarthy J. What is artificial intelligence? November 12, 2007. https://www-formal.stanford.edu/jmc/whatisai.pdf. Accessed 14 Sept 2024.
12. Choi J, Aghaeepour N, Becker M. Machine learning techniques. In: Ceresoli M, Abu-Zidan FM, Staudenmayer KL, Catena F, Coccolini F, editors. Statistics and research methods for acute care and general surgeons. 1st ed. Cham: Springer Nature; 2022. p. 147–64.
13. Al Kuwaiti A, Nazer K, Al-Reedy A, Al-Shehri S, Al-Muhanna A, Subbarayalu AV, Al Muhanna D, Al-Muhanna FA. A review of the role of artificial intelligence in healthcare. J Pers Med. 2023;13(6):951.
14. Scali ST, Stone DH. The role of big data, risk prediction, simulation, and centralization for emergency vascular problems: lessons learned and future directions. Semin Vasc Surg. 2023;36(2):380–91.
15. Javaid M, Haleem A, Singh RP, Suman R, Rab S. Significance of machine learning in healthcare: features, pillars and applications. Int J Intell Netw. 2022;3:58–73.
16. Sadiku MNO, Zhou Y, Musa SM. Natural language processing. Int J Adv Sci Res Eng. 2018;4:68–70.
17. Kuo RYL, Harrison C, Curran TA, et al. Artificial intelligence in fracture detection: a systematic review and meta-analysis. Radiology. 2022;304(1):50–62.
18. Madhuri J, Indiramma M. Artificial neural networks based integrated crop recommendation system using soil and climatic parameters. Indian J Sci Technol. 2021;14:1587–97.
19. Feng J, Lu S. Performance analysis of various activation functions in artificial neural networks. J Phys Conf Ser. 2019;1237:022030.
20. Team GL. What is artificial intelligence in 2024? Types, trends, and future of it? Great learning blog: free resources what matters to shape your career! Published November 8, 2023. https://www.mygreatlearning.com/blog/what-is-artificial-intelligence/. Accessed 21 Feb 2024.
21. Dicuonzo G, Galeone G, Shini M, Massari A. Towards the use of Big Data in healthcare: a literature review. Healthcare (Basel). 2022;10(7):1232.
22. Tse G, Lee Q, Chou OHI, Chung CT, Lee S, Chan JSK, et al. Healthcare Big Data in Hong Kong: development and implementation of artificial intelligence-enhanced predictive models for risk stratification. Curr Probl Cardiol. 2024;49(1 Pt B):102168.
23. Mao Z, Liu C, Li Q, Cui Y, Zhou F. Intelligent intensive care unit: current and future trends. Intensive Care Res. 2023:1–7. https://doi.org/10.1007/s44231-023-00036-5.
24. Cicek D, Kantarci B. Use of mobile Crowdsensing in disaster management: a systematic review, challenges, and open issues. Sensors (Basel). 2023;23(3):1699.
25. Li S, Yi H, Leng Q, Wu Y, Mao Y. New perspectives on cancer clinical research in the era of big data and machine learning. Surg Oncol. 2024;52:102009. https://doi.org/10.1016/j.suronc.2023.102009.
26. Kondylakis H, Kalokyri V, Sfakianakis S, Marias K, Tsiknakis M, Jimenez-Pastor A, et al. Data infrastructures for AI in medical imaging: a report on the experiences of five EU projects. Eur Radiol Exp. 2023;7(1):20.
27. Global Forum for Health Research. The 10/90 report on Health Research 2003–2004. Geneva: Global Forum for Health Research; 2004. https://www.files.ethz.ch/isn/17141/1090.04.pdf. Accessed 24 Sept 2024.
28. Walsh G, Stogiannos N, van de Venter R, Rainey C, Tam W, McFadden S, et al. Responsible AI practice and AI education are central to AI implementation: a rapid review for all medical imaging professionals in Europe. BJR Open. 2023;5(1):20230033.
29. Khalid N, Qayyum A, Bilal M, Al-Fuqaha A, Qadir J. Privacy-preserving artificial intelligence in healthcare: techniques and applications. Comput Biol Med. 2023;158:106848.